SPECIAL THANKS

To my parents, Dorothy and Tom, for my education and values.
To my wife, Kristine, for her love and constant support.
To my children, Sarah, Patrick, and Katy, for their patience.

Preface

We designed this text to cover a particular area of critical care: the postoperative course. Such patients present unique problems and issues. They often have multiple-interacting system involvement that requires rapid and directed attention. One hopes that the desired response quickly follows. At a minimum, the correct treatment path prevents or minimizes long-term consequences.

The information assembled here provides practical and state-of-the-art information to care for the critically ill postoperative patient. The case reports help to introduce the material in the accompanying chapter, and the margin notes highlight the most important information. The index should easily direct one to specific information. We hope that the reader will find this a practical and useful addition to his or her library.

I would like to add a special thanks to my secretary, Poppy Smith, for her editorial assistance.

Gainesville, Florida *T. James Gallagher*

Contributors

William S. Blau, M.D., Ph.D.
Assistant Professor of Anesthesiology
University of North Carolina School of Medicine
Chapel Hill, North Carolina

Frederick R. Bode, M.D.
Associate Professor of Clinical Medicine
Division of Pulmonary and Critical Care
University of Missouri-Columbia School of Medicine
Columbia, Missouri

Philip G. Boysen, M.D.
Professor and Chairman
Department of Anesthesiology
School of Medicine
University of North Carolina
Chapel Hill, North Carolina

Bart Chernow, M.D.
Professor of Medicine, Anesthesia, and Critical Care
Johns Hopkins University School of Medicine
Physician-in-Chief
Sinai Hospital of Baltimore
Baltimore, Maryland

R. Phillip Dellinger, M.D.
Professor and Director of Pulmonary and Critical Care Medicine
University of Missouri-Columbia School of Medicine
Columbia, Missouri

John B. Downs, M.D.
Professor and Chairman of Anesthesiology
University of South Florida College of Medicine
Tampa, Florida

Steven R. Ford, M.D.
Assistant Professor of Anesthesiology
University of Texas Medical Branch
Galveston, Texas

Mark L. Franklin, M.D.
Instructor in Clinical Anesthesia
Northwestern University Medical School
Assistant Medical Director, Respiratory and Critical Care
Chicago, Illinois

Andrea Gabrielli, M.D.
Assistant Professor
Department of Anesthesiology
University of Texas
Houston, Texas

T. James Gallagher, M.D.
Professor of Anesthesiology and Surgery
Chief of Critical Care Medicine
University of Florida College of Medicine
Gainesville, Florida

Scott B. Groudine, M.D.
Assistant Professor of Anesthesiology
Albany Medical College
Albany, New York

Craig S. Kitchens, M.D.
Professor of Medicine
University of Florida College of Medicine
Chief, Medical Service
Veterans Affairs Medical Center
Gainesville, Florida

A. Joseph Layon, M.D.
Associate Professor of Anesthesiology and Medicine
University of Florida College of Medicine
Gainesville, Florida

Philip D. Lumb, M.D.
Professor of Anesthesiology and Surgery
Chairman of Anesthesiology
Albany Medical College
Albany, New York

Loren D. Nelson, M.D.
Associate Professor of Surgery and Anesthesiology
Director of Surgical Critical Care Service
Vanderbilt University Medical Center
Nashville, Tennessee

Kent S. Pearson, M.D.
Associate Director
Surgical Intensive Care Unit
Associate Professor of Anesthesia
University of Iowa College of Medicine
Iowa City, Iowa

Carl J. Pepine, M.D.
Professor of Medicine
Co-Director, Division of Cardiology
University of Florida College of Medicine
Gainesville, Florida

Donald S. Prough, M.D.
Professor and Chair of Anesthesiology
University of Texas Medical Branch
Galveston, Texas

Jukka Räsänen, M.D.
Associate Professor of Anesthesiology
University of South Florida College of Medicine
Tampa, Florida

Robert J. Schultz, M.D.
Instructor, Department of Anesthesiology
University of Alabama at Birmingham
Birmingham, Alabama

Jeffrey S. Vender, M.D.
Associate Professor of Clinical Anesthesia
Northwestern University Medical School
Chicago, Illinois
Director, Medical-Surgical Intensive Care Unit
Evanston Hospital
Evanston, Illinois

Robert F. Wilson, M.D.
Professor, Department of Surgery
Wayne State University School of Medicine
Detroit, Michigan

Contents

CHAPTER 1

Immediate Needs of the Postoperative Patient

T. James Gallagher

Case Report

Mr. H was a 5′10″, 210-pound, 69-year-old man. He entered the emergency room with a complaint of severe abdominal pain. Physical examination revealed a blood pressure of 80/58 mm Hg and a pulse rate of 116/min. The patient's abdomen was tender and distended, and a pulsatile mass was noted. Large-bore IV access was obtained, and the patient was rapidly transferred to the operating room with a diagnosis of ruptured intra-abdominal aneurysm.

On arrival in the operating room, the patient underwent a rapid sequence induction following attachment to the usual monitors. The operative procedure itself was difficult and lasted approximately $5\frac{1}{2}$ hours. Initially, while the surgical team attempted to gain control of the aorta, the patient had a 25-minute period of blood pressures in the range of 60 to 70 mm Hg. For the duration of the procedure, the patient had an average urine output of 30 ml/hr. Intraoperative blood gas ($F_{I}O_2$ = 1.0) was PaO_2, 80 mm Hg; $PaCO_2$, 48 mm Hg; and pH, 7.28. Attempts to increase the PaO_2, including positive end-expiratory pressure (PEEP) and manipulation of the tube, were unsuccessful.

During the procedure, the patient received 13 units of packed red blood cells, 8 units of fresh frozen plasma, and 20 units of platelet. In addition, he received 16 L of normal saline and Ringer's lactate.

On arrival in the intensive care unit (ICU), the patient was intubated, and his abdomen was noted to be grossly distended with the dressing in place. Initial vital signs included blood pressure of 100/60 mm Hg and heart rate of 115/min. His temperature was 33°C, and he was shivering. The electrocardiogram revealed occasional premature ventricular contractions (PVCs). Central venous pressure was 6 mm Hg. During the first hour, the patient made 28 ml of urine.

Further initial data collection included an electrocardiogram, which revealed ST-segment depression over the lateral chest leads, as well as inverted T waves. A chest radiograph revealed a right main stem intubation with left lower lobe collapse. Laboratory studies included hematocrit and hemoglobin, clotting studies, and electrolyte determinations. Because of the intraoperative hypotension and changes in the electrocardiogram, cardiac enzyme studies were ordered, to evaluate the possibility of myocardial infarction.

The patient initially received 2 more units of packed red blood cells and 1 L of Ringer's lactate. A warming blanket was utilized. Because of shivering and increased oxygen consumption, he was paralyzed with 10 mg vecuronium.

The endotracheal tube was pulled back and verified to be above the carina. A bronchoscope was utilized to remove inspissated secretions from the left lower lobe. Subsequent chest radiographs revealed reexpansion. Because of low urine output and hypotension, a pulmonary artery catheter was placed. Initial data revealed a cardiac output of 3.2 L/min and a wedge pressure of 16 mm Hg. Systemic vascular resistance was calculated at 1700 dynes $\times$ sec $\times$ cm^{-5}. Dopamine, which had been originally administered at a rate of 3 μg/kg/min, was increased to 10 μg/kg/min. Cardiac output increased to 6.1 L/min.

Laboratory data revealed a potassium of 3.1 mEq/L and a blood glucose of 294 mg/dl. The prothrombin time (PT) was 15.3/11.8 seconds, and the partial thromboplastin time (PTT) was 43 seconds. The platelet count was 89,000. Two more units of fresh frozen plasma were given, 60 mEq of potassium were infused over 3 hours, and the glucose concentration was controlled with 8 units of intravenous insulin.

Eight hours after the patient's arrival in the ICU, his temperature had increased to 36.5°C, and cardiac output was 6.8 L/min. The patient was awake and followed commands.

The anesthesiologist has multiple treatment goals for the patient. Provision of physiologic stability during the operative procedure must always serve as the most important principle. This includes a deft balance of anesthetic agents that, in their own right, may have detrimental effects on the cardiovascular and pulmonary systems. The need to provide normal physiologic balance may at times preclude the second goal of the anesthesiologist—that of absence of pain and provision of amnesia. Although these are laudable goals, and perhaps to the lay public most important, they take secondary precedence to the maintenance of homeostasis. The surgeon also requires a quiet operative field. This not only permits the procedure to be accomplished readily, but also may help to mitigate complications of the procedure, as well as time requirements.

Several factors during the discontinuation and wakeup phases of anesthesia can contribute to myocardial problems. The wakeup process usually takes place relatively rapidly. As such, the anesthesiologist most often uses minimal amounts of sedatives and analgesics. The introduction of more of these agents at this point would simply delay and confuse the emergence state. However, the absence of these agents obviously can contribute to hypertension, hypercarbia, catecholamine release, and agitation.

The extubation phase of anesthesia can present serious complications that result in hypoxemia. These have been previously discussed and include failure to breathe, aspiration, and upper airway edema. Furthermore, any development of hypercarbia in a brain-injured patient may contribute to an increased blood brain flow and elevated intracranial pressure.

Once the patient is awake, the transport process to the ICU can further exacerbate the situation. The patient may be moved from the operating table to a stretcher and finally onto a bed in the ICU. The movement itself, with its potential for bumps, banging into walls, and elevator trips, can aggravate pain and agitation. The greater number of floors to be traversed, the greater the risk to the patient and the more difficult to control hemodynamics during this period.

ANESTHETIC EMERGENCE IN THE ICU

We advocate that critically ill patients not be awakened in the operating room, but rather in the ICU. This means that the anesthetic delivery continues right up until the patient actually leaves the operating room. Combined with a minimal transport time, this procedure should ensure that the patient will arrive in the ICU still well anesthetized. This procedure minimizes the risk involved in the rapid awakening usually required in the operating room. In the ICU, the patient can be awakened at a rate that is most advantageous to the maintenance of homeostasis. If events begin to get out of control and hypertension or tachycardia develops, it can be treated and the patient reanesthetized. All in all, the process allows much tighter control of vital signs.

- *Anesthetic emergence in the ICU usually results in a more stable, viable patient.*

Emergence in the ICU also ensures that the pulmonary status can be better evaluated. Often, pulmonary assessment in the operating room includes pulse oximetry. In the ICU, not only can blood gases be evaluated for more information about pulmonary status, but also a chest film can be taken. These steps often preclude premature extubation of the patient with early deterioration of lung function.

TRANSPORT PROCESS

• Physicians and other personnel notoriously overventilate patients when they use a hand ventilation system. They also often cause extremely high airway pressures.

• The degree of monitoring during transport should be influenced by the stability or instability of the patient.

All patients during transport require basic equipment (Table 1–1). Oxygen is the first consideration. If the patient is extubated, face masks may be sufficient; otherwise, patients should be attached to a self-inflating or Mapelson circuit[1] to provide positive pressure breathing during the transport process. PEEP can be applied as necessary. A pressure monitor should be attached to the circuit so the anesthesiologist can gauge the pressure during the positive pressure and level of PEEP. At the very least, pulse oximetry should be employed. All pulse oximeters are portable and can easily be accommodated during the process.

A heart rate monitor should accompany the patient. This will alert the clinician not only to any changes in heart rate, but also to the development of arrhythmias. Blood pressure should also be monitored indirectly or by invasive methods. If an arterial line has been placed in the operating room, it should be attached to the monitor during transport. Often, on arrival in the ICU, valuable time is wasted while patients are being attached to various monitors. By the time vital signs such as blood pressure are actually checked, they may be extremely abnormal.

One must ensure that any equipment necessary to treat emergencies accompanies the patient. This includes drugs to treat hypo- and hypertension and arrhythmias. A laryngoscope and extra endotracheal tubes should also be available. One should not count on having the equipment available at the other end of the transport.

All equipment necessary for the patient should be in the ICU prior to the patient's arrival. This includes mechanical ventilators and any vasoactive infusions that may be necessary. The communication process should have advised the ICU of the types of drips and current infusion rates. Provided the patient is still anesthetized, there should be little need initially to change rates. Respiratory therapists should be on hand to attach the mechanical ventilator and to initiate ventilation.

The patient should not be transported from the operating room if any evidence of instability exists. This includes the use of intermittent drugs to treat hyper- or hypotension within the last 10 minutes or hypoxemia. In addition, any ventricular arrhythmias that re-

Table 1–1.
Equipment for Patient Transport

Self-inflating or Mapelson circuit
Pulse oximeter
Blood pressure monitor
Laryngoscope
Assortment of endotracheal tubes
Vasoactive drugs
Antiarrhythmic agents
ECG

quired treatment should no longer be present. Therapy for any of these problems can be initiated in the operating room, and there is little need to make a rapid and probably unsafe trip to the ICU at that time; 10 to 15 minutes of stability should provide sufficient assurance that it is safe to transport the patient.

GENERAL EVALUATION

When the critically ill postoperative patient first arrives in the ICU, several goals need to be accomplished almost simultaneously. These include immediate assessment of vital signs, including heart rate, blood pressure, cardiac rhythm, and neurologic status, to ensure a degree of stability. Simultaneously, blood samples must be sent to the laboratory, to develop baseline information. Furthermore, any instabilities require rapid correction. All this follows the philosophy that maintenance of homeostasis contribute to the patient's safe and rapid recovery. Therefore, the goal remains always to attempt to normalize function.

• *When the patient arrives in the ICU following surgery, all new laboratory data should be obtained to develop a base of information for the patient. Previous history or data may be of little help following the latest operative procedure.*

It may be difficult to detect most postoperative myocardial ischemia. This includes the period of emergence in the operating room, as well as the transport process and initial recovery in the ICU. Reports indicate that as many as 60% of ischemic events may not be readily apparent.[2] This no doubt has to do with placement of various electrodes and monitors used in the operating room and during the transport process. The clinician will find it necessary to take all measures to minimize any factors known to contribute to ischemia.

A standard 12-lead electrocardiogram should be recorded on all postoperative patients who are at risk for or have coronary artery disease. In general, this includes all patients, male and female, over the age of 50 years. Similarly, any patient who has developed even transient ischemia intraoperatively or an episode of severe hypotension should also have an electrocardiogram. Ischemia or injury patterns evident in the ST-T wave segment should be searched for and treatment rapidly initiated. Often, the only findings are subtle changes not apparent on a preoperative electrocardiogram. These may include flattening of T waves or inversion, as well as ST-T wave segment elevation or depression (Fig. 1–1). If abnormalities are noted and treatment instituted, then follow-up electrocardiograms should be performed at regular intervals to ensure that therapy has actually corrected the problem.

A chest film should be obtained on all patients who return to the ICU following surgery. This study will rule out significant atelectasis, barotrauma, or other pulmonary derangements that might occur during the operative procedure. For patients who are still intubated, the chest film also confirms appropriate tube position. In many instances, central line or pulmonary artery catheter placement in the operating room is not followed up with a chest film to ensure appropriate positioning and absence of barotrauma. This needs to be carried out in the immediate postoperative period.

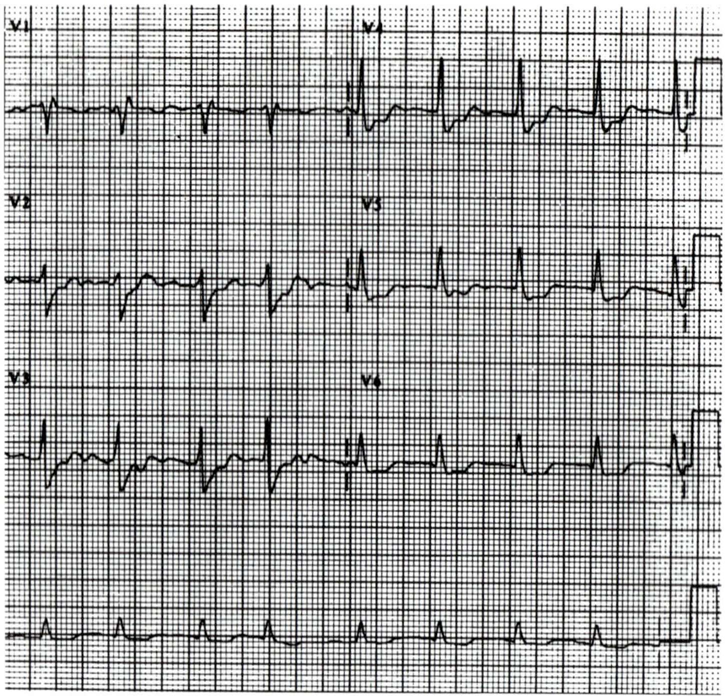

Figure 1–1.
ST-T wave depression. At the time of admission, the patient was in septic shock and had a heart rate greater than 125/min.

Hematocrit and hemoglobin provide a baseline indication of the oxygen carrying capacity. Significant hemodilution may occur secondary to fluid therapy, particularly if little or no blood was given.[3] Based on the clinical situation, as well as on hemoglobin/hematocrit, blood transfusion may be indicated. For patients with known or suspected intra-abdominal sepsis, multiple system trauma, or myocardial ischemia, or in those patients who have undergone a complicated procedure such as aortic aneurysmectomy, we prefer to maintain hemoglobin at 11 to 12 g/dl.[4] In other, more stable situations, and in younger patients, a hemoglobin as low as 8 g/dl may be sufficient. As a non-newtonian fluid, and in normothermic patients, hemoglobin values as high as 15 g/dl will not cause any alterations in viscosity.[5] If anything, the myocardium will not need to work as hard to maintain oxygen delivery, and microcirculatory flow will certainly not be affected.

• *To ensure adequate oxygen delivery, most critically ill patients require hemoglobin levels in the delivery range of 12 to 13 g/dl.*

METABOLIC EVALUATION

Most patients receive minimal if any potassium replacement during surgery and anesthesia. In fact, unless Ringer's lactate solution is used, most patients receive no potassium. Hypokalemia, commonly secondary to hemodilution, develops in the postoperative period. Hyperventilation may also contribute. Potassium may also be lost in urine. Many postoperative arrhythmias are secondary to low or relatively low potassium values.

Hypokalemia in the critically ill should be defined as a value lower than 4.5 mEq/L. Because total body potassium approaches 3000 mEq/L and is in equilibrium, serum values do not have to change substantially to reflect major increases or decreases in total body values. Levels lower than 4.5 mEq/L are associated with an increased risk of severe ventricular arrhythmias, probably in part as a result of low cardiac tissue values. The risk of such arrhythmias increases with hypothermia. Hypokalemia almost surely follows the administration of any loop diuretic and should be anticipated and treated early before symptoms such as arrhythmias develop. Hypokalemia can also develop, at least transiently, following hyperventilation and the associated respiratory alkalosis.

- *The majority of postoperative arrhythmias represent relative or true hypokalemia.*

Intraoperative hypertonic saline infusions are increasingly popular, but they can result in significant hypernatremia.[6,7] Usually, less volume is required, compared to more dilute solutions such as Ringer's lactate. Depending on the particular solution, sodium concentrations can range from 154 to 462 mEq/L. Sodium values should be checked in the immediate postoperative period. Serum sodium levels up to 155 mEq/L do not require any specific therapy other than avoidance of more salt; however, the patient's sodium level should be followed closely. Levels above 155 mEq/L may cause brain water shifts and should be treated.[8] Treatment normally consists of dilute fluid therapy such as D5W or 0.25 normal saline. Total body water (60% of body weight) must be taken into account to determine the amount of fluid required. Sodium distributes over total body water. Correction of serum sodium to below 155 mEq/L should occur over 8 to 12 hours. On occasion, a loop diuretic can be employed. Despite water loss, such therapy can significantly reduce total body sodium. Serum levels further decrease during free water replacement.

- *Without careful attention to detail, the use of hypertonic saline can result in serious electrolyte abnormalities, usually hypernatremia.*

Solutions such as Ringer's lactate and other dilute solutions almost always result in mild hyponatremia, with values ranging between 130 and 136 mEq/L. The exaggerated antidiuretic hormone (ADH) secretion that normally follows surgery and trauma also contributes to such results.[9] Values within this range rarely require correction.

We have noted that, with the increased use of hypertonic-containing solutions, hyperchloremia is present in the postoperative period. This causes metabolic acidosis. Simplistically, the increased chloride anion exchanges with bicarbonate in the distal tubules. This nonanion gap acidosis, once diagnosed, usually requires no specific therapy; however, other causes of acidosis including lactic acidosis and ketoacidosis must also then be searched for and ruled out or treated. Postoperative lactic acidosis may follow a period of prolonged hypoperfusion, use of a tourniquet, or hypothermia. Most such situations are self-limited and respond to adequate volume restoration and improvement of cardiac output. Another common cause of acidosis in postoperative patients is renal tubular acidosis in patients with renal dysfunction or failure.

- *Almost all postoperative acidosis represents hyperchloremia or excess lactate secondary to hypoperfusion.*

Magnesium, phosphorus, and ionized calcium often decrease to abnormally low levels following surgery and anesthesia. This probably represents dilution and minimal replacement, if any, during the operative procedure. Low ionized calcium levels contribute to a decrease in cardiac contractility. Respiratory and metabolic alkalosis can lower values even further. When patients exhibit hemodynamic instability, or when values are less than 1.8 mEq/L, replacement should be standard. Calcium chloride has three times the number of available calcium ions as calcium gluconate. Up to 1 g of calcium chloride can be given slowly over 4 to 5 minutes via a central line; 2 g are often sufficient to raise ionized calcium to acceptable levels. Care should be taken because severe arrhythmias can develop if the drug is given too rapidly or if administered to hypokalemic or hypothermic patients.

- *Disproportionate rises of the BUN to creatinine occur when the gut or abdomen resorbs old blood.*

Blood urea nitrogen (BUN) and creatinine should also be measured. Not only do the data help to delineate baseline renal function, but also changes in BUN can help to assess the state of hydration. Blood resorption from the gastrointestinal tract can elevate BUN, however, and may further confuse the picture. Creatinine clearance can significantly decrease without any apparent change in serum creatinine.[10] Creatinine clearance values of 50 ml/min may still be associated with normal serum creatinine levels. Patients with decreased peripheral musculature may also have normal or low serum creatinine levels despite altered renal function. Today, few patients develop total renal shutdown and anuria. More commonly, renal dysfunction manifests itself with elevated BUN and creatinine, but

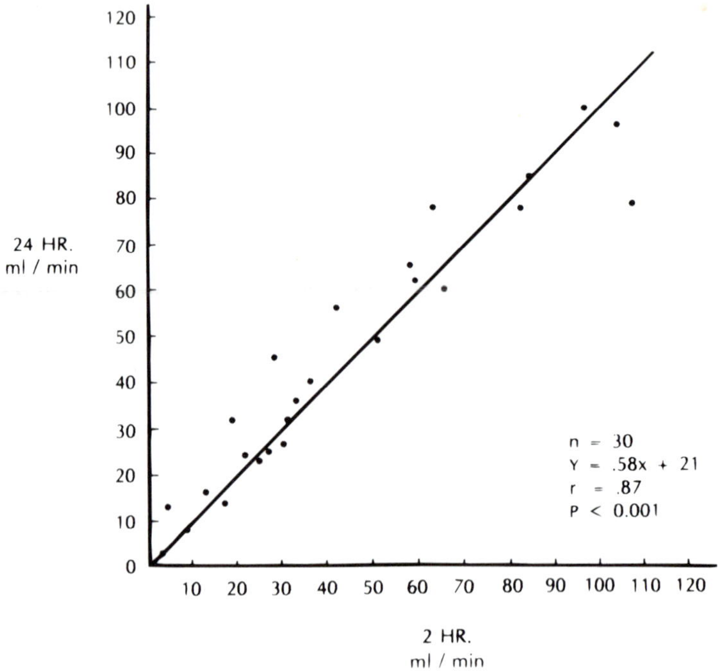

Figure 1–2.
Correlation between 24-hour and 2-hour creatinine clearance.

urine volume is not often affected. Renal function can be rapidly analyzed by performance of a 2-hour creatinine clearance (Fig. 1–2). This test provides the same information as a 24-hour study and has been well validated.[11] Also, loop diuretic therapy does not interfere with the results.

One can count on hyperglycemia being present in almost every postoperative patient. This is a normal stress response due to increased insulin release and altered uptake following surgery or trauma. Most patients have glucose levels that approximate 250 mg/dl. Clearly, this level can be higher in diabetics. Hyperglycemia may result in glucosuria, which can confuse the evaluation of the intravascular volume status and organ perfusion. We attempt to maintain glucose levels below 250 mg/dl. Data suggest that, in acutely brain-injured patients, elevated blood glucose levels are associated with a worsened outcome.[12] Therefore, in brain-injured patients we require even closer control to maintain glucose levels below 150 mg/dl. Most patients' glucose levels can be managed with intermittent insulin infusions based on a sliding scale. Subcutaneous administration of insulin should be avoided in the postoperative patient. The unpredictability of uptake due to blood flow alterations makes this route undesirable. However, when glucose levels remain above 300 mg/dl and do not readily respond to intermittent insulin administration, we begin a continuous IV infusion of insulin. This must be coupled with hourly measurements of blood glucose levels so the insulin infusion can be adjusted accordingly. Glucose dipsticks are inadequate to maintain appropriate control.

• *Control of glucose usually results in fewer complications, better wound healing, and an overall better outcome.*

CLOTTING EVALUATION

In the immediate postoperative period, we almost always measure prothrombin time (PT) and partial thromboplastin (PTT) values, as well as platelet count. The information provides an initial baseline to judge the patient's ability to clot. For instance, continued oozing or bleeding postoperatively in a patient with normal values, including bleeding time, almost always indicates surgical bleeding.[13] Large-volume blood transfusion therapy of 8 units or more dilutes platelets.[14] However, bleeding does usually not occur until values fall between 20,000 to 50,000. An abnormal PT, in addition to its role as an indicator of clotting factor dilution, particularly V and VIII, may also herald early liver dysfunction. Although elevated liver enzymes and bilirubin can develop for multiple reasons, an uncorrectable PT has ominous implications and can indicate end-stage liver disease.

• *Correction of clotting problems in the postoperative period should be guided by the PTT, PT, and platelet count. Therapy should be continued with appropriate products at least until these tests reach acceptable ranges.*

Whereas the PT and PTT may be mildly elevated postoperatively, this does not necessarily indicate either a potential for rebleeding or a need for therapy. Most times, an elevation of PT by 1.0 to 1.5 seconds and PTT by 5 seconds without evidence of active bleeding can be followed, and fresh frozen plasma or cryoprecipitate with their attendant infectious complications can be avoided.[15,16]

CARDIOVASCULAR ISSUES

Upon the patient's emergence from anesthesia, major goals include prevention of myocardial ischemia and improvement of oxygen delivery and, by inference, cardiac output. During general anesthesia, most agents provide a mild cardioprotective effect. This evolves because of the reduction in metabolic demands during general anesthesia. Similarly, almost all agents suppress cardiac output and therefore oxygen delivery.[17] The reduced metabolic needs create a balance with reduced oxygen delivery. Several factors in the postoperative period contribute to the development of mild cardiac ischemia (Table 1–2). Data suggest that despite the use of analgesics, catecholamine increases persist for hours immediately following surgery.[18] This can result in increased myocardial work in excess of available oxygen. Pain, anxiety, and agitation all increase myocardial oxygen demands.

Tachycardia

Tachycardia at rates greater than 100/min may cause ischemia in older patients, or even in younger ones with underlying coronary artery disease.[19] To ensure that tachycardia does not cause ischemia due to increased myocardial oxygen demands, heart rates should be maintained below 90/min. Patients who have had cardiac surgery demonstrate ischemia up to 18 hours postoperatively,[20] despite attempts to reduce myocardial oxygen demands.

Potential causes of tachycardia include rapid emergence from anesthesia with acute onset of pain or awareness, particularly if an inhalation anesthetic was used alone without any narcotics. Often, narcotics given near the end of the procedure can blunt this response. Agitation may also contribute to tachycardia. At times, this can develop as an idiosyncratic response either to anesthetic agents or to drugs given preoperatively. An example includes a possible adverse psychotic response to ketamine. Hypovolemia will often be manifested by tachycardia. Clinicians should also recognize that unsuspected hypoxemia and hypercarbia can both contribute to a tachycardia. Textbooks often discuss the bradycardia consistent with hypoxemia. However, tachycardia develops more often.

• *In the critically ill older patient, a slow heart rate is preferred and results in less overall ischemia.*

Obviously, hypovolemic-induced tachycardia requires fluid or blood. Even after administration of adequate analgesia, pain-induced tachycardia may persist.

Table 1–2.
Cause of Postoperative Myocardial Ischemia

Tachycardia
Hypertension: elevated systemic vascular resistance
Pain
Hypotension

Table 1–3.
Postoperative Drugs to Reduce Heart Rate

Esmolol
Propranalol
Labetalol
Verapamil
Adenosine

Tachycardia can be treated with beta or calcium channel blockers (Table 1–3). The two most appropriate beta blockers for this task are propranolol and esmolol. Propranolol, in incremental doses of 1 mg up to a total of 6 mg, decreases heart rate, but it usually does not affect contractility or blood pressure. If patients have a pulmonary artery catheter in place, this can be effectively demonstrated by measurement of stroke volume before and after infusion. The effects of the drug may last several minutes to several hours. Readministration may be necessary. Esmolol can be given in a 50-mg bolus or as a continuous infusion of 50 to 300 μg/kg/min. Unfortunately, this drug exhibits both inotropic and chronotropic activity. Much more often, we have seen a reduction in stroke volume when this agent has been used. This reflects a decrease in cardiac contractility. However, both agents effectively lower heart rate.

Adenosine can be effectively used in patients with supraventricular tachycardia.[21] While rarely therapeutic, the agent often facilitates diagnosis because of its ability to induce atrioventricular (AV) nodal block. A dose of 6 mg is usually sufficient. Heart rates may vary transiently decreasing to as low as 20/min.

Some calcium channel blockers can effectively reduce heart rate. Unlike beta blockers, they do not cause bronchoconstriction. We have found diltiazem effective in bolus doses of 10 mg, followed by a continuous infusion up to 25 mg/hr. Unlike beta blockers, diltiazem has little if any effect on cardiac contractility. However, if patients are hypovolemic, its vasodilatory properties can cause mild hypotension. Verapamil has also been utilized to reduce heart rate, but it is usually reserved for cases of atrial fibrillation coupled with a rapid ventricular rate. Unlike diltiazem, verapamil is more likely to cause systemic hypotension. In fact, it should not be used if the atrial fibrillation has caused systemic hypotension.

- *Calcium blockers can reduce heart rate without the debilitating negative inotropic effects of beta blockers.*

Many postoperative patients have a combination of tachycardia and hypertension. Labetalol can be a most effective drug under these circumstances. Its beta blockade effects reduce heart rate, and its peripheral vasodilator properties effectively treat hypertension. In the postoperative patient, doses should initially be small, usually 5 mg. The dose can then be increased, based on the patient's initial response. We have effectively used this drug as a continuous infusion up to 80 mg/hr both for heart rate reduction and as an antihypertensive.

Bradycardia

Bradycardia is usually defined as a heart rate lower than 60/min. By itself, it is not a problem and is often seen in well-trained athletes. Bradycardia may result in low blood pressure in patients unable to maintain an adequate stroke volume. Such low heart rates may also make the patient more predisposed to ventricular arrhythmias such as premature contractions.

Causes of bradycardia include nodal rhythm, hypothermia, sick sinus syndrome, beta blockade, and occasionally hypoxemia. Myocardial ischemia can present as a sinus or nodal bradycardia. Bradycardia usually develops as core temperature decreases below 35.0°C. Sick sinus syndrome may alternate between brady- and tachyarrhythmias. Patients on long-term beta-blocker therapy may take a day or so before the tissue levels are low enough that heart rate will actually increase. Most patients with bradycardia respond to atropine at doses of 1.0 to 2.0 mg. Glycopyrrolate (Robinul, 5 mg) has also been effective. We reserve this therapy for bradycardia accompanied by either hypotension or ventricular arrhythmias.

Persistently low heart rates of 40/min or less or those associated with arrhythmias may require cardiac pacing. External pacing can be carried out with electrodes placed on the anterior and posterior surfaces of the chest. These devices permit heart rate monitoring with sensors able to initiate pacing when rates drop below the predefined range. This can be somewhat painful to the patient. However, external pacing is an effective method when venous access is not available. Invasive temporary pacing can be carried out with a balloon-tip pacer floated into the right ventricle and lodged within the trabeculae. This catheter is often difficult to place and should be located before the patient develops any problems requiring its use. The Paceport (Baxter Edwards, Critical Care Division, Santa Ana, CA) version of the pulmonary artery catheter has a lumen that, when the catheter is in the appropriate position, opens into the right ventricle (Fig. 1–3). A pacing wire can then be inserted through this lumen and lodged within the ventricular trabeculae. A pacer box can then be attached and ventricular pacing initiated. A temporary pacer does not always stay in the correct position and therefore should be evaluated from time to time to ensure that it will still capture when required. Often, pacing is momentarily lost during delivery of a positive pressure breath. No doubt the increased airway pressure causes ventricular dilation, and the pacing wire loses contact with the chest wall. Placement is adequate when the amperage required to initiate pacing is 5 mA or less. Requirement of higher levels indicates nonideal wire placement and a greater likelihood of failure if pacing becomes necessary. Once a pacing wire is placed, it seems logical to maintain the pacing box in the sensing mode.

• *It is far easier to place a pacemaker prophylactically for suspected bradycardia than to wait until it is actually needed.*

Hypertension

Postoperative hypertension usually develops in patients with inadequate analgesia or in those who become agitated. The greatest prob-

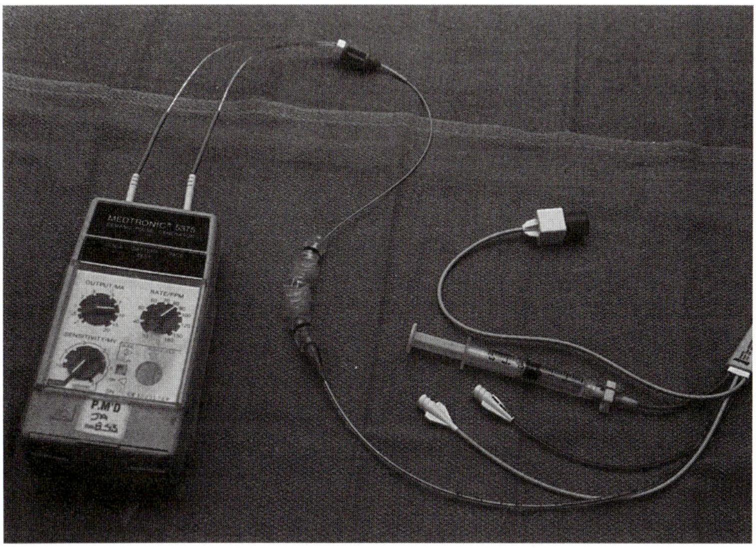

Figure 1–3.
The Paceport pulmonary artery catheter. When properly placed, the wire port provides access to the right ventricle. This usually ensures adequate contact, even during right heart dilation following delivery of a positive pressure breath. (Courtesy of Baxter Edwards, Critical Care Division, Santa Ana, CA, and Medtronic, Minneapolis, MN.)

lems arise in patients who were hypertensive preoperatively or were already on antihypertensive therapy. Rarely does hypervolemia cause hypertension.

Hypertension can have several detrimental effects. It increases impedance to the left ventricle. In turn, the heart must increase wall tension, which in effect increases left ventricular afterload. This can cause myocardial ischemia. A compromised heart may worsen its degree of failure. Hypertension can place undue stress on vascular suture lines or may even dislodge a clot in a vessel. Severe unchecked hypertension can lead to an intracranial bleeding or rupture of an unsuspected aneurysm. Patients who have undergone removal of a cerebral arteriovenous malformation may be at risk of bleeding even if pressures are kept in what is usually a normal range. The many vessel perforators left behind are likely to bleed if the patient becomes hypertensive.

Hypertension can be treated with either continuous or intermittent therapy (Table 1–4). Labetalol can be given in 5- to 10-mg increments to provide short-term control. However, for longer term therapy up to 24 hours, sodium nitroprusside works best. The drug should be administered through a central line. The usual dosages are 0.5 to 6.0 mg/kg/min. The rapid onset and dissipation of action following discontinuance provides excellent control. Generally, in adults, cyanide toxicity is a theoretic rather than a real consideration. Signs include tachyphylaxis, acidosis, and increased venous oxygen content. On the other hand, cyanate toxicity happens much more frequently. Major symptoms include confusion and agitation.[22]

• *Sodium nitroprusside rarely, if ever, causes cyanide toxicity.*

Table 1–4.
Postoperative Drugs to Treat Hypertension

Drug	Dosage
Labetalol	5–15 mg IV bolus 10–80 mg/hr
Nitroprusside	0.5–5.0 μg/kg/min
Nitroglycerin	0.5–4.0 μg/kg/min
Nicardipine	5–25 mg/hr

Although nitroglycerin primarily dilates the venous bed, it does have mild arterial dilating capabilities. In the elderly, these effects are more profound. Dosages vary between 0.5 and 4.0 mg/kg/min to treat hypertension.

If patients require antihypertensive therapy beyond the first 24 hours, it may be advisable to select other agents, so nitroprusside in particular can be discontinued. Labetalol can be added as a continuous infusion up to 80 mg/hr. This agent can also be administered on an intermittent basis. Nicardipine, a calcium blocker antihypertensive agent, can also be administered on a continuous basis. Other popular agents include enalapril, an angiotensin converting enzyme (ACE) inhibitor, and sublingual nifedipine, a calcium blocker. Patients on preoperative antihypertensive agents should be restarted on these drugs as soon as feasible.

Hypotension

Postoperative hypotension requires immediate treatment and diagnosis. Attempts to restore blood pressure should begin while simultaneous efforts are undertaken to make a diagnosis.

Unsuspected pneumothorax can cause hypotension, particularly if it is a tension pneumothorax (Fig. 1–4). Rapid relief of the pneumothorax almost always restores blood pressure. In cases of severe, life-threatening hypotension and physical signs consistent with pneumothorax, a chest tube should be rapidly placed. These signs include a tympanitic (noted on percussion) chest sound, a deviated trachea, decreased breath sounds on one side, and subcutaneous air, particularly in the neck and supraclavicular areas. Pneumothorax presents with all variations and combinations of these findings. It can even exist in the absence of any of these findings. A chest radiograph should always be obtained if hypotension develops in a patient who requires mechanical ventilation or who has recently had a central line placement. Pneumothorax following central line placement can have a delayed onset. Therefore, any earlier chest film following line placement does not rule out the diagnosis. The likelihood increases if the patient has had a central line placement or attempt on the same side as the apparent signs.

- *On occasion, pneumothorax is not diagnosed even on a chest film. It is almost always noted on a CT scan.*

A 14-gauge needle placed in the intrathoracic space is not appropriate therapy for suspected pneumothorax. Once the needle is

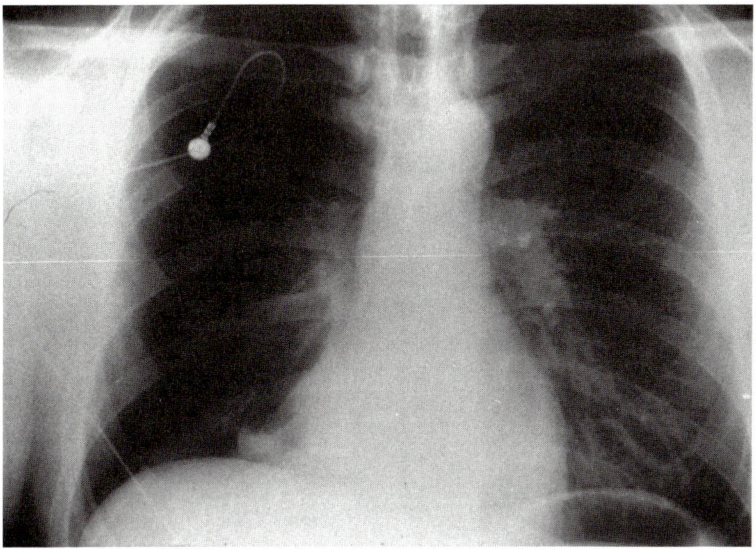

Figure 1–4.
Pneumothorax. Despite an almost complete pneumothorax, this patient did not demonstrate any evidence of hemodynamic compromise.

placed, a chest tube will ultimately be needed. In addition, the small diameter needle does not usually relieve enough air to restore blood pressure to the normal range. Furthermore, if the needle penetrates lung tissue, air will be aspirated even if a pneumothorax is not present. In skilled hands, a chest tube can be placed almost as rapidly as a 14-gauge needle. In the supine patient, all the air will be anterior. To rapidly relieve the pneumothorax, make a 1.5- to 2-inch incision over the third or fourth rib down to the level of the rib itself. The incision should be in the midclavicular line to avoid potential injury to the internal mammary artery, which lies close to the sternal border. Then rapidly advance a hemostat or Kelly clamp over the top of the rib to puncture the pleura. Once the pleura is entered and the tissue is spread, air will rapidly evacuate, even before the tube is placed. At this point, the emergency should be over. Then, under a more controlled situation, the chest tube can be advanced and angled cephalad. When emergency chest tube placement is required for relief of a pneumothorax, one should not worry about cosmetics and attempt to make lateral incisions or tunnel the chest tube over one or more rib interspaces. Speed is of the essence.

Hypovolemia probably represents the most common cause of postoperative hypotension. Treatment consists of rapid fluid replacement. Administer fluid as a bolus in the form of 500 ml of balanced electrolyte solution, such as normal saline or Ringer's lactate, or 250 ml of a colloid solution such as 5% albumin. Crystalloids are obviously cheaper, but they require larger volumes than colloids to increase intravascular volume. Large-bore IV access should be made readily available. This is best accomplished with introducers such as those used for pulmonary artery catheter placement, placed in the antecubital veins. The location and size of the

• *A trauma patient's IV site selection should be based on ability to deliver fluids to the heart without traversing injured or leaking vessels.*

femoral vein makes it an easy target in hypovolemic patients when other sites are difficult to cannulate. Long central lines should usually be avoided for rapid volume replacement. They take longer to place, and their length and diameter significantly increase the resistance to flow. Fluid may need to be administered under pressure. In the case of colloids, which ordinarily come in glass bottles, the fluid can be rapidly infused by interfacing a stopcock into the IV line. The fluid can then be drawn up from the bottle into a 50-ml syringe and then rapidly pushed into the patient. Hypertonic saline solutions including 3% normal saline also restore intravascular volume. When given rapidly or as a bolus, however, such fluids can cause transient increases in serum sodium levels with consequent cerebral and other metabolic derangements.[23]

• *For hypovolemic, hypotensive patients, rapid fluid replacement, rather than the specific solution, ultimately becomes important in volume restoration.*

The need for bolus fluid administration requires assessment of the adequacy of current cardiovascular monitoring. If a central line is not in place, one will likely be needed, particularly if the patient does not respond to the first bolus. Although central venous pressure determinations may be of some help, a pulmonary artery catheter obviously provides more information. It does take slightly longer to place the pulmonary artery catheter. The catheter's utility depends on the physician's and the unit's ability to rapidly prepare and have the equipment on hand to place the catheter. The response time should certainly enter into the clinician's decision in regard to the appropriate monitor under these circumstances.

Although hypovolemia may be the cause of hypotension and fluid administration may be appropriate, blood pressure may not rapidly increase. Similarly, other causes of hypotension may exist. In these circumstances, pressor agents should be started. Vasopressors should be utilized when inadequate myocardial perfusion risks development of ischemia.

In certain instances, hypotension is a direct result of peripheral vasodilatation, such as following spinal cord injury or after overenthusiastic administration of vasodilators including sodium nitroprusside. Sepsis also causes peripheral vasodilation and hypotension. If systolic pressures are less than 60 mm Hg, myocardial ischemia will likely develop. Agents such as phenylephrine and norepinephrine have primarily alpha effects. This means that they do not directly improve contractility but simply increase vasoconstriction. These drugs may be appropriate to restore perfusion pressure, particularly if myocardial ischemia coexists. They do not directly increase heart rate.

• *Severe hypotension should be rapidly corrected even with alpha agonists if necessary.*

Hypotension secondary to a low cardiac output state usually requires an agent with inotropic activities. Such agents include epinephrine, dopamine, and dobutamine (Table 1–5). Although the most apparent clinical manifestation of this condition is low blood pressure, the real cause resides in altered cardiac contractility. These agents increase contractility and thereby cardiac output and blood pressure. In low doses, epinephrine has some peripheral vasodilatator effects. In most clinical dosage ranges, however, it simply increases systemic blood pressure by vasoconstriction and improved contractility. Dosages range from 0.01 to 1.0 μg/kg/min. Dopamine

Table 1–5.
Vasoactive Drugs

Drug	Inotrope	Vasopressor
Epinephrine	yes	yes
Dopamine	yes	in high dose
Dobutamine	yes	no
Neo-Synephrine	no	yes
Phenylephrine	no	yes

probably has vasodilating effects up to 10 μg/kg/min, but this range varies for each patient. In the elderly, the alpha effects may be seen even at low dosage ranges of 2 to 5 μg/kg/min. Even with the use of vasopressors, dopamine in low doses (2 to 5 μg/kg/min) preserves renal blood flow secondary to its dopaminergic properties.[24,25] Dobutamine, in the usual clinical range of 5 to 15 μg/kg/min, primarily causes vasodilatation while it enhances contractility. This drug can also have a pressor response. Despite claims to the contrary, dobutamine, like the other agents, can increase heart rate.

In an emergency, epinephrine is often available for bolus administration. However, if it is used this way, one should begin with small incremental doses. In some circumstances, such as hypotension secondary to nitroprusside, a large bolus of epinephrine can cause severe increases in blood pressure, as high as 300 mm Hg. Begin with 0.1 mg or less and increase the dose until the desired response is attained.

Arrhythmias

Postoperative ventricular arrhythmias such as premature ventricular contractions and ventricular tachycardia are generally a result of ischemia, hypokalemia, or hypothermia. When present, any of these conditions should be rapidly reversed. If potassium levels are lower than 2.5 mEq/L and life-threatening ventricular arrhythmias develop, the patient should be treated with an infusion of 2 to 3 mEq potassium chloride, given directly by the physician. Otherwise, the drug should be administered by continuous infusion with a maximum dosage of 30 mEq/hr. The propensity for arrhythmias significantly increases when serum potassium remains below 4.5 mEq/L.

Hypothermia below 34°C also contributes to arrhythmia generation. These arrhythmias usually consist of bradycardia or premature ventricular contractions.[26]

Treatment of ventricular arrhythmias includes a lidocaine infusion up to 4 mg/hr. Ventricular tachycardia can be treated with external electrical countershock. This should be done at the maximum dosage of 360 joules. Care should be taken to place the paddles so the current actually moves across the heart (Fig. 1–5). This requires placement of the second paddle as far posterior on the chest wall as possible. In many situations, the paddles are placed so close together that the current does not flow across the myocardium.

- *Prior to cardioversion, the physician should know how to operate the defibrillator. Synchronization is not necessary during ventricular fibrillation or tachycardia.*

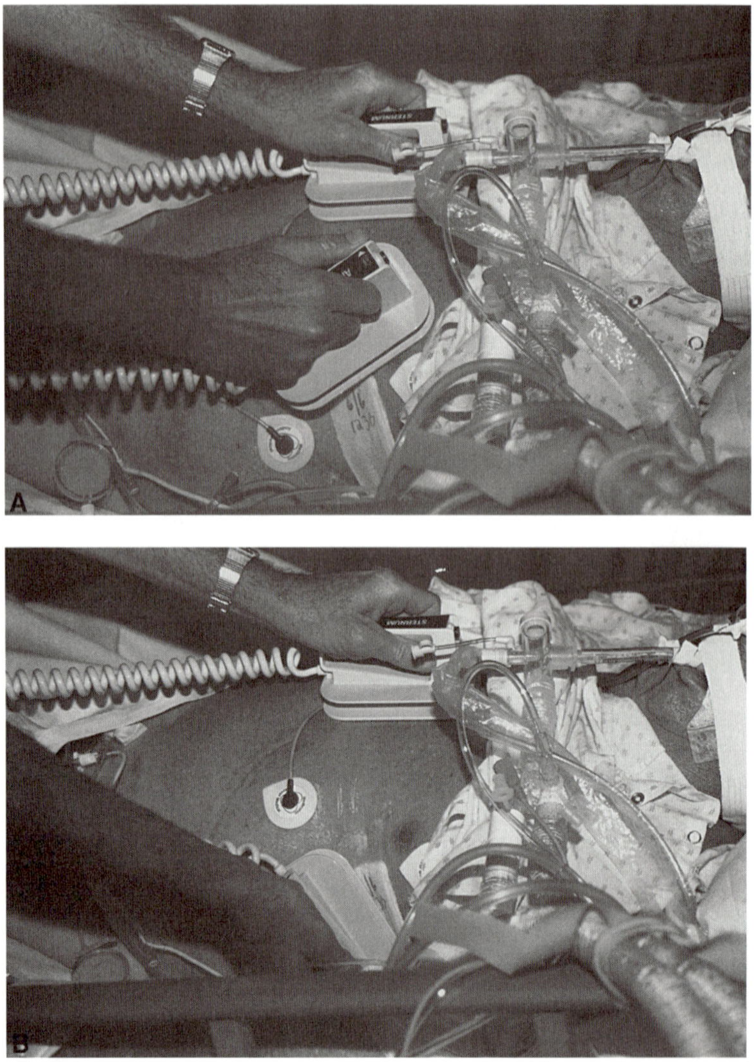

Figure 1–5.
A, Incorrect placement of paddles for defibrillation. B, Correct placement of paddles for defibrillation. The greater the anterior-posterior difference between the paddles, the greater the energy delivery to the heart.

Supraventricular tachycardia or sinus tachycardia can be treated as previously described. This involves the use of calcium channel blockers, beta blockers, and, when necessary, adequate pain control.

PULMONARY CONSIDERATIONS

Major pulmonary problems that develop on emergence from anesthesia relate to hypoxemia. Aspiration is often cited as the most likely cause of postoperative hypoxemia, and it is almost always part of the differential diagnosis. Unfortunately, it can rarely be completely excluded. Obviously, if the patient vomits during induction of anesthesia or if gastric contents are found in the posterior pharynx, then a higher index of suspicion for aspiration should exist.

Premature endotracheal tube removal in the immediate postoperative period, before the patient is fully awake or before neuromuscular blockade is adequately reversed and the patient is able to protect the airway, can lead to vomiting and aspiration. Several steps can help reduce the occurrence of this problem. One is to allow the patient to be fully awake before extubation. Only when the patient shows signs of swallowing and the gag reflex returns can the anesthesiologist believe that the likelihood of aspiration has been minimized.

Patients with known or suspected full stomachs should have a nasal or oral gastric tube passed during the operative procedure. H_2 blockers, given preoperatively, reduce gastric fluid volumes and thereby limit the potential of aspiration. Although H_2 blockers may also elevate pH, it has become less clear that this is of major benefit. In fact, long-term use of H_2 blockers has actually been associated with an increase in airway colonization, demonstrated by recovery of bacteria from the gastric contents, posterior pharynx, and lungs of such patients.[27,28]

- *The role of H_2 blockers in postoperative care may diminish.*

Negative pressure pulmonary edema can develop following extubation and can lead to significant desaturation.[29] Ordinarily, such a situation develops after significant upper airway obstruction heralded by stridor, laryngeal edema, or discoordinate breathing. Young, healthy patients in particular can develop significant intrathoracic pressures. It is not unusual for intrathoracic pressures to exceed -100 cm H_2O. The large increase in negative pressure affects the pulmonary interstitium, which also develops a negative pressure. This results in a significant imbalance of the Starling forces with the accumulation of fluid in the interstitial space at a rate more rapid than can be removed by lymphatic drainage.[30] Fortunately, reinstitution of positive pressure ventilation and diuresis will reverse hypoxemia and contribute to fluid removal from the lung.

Other mechanisms in the development of negative pressure pulmonary edema include the generation by large intrathoracic pressures of significant increases in pulmonary venous return. This volume increase of the pulmonary vascular system leads to elevated intravascular pulmonary artery pressures. This shifts fluid from the vascular to the interstitial space.

Overzealous intraoperative fluid administration can lead to the development of postoperative pulmonary edema and respiratory insufficiency. Technically, this does not represent adult respiratory distress syndrome, but merely fluid overload.

In patients without central venous pressure or capillary wedge pressure monitoring, fluid administration is often guided by blood pressure response and urinary output. However, both are imprecise indicators of intravascular volume status. Furthermore, they can be altered by effects unrelated to intravascular volume. Blood pressure may increase following the onset or awareness of pain. Urine output can be affected by such factors as glucosuria and osmotic diuretics.

Therefore, fluid administration that seems in excess of normal maintenance requirements or those designed to replace interoperative blood loss can contribute to postoperative hypoxemia. At times, an overdosage of anesthetics that results in a blood pressure drop may be treated with large volumes of fluid rather than with a reduction of the anesthetic agent. Overestimates of blood loss may also lead to excess fluid administration.

In general, the longer the operation, the more difficult to judge actual fluid and blood losses and the greater the possibility of fluid overload. Fluid loss during an intra-abdominal or intrathoracic procedure approaches 6 ml/kg/hr. Textbooks often state that peripheral procedures result in a fluid loss of 3 ml/kg/hr.[31,32] This estimate often proves excessive. Moreover, most operating room environments are cool to cold. As the patient becomes hypothermic, intravascular volume and requirements decrease, a factor not often taken into account.

Mechanical factors during delivery of the anesthetic can also cause hypoxemia. These include hypoventilation with the development of atelectasis as well as main stem intubation. The utilization of small tidal volumes without PEEP enhances the likelihood of such developments.

Prevention of Hypercapnia

• Patients with chronic lung disease who have received narcotics have an altered CO_2 response curve and are more likely to retain CO_2.

Hypercapnia also often develops in the postoperative period (Table 1–6). Hypercapnia can develop secondary to either residual anesthetics or failure to ventilate patients adequately postoperatively. Often, at or near the end of an operation, the anesthesiologist permits the patient to breath spontaneously. However, residual anesthetics may contribute to a decrease in overall minute volume, with resultant hypercapnia. Narcotics, if used intraoperatively or preoperatively, may still be present and may further contribute to respiratory depression. Even fentanyl, a short-acting narcotic, may exert such effects up to 4 hours after its last administration. Patients who exhibit signs of narcosis such as constricted pupils often respond to reversal agents such as naloxone. Hyperventilation with fresh gases, including 100% oxygen, usually rapidly eliminates any residual inhalation agents.

Residual neuromuscular blockade causes postoperative hypercapnia. One cannot always adequately judge the degree of reversal of muscle paralysis with a blockade monitor. The textbooks indicate

Table 1–6.
Causes of Hypercapnia

Residual anesthetics
Residual neuromuscular blockade
Narcotic analgesics, including epidural
Chronic lung disease
Upper abdominal or chest surgery

that three out of four or four out of four of a train of four are adequate for extubation. In fact, such patients may have as many as 70% of their neuromuscular receptors still blocked.[33] Under these circumstances, the patient may be able to maintain tidal ventilation but will not have any reserves to generate a cough or to mobilize secretions. The ability to hold the head up from the supine position for more than 5 seconds actually represents a better clinical indicator of the adequacy of neuromuscular blockade reversal. At least 50% of receptors are unblocked if the patient can perform such a maneuver.[34] These patients will be able to sustain a cough and deep breath. Patients may often look as though neuromuscular blockade has been reversed in the operating room, but because of hypothermia, they may again develop signs of paralysis. Attempts to reverse neuromuscular blockade in patients with a temperature of less than 35.5°C often result in such clinical situations. In addition, patients who are severely acidotic, with a pH lower than 7.20, may not respond in the anticipated way to neuromuscular blockade reversal.[35]

- *A blockade monitor by itself cannot accurately predict when the effects of a neuromuscular blocking agent have been adequately reversed.*

Certain surgical procedures, by their nature, may contribute to hypoventilation postoperatively. Upper abdominal or thoracic procedures, because of pain and the impact of the procedure, cause a decrease in functional residual capacity (FRC) and lead to hypoventilation and CO_2 retention. Patients with muscle splitting incisions, such as for thoracotomy or a chevron-type incision in the abdomen, may experience significant amounts of pain and may therefore splint and hypoventilate and in general not breathe well postoperatively. The markedly obese patient, particularly after abdominal surgery, may breath inadequately and may develop CO_2 retention.

Epidural narcotics can contribute to hypercapnia. Systemic uptake can cause narcotization similar to that produced by systemically administered agents.[36] The usual clinical signs of pinpoint pupils and altered level of consciousness are evident.

RENAL PROBLEMS

Oliguria and anuria are among the most common problems seen postoperatively. Causes include hypovolemia or low cardiac output despite adequate intravascular volume. Other causes can include an obstructed catheter, acute renal failure or damage to the collecting system such as ureteral obstruction, and bladder perforation and leak.

Acute renal failure can follow suprarenal cross clamping of the aorta. Severe or prolonged intraoperative hypotension can also be the culprit. Acute renal artery thrombosis is rare, but occasionally occurs; a renal scan will demonstrate the absence of blood flow.

At times, urine will drain from sites other than the bladder catheter. Sites include ureteral stents, nephrostomy tubes, or an ileal conduit. The clinician should know where to expect the urine to drain. This may involve a conversation with the surgeon, to understand the actual procedure performed.

The diagnosis of hypovolemia can be made on clinical signs.

Findings include reduced urine volume, a urine specific gravity greater than 1.020, and, when available, low central venous or pulmonary capillary wedge pressure. Hypovolemia reduces cardiac output. A fluid challenge of 500 to 2000 ml of balanced electrolyte solution or 250 ml of plasma protein fraction can serve as a diagnostic intervention. Other diagnostic methods include irrigation of the catheter and measurement of BUN and creatinine, particularly in patients with significant muscle wasting. A rapid elevation of BUN or creatinine from preoperative levels may indicate leakage into the peritoneal cavity. Urine can also leak through other abdominal drains. Analysis of such fluid usually resolves the problem. Abdominal ultrasound can allow one to make the diagnosis of acute obstruction of the urinary drainage system. Intravenous pyelography is usually of little help as a determinant of the cause of acute postoperative renal failure.

• *Oliguria in the postoperative period is almost always due to hypovolemia. A small percentage of patients who are receiving long-term diuretic therapy may require small doses of a loop diuretic to initiate urine flow.*

Treatment of low urine output can sometimes consist of a simple intervention such as placement of a new catheter. When appropriate, volume expansion should be carried out as described in Chapter 6. A low cardiac output requires intervention to restore cardiac output, including inotropes.

For reasons not completely understood, despite adequate intravascular volume and cardiac output, some postoperative patients may have a redirection of blood flow away from the kidney. Low-dose dopamine (3 to 5 μg/kg/min) will stimulate dopaminergic receptors within the renal vascular bed and improve renal blood flow and urinary output. Low-dose dopamine is also effective in the maintenance of renal blood flow in patients receiving alpha-adrenergic therapy. Patients on long-term diuretic therapy may require reinstitution of diuretics. Occasionally, in patients who have adequate volume but minimal urine, a small dose of loop diuretic (5 mg furosemide) may initiate urine flow.

Diabetes insipidus can develop in the patient with a severe head injury or after operative procedures including hypophysectomy. Urine output usually exceeds 200 ml/hr. Specific gravity ranges between 1:000 and 1:004. If measured, urine sodium is less than 20 mEq/L. The main dangers consist of dehydration, hypernatremia, hyperosmolarity, and risk of further brain injury.

NEUROLOGIC EVALUATION

Chapter 14 describes in detail the evaluation and therapy for the obtunded patient. Obviously, mental status can be clouded by residual anesthetics, premedications, and analgesics. Incomplete reversal of neuromuscular blockade interferes with the neurologic examination. Patients with liver or renal dysfunction may clear drugs at a much lower rate than normal. Table 1–7 is a list of causes of postoperative neurologic changes.

Hypoxia can alter mental status. When hypoxia is ongoing, the patient's status may vary between agitation and confusion and may progress to unresponsive coma. Failure to awaken following hypox-

Table 1–7.
Causes of Postoperative Neurologic Changes

Hypotension
Stroke
Electrolyte disturbance
Intracranial bleed
Oversedation
Residual paralysis
Hyper- or hypoglycemia

emia does not auger well, particularly if this persists beyond 24 hours.

Patients can suffer an intraoperative stroke. These strokes may be embolic following carotid artery surgery, or they may be caused by a thrombus from a fibrillating left atrium. Sustained, severe hypotension can also cause stoke. The answers may be found in the anesthesiologist's record.

Rapid hemodilution and a serum sodium decrease to less than 120 mEq/L can lead to significant intracerebral fluid shifts, edema, and profound alteration of mental status.[37] Such changes relate to rapidity of the serum sodium decrease. The most likely surgery-related cause is water uptake during transurethral resection of the prostate.

Neurosurgical procedures themselves can cause severe postoperative edema and altered mental status. A patient admitted for trauma may only have an initial cursory examination before surgery for other more immediate problems. Meantime, the head injury may continue to worsen and only become apparent following admission to the ICU.

Patients can bleed following neurosurgical procedures. Uncontrolled hypertension, particularly during emergencies, could conceivably lead to intracranial bleeding or rupture of an unknown aneurysm.

Cerebral vasospasm can develop following clipping of an intracranial aneurysm.[38] However, this complications usually develops several days postoperatively and is related to the amount of blood in the cisterns. The first sign may be a depressed level of consciousness.

Failure to move the extremities can result from operating room problems. These can include positioning or spinal cord distraction during certain procedures. Aneurysm surgery, particularly for repair of thoracoabdominal aneurysms, can result in interrupted blood flow and paralysis or paresis.[39] Epidural hematoma can follow successful or unsuccessful epidural or spinal block or catheter placement.[40]

Evaluation of altered mental status includes discontinuation or reversal of all possible causal agents. The anesthesiologist should be questioned and the anesthetic record reviewed.

Physician examinations include evaluation of the patient's level of consciousness and ability to follow commands. Motor function

• *Postoperative patients with altered neurologic findings usually require an emergency CT scan.*

and strength must also be checked. Localized findings more often point to a structural defect. More generalized responses usually indicate global injury.

Laboratory studies should be based on what is likely to cause the observed findings. These studies include blood gas analysis, serum sodium, osmolarity, phosphate levels, and BUN. Rarely do other chemical abnormalities cause mental status changes. Obviously, unsuspected liver failure must be ruled out; however, in liver failure the patient is usually jaundiced.

A computed tomographic (CT) scan can demonstrate bleeding or increased intracranial pressure. The radiolucencies indicative of stroke usually do not appear for several days (Fig. 1–6).

Once evident, any correctable abnormalities should be attended to as rapidly as possible.

Treatment of diabetes insipidus initially consists of efforts to maintain normal intravascular volume and serum sodium. Awake, extubated patients can often simply drink enough fluids to keep up with fluid loss. These patients should avoid drinks with sugar because of the risk of hyperglycemia. Patients unable to drink require replacement of urine with dilute solutions of D5W or 0.25 saline. Urine should not be replaced on a milliliter-for-milliliter basis. This only contributes to continued increased urine volume. Usually, replacement on a basis of 0.5 or 0.75 ml to 1.0 ml is sufficient to

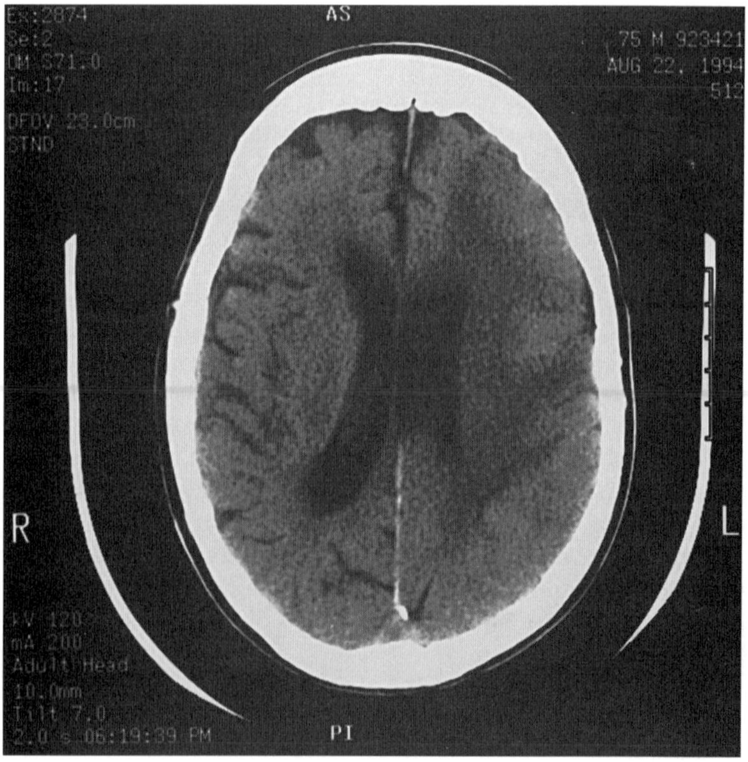

Figure 1–6.
CT evidence of an occlusive stroke involving the middle cerebral artery.

maintain acceptable serum sodium levels of less than 155 mEq/L. A solution of 0.25 saline does not pose any problems with hyperglycemia and provides some salt to help preserve renal concentrating mechanisms.

We reserve vasopressin[41] or DDAVP[42] for situations when urine volume exceeds 400 ml/hr. Vasopressin (Pitressin, 5 units IV) has the advantage of a short duration of action and is less likely to cause the syndrome of inappropriate antidiuretic hormone (SIADH) secretion. DDAVP (5 units) provides long-term control.

SIADH usually occurs in patients with head injury or following neurosurgical procedures.[42] The first indication is a decrease in serum sodium, usually to less than 130 mEq/L. Urine volume, sodium concentration, and specific gravity provide minimal diagnostic help. A low serum osmolarity (< 280 mOsm) and high urine osmolarity (> 400 mOsm) help to make the diagnosis. The major therapy in medical patients consists of fluid restriction. This is usually not possible in surgical patients. Therefore, when serum sodium decreases below 130 mEq/L, we maintain a continuous infusion of 3% saline and monitor serum sodium regularly. Particularly in patients with head injuries, low serum sodium can lead to an increase in brain water.

HYPOTHERMIA

Postoperative hypothermia can cause significant problems in the critically ill patient. The usual causes of hypothermia include a relatively cool operating room and failure to keep the patient warm. This situation is further aggravated by the use of the fluids kept at room temperature. These fluids include crystalloids, colloids, and blood. Paralysis prevents heat generation by muscle shivering. Trauma patients may already be hypothermic even before their arrival in the operating room.

Several different methods can be used to measure core temperature. The most obvious and common is the temperature obtained from a pulmonary artery catheter. The thermistors are accurate in this regard. Rectal temperatures have an offset of about 1°C when compared with pulmonary artery catheter determination of core temperature. Some bladder catheters now allow measurement of bladder urine temperature. Again, this seems to correlate well with other accepted methods of core determination. Infrared technology has been introduced to measure tympanic membrane temperatures. Although this method requires accurate placement of the probe within the ear canal, it can give highly accurate and reliable determinations of core temperature.[43] In general, we avoid the use of oral and axillary temperatures in critically ill patients.

- *Tympanic membrane temperatures require accurate placement of the probe so as to not record ear canal temperature.*

Hypothermia can cause or lead to significant complications. For example, data suggest that hypothermia interferes with normal function of the coagulation cascade. As body temperature decreases, elevation of both prothrombin and partial thromboplastin develops.[44] This will happen despite a normal amount of coagulation factors present in blood. Moreover, because most coagulation tests are performed at 37°C, this type of dysfunction may not be immediately detectable by the usual laboratory methods. Therefore, despite a normal PT or PTT, we cannot rule out coagulopathy in a bleeding patient who remains hypothermic.

Platelet function is also significantly altered at reduced body temperatures. Because platelets are normally stored at 4°C, some time must be allowed after infusion before one can expect platelets to function normally.[45] Therefore, when platelets are given to a hypothermic patient, their maximal impact may not be realized. All these factors become further magnified at body temperatures below 35°C.

Cardiovascular function may also be compromised by hypothermia.[46] Hypotension that develops when the temperature falls below 33°C probably follows reduced cardiac function and output. A J wave usually appears on the electrocardiogram between the QRS and T-wave segments. While not pathognomonic, it is often present at temperatures of 30 to 32°C. Next, bradycardia develops, and other arrhythmias include atrial and ventricular fibrillation.

The intense vasoconstriction that accompanies hypothermia often causes postoperative management complications. For example, these patients can demonstrate significant hypertension. Attempts to reduce blood pressure with vasodilators can lead to profound vasodilatation and hypotension because of the diminished intravascular volume. The problem will continue during the rewarming process if inadequate fluid resuscitation accompanies the vasodilatation.

Rewarming can result in metabolic acidosis with increased serum lactate. This so-called rewarming acidosis develops because of hypoperfusion due to the intense vasoconstriction. As temperature increases, or as intravascular volume expands, perfusion reestablishes itself through these previously anaerobic areas. The washout of the products of anaerobic metabolism, if of sufficient volume, can overcome the usual buffer mechanisms and can lead to at least a transit metabolic acidosis. Hypothermia can cause significant alteration in oxygen delivery and consumption.

Cold temperatures can directly affect cardiac output and result in a reduction in oxygen delivery. The reduced body temperatures cause a leftward shift of the oxyhemoglobin dissociation curve. The increased hemoglobin affinity for oxygen reduces its availability at peripheral tissues. Extraction is impaired, and the likelihood of increased oxygen extraction or metabolic acidosis increases.[47]

Shivering generally begins at temperatures between 35 and 36°C. Shivering can dramatically increase oxygen consumption by as much as 200 to 300%.[48] This is usually far in excess of what can be made up by utilizing the oxygen reserves, particularly when oxygen delivery and cardiac output are impaired.

Neurologic function also suffers during hypothermia. Cerebral blood flow decreases by 6 to 7% for every 1°C drop in temperature.[49] Confusion and disorientation begin at temperatures below 35°C. Dilated pupils can be noted as the temperature drops below

32°C, and voluntary movements cease at temperatures lower than 28°C. Furthermore, animal studies have suggested that hypothermia may result in a reduction in cerebral blood flow that does not return to normal values despite rewarming.[50] This could theoretically result in altered neurologic function and might possibly explain some of the changes seen after cardiopulmonary bypass.

Data seem to suggest that hypothermia in general reduces the body's immune system.[51] Studies have suggested that survival decreases in patients with sepsis or trauma and accompanying hypothermia. To date, it is unclear how hypothermia interferes with the normal immune response. Among other factors, hypothermia is associated with granulocytopenia and interference with normal cytokine release. Therefore, in such situations, hypothermia combined with a bacterial inoculum such as following a prolonged intra-abdominal procedure or trauma can lead to a high incidence of sepsis and septic complications in such patients.

Hypothermia depresses liver function, including drug elimination. Pancreatic inhibition causes inadequate insulin release. Hyperglycemia ensues. If exogenous insulin has been administered, during rewarming, hypoglycemia can potentially occur because of increased endogenous insulin release.

The best treatment for hypothermia is prevention or minimization of its development. In the operating room, this should include maintenance of high ambient temperatures. This may cause discomfort for the surgeons, but the patient's needs take precedence. All body parts not in the operative field should be covered. Several new devices on the market provide surface warming. The head has a large surface vascular supply. Therefore, the patient's head should be covered and kept warm during the operation. All fluids should be delivered at a normothermic body temperature (37°C). These fluids can be kept in a heater until they are needed. Gases from the ventilator should be heated to maximum values, usually 39°C. By the time they reach the patient's airway, they will have cooled to about 37°C. If the patient begins to develop hypothermia, warm fluids can be used to irrigate the abdomen and chest. The anesthesiologist should ensure that the patient does not lie on surfaces wet from either dripping blood or fluids.

- *Continued physical evaluation and/or line placement in the hypothermic patient contributes to the inability to raise core temperature.*

Postoperatively, hypothermia requires aggressive therapy. The patient should be completely covered with warming blankets. Blankets that use circulating water to warm the patient can be placed above and below the patient. Warming blankets with forced hot air can be placed above the patient. The patient's exposed body surfaces should be covered, including the head. Nursing personnel should ensure that the patient is kept covered and should promptly replace blankets after physical examinations have been performed. All fluids should be delivered through warmers. External heat lamps can also be utilized to help warm the patient. Care should be taken that they are kept at the correct distance so as not to burn the patient's skin. These lamps can be helpful for temperature preservation when the patient's covers must be removed to perform a procedure.

If intravascular volume is adequate, sodium nitroprusside can dramatically aid in the warming process. Its vasodilating properties increase skin blood flow, which then acts as a heat exchanger. Care should be taken because intravascular volume depletion can lead to significant hypotension.

Hypothermia can be therapeutic when patients have suffered brain injury. Mild hypothermia to 34°C can result in a significant decrease in brain oxygen requirements. Injured areas with reduced oxygen delivery may be better able to withstand the immediate post-insult/injury period if the metabolic demands can be reduced.[52] Problems in the past were primarily related to a high incidence of septic complications. Now, however, with a better understanding of how to prevent sepsis with appropriate antibiotic usage and prevention of central line sepsis, this therapy may still prove beneficial to such patients.

REFERENCES

1. Bain JA, Spoerel WE: Flow requirements for a modified Mapleson D system during controlled ventilation. Can Anaesth Soc J 1973; 20:629.
2. Mangano DT, Browner WS, Hollenberg et al: Association of perioperative myocardial ischemia with cardiac morbidity and mortality in men undergoing noncardiac surgery. N Engl J Med 1990; 323;1781–1788.
3. Cervera AL, Moss G: Crystalloid distribution following hemorrhage and hemodilution: mathematical model and prediction of optimum volumes for equilibration at normovolemia. J Trauma 1974; 14: 506–520.
4. Lorente JA, Landin L, DePablo R et al: Effects of blood transfusion on oxygen transport variables in severe sepsis. Crit Care Med 1993; 21:1312–1318.
5. Jobes DR, Gallagher J: Acute normovolemic hemodilution. Intern Anesthesiol Clin 1982; 20:77–95.
6. Traverso LW, Bellamy RF, Hollenbach SJ, Witcher LD: Hypertonic sodium chloride solutions: effect on hemodynamics and survival after hemorrhage in swine. J Trauma 1987; 27:32–39.
7. Holcroft JW, Vassar MJ, Turber JE et al: 3% NaCl and 7.5% NaCl/ Dextran 70 in the resuscitation of severely injured patients. Ann Surg 1987; 206:279–288.
8. Kaieda R, Todd MM, Cook LN et al: Acute effects of changing plasma osmolality colloid oncotic pressure on the formation of brain edema after cryogenic injury. Neurosurgery 1989; 24:671–678.
9. Dudley HF, Boling EA, LeQuesne LP et al: Studies on antidiuresis in surgery: effects of anesthesia, surgery and posterior pituitary antidiuretic hormone on water metabolism in man. Ann Surg 1954; 140: 354–367.
10. Schrier RW: Acute renal failure. JAMA 1982; 247:2518–2525.
11. Wilson RF, Soullier G: The validity of two hour creatinine clearance studies in critically ill patients. Crit Care Med 1980; 8:281–284.
12. Andrews BT: The intensive care management of patients with head injury in neurosurgery intensive care. Andrews BT, ed, New York, McGraw-Hill 1993; pp. 227–232.
13. Fischbach DP, Fogdell RT, eds: Coagulation: the essentials. Baltimore, Williams & Wilkins, 1981.
14. National Institutes of Health Consensus Development Conference

Statement: Platelet transfusion therapy. JAMA 1987; 257:1777–1780.
15. Surgenor DM, Wallace EL, Hao S et al: Collection and transfusion of blood in the United States, 1982–1988. N Engl J Med 1990; 322: 1646–1651.
16. Bove JR: Transfusion-associated hepatitis and AIDS. What is the risk? N Engl J Med 1987; 317:242–245.
17. Pavlin EG, Su JU: Cardiopulmonary pharmacology anesthesia, 3rd ed. Miller RD, ed, New York, Churchill Livingstone, 1990; pp. 105–134.
18. Chiolero R, Flatt JP, Revelly JP et al: Effects of catecholamines on oxygen consumption and oxygen delivery in critically ill patients. Chest 1991; 100:1676–1684.
19. Slogoff S, Keats AS: Randomized trial of primary anesthetic agents on outcome of coronary artery bypass operations. Anesthesiology 1989; 70:179–188.
20. Mangano DT, Browner WS, Hollenberg M et al: Long term cardiac prognosis following noncardiac surgery. JAMA 1982; 268:233–239.
21. Gatell JA, Barner HB, Shevde K: Adenosine and myocardial protection. J Cardiothorac Vasc Anesth 1993; 7:466–480.
22. Pasch T, Schulz V, Hoppelshauser G: Nitroprusside-induced formation of cyanide and its pharmacol. J Cardiovasc Pharmacol 1983; 5: 77–85.
23. Layon AJ, Duncan D, Gallagher TJ et al: Hypertonic saline as a resuscitation solution in hemorrhagic shock: effects on extravascular lung water and cardiopulmonary resuscitation. Anesth Analg 1987; 66: 154–158.
24. Swygert TH, Roberts LC, Valek TR et al: Effect of intraoperative low-dose dopamine on renal function in liver transplant recipients. Anesthesiology 1991; 75;571–576.
25. Conte G, Canton AD, Sabbatini M et al: Acute cyclosporine renal dysfunction reversed by dopamine infusion in healthy subjects. Kidney Int 1989; 36:1086–1092.
26. Reuler J: Hypothermia, pathophysiology, clinical settings and management. Ann Intern Med 1978; 89:519.
27. Priebe HJ, Skillman JJ, Bushness LS et al: Antacid versus cimetidine in preventing acute gastrointestinal bleeding: a randomized trial in 75 critically ill patients. N Engl J Med 1980; 302;426–430.
28. Driks MR, Craven DE, Celli BR et al: Nosocomial pneumonia in intubated patients given sucralfate as compared with antacids or histamine type 2 blockers: the gastric colonization. N Engl J Med 1987; 317: 1376–1382.
29. Lang SA, Duncan PG, Shephard DAE et al: Pulmonary oedema associated with airway obstruction. Can J Anaesth 1990; 37:210–218.
30. Starling EH: On the absorption of fluids from the connective tissue spaces. J Physiol 1986; 19:312–326.
31. Traverso LW: Fluid resuscitation after an otherwise fatal hemorrhage. I. Crystalloid solutions. J Trauma 1986; 26:168–175.
32. Cervera AL, Moss G: Crystalloid distribution following hemorrhage and hemodiluting: mathematical model and prediction of optimum volumes for equilibration at normovolemia. J Trauma 1974; 14; 506–520.
33. O'Connor NF, Roizen MF: Use of muscle relaxants in the intensive care unit. J Intens Care Med 1993; 8:34–46.
34. Partridge BL, Abrams JH, Bazemore C et al: Prolonged neuromuscular blockade after long-term infusion of vecuronium bromide in the intensive care unit. Crit Care Med 1990; 18:1177–1179.

35. Pavlin EG, Holle RH, Schoene RB: Recovery of airway protection compared with ventilation in humans after paralysis with curare. Anesthesiology 1989; 70:381–385.
36. Watson J, Morre A, McQuay H et al: Plasma morphine concentrations in analgesic effects of lumbar extradural morphine and heroin. Anesth Analg 1984; 63:629–634.
37. Sterns RH: Severe hyponatremia: the case for conservative management. Crit Care Med 1992; 20:534–539.
38. Adams HP, Kassell NF, Torner JC et al: Predicting cerebral ischemia after aneurysmal subarachnoid hemorrhage: influences of ctitical condition, CT results and antifibrinolytic therapy. Neurology 1987; 37: 1586.
39. Shenaq SA, Svensson LG: Paraplegia following aortic surgery. J Cardiothorac Vasc Anesth 1993; 7:81–94.
40. Rao TKL, El-Etr A: Anticoagulation following placement of epidural and subarachnoid catheters: an evaluation of neurologic sequelae. Anesthesiology 1981; 55:618–620.
41. Hall J, Robertson G: Diabetes insipidus. Crit Care Med 1990; 4:342.
42. Moses AML, Notman DD: Diabetes insipidus and syndrome of inappropriate antidiuretic hormone secretion (SIADH). Adv Intern Med 1982; 27:73–100.
43. Chamberlain JM, Grandner J, Rubinoff JL, et al: Comparison of tympanic thermometer to rectal and oral thermometers in a pediatric emergency department. Clin Pediatr 1991; 30:24–29.
44. Woodhouse P, Keating WR, Coleshaw SR: Factors associated with hypothermia in patients admitted to a group of inner city hospitals. Lancet 1989; 2:1201.
45. Bogdonoff DL, Williams ME, Stone DJ: Thrombocytopenia in the critically ill patient. J Crit Care 1990; 5:1186–1205.
46. Frank SM, Beattie C, Christopherson R et al: Unintentional hypothermia is associated with postoperative myocardial ischemia. Anesthesiology 1993; 78:468–476.
47. Shapiro BA, Perussi WT: Blood gas analysis in critical care. Civetta JM, Kirby RR, Taylor RW, eds, Philadelphia, JB Lippincott, 1992; pp. 326–329.
48. Guffin A, Girard D, Kaplan JA: Shivering following cardiac surgery: hemodynamic changes and reversal. J Cardiothorac Anesth 1987; 1: 24–28.
49. Williams GR, Spencer FC: The clinical use of hypothermia following cardiac arrest. Ann Surg 1958; 148:462.
50. Clifton GL, Jiang JY, Lyeth BG et al: Marked protection by moderate hypothermia after experimental traumatic brain injury. J Cereb Blood Flow Metab 1991; 11:114–121.
51. Kramer MR, Vandij KJ, Rosin AJ: Mortality in elderly patients with thermoregulatory failure. Arch Intern Med 1989; 149:1521.
52. Natale JE, D'Alecy LG: Protection from cerebral ischemia by brain cooling without reduced lactate accumulation in dogs. Stroke 1989; 20:770–777.

CHAPTER 2

Selection of Appropriate Monitoring Techniques

T. James Gallagher

Case Report

The patient was a 43-year-old woman admitted to the intensive care unit (ICU) following acute decompensation in the surgical ward. The patient had been operated on 3 days before for removal of a recurrent malignant brain tumor. She had become progressively hypoxemic, and a blood gas reading in the surgical ward revealed a PaO_2 of 28 mm Hg and $PaCO_2$ of 34 mm Hg. The patient was combative. She was intubated on the scene with the aid of thiopental sodium (Pentothal) and succinylcholine and was rapidly transferred to the surgical ICU.

On arrival in the ICU, the patient had signs of altered mental status and elevated intracranial pressure (ICP). An ICP monitor was placed as well as an arterial line. The chest radiograph taken following intubation showed diffuse bilateral pulmonary edema. Laboratory data on admission revealed a serum sodium of 128 mEq/L and potassium of 3.8 mEq/L.

The patient was placed on 100% oxygen with a positive end-expiratory pressure (PEEP) of 15 cm H_2O. The ventilator rate was 10/min; PaO_2 was 130 mm Hg, $PaCO_2$ was 38 mm Hg, pH 7.29. Because of the pulmonary edema, a pulmonary catheter was placed both for diagnosis and for intended therapy.

Respiratory monitoring included pulse oximetry and intermittent arterial blood gases. The peak inflation pressures during mechanical ventilation were less than 55 cm H_2O. The ICP was continuously monitored. Initial values were 24 mm Hg. Hyperventilation was instituted to reduce ICP. An end-tidal CO_2

monitor was placed inline and calibrated with the initial blood gases.

In addition to ICP, cerebral perfusion pressure (CPP) was also monitored. This included the arterial line zeroed at the carotid bifurcation to obtain accurate assessment of cerebral blood pressure. PEEP and the FiO_2 were weaned by intermittent blood gas analysis or by monitoring the pulse oximeter.

Steps were then taken to correct the metabolic abnormalities. The patient weighed 60 kg, and total body water was calibrated to be 36 L. The ideal sodium was judged to be 145 mEq/L. Therefore, the patient was calculated to have a sodium deficit of 16 mEq/L or a total of 576 mEq/L. During the first 4 hours in the ICU, the average urine output was 100 ml/hr. The initial urine sodium concentration was 354 mEq/L. This was estimated as a 849 mEq/L sodium loss per day. Plans were made to replace the initial sodium deficit of 576 mEq/L over 2 days. Therefore, it was judged that the patient required 280 mEq/L plus the 849 mEq/L of sodium lost each day. This totaled 1029 mEq/L per day. It was further calculated that with an infusion of 3% saline, this would require approximately 2.2 L per day 3% saline to make up the sodium loss. It was elected to monitor the serum and urine sodium values on a 4-hour basis so the adjustments in the sodium concentration infusion rates could be made as necessary. Two and a half days later, serum sodium was 142 mEq/L and ICP had stabilized at 18 mm Hg.

GENERAL PHILOSOPHY

At its most basic, monitoring consists primarily of observation. Nurses and physicians observe the patient for changes in mental status, vital signs, peripheral perfusion, and the like. Respiratory and physical therapists observe the patient's response to their various interventions. Has the patient been able to increase range of motion? Are the pressures in the airway lower now during mechanical ventilation? Families can be particularly helpful in regard to the patient's mental status. Often they are the first to recognize either deterioration or a return to baseline levels.

• *At its simplest, monitoring includes observation of the patient. In addition to vital signs, factors include color, level of consciousness, and general appearance.*

We can monitor the progress or deterioration of the patient in any number of ways. Simple observation can and does provide more information than might first be thought, particularly in this age of high technology. For example, the patient with blue kneecaps following a major surgical procedure usually has low cardiac output and decreased intravascular volume. Pallor may indicate underlying anemia. Cyanosis can be easily observed in many patients. Agitation can be an indication of many problems including hypoxemia or inadequately treated pain. The level of awareness of the patient can indicate the degree of cerebral perfusion. Simple observation can determine the adequacy of urine output based on volume and the apparent concentration.

The family at the patient's bedside can often provide much useful information. To the average clinician, the patient may look awake, alert, and of normal mental status. Often, however, the behavior is quite different from the patient's usual reactions. This information can provide help to assess the degree of mental status changes secondary to perfusion or trauma. Obviously, respiratory therapists can be helpful in pointing out pulmonary problems. When the clinician is by the bedside, the patient may look stable and comfortable during mechanical ventilation. The quality and quantity of secretions as well as the frequency of suctioning can all provide information useful for monitoring and for determination of the patient's ability to be extubated. Physical therapists might detect an enlarged leg circumference indicative of thromboembolism. They are usually the first to recognize a foot drop and the need for splinting.

All those who come by the bedside can help. The clinician must learn to use the eyes and ears of all involved and to act accordingly. Most physicians do not take the time to read nursing notes. At the very least, they ought to discuss with the nurse what has occurred in their absence and perhaps take it a step further and read the nursing notes. In my opinion, most nursing notes are not read except by the expert witness at the time of a malpractice case.

Secondarily, monitoring involves recording of the observed information. Today, most intensive care units (ICU) use a bedside flow sheet. This provides spaces to record vital signs, fluid infusion, outputs, and laboratory test results performed throughout the day. Such systems are subjective and are prone to recording errors. The frequency of input varies, depending on the time available to the bedside nurse and the patient's acuity level. Some information may actually be forgotten or discarded before it can be entered into the flow sheet.

Computerized data acquisition systems have been installed in some intensive care units.[1] These systems input information directly from the bedside monitor. They also integrate data from other information systems within the hospital such as the laboratory, pharmacy, and radiology departments. The data acquisition system then manipulates all the collected data and displays the information in a series of predesigned screens. These screens can be customized for each particular unit and in some cases for individual physicians. Obviously, such systems increase the speed of data collection and have decidedly fewer errors. Their use in intensive care units will continue to increase as the systems mature.

The new automated records systems have been slow to develop because of numerous technical problems. However, they ought to be able to replace some of the common problems of handwritten records. For example, current methods of blood pressure recording subjectively determine which pieces of information will be selected and recorded by the nurse. Moreover, frequency of data collection may vary. Even though blood pressure and pulse rate may have been ordered to be recorded every hour, this may not necessarily occur at the specific time ordered because of other duties of the bedside nurse. Often information is recorded on various scraps of paper during the course of care for a difficult patient and is only later entered into the permanent record. Unfortunately, such information can be lost forever. Handwritten records essentially prevent continuous gathering of information that may be useful to help determine a sequence of events. Furthermore, we are limited in how that information can be displayed in the most useful way. On occasion, bar grafts may provide more readily apparent information than other forms of data displays, such as tables or line graphs.

The automated system will eventually give the bedside nurse more time for actual hands-on nursing care. The data will be collected as often as necessary and for as long as might be required. Certain potential problems can develop with these new automated systems. Data are recorded at the indicated time regardless of any other factors. If problems have occurred with invasive monitoring, such as damping of an arterial line, that pressure will still be recorded as the actual pressure. Fortunately, most systems have an override, so the data can be edited and corrected as necessary. Although such systems save time, to date they have generated more paper than the simple, handwritten flow sheet. Until familiarity and comfort with such systems increase the introduction rate will most likely continue to be slow.

• *Bedside data acquisition systems provide more time for bedside nursing.*

Data collection should be ordered as frequently as is thought necessary to aid in the management and treatment of a particular problem. The intervals between should coincide with the safest amount of time that the patient may be judged to tolerate any potential abnormalities intended to be monitored.

Most often, patients in an ICU all have the same type of monitoring. As we become more cost efficient, we need to be more selective and only apply the specific degree of monitoring absolutely required. For example, it seems to be almost an unwritten rule that all patients in the ICU have vital signs recorded every hour. In some patients, this may not be often enough, but in many patients it is probably all too frequent. Other than an increased nursing workload, and more blanks filled in on the flow sheet, it is doubtful such practice impacts on patient outcomes.

Information should be centrally located. At this time, while most units still use handwritten flow sheets, it tends to simplify things if all data are found on the flow sheet. Multiple pieces of paper at the bedside generally add to the confusion and make it difficult to organize and interpret disparate pieces of information. Such data are also more likely to become lost. In the future, with microprocessor-controlled systems, data will be manipulated in multiple ways to allow better comparison among different types of information and a greater indepth understanding of what is going on with the patient.

Monitoring frequency varies with each clinical situation and individual patient. Depending on stability, vital sign recordings may occur every 1 or 5 minutes up to intervals of 2 to 4 hours. Laboratory data collection rates will also vary with the patients' illness and severity index.

ROUTINE MONITORING

All patients admitted to the ICU require the same basic monitoring. Beyond that, the individual clinical situation will dictate further needs. Even the most unsophisticated unit has electrocardiogram (ECG) monitoring available. Most current monitors provide information on heart rate and arrhythmias. Newer systems incorporate software to provide ischemia analysis. However, such information requires consistent and reproducible lead placement. For surgical patients with dressings, it may not be possible to place leads in the appropriate position. Therefore, the ST-T wave segment analysis may not be accurate. The nurse and the clinician should also discipline themselves to observe the actual tracing rather than the digital display of heart rate. Monitors can misinterpret elevated T waves as QRS complexes. The digital display of heart rate may be double the actual rate. This can also occur when pacemaker spikes are counted as QRS complexes.

The patient must be placed in the ICU where he or she can be seen at all times by the nursing staff. Unfortunately, many units are designed so nurses at the central station cannot directly observe the patients. Attempts to make up for this design flaw include central monitors, but monitors may not tell the entire story. Many a time a patient has had cardiac arrest caused by disconnection from the mechanical ventilator, and a long period has elapsed before any monitor alarms have gone off. In addition, observation of the bedside monitor even if vital signs are not being recorded provides continuous online assessment of the patient's progress. Such things as patient agitation, attempts to remove lines, and color are not currently monitored by special methods. They require the nurse or some other caregiver to make the assessment.

- *ICU design should allow all patients to be visualized from anywhere within the unit.*

All critically ill patients need intravascular volume status and intake and output regularly observed. Urinary output should be quantitated on a regular basis. This provides indirect information on renal perfusion as well as on the overall fluid status of the patient. Almost all modern ICUs deliver all fluids and medications through infusion pumps. Unless one directly observes the pump, it may be difficult to know whether the pump is actually infusing as presumed. Most readers of this chapter have probably had the experience of presuming that a drug infusion is underway, particularly a vasoactive agent, when in fact the drug has been delivered into the bed and not into the patient.

Nowadays, blood pressure measurements can be determined using Korotkoff sounds or by automated oscillometric methods.[2] Korotkoff sounds rely on sound generated by blood flow when the cuff pressure falls slightly below the arterial pressure. The diastolic pressure determination requires interpretation of a change in sound. Errors with this method include an inability to detect the first faint sound consistent with systolic blood pressure. The size and deflation rate of the cuff and the patient's heart rate can all obviously introduce errors in these measurements. Some individuals may have a 20-mm Hg difference between arms.

Most oscillometric or automated systems utilize the signal-to-noise ratio to record pressure. Some systems may identify the highest signal-to-noise ratio as the mean arterial pressure. Once identified, the memory is searched to identify the first signal, which is labeled the systolic blood pressure. Once systolic and mean arterial pressure are known, diastolic pressure can be calculated. The frequent inflation of automated systems has caused thrombotic problems in some patients' arms.[3] The system should not ordinarily be cycled more than once every 5 minutes except in emergency situations.

The most basic pulmonary monitoring system consists of patient observation. For example, a respiratory rate greater than 30/min usually indicates a problem. Possibilities include hypoxemia or increased CO_2 production.[4,5] Fever can elevate the metabolic rate, as can shivering.[6,7] Pulmonary edema can develop secondary to adult respiratory distress syndrome (ARDS) or overenthusiastic fluid administration. A normal respiratory rate ranges between 12 and 20 breaths/min. Lower rates may indicate depression secondary to either narcotics or sedatives.

• *An apparently adequate PaO_2 may represent instability if a high FIO_2 is required.*

Asynchronous motion of the chest and abdomen during respiration often means upper airway obstruction. Such discoordinate breathing may also develop during recovery from neuromuscular blockade. Patients with upper airway obstruction may also exhibit auditory stridor. At its most basic, respiratory monitoring also includes observation of the FIO_2. This is required to interpret blood gas results or pulse oximetry. A PaO_2 of 100 mm Hg on an FIO_2 of 0.9 indicates far more derangement than the same PaO_2 on an FIO_2 of 0.4. The presence of rhonchi indicates fluid in the lower airways. Rales may be indicative of pulmonary edema. Unequal breath sounds or the absence on one side can indicate collapse or pneumothorax.

Urinary output provides indirect information on overall organ perfusion. Initially, output should be monitored on an hourly basis. Most clinicians agree that acceptable urinary output should exceed 0.5 ml/kg/hr. The urine should also be checked for presence of glucose, ketones, and specific gravity. Urine volume may be falsely elevated by the presence of glucose or the previous use of diuretics in the operating room. Diuretics may manifest their effects for several hours following their administration. Myoglobin must be searched for in the urine of patients who have had prolonged hypoperfusion events or crush injuries.

All ICUs should regularly monitor the patient's temperature, particularly on admission. Hypothermia can occur following prolonged operative procedures. Often, the problem reflects the massive fluid and blood given during the procedure.[8] A cold operating room and an uncovered patient contribute to hypothermia. Hyperthermia most often represents infection.[9] Temperature may be also elevated by drug, fever, or blood in the subarachnoid space. Rarely, malignant hyperthermia first manifests itself in the postoperative period.[10]

• *Core temperatures can best be measured through a pulmonary artery catheter or tympanic membrane scanner.*

The pulmonary artery temperatures provide the most accurate core readings.[11] Recent data suggest that measurement of bladder temperature via a Foley catheter can also provide temperature read-

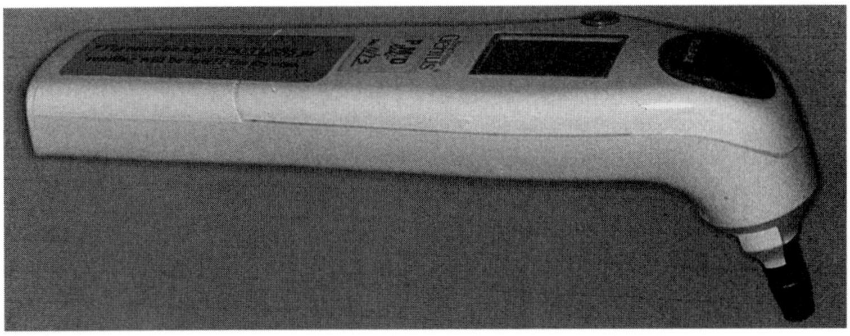

Figure 2–1.
The tympanic membrane probe must be positioned in the ear so it records tympanic membrane temperature, not temperature from the ear canal.

ings close to core values. Rectal temperatures have about a 1°C offset from core temperatures. During mechanical ventilation, oral temperatures become unreliable because of the passage of cold gases past the thermometer. Similarly, axillary temperatures provide little meaningful information in critically ill patients. Recently, devices have appeared on the market that measure tympanic membrane temperature (Fig. 2–1).[12] The data would suggest that when these devices are correctly focused on the ear drum, they can accurately reflect core temperatures.

The basic neurologic examination consists of the evaluation of the patient's level of consciousness. This includes the ability to follow simple and complex commands. The movement of extremities in response to various commands is also part of the neurologic examination. Many units utilize the Glasgow coma score as an objective method to follow neurologic status (Table 2–1).

Examination of the abdomen in surgical patients should be part of routine monitoring. This includes assessment of bowel sounds and the degree of distention. Is the abdomen soft or hard? Have

Table 2–1.
Glasgow Coma Score

Area Tested	Response	Score
Eyes Open	none	1
	to pain	2
	to voice	3
	spontaneously	4
Verbal	none	1
	not comprehensible	2
	garbled	3
	confused speech	4
	oriented speech	5
Motor	flaccid	1
	abnormal extension	2
	abnormal flexion	3
	normal flexion	4
	localizes to pain	5
	follows commands	6

changes occurred? New onset of right upper quadrant tenderness in a debilitated patient can indicate acalculous cholecystitis, particularly if the alkaline phosphatase is elevated. Distention or the absence of bowel sounds may indicate worsening peritonitis, bleeding, or other catastrophic problems.

Finally, monitoring includes observation of wounds for bleeding or suture disruption. Any drainage systems including chest tubes or abdominal drains should be observed for the volume of output as well as for any signs of new or continued bleeding. On occasion, this may include measurement of hematocrit from the drains. Discontinuation of drainage may indicate a mechanical problem such as obstruction of the drain.

SPECIALIZED MONITORING

Cardiovascular Monitoring

Indwelling arterial catheters allow precise minute-to-minute or more frequent determination of blood pressure. Indications for catheter placement include unstable blood pressure, the use of vasoactive agents, and frequent blood sampling, particularly for blood gas analysis.

- *The brachial artery is contraindicated for invasive arterial monitoring.*

Arterial cannulation sites should not be end vessels. This would preclude use of the brachial artery. The most common sites are the radial, axillary, femoral, and dorsalis pedis arteries.[13] The superficial temporal artery can also be cannulated. Similarly, the radial or ulnar artery should only be used if flow has been demonstrated in its companion vessel. The best method for determining flow is a Doppler probe placed directly over the artery. This eliminates the need for the so-called Allen's test. Particularly when other sites are not available, the femoral artery may be the easiest to palpate and to catheterize. A 6-inch 20-gauge catheter commonly used for pediatric central venous pressure monitoring works quite well for this site.

The axillary artery provides an excellent alternative for line placement. Enough collateral flow exits to ensure perfusions of the extremity. The same catheter described for femoral artery placement can be used in the axillary artery. The site of entry is similar to that used for axillary block. The artery is palpated when the arm has been abducted 180°. Entry is aided by maintenance of the needle in the same plane as the upper arm.

- *When overshoot is noted on the monitor, "the return to flow" method provides the best measurement of systolic blood pressure.*

On occasion, the arterial trace may display "overshoot." In such a situation, the systolic pressure may exceed that recorded by cuff, often by 20 mm Hg or more. This situation primarily develops in patients with arteriosclerotic disease.[14] The nonelastic, noncompliant vessels transmit more of the pressure wave that results from ejected blood hitting the wall of the aorta. The nonelastic vascular system then transmits this nondampened pressure wave to the monitoring site. This phenomenon can be readily noted on the arterial pressure wave form as a narrow area under the peak of the pressure trace. In other words little if any flow exists at this pressure

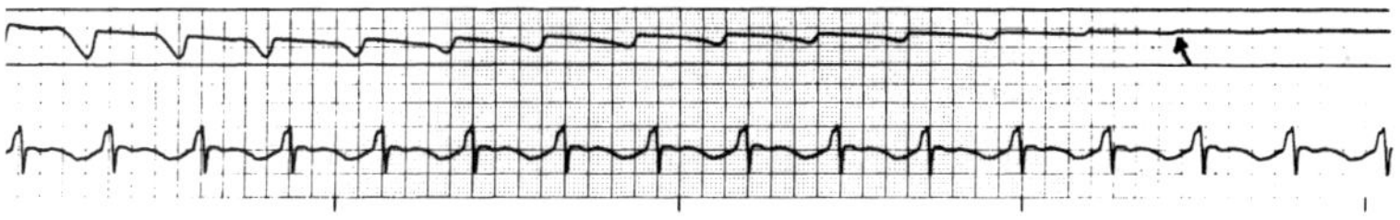

Figure 2–2.
The return to flow method of blood pressure analysis. Cuff inflation has eliminated the arterial pressure trace. The arrow depicts the first evident pressure wave, indicative of flow. The mercury manometer pressure noted at this time corresponds to the return to flow systolic blood pressure.

level. The best way to rectify the difference in observed pressures between cuff and arterial line is the "return to flow" method (Fig. 2–2). A blood pressure cuff is placed on the extremity proximal to the cannulation site. The cuff is then inflated to a pressure that occludes the arterial trace on the monitor. Reduction of the cuff pressure ultimately results in the reappearance of the wave form on the monitor. The cuff pressure at which the wave form first reappears is called the "return to flow" pressure. This coincides with the systolic pressure and represents the most accurate blood pressure.

- *Central venous pressure does not provide information on intravascular volume status.*

Central venous pressure can provide information about intravascular volume and right heart function. However, one must recognize the nonlinear relationship between central venous pressure and intravascular volume.[15] The clinician can follow the trend of the central venous pressure and combine that with the clinical situation to develop an understanding of the patient's current intravascular status. Central venous pressures are accurate only if the tip of the catheter resides in the superior vena cava. Therefore, attempts to measure central venous pressure with introducers in the subclavian or internal jugular veins may not provide accurate information.

Central venous catheters can and are readily used for infusion of various vasoactive drugs. This use permits central delivery of the agents and a more accurate and predictable response. The narrow lumen of most central venous catheters develops significant resistant to rapid flow of various fluids. As a result, such catheters are not advised for large-volume fluid administration, which requires rapid infusion rates. Although few data currently exist, there may be some difficulties with the popular pigtail-tip catheters and their ability to measure pressure adequately, because they are pointed upstream instead of downstream. This may explain some of the discrepancies in central venous pressure when a central venous pressure catheter replaces a pulmonary artery catheter that has also been used to monitor central venous pressure.

Pulmonary artery catheters not only measure pulmonary capillary wedge pressure and cardiac output, but also offer other desirable clinical information.[16] When the patient's intravascular status is in question, pulmonary artery and wedge pressures can provide information to help solve the dilemma. Catheters can readily enable one to discern whether the problem is one of inadequate volume, low cardiac output, or elevated systemic vascular resistance (SVR). It is generally accepted that patients with a known ejection fraction of $<40\%$ have enough compromise that the ability to measure, understand, and manipulate the cardiovascular system with the use of a pulmonary artery catheter is warranted. Data suggest that in "high-risk" patients including those with severe, ongoing sepsis, a threshold level of oxygen delivery seems to correlate with survival.[17,18] This clinical status can best be treated with pulmonary artery catheterization. Patients whose intravascular volume and cardiac status are questionable and who do not respond to a reasonable amount of fluids (usually between 1 and 2 L) usually require pulmonary artery catheterization and monitoring.

• *Despite its usefulness in the operating room, transesophageal echocardiography does not provide adequate monitoring in the ICU.*

We see patients today who have significant cardiac dysfunction and who in the past would have been candidates for intraoperative pulmonary artery catheterization. Many of them are now monitored with the use of transesophageal echocardiography during surgery and anesthesia. In the anesthetized patient, this device can provide useful details about intravascular volume and the degree of contractility. However, the same patients in the postoperative period additionally undergo certain metabolic derangements that involve oxygen delivery and utilization. Because of the intermittent availability and subjectivity of results, echocardiography does not yet play a major role in the postoperative care of such patients. A pulmonary artery catheter provides more diverse and detailed information during the recovery period (Table 2–2).

As we advance our understanding of the critically ill patient, it has become clear that knowledge of the patient's metabolic status provides a key to outcome. Information on oxygen delivery, oxygen consumption, and the oxygen extraction ratio provide important clinical information about the patient's metabolic status.[19] Oxygen delivery requires knowledge of cardiac output, hemoglobin, and oxygen saturation. Oxygen consumption calculations use knowledge of mixed venous and arterial oxygen contents as well as cardiac

Table 2–2.
Information Available from a Pulmonary Artery Catheter

Cardiac output/index
Pulmonary capillary wedge pressure
Central venous pressure
Pulmonary artery pressure
Stroke volume
Right and left ventricular stroke work/index
End diastolic volume/index
Ejection fraction
Systemic and pulmonary vascular resistance/index
Oxygen delivery/index
Oxygen consumption/index
Arterial-venous oxygen content difference
Mixed venous oxygen tension (SvO_2)
Mixed venous oxygen saturation
Pulmonary venous admixture (Qsp/Qt)

output. Both measurements require mixed venous blood from the pulmonary artery.

Arterial oxygen content (CaO_2)

$$CaO_2 = [(Hgb \times 1.34) \times (Art\ O_2\ Sat)] + [(.0031 \times PaO_2)]$$

Venous oxygen content (CvO_2)

$$CvO_2 = [(Hgb \times 1.34) \times (Ven\ O_2\ Sat)] + [(.0031 \times PvO_2)]$$

$$PvO_2 = \text{mixed venous } PO_2$$

Oxygen delivery (DO_2)

$$DO_2 = C.O. \times CaO_2$$

Oxygen consumption (VO_2)

$$VO_2 = C.O. (CaO_2 - CvO_2)$$

Several innovations of the pulmonary artery catheter are now in clinical use. Continuous monitoring of the venous oxygen saturation provides indirect information on the patient's metabolic state (Fig. 2–3).[20] In general, a decrease in venous saturation (SvO_2) indicates either inadequate oxygen delivery or an increase in oxygen consumption, or sometimes both. Critically ill patients can often change oxygen consumption without a concomitant increase in oxygen delivery.[21] Changes in SvO_2 provide an early warning system to the clinician and indicate the need to search for and to determine the cause of the change in the patient's metabolic status.

• *Pulmonary artery catheterization has evolved into monitoring of the metabolic state of the patient, including the oxygen delivery and demand.*

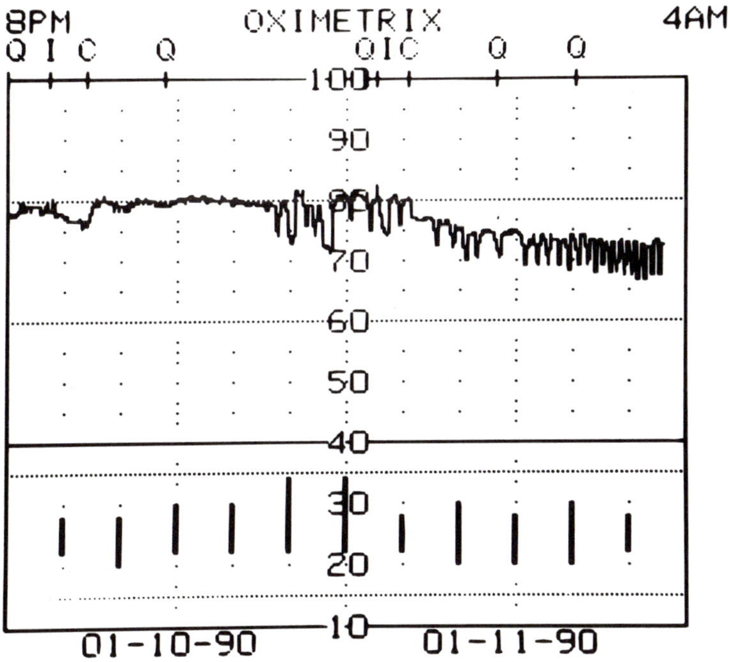

Figure 2–3.
SvO_2 monitoring. Note the decrease in SvO_2 following the onset of fibrillation and a concomitant drop in cardiac output and oxygen delivery.

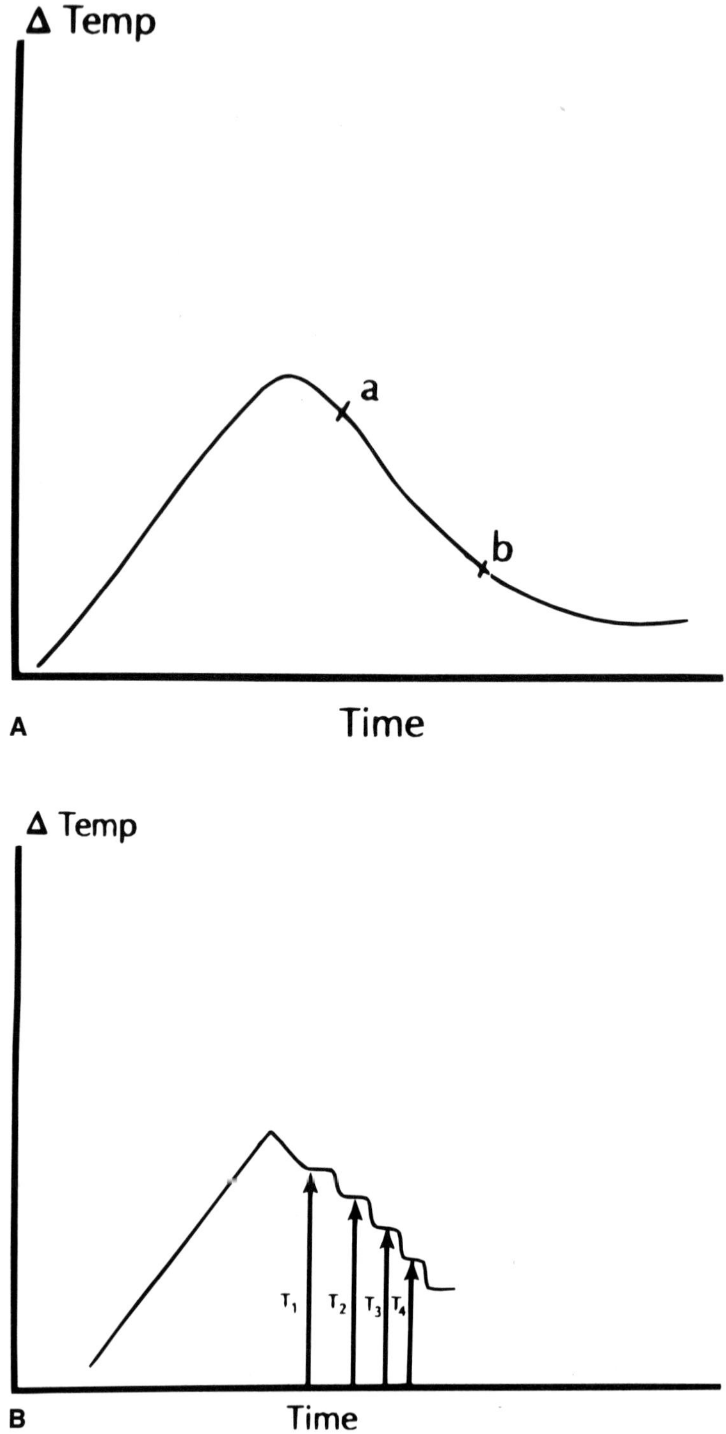

Figure 2–4.
Calculation of end-diastolic volume. A, Normal pulmonary artery catheters integrate the curve from a to b to derive cardiac output. This occurs over several heart beats. B, To measure end-diastolic volume, the thermistor must have a rapid response and be able to demonstrate the temperature change on a beat-to-beat basis.

New advances in thermistor design now provide calculation of end-diastolic volume (Fig. 2–4).[22] Data have demonstrated the accurate correlation between thermodilution determination of end-diastolic volume and that calculated by echocardiography.[23] Further, data suggest that end-diastolic volume correlates more accurately with stroke volume than does pulmonary capillary wedge pressure.[24]

Other developments with pulmonary artery catheters include continuous determinations.[25] Several different technologies have been used. It is unclear whether such data add useful information for the management of these patients.

Devices that utilize plethysmography to measure intravascular volume had met with minimal success.[26] Currently, such devices do not appear to play a role in the management of the critically ill.

Indwelling intravascular sensors are now available to provide online determinations of PaO_2, $PaCO_2$, and pH (Fig. 2–5). These sensors are threaded through the arterial catheter directly into the artery.[27] Their high cost precludes routine use in all patients. However, if critically ill patients require frequent manipulations of the

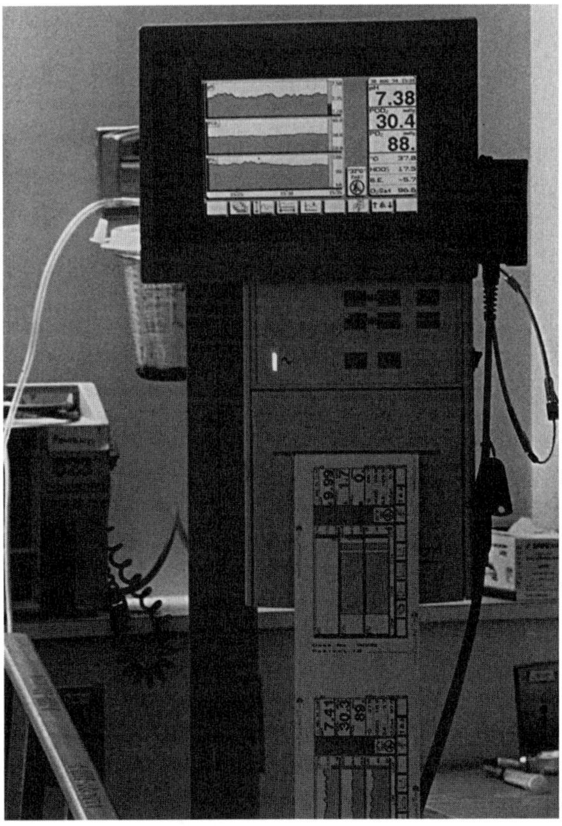

Figure 2–5.
A bedside monitor that allows continuous online determination of PO_2, PCO_2, and pH. Because of the current high cost, patients require multiple daily blood gas determinations to make this device cost effective. (Courtesy of Biomedical Systems, Inc., Malvern, PA.)

mechanical ventilator, such sensors can provide instantaneous feedback and can minimize or eliminate the need for laboratory determination of blood gas values.

Pulmonary Monitoring

Today, almost all critically ill patients have pulse oximetry measurements. In fact, it is a standard for the operating room. This simple, noninvasive procedure provides valuable information on the patient's pulmonary status. However, because of the shape of the oxygen dissociation curve, a patient may have a significant change in PaO_2 without any change in oxygen saturation. For example, PaO_2 will fall from 200 to 100 mm Hg without any change in oxygen saturation by pulse oximetry. Although such a change represents a significant alteration of pulmonary function, it would not be evident simply by following oxygen saturation.

During mechanical ventilation, certain parameters require monitoring. These include the peak inflation pressure (PIP), FIO_2, and PEEP. In addition, tidal volume from the mechanical ventilator as well as that during spontaneous ventilation or with a pressure support breath are monitored. In addition, the mechanical rate should be noted. When a specialized technique such as pressure control ventilation is used, the pressure differential between the peak pressure and PEEP should also be followed (Fig. 2–6).

As increase in PIP may indicate reduced lung compliance due to increased fluid accumulation, atelectasis, or pneumothorax.[28] PIP may also increase because of a circuit obstruction due to blood or secretions. If the tidal volume during pressure support ventilation increases, this may indicate overall improvement in compliance. A reduction in PIP with the same tidal volume also indicates improved compliance.

• *Today, many advocate minimization of peak inflation pressures during mechanical ventilation. This should result in an overall reduction of barotrauma.*

Pulmonary barotrauma results from both high inflation pressures and large tidal volumes. Many authorities now advocate that peak inflation pressures be limited to between 40 and 60 cm H_2O.[29] Instead of the large tidal volumes previously recommended, volumes in the range of 7 to 10 ml/kg may be more appropriate.[30] Because almost all physicians use at least a low level of PEEP during mechanical ventilation, the chances of atelectasis from small tidal volumes seems minimal.

The spontaneous respiratory rate also provides useful information. A rapid rate (>30/min) can indicate hypoxemia. Moreover,

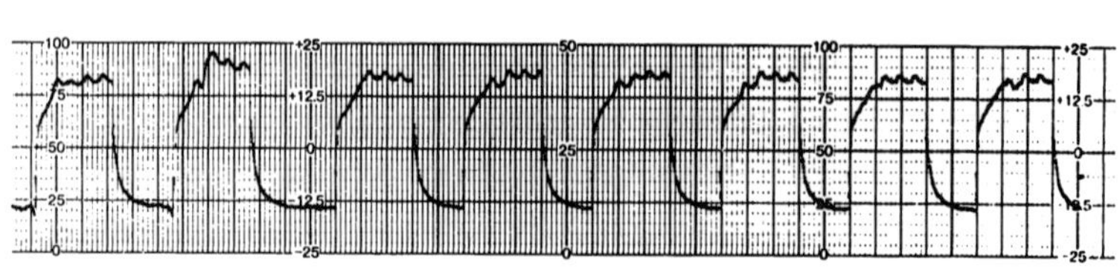

Figure 2–6.
Airway tracing during pressure control ventilation. The patient has attempted spontaneous respiration during delivery of the positive pressure breath. The duration as well as the pressure limit are preset on the ventilator.

patients also increase rate and simultaneously decrease tidal volume in response to factors that can increase the work of breathing. These can include reduced compliance or a poorly engineered ventilator circuit. A small-diameter endotracheal tube can also add to the breathing workload.

Not all patients in an ICU require a chest radiograph, but the immediate postoperative patient should have one on arrival in the ICU. This will allow the physician to determine not only the adequacy of any central line placement, but also the position of the endotracheal tube tip. When the tip resides above the clavicular heads, neck extension can actually dislodge the tube. If at the carina, the tip can migrate into a main stem bronchus during neck flexion. The chest film also serves as baseline for further evaluation of the patient's radiographic progress.

If close control of $PaCO_2$ is desired end-tidal CO_2 ($ETCO_2$) monitoring may help.[31] This noninvasive method provides continuous feedback. Normally, a gradient exists between $PaCO_2$ and $ETCO_2$. The difference represents the anatomic dead space that makes up part of the expired gas sample. The usual gradient measures 5 to 10 mm Hg. A larger gradient may indicate increased dead space. This could result from atelectasis, pulmonary embolism, and even excessive PEEP. The wave form during capnography can also provide useful information (Fig. 2–7). Failure to reach a plateau may indicate bronchial constriction. A leak in the ventilator circuit may present as a reduced $ETCO_2$. Spontaneous breathing may also be noted by capnography.

- *Ventilator circuits including the endotracheal tube can significantly increase the work of breathing during mechanical ventilation.*

When patients breath spontaneously during mechanical ventilation, the work of breathing reflects the effects of chest wall and lung compliance as well as the imposed work from the ventilator circuit and endotracheal tube.[32] Compliance can be improved by increased PEEP, correction of atelectasis, or diuresis to remove lung water. Once compliance has been maximized and, when possible, the patient placed in a more upright position, the clinician can do little further to change the lung and chest wall components of the work of breathing. However, the imposed work can and should be minimized. The smaller the diameter of the endotracheal tube, the greater the work of breathing.[32] Pressure support ventilation can minimize the overall work of breathing and completely eliminate the imposed work.[33] This may be desirable when patients are critically ill and oxygen delivery minimally meets metabolic demands. Work of breathing can often be clinically noted by the increased spontaneous rate of the patient. However, sedatives and narcotics can mask the increased rate even if breathing work has increased. Devices are now available that measure esophageal and intragastric pressure and can provide on-line continuous readouts of work of breathing (Fig. 2–8).[34] With the same device, a catheter tip placed at the proximal end of the endotracheal tube can utilize the pressure differential across the endotracheal tube to measure the imposed work of breathing.

The introduction of both pulse oximetry and capnography and observation of the patient's spontaneous respiratory rate have con-

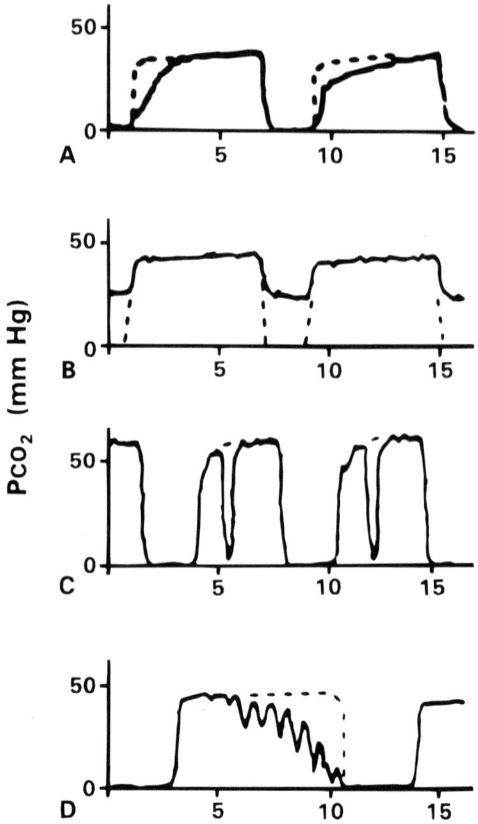

Figure 2–7.
End-tidal CO_2 response curves. A, The slow rise in the initial curve. This indicates some degree of airway obstruction. B, The end-tidal CO_2 does not return to zero. This normally indicates rebreathing. C, This curve indicates spontaneous breaths during delivery of a positive pressure breath. D, The decay in this curve represents gas coming from an organ other than the lungs, in this case, intubation of the esophagus.

tributed to a decrease in the number of blood gas determinations. Rather than measurements at predetermined intervals, blood gases can be determined on an as-needed basis, such as to assess a change in apparent clinical status or unexplained oxygen saturation or $ETCO_2$ change. Blood gas measurements may not be necessary after each ventilator change, but they still provide the only window to the acid-base status of the patient.

Neurologic Monitoring

• *The cerebral perfusion pressure may provide more information on the patient's likelihood of recovery than intracranial pressure.*

Monitoring the level of consciousness, response to commands, and Glasgow coma scale permits close bedside observation of the critically ill patient with neurologic injury or following intracranial surgery. Additionally, the most common parameter measured has always been intracranial pressure (ICP). To date, a Glasgow coma score less than 8 and an intracranial pressure above 25 mm Hg have

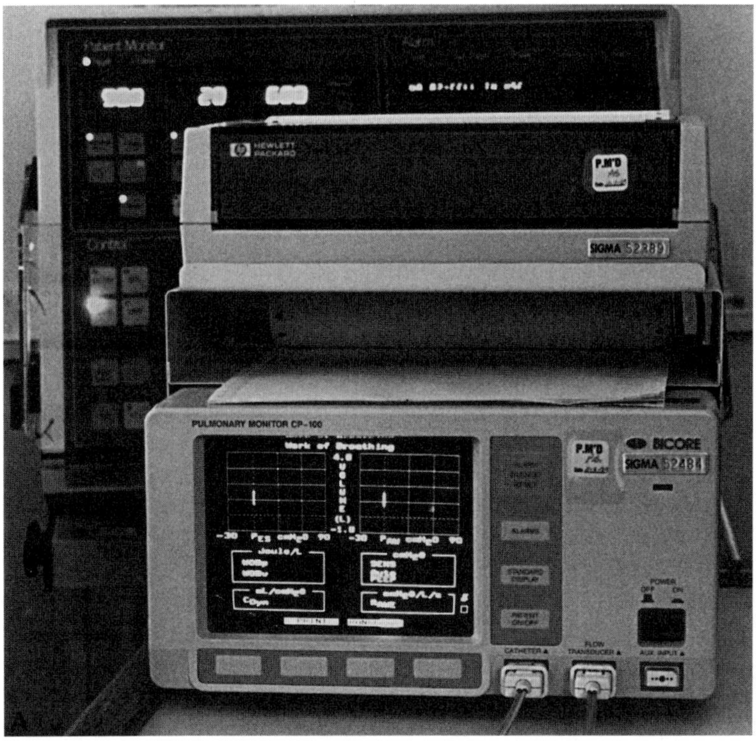

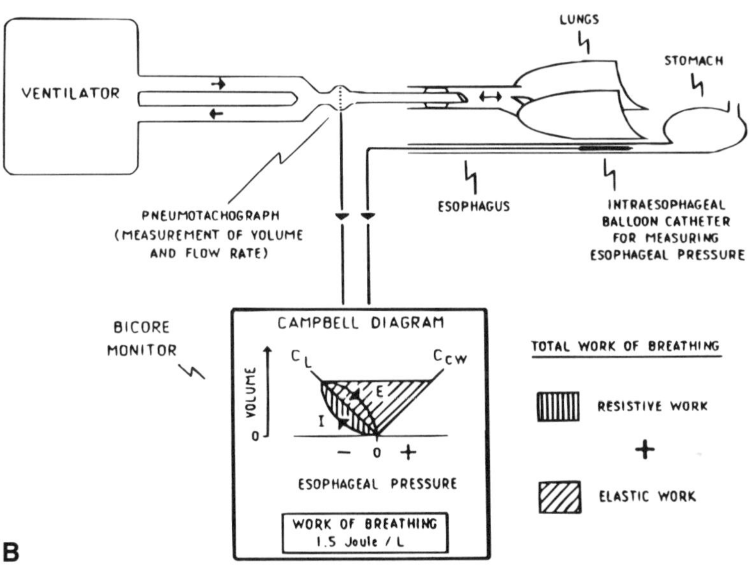

B

Figure 2–8.
A, A bedside device for measurement of work of breathing. (Courtesy of Bicore, Inc., Irvine, CA.) B, Clinical method of measuring the work of breathing performed by the patient (including physiologic plus imposed work) is illustrated. Work is computed using the Campbell diagram, which shows the change in volume plotted over the change in esophageal pressure (inference of intrapleural pressure) during spontaneous inhalation (I) and exhalation (E). Inspiratory resistive work of breathing includes the physiologic resistive work on the airways and the resistive work imposed by the breathing apparatus (vertical lines). Elastic work of breathing is the triangular shaped area subtended by the lung and chest wall compliance curves (diagonal lines). Total measured work of breathing, the sum of resistive and elastic work, is 1.5 J/L in this example.

been associated with poor outcome.[35] Attempts to reduce intracranial pressure have usually utilized hyperventilation to reduce blood flow to the brain, head elevation, and, when appropriate, diuretics.[36,37] However, intracranial pressure by itself only represents part of the story. The more important factor is cerebral perfusion pressure (CPP).[38] Mean arterial pressure minus ICP equals CPP. In fact, the arterial transducer should be zeroed to the level of the carotid bifurcation to provide accurate data on brain perfusion pressures. Even in the face of an elevated ICP, a CPP above 80 to 100 mm Hg can ensure adequate brain blood flow. Therefore, CPP must be calculated and always coupled with displays of ICP. In fact, elevations of ICP may require elevation of arterial pressure to maintain adequate CPP. Traditional methods of reducing ICP such as hyperventilation work by vasoconstriction, which reduces blood brain flow; however, this hypoperfusion can create cerebral ischemia and potential brain acidosis.[39]

• *When the CT scan does not demonstrate edema or bleeding, postoperative vasospasm can be diagnosed without an angiogram.*

The critically ill patient with known brain injury or following intracranial procedures will require prompt attention if any changes develop. A major alteration in mental status or localizing signs usually requires a computed tomographic (CT) scan once any laboratory-aided diagnosis such as hypoxia or hypoglycemia has been ruled out. The CT scan can enable one to differentiate between a mass lesion, such as hemorrhage, and brain edema. Following intracranial aneurysm surgery, alteration of mental status without an accompanying change in the CT scan usually indicates vasospasm. Ischemic injury to the brain coupled with stroke does not appear as an acute change on the CT scan. These findings may not be evident for as long as 7 days following the event. In the immediate postoperative period, there is usually little need for magnetic resonance imaging (MRI).

Transcranial Doppler flow studies have shown some evidence as an aid in the management of the critically ill patient.[40] When operated properly, the transcranial Doppler study can indicate vasospasm. At times, it can also demonstrate the complete absence of brain blood flow. This can be helpful in the determination of brain death. Technetium-labeled studies can determine brain death by the absence of intracranial blood flow.

A critically ill postoperative patient on occasion may require a lumbar puncture in addition to other diagnostic studies. An elevated ICP must first be ruled out. This can be done by ICP monitoring or evaluation of the CT scan. Although not used as frequently today, the electroencephalography (EEG) monitor may be of benefit during therapy. It can often provide information on the presence of seizure activity, particularly in the comatose, sedated, or paralyzed patient. When barbiturate therapy is undertaken, an isoelectric EEG serves as the therapeutic goal.[41] Simplified EEG monitors now available can be used at the bedside.[42] Evoked potential monitoring has become a useful bedside tool.[43] It is easier to use than the EEG and provides reliable reproducible information on brain function. Sensory evoked potentials can indicate brain viability when other factors are no longer available.

Specific complications following neurologic injuries or surgery include diabetes insipidus (DI) and the syndrome of inappropriate antidiuretic hormone release (SIADH). These must be continually monitored for to determine their presence. Patients with DI present with a urine output greater than 200 ml/hr. Because this is primarily free water, serum sodium will increase usually to levels of 150 mEq/L or higher. In addition, urine specific gravity varies between 1.000 and 1.004. If this condition is undiagnosed or untreated, severe hypernatremia can develop.

SIADH presents in a more subtle manner. There are often no apparent changes in urine volume. Serum sodium decreases because of the accumulation of free water. The syndrome first becomes apparent when serum sodium begins to decline to or below 130 mEq/L. Serum osmolarity decreases to below 280 mOsm, and urine osmolarity exceeds 400 mOsm. In such patients, serum sodium should be followed on a frequent basis. The resultant reduction in serum osmolarity can influence brain water accumulation.

Blood and Fluids

Often patients require blood in the postoperative period. When hypotension accompanies the blood requirements, it is usually obvious that a severe problem is at hand and everyone's attention becomes focused. However, if the patient's vital signs remain stable despite a falling hematocrit, and if the patient continues to receive blood intermittently, evidence of continued bleeding may not be so readily apparent. In fact, several hours may elapse before anyone recognizes that the patient has received a further 6 to 8 units of blood and most likely requires operative intervention. Close attention must be paid not only to the hematocrit and hemoglobin, but also to the volume and rate of blood replacement.

Clotting abnormalities usually develop secondary to hemodilution following massive transfusion therapy.[44] Platelet transfusions are begun when platelet counts fall below 50,000 in a patient with obvious bleeding. If severe bleeding persists, platelet counts below 100,000 may be an indication for more platelets, particularly if a bleeding time cannot be performed. The platelet count should be monitored on a regular basis (every 4 to 6 hours) to guide further therapy. Often, bleeding time shows a qualitative deficit when the total platelet count appears normal. Similarly, the prothrombin (PT) and partial thromboplastin (PTT) times will guide fresh frozen plasma or cryoprecipitate therapy to restore factors V and VIII. The return of clotting studies to normal serves as the end point for all factor replacement therapy.

• *Despite platelet counts above 50,000, patients who continue to bleed postoperatively should receive further platelet transfusions.*

Crystalloid therapy should also be closely followed. Fluid balance cannot help to delineate the need for diuresis. Moreover, a decreased hematocrit can represent hemodilution, as opposed to active bleeding. The rate of blood loss through a chest tube aids in the determination of the need for operative intervention.

Nutrition

• *Critically ill patients require adequate protein replacement. This should be in amounts of 2 g/kg/day in the form of amino acids.*

Nutritional changes in the acutely ill patient can be found regularly. Recent data suggest that total caloric replacement may not be absolutely necessary.[45] It may be better to underfeed these patients slightly. However, they do require substantial protein replacement. This usually is between 1.5 and 2 g/kg/day for acutely ill patients.[46] The adequacy of protein replacement can be determined by transferrin levels. Because transferrin requires 3 to 4 days to respond to changes in therapy, the levels can be followed at that same frequency. Other estimates for protein replacement include a 24-hour nitrogen balance study. Monitoring with bedside metabolic carts can determine both oxygen consumption and CO_2 production and estimate caloric needs.[47] The clinician must remember that oxygen consumption may change by as much as 20% throughout the day.[48] During nutritional support therapy, other factors require observation. Triglyceride levels should be checked following initial lipid infusion. An elevated level signals the need for a decreased volume and infusion rate. Hypophosphatemia and hypomagnesemia can develop secondary to protein synthesis. Low phosphate levels can decrease mental status. Reduced magnesium values interfere with neuromuscular function. All electrolytes should be analyzed daily.

Hyperglycemia is the most common complication of nutritional support. Even in diabetics, not overfed, the stress state can interfere with normal pancreatic and insulin function. Blood glucose must be monitored closely. If levels can be controlled by a sliding scale, this may mean determinations every 4 or 6 hours. If a continuous insulin infusion is used, blood glucose levels should be checked every 1 to 2 hours. Glucosuria negates urine output as an indicator of organ perfusion.

Sepsis

Signs of sepsis include hyper- (<38.5°C) or hypo- (>35°C) thermia, and an elevated (>12,000) or depressed (<4000) white blood cell count. The immature band cells on the differential count almost always exceed 10%. Cardiovascular and respiratory changes are usually nonspecific. They can include tachycardia, hypotension, tachypnea, and relative hypoxemia. Mental confusion often precedes other evidence of sepsis.

Obviously, the patient with known bowel perforation or pancreatitis has a high risk of developing sepsis with the accompanying signs and symptoms. Maxillary sinusitis frequently follows nasal intubation and can cause fever and other findings common with sepsis.[49] On occasion, retained tampons, epididymitis, or a perirectal abscess can be the source. Central venous lines can become infected or colonized and lead to sepsis. Many protocols call for line replacement or change on a regular basis.[50] Currently, we change central lines every sixth day. We place the new line with a fresh stick. These practices are altered in patients with coagulopathy or in the absence of sites, such as in a burn patient. Then the line may be replaced over a guide wire. Rarely is a cerebrospinal fluid (CSF) infection the cause of fever in the postoperative period.

In addition to frequent vital signs, the patient's white blood cell count should be monitored daily. Blood, urine, and sputum cultures should be performed during each fever spike above 38.5°C. Ideally, cultures should be drawn prior to the fever, but this never happens.

In high-risk patients, we perform daily surveillance cultures of blood, urine, and sputum. Often such patients are on antibiotic therapy already or may not manifest a fever to serve as an indicator for culture. Daily cultures can enable one to diagnose an occult infection as well as changing flora or development of antibiotic resistance. One should not ignore positive yeast cultures. Candida is now a frequent cause of nosocomial pneumonia.[51]

Drugs such as vancomycin and aminoglycoside can cause renal damage.[52] The kidney primarily excretes these agents. Therefore, drug levels should be monitored on a regular basis, particularly if renal function deteriorates. Peak and trough levels of antibiotics provide important information. We usually obtain these after the third dose of the aminoglycoside antibiotic. Current practice indicates longer frequencies between drugs. This will allow higher initial dosages with higher drug concentrations and better bacterial killing properties.[53] Appropriate dosing intervals prevents accumulation, with possible renal toxicity.

- *Antibiotic levels can help guide therapy to prevent renal toxicity. Trough drug levels provide minimal information on the killing power of the drugs.*

Renal and Hepatic Function

Renal and hepatic function require monitoring in the postoperative period. Changes in urine volume provide rapid assessment of perfusion. Usually, a sudden decrease represents decreased intravascular volume or low cardiac output. An abrupt discontinuation of urine may result from vascular occlusion or an obstructive phenomenon. Occasionally, the bladder catheter may become obstructed.

On a daily basis, blood urea nitrogen (BUN) and creatinine provide useful information. Elevations of both indicate acute renal failure, usually secondary to hypoperfusion, sepsis, or some toxin such as aminoglycosides. Creatinine clearance indicates glomerular filtration. A 2-hour study is as reliable as a 24-hour collection. Loop diuretics do not interfere with this determination. The fractional excretion of sodium also aids in the diagnosis of renal failure; however, its results are altered by diuretic therapy.

Other problems such as absorption of blood from the gastrointestinal tract can elevate the BUN. Amino acid administration during hyperalimentation can also raise the BUN.

Most changes in liver function develop slowly. Therefore, liver function studies need only be collected daily, at most. Hepatocellular dysfunction in the critically ill patient usually results in a mildly elevated bilirubin in the range of 4 to 6 mg/dl. LDH values are too nonspecific to be of much benefit. The enzymes SGOT and SGPT rarely increase except in hepatitis or acute ischemic injury. Hepatic resection or trauma may cause a transient enzyme elevation.

Critically ill patients, particularly if not fed, can develop acalculous cholecystitis.[54] Signs and symptoms include right upper quadrant tenderness, elevated bilirubin, and a rising alkaline phosphatase level. Ultrasound or CT provides the definitive diagnosis based on sludge in the gallbladder and a thickened wall. Initial treatment involves percutaneous cholecystostomy.

In general, monitoring should be selective for each patient. This includes not only the specifics, but also the frequency. In conclusion, it seems easy to order a specific test, but discontinuation or cancellation is always far more difficult. Yet, laboratory testing may be the area of critical care medicine in which we can have the greatest impact on cost effectiveness.

REFERENCES

1. Kavila LS, Shabot MM: Keys to successful implementation of an ICU patient data management system. Int J Clin Monit Comput 1988; 5: 15–25.
2. Ramsey M III: Blood pressure monitoring: Automated oscillometric devices. J Clin Monit 1991; 7:56–67.
3. Kennedy HL, Horan MJ, Sprague MK et al: Ambulatory blood pressure in healthy normotensive males. Am Heart J 1983; 106:717–722.
4. Askanazi J, Rosenvau SH, Hyman AL et al: Respiratory changes induced by the large glucose loads of parenteral nutrition. JAMA 1980; 245:1444–1447.
5. Cherniack NS, von Euar C: Central neuro reflex control of breathing. In: Fishman AP, ed: Pulmonary diseases and disorders. New York, Newer-McGraw-Hill, 1980; p. 278.
6. Leibschutz DC, Blutros AR, Printen KJ: Metabolic response to hyperthermia. Surg Gynecol Obstet 1974; 139:403–405.
7. Pflug AE, Aashiem JM, Foster C et al: Prevention of post-anesthesia shivering. Can Anaesth Soc J 1978; 25:43–49.
8. Pavlin EG: Hypothermia in traumatized patients. In: Grande CN, ed: Trauma, anesthesia and critical care. St. Louis, CV Mosby, 1993; pp. 1131–1132.
9. Dinarello CA, Cannon JG, Wolff SN: New concepts on the pathogenesis of fever. Rev Infect Dis 1988; 10:168–189.
10. Gronert GA: Malignant hyperthermia. In: RD Miller, ed: Anesthesia. New York, Churchill-Livingstone, 1986; pp. 1971–1984.
11. Shoemaker WC, Ayres S, Grenvik A et al, eds: Textbook of critical care, 2nd ed. Philadelphia, WB Saunders, 1989; p. 148.
12. Shinozaki T, Deane R, Perkins FM: Infrared tympanic thermometer: evaluation of a new clinical thermometer. Crit Care Med 1988; 16: 148–150.
13. DeAngelis J: Axillary arterial monitoring. Crit Care Med 1976; 4: 205–214.
14. Gardner RM, Hollingsworth KW: Optimizing ECG and pressure monitoring. Crit Care Med 1986; 14:651.
15. Matthay MA: Invasive hemodynamic monitoring in critically ill patients. Clin Chest Med 1983; 4:233–249.
16. Venderjas JS: Pulmonary artery catheter monitoring. Anesth Clin North Am 1988; 6:743–767.
17. Yu M, Levy MM, Smith P et al: Effect of maximizing oxygen delivery

on morbidity and mortality rates in critically ill patients: a prospective, randomized, controlled study. Crit Care Med 1993; 21:830–838.
18. Tuchschmidt J, Fried J, Astiz M et al: Elevation of cardiac output and oxygen delivery improves outcome in septic shock. Chest 1992; 102: 216–220.
19. Mahette CK, Jaffe MB, Sasse SA et al: Relationship of thermodilution cardiac output to metabolic measurements and mixed venous oxygen saturation. Chest 1993; 104:1236–1242.
20. Nelson LD: Continuous venous oximetry in surgical patients. Ann Surg 1988; 203:329–333.
21. Ronco JJ, Phang PP, Walley KR et al: Oxygen consumption is independent of changes in oxygen delivery in severe adult respiratory distress syndrome. Am Rev Respir Dis 1991; 143:1267–1273.
22. Vincent JL, Thirion M, Brimioulle S et al: Thermodilution measurement of right ventricular ejection fraction with a modified pulmonary artery catheter. Intensive Care Med 1986; 12:33–38.
23. Jardin F, Brun ND, Hardy A et al: Combined thermodilution and two-dimensional echocardiographic evaluation of right ventricular function during respiratory support with PEEP. Chest 1991; 99:162–168.
24. Diebel LN, Wilson RF, Tagett MG et al: End diastolic volume: a better predictor of preload in the critically ill. Arch Surg 1992; 127:817.
25. Segal J, Gaudiani V, Nishimura T: Continuous determination of cardiac output using a flow-directed Doppler pulmonary artery catheter. J Cardiothorac Vasc Anesth 1991; 5:309–315.
26. Wong DH, Tremper KK, Stemmer EA: Noninvasive cardiac output: simultaneous comparison of two different methods with thermodilution. Anesthesiology 1990; 72:784.
27. Zimmerman JL, Dellinger RP: Initial evaluation of a new intra-arterial blood gas system in humans. Crit Care Med 1993; 21:495–500.
28. Marcy TW, Marini JJ: Inverse ratio ventilation in ARDS: rationale and implimentation. Chest 1991; 100:494–504.
29. Marini JJ: Lung mechanics in adult respiratory distress syndrome: recent conceptual advances and implications for management. Clin Chest Med 1990; 11:673–690.
30. Slutsky AS, et al: Mechanical ventilation: ACCP Consensus Conference. Chest 1993; 104:1833–1859.
31. Swedlow DB: Capnometry and capnography: the anesthesia disaster early warning system. Semin Anesth 1986; 5:194–205.
32. Bersten AD, Rutten AJ, Vedig AE et al: Additional work of breathing imposed by endotracheal tubes, breathing circuits, and intensive care ventilators. Crit Care Med 1989; 17:671–677.
33. Kacmarek RM: The role of pressure support ventilation in reducing clinical work of breathing. Resp Care 1988; 33:99–120.
34. Banner MJ, Kirby RR, Blanch P et al: Decreasing imposed work of a breathing apparatus to zero using pressure support ventilation. Crit Care Med 1993; 21:1333–1338.
35. Pons PT: Head Trauma. In: Rosen P, Barkin R, eds: Emergency medicine concepts and clinical practice. St. Louis, Mosby-Yearbook, 1992; pp. 338–354.
36. White RJ, Likavec MJ: The diagnosis and initial management of head injury. N Engl J Med 1992; 327:1507–1511.
37. Olshaker JS, DePriest WW: Head trauma. Emerg Med Clin North Am 1993; 11:165–186.
38. Rosner MJ: Pathophysiology and management of increased intracranial pressure in neurosurgical intensive care. In: Andres BT, ed: *Neurosurgical intensive care.* New York, McGraw-Hill, 1993; pp. 57–112.

39. Rosner MJ, Becker DP: Experimental brain injury: successful therapy with the weak-base tromethamine (with a review of CNS acidosis). J Neurosurg 1984; 60:961.
40. Martin NA, Doberstein C, Zane C et al: Post-traumatic cerebral arterial spasm: transcranial doppler ultrasound, cerebral blood flow, and angiographic findings. J Neurosurg 1992; 77:575–583.
41. Eisenberg HM, Frankowski RF, Conant CF et al: High-dose barbiturate: their control of elevated intracranial pressure in patients with severe head injury. J Neurosurg 1988; 69:15.
42. Bickford RG, Billinger TW, Fleming NI et al: The compressed spectral array. Proc San Diego Biomed Symp 1975; 11:365.
43. Aminoff MJ: The use of somatosensory evoked potentials in the evaluations of the central nervous system. Neurol Clin 1988; 6:809–823.
44. Saito H: Normal hemostatic mechanisms: disorders of hemostasis. In: Ratnoff OD, ed: Disorders of hemostasis. Philadelphia, WB Saunders, 1991; pp. 18–47.
45. Gianotti L, Alexander JW, Nelson JL et al: Role of early enteral feeding and acute starvation on bacterial translocation and host-defense: prospective randomized trials. Crit Care Med 1994; 22:265–272.
46. Cerra FB: How nutrition intervention changes what getting sick means. JPEN J Parenter Enteral Nutr 1990; 14:164S–169S.
47. Browning JA, Linberg SA, Turney SZ et al: The effect of a fluctuating FIO_2 on metabolic measurements in mechically ventilated patients. Crit Care Med 1982; 10:82–85.
48. Field S, Kelly SM, Macklem PT: The oxygen cost of breathing in patients with cardiorespiratory disease. Am Rev Respir Dis 1982; 126: 9.
49. Gallagher TJ, Civetta JM: Acute maxillary sinusitis complicating nasotracheal intubation: a case report. Anesth Analg 1976; 55:885–886.
50. Eyer S, Brummitt C, Crossley K et al: Catheter-related sepsis: prospective, randomized study of three methods of longterm catheter maintenance. Crit Care Med 1990; 18:1073–1079.
51. Frankin C, Netry N: Life threatening candida infections in the intensive care unit. J Intensive Care Med 1992; 7:127–137.
52. Bennett WN, Aronoff G, Golper TA et al: Drug prescribing in renal failure: dosing guidelines for adults, 2nd ed. Philadelphia, American College of Physicians, 1991.
53. Kapusink JE, Sand MV: Challenging conventional aminoglycide dose regimens. Am J Med 1986; 80:908.
54. Fox MS, Wilk DJ, Weissman HS et al: Acute acalculous cholecystitis. Surg Gynecol Obstet 1984; 159:13.

CHAPTER 3

The Perioperative Stress Response and Its Relationship to Perioperative Endocrine and Electrolyte Disorders

Bart Chernow

Case Report

A 48-year-old female patient was admitted to the emergency room with an acute abdomen. The patient had been receiving long-term steroid therapy, prednisone 60 mg/day, for Crohn's disease. She had not felt well over the last 2 days and had temperatures up to 99°F. After developing progressive lethargy, she was brought to the emergency room.

Evaluation in the emergency room indicated an acute abdomen with free air noted on the lateral abdominal film. At operation, the patient had frank fecal soiling. The perforated area was isolated and a loop colostomy performed. Drains were placed, and the patient was taken to the intensive care unit (ICU) following surgery. In the operating room, the patient's blood pressure had remained at 75 to 80 mm Hg. Urine output was 35 ml for the 2-hour procedure. In the ICU, the patient was maintained on mechanical ventilation. A pulmonary artery catheter was passed to aid in management of hypotension and fluid replacement. Pulmonary capillary wedge pressure, which was originally 7 mm Hg, was increased to 15 mm Hg with crystalloid balanced electrolyte solutions and 1 unit of packed red blood cells. Despite this therapy, the patient's blood pressure remained in the range of 90 mm Hg, and cardiac output was 3.7 L/min. The patient's oxygen delivery was in the range of 420 ml/min/m^2.

A dopamine infusion was begun with infusion rates up to 14 μg/kg/min. However, this therapy resulted in minimal change in blood pressure or cardiac output. The patient was then started on an epinephrine infusion at rates up to 0.3 μg/kg/min. Blood pressure increased to 110 mm Hg and cardiac output to 5.8 L/min. Oxygen delivery also improved to 590 ml/min/m^2. She was also started on hydrocortisone at 100 mg/8 hr. Because of the hypotension, the patient was given a bolus dose of 50 mg of the drug in addition to a continuous infusion.

Endocrine systems mediate the body's responses to surgical or traumatic stress. The endocrine glands are linked in this important function to stress-related responses in the central nervous system and immune system network. The most recent evidence of these interrelationships prompts us now to refer to the importance of the "neuroendocrine-immune axis" in the perioperative stress response.[1] Understanding these stress responses and the functions of this multisystem axis provides a key foundation to build strategic approaches for the prevention, diagnosis, and treatment of several common perioperative endocrine and electrolyte disorders.

NEUROENDOCRINE-IMMUNE AXIS

The biology of the endocrine glands is well known. Use of the hypothalamic-pituitary-adrenal gland interactions as a prototype makes it easy to describe the mechanisms of trophic hormone stimulation on target gland tissues and the negative feedback loops that help to regulate hormonal release.[2] The degree of hormonal response (in this case, cortisol) to clinically important stress has been described for adults and children who undergo surgery and in patients with severe stress due to septic shock.[3–5] Chrousos has identified corticotropin-releasing hormone and the locus ceruleus-norepinephrine systems in the nervous system as the principal "effectors" of the stress response.[6] The interactions between the neuroendocrine system and the immune system have been detailed by Holaday and Reichlin.[1,7]

• *Glucocorticoids inhibit immune function, while growth hormone stimulates the immune system. The timing of the immune response to sepsis has not been delineated.*

Certain hormones such as glucocorticoids and somatostatin may inhibit immune functions, while other hormones such as growth hormone and prolactin stimulate immune functions. Similarly, the evidence is convincing that macrophage/monocyte-generated cytokines, such as interleukin-1 and tumor necrosis factor, influence and probably help to regulate stress hormone responses.[8–14] Circulating cytokine concentrations correlate with the severity of illness in the same way that stress hormones vary with the degree of illness.[15–17] The timing of the neuroendocrine responses to surgical stress and the potential complications of surgery also take on importance. Although we understand the timing of the early hormonal responses to surgery, we know much less about the immune system and its timing to response.[3,18] The timing of the immune changes (e.g., cytokine alterations) has particular importance as we apply tools from molecular biology (i.e., monoclonal antibodies, cytokine receptor antagonists) at the postoperative patient's bedside. The lack of knowledge about the timing of the immune response may limit the success of future anticytokine therapy.[19,20]

New insights into the regulation and importance of the body's stress responses continue to unfold. We now have some understanding of the role played by heat shock proteins in the activation of the stress response at the molecular level.[21] In critically ill patients, the responsiveness of the neuroendocrine-immune axis may be altered, and plasma hormone concentrations may provide predictive information.[22,23]

Clinical Implications in the Postoperative Period

Going beyond the prototype of cortisol as a stress hormone leads us to consider the broader stress response (Table 3–1). Among the

Table 3–1.
Components of the Stress Response

Classic Stress Hormones
Corticotropin releasing hormone
Adrenocorticotropic hormone
Cortisol
Epinephrine
Norepinephrine
Prolactin
Growth hormone
Glucagon
Other Hormones Affected by Stress
Insulin
Testosterone
? Estrogen
Luteinizing hormone
Follicle stimulating hormone
? Melanocyte stimulating hormone
Thyrotropin releasing hormone
Thyrotropin
Thyroxine
Triiodothyronine
? Somatostatin
Parathyroid hormone
? Calcitonin
Dopamine
Endocrine-Immune Related Factors in Stress
Interleukins
Tumor necrosis factor
Interons
Free fatty acids
Heat shock proteins
Calcium, vitamin D

vast array of stress components, it quickly becomes clear that the stress response accounts for, or at least contributes to, numerous postoperative endocrine and electrolyte problems, as discussed in the following sections.

Cortisol

Most patients who undergo surgery have no problem with the minimal increases in circulating cortisol concentrations that are a consequence of the stress response to surgery. However, occasionally a patient with subclinical adrenal insufficiency develops postoperative hypotension, hypothermia, hyperkalemia, or other manifestations of this deficiency state. An important clue that the patient may have adrenal insufficiency is the finding of eosinophilia in the peripheral blood analysis. A second indication that adrenal insufficiency may be a concern is the finding of hyperpigmentation. This latter sign is consistent with primary adrenal insufficiency. In secondary adrenal insufficiency, in which the hypothalamus and/or pituitary glands are dysfunctional, hyperpigmentation does not develop. If a patient has received glucocorticoid therapy, it is important to consider whether replacement therapy has been adequate.

- *Postoperative adrenal insufficiency is manifested by hypotension, hypothermia, hyperkalemia, and eosinophilia.*

If there is a concern that a hypotensive postoperative patient may have adrenal insufficiency, the clinician should perform a corticotropin (ACTH) stimulation test. In this diagnostic procedure, a small dose of $\alpha 1-24$ corticotropin is administered, and the plasma cortisol concentration is measured immediately before and 30 minutes after ACTH administration. Normally, plasma cortisol concentration increases by more than 7 μg/dl from baseline, and the absolute plasma cortisol level must increase to more than 18 μg/dl. In critically ill patients, the plasma cortisol level may be greater than 18 μg/dl at baseline, and the increment may be less than 7 μg/dl. These findings are still consistent with a normal hypothalamic-pituitary-adrenal axis. While waiting for the results of the ACTH stimulation test, it is reasonable to administer 1 or 2 mg of dexamethasone every 8 to 12 hours.

- *The ACTH stimulation test enables one to diagnose postoperative adrenal insufficiency. Normally, the plasma cortisol level increases to greater than 18 μg/dl.*

In the glucocorticoid-treated patient, perioperative steroid coverage is an important concern. My colleagues and I have recently summarized the important considerations in the provision of perioperative glucocorticoid coverage.[24] Our conclusions, which supported the work of others, indicated that the amount of glucocorticoid replacement therapy that we have traditionally given to steroid-dependent patients is excessive.[25] Indeed, the traditional approach of 100 mg of hydrocortisone preoperatively, 100 mg of hydrocortisone intraoperatively, and 100 mg of hydrocortisone postoperatively exceeds the needs of most patients. We now believe that the amount of glucocorticoid replacement therapy should be based on three variables: (1) the amount of glucocorticoid that the patient has been receiving; (2) the duration of previous glucocorticoid therapy; and (3) the length and nature of the surgical case.

- *Patients who receive steroid therapy prior to surgery should have their pre- and postoperative steroid dosage adjusted based on the previous dosage rates, as well as the stress likely to be evoked by the particular operative procedure.*

Thus, for example, a patient receiving 5 mg of prednisone every other day for a problem such as asthma and who undergoes a minor procedure such as an inguinal hernia repair might require only 5 mg of prednisone as an orally administered preoperative steroid dose and 5 mg of methylprednisolone intraoperatively. The following day, the patient should likely receive 5 mg of oral prednisone again. In fact, if the inguinal hernia repair is done under local anesthesia, the patient may only require the 5-mg preoperative dose of prednisone (the preoperative dose to be administered within 2 hours of the start of the case). For a more advanced procedure in a patient who has been receiving a larger dose of glucocorticoid, the amount of perioperative steroid coverage should increase. As an example, a patient who has inflammatory bowel disease and has been receiving 60 mg of prednisone for many years and who now requires a colectomy would likely benefit from 100 mg of hydrocortisone preoperatively, intraoperatively, and postoperatively.

Glucocorticoids may have negative effects on immune function. We know that glucocorticoids suppress immunity, and the mechanisms are probably multifactorial. Certainly, elegant data have been presented that indicate that glucocorticoids have important effects on B cells and potentially suppress the antimicrobial activity of human macrophages.[26,27] Because of these type of actions, potential modulation of the stress response may be beneficial. Anesthesiologists have attempted to limit the physiologic and hormonal responses following major sugical procedures. If a glucocorticoid is chosen for administration, clinicians should be aware that dexamethasone and methylprednisolone are less likely to cause a steroid-induced metabolic alkalosis than hydrocortisone. Hydrocortisone is probably the drug of choice for treatment of patients with perioperative adrenal insufficiency. Dexamethasone and methylprednisolone are the choice for the treatment of a glucocorticoid-responsive cause of respiratory failure or tumor-associated cerebral edema.[28] Some anesthetic techniques may decrease the glucocorticoid response to surgery. Epidural postoperative analgesia achieves that goal.[29] Certain medications may contribute to adrenal insufficiency. High-dose ketoconazole therapy can occasionally cause such a problem.[30]

- *Glucocorticoids affect B-cell function, as well as macrophages. Epidural analgesia can suppress the glucocorticoid response following surgery.*

Growth Hormone

Growth hormone is indicated for the treatment of growth hormone deficiency leading to short stature. However, growth hormone has also been administered to elderly men to possibly aid in quality of life. In addition, growth hormone has been used in malnourished surgical patients in an attempt to decrease negative nitrogen balance. A number of studies in experimental situations have indicated that growth hormone administration improves weight gain and wound healing. This may have relevance to perioperative patients.[31]

- *Growth hormone may promote wound healing.*

Glucagon

Glucagon deficiency is rare, and glucagon excess (glucagonoma) is similarly unusual. Glucagon does have relevance, however, in the perioperative patient in that glucagon is, in my opinion, the drug of choice for treatment of inadvertent beta-adrenergic receptor overdose. It can also be used to treat calcium channel blocker overdose. Glucagon can also act as a potential inotropic agent when adrenergic agents fail.[31] Glucagon may also be useful in the treatment of perioperative hypoglycemia.

Norepinephrine and Epinephrine

• Continued or long-term use of catecholamines may ultimately cause a decrease in adrenergic receptor function.

Obviously, one important issue in regard to catecholamines in the perioperative period is the potential of a patient with pheochromocytoma. Such an individual may have a severe perioperative hypertensive crisis. Fortunately, this situation remains rare since most patients with hypertension are screened for the presence of pheochromocytoma with the initiation of their therapy. Some elderly patients who have postoperative orthostatic hypotension may actually suffer from autonomic nervous system dysfunction. If patients fail to respond to volume repletion, one of these autonomic dysfunctional syndromes should be considered. If patients develop hypotension (for example, due to sepsis), prolonged catecholamine therapy may similarly lead to decreased adrenergic receptor responsiveness. In this type of situation, it is appropriate to switch to a nonadrenergic inotropic or vasopressor agent in an attempt to reconstitute normal adrenergic receptor function.

Prolactin

• Dopamine can induce hypoprolactinemia, which in turn interferes with T-lymphocyte function. It may have implications in a septic patient.

As indicated earlier in this chapter, prolactin may be an important stress hormone. Prolactin likely serves as an immunomodulator or immunostimulant hormone. Postoperative patients who receive dopamine or dopamine receptor agonists may develop hypoprolactinemia, which can impair the ability of T lymphocytes to respond to mitogenic stimulation. This area of interest has expanded and is a focus of ongoing investigation. The reader is cautioned that we are early in our data base about this particular subject, and for that reason, physicians should not stop using dopamine in the perioperative period. However, one must stay abreast of new information in regard to this subject.[1]

Heat Shock Protein

• Elevated temperatures in a septic patient may play an important role in the patient's ability to combat infection.

Recent data have provided important information on heat shock proteins and outcome from experimental septic shock.[32,33] In that work, the induction of heat shock proteins either by hyperthermia or pharmacologic induction (with the use of sodium arsenite) reduced the mortality rate following the induction of experimental sepsis. These important contributions suggest that perioperative temperature increases may actually play an important adaptive role in the induction of these heat shock proteins. The mechanisms by which heat shock proteins improve outcome are not totally defined. However, these recent contributions suggest the possibility that it may not necessarily be beneficial to treat temperature increases with antipyretic agents. Another alternative would be to consider whether the administration of heat shock protein inducers would help to reduce the mortality rate from postoperative septic shock. This area is also an important focus of ongoing investigation.[34]

Sex Steroids

Parker and associates in 1985 provided evidence for adrenocortical adaptation to various forms of severe illness.[35] In that work, these investigators demonstrated a decrease in sex steroid formation in parallel with illness-associated increases in glucocorticoid and mineralocorticoid production. More recently, Spratt and colleagues demonstrated that there is suppression of the reproductive axis, and it is directly related to disease severity.[36] Following discharge from the ICU and the hospital, former patients may have diminished libido and/or the potential for diminished sexual function. For many postoperative patients, this area, which we rarely discuss with patients, may hold great importance.

Thyroid Dysfunction

Dopamine and cortisol both inhibit the release of thyroid-stimulating hormone (TSH) from the pituitary gland. Critically ill patients following surgery who have increases in endogenous circulating concentrations of dopamine and cortisol may have falsely low plasma TSH concentrations despite the presence of primary hypothyroidism. Therefore, the clinician who assesses thyroid function in postoperative critically ill patients should recognize that even slight increases above the normal range in the circulating TSH concentration may reflect clinically important hypothyroidism. Indeed, the measurement of the circulating TSH concentrations is probably the best test to determine whether a patient has hypothyroidism. We and others have determined that following surgery there are marked (35 to 70%) decreases in circulating thyroxine (T_4) and triiodothyronine (T_3) concentrations.[37] These T_4 and T_3 decreases are found in the sick euthyroid syndrome. Thus, if clinicians only assess T_4 and T_3 levels, they may be misled into thinking that the patient has hypothyroidism when, indeed, the patient has the sick euthyroid syndrome. For that reason, the circulating TSH concentration is the more important variable to measure.

- *Critically ill patients who have even slight elevations in TSH may in fact have clinical hypothyroidism. TSH, and not T_4 or T_3, will best diagnose hypothyroidism.*

We worry about postoperative hypothyroidism in patients who have hypothermia, who cannot be weaned from mechanical ventilatory support, or who have unexplained increases in circulating creatine kinase concentrations or hypercholesterolemia. Such patients may also have delayed return in deep tendon reflexes. Patients with hypothyroidism in the postoperative period may develop clinically important serous effusions (ascites, pleural effusions, pericardial effusions) and hypothermia (with alterations in central thermoregulation and impairment in shivering thermogenesis). They also have impairments of the ventilatory responses to hypoxia and hypercap-

- *Hypothyroidism can prevent patients from weaning off the mechanical ventilator.*

nia (this latter concern can potentially lead to an inability to be weaned from mechanical ventilatory support). These problems associated with hypothyroidism may be accentuated in patients who have prolonged nutritional deficiency and/or in those patients receiving benzodiazepenes and opiates in the postoperative period.[38]

ALTERING THE STRESS RESPONSE

• *The stress response actually enhances immune function.*

Dr. Douglas Wilmore has suggested three strategies that may be important to enhance recovery from catabolic illnesses. These strategies are (1) reduction of the inflammatory response; (2) provision of specific nutrients to support tissue requirements during catabolic illness; and (3) potential administration of growth factors that might improve tissue repair in protein synthesis. All of these strategies may help to improve outcome following surgery in certain patient populations.[39]

As previously mentioned, the administration of growth hormone may contribute to improvement in postoperative positive nitrogen balance.[40] We have begun to understand how to modulate the inflammatory response. The stress response is not all bad. We know, for example, that the body is designed to activate immune functions to fight microorganisms that have entered the body. Some investigators have been concerned that modulation of these immune mechanisms may be more detrimental than helpful. The next few years should help us to discover whether these concerns are justified. With advances in molecular biology, we now have the tools to inactivate macrophage-generated cytokines, as an example, that may serve important primary roles in the stress response.

In addition to the hormonally mediated alterations in the postoperative patient, certain electrolytes are also abnormal in the postoperative period. These electrolyte abnormalities reflect other components of the stress response. An example is hypocalcemia. We have determined that hypocalcemia is common in postoperative patients,[41,42] and we know the causes are multifactorial.[43,44] Hypocalcemia is a consequence of illness-associated hypoparathyroidism and alterations in vitamin D metabolism. In addition, illness-induced increases in catecholamines lead to lipolysis, which contributes to an augmentation of calcium binding to protein. Hypocalcemia may occur as a consequence of postoperative hypomagnesemia, and it may also be due to intracellular shifts of calcium as a consequence of numerous factors including changes in acid-base status. These types of illness-associated changes in calcium metabolism are also seen with magnesium. Clinicians should recognize that the greater the hormone or electrolyte abnormality, the more likely it is to be clinically important. The closer the concentrations of hormones and electrolytes are to normal, the less clinical importance the abnormality has. Normalization of postoperative abnormalities in hormone and electrolyte concentrations may not be justified. There have been few studies to analyze whether it is efficacious to normalize mildly decreased concentrations of hor-

• *Minor variations from normal values of hormones or electrolytes may not necessarily need correction.*

mones or electrolytes in the postoperative period. For that reason, at the present time, replacement therapy is usually restricted to patients with known deficiency states, those patients with clearly, clinically defined hypofunctional endocrine glands, and those patients with progressive or marked reductions in various electrolytes such as calcium and magnesium.

STRESS HYPERGLYCEMIA

The classic stress hormones (norepinephrine, epinephrine, growth hormone, cortisol, and glucagon) are all counterregulatory hormones that antagonize or inhibit insulin's action and help to mobilize glucose into the circulation. Therefore, stress hyperglycemia is common in the postoperative critically ill patient. Usually, the hyperglycemia seen in this patient population is mild to moderate (values of between 120 and 200 mg/dl). However, in occasional patients, the blood glucose concentration may exceed 200 mg/dl, which leads to glucosuria and potentially to changes in circulating osmolality. This severe stress hyperglycemic response is especially common in patients with diabetes mellitus. Recent evidence would suggest that tight control of glucose concentrations in diabetic patients is efficacious in preventing long-term complications.[45] However, little evidence exists in regard to tight control of diabetes mellitus in critically ill patients.

- *Elimination of hyperglycemia may aid both white blood cell function and wound healing.*

I believe that control of hyperglycemia is useful in several situations: (1) in patients with hyperglycemia-induced glucosuria, glucosuria impairs the ability of the clinician to follow the urine output as an index of renal tissue perfusion; (2) when the serum osmolality exceeds 300 mOsm/L as a consequence of hyperglycemia, a lowered circulating glucose concentration helps to control this hyperosmolar response; (3) in patients with postoperative infection, tighter control of glucose metabolism may aid white blood cell function; and (4) control of severe stress hyperglycemia may aid wound healing.

OTHER ENDOCRINE METABOLIC IMPLICATIONS OF THE STRESS RESPONSE

There are several clinical advantages to knowledge about the stress response. First, circulating concentrations of prolactin (a stress hormone) may be potentially reflective of a seizure disorder (versus a pseudoseizure disorder in the postoperative period). A second point has to do with the molecular scientific approach that we are currently undertaking to modulate the stress response with the use of monoclonal antibodies. A good discussion of this process using tumor necrosis factor as a prototype is contained in an article by Giroir.[46] A third clinical situation refers to the adequacy of sedation reflected by changes in heart rate. We believe that inadequate sedation may be reflected by tachycardia that would occur as a consequence of stress-induced release of epinephrine and norepinephrine, which then modulate this hemodynamic response.

In conclusion, the stress response serves as a vital and protective mechanism that the body uses to deal with critical illnesses, trauma, and serious infection. Since many of our postoperative patients face the complications of infection, problems with wound healing, and the possibility of organ dysfunction, knowledge of the stress response assumes clinical importance. The classic "fight or flight" hormones have been markedly extended to include many other hormones that are altered in their concentrations under a variety of stressful situations. The endocrine-immune linkage has become increasingly clear, and a number of novel pharmacologic approaches may be achieved as we expand the data base in this important area.

REFERENCES

1. Holaday JW: Anterior pituitary hormones and critical illness. In: Chernow B, ed: The pharmacologic approach to the critically ill patient, 3rd ed. Baltimore, Williams & Wilkins, 1994; pp. 890–900.
2. Federman D: The adrenal. In: Rubenstein E, Federman D, eds: Scientific American medicine. New York, Scientific American Press, 1994; Section 3 (IV), pp. 1–17.
3. Chernow B, Alexander HR, Smallridge RC et al: Hormonal responses to graded surgical stress. Arch Intern Med 1987; 147:1273–1278.
4. Khilnani P, Munoz R, Salem M et al: Hormonal responses to surgical stress in children. J Pediatr Surg 1993; 28:1–4.
5. Schein RMH, Sprung CL, Marcial E et al: Plasma cortisol levels in patients with septic shock. Crit Care Med 1990; 18:259–263.
6. Chrousos GP: Molecular and endocrine mechanisms of the stress response. In: Sternberg EM, moderator: The stress response and the regulation of inflammatory disease. Ann Intern Med 1992; 117:854–857.
7. Reichlin S: Neuroendocrine-immune interactions. N Engl J Med 1993; 329:1246–1253.
8. Bernton EW, Beach JE, Holaday JW et al: Release of multiple hormones by a direct action of interleukin-1 on pituitary cells. Science 1987; 238: 519–521.
9. Stenzel-Poore M, Vale WW, Rivier C: Relationship between antigen-induced immune stimulation and activation of the hypothalamic-pituitary-adrenal axis in the rat. Endocrinology 1993; 132:1313–1318.
10. Breder CD, Dinarello CA, Saper CB: Interleukin-1 immunoreactive innervation of the human hypothalamus. Science 1988; 240:321–324.
11. Sharp BM, Matta SG, Peterson PK et al: Tumor necrosis factor-α is a potent ACTH secretagogue: comparison to interleukin-1β. Endocrinology 1989; 124:3131–3133.
12. Darling G, Goldstein DS, Stull R et al: Tumor necrosis factor-immune endocrine interaction. Surgery 1989; 106:1155–1160.
13. Woloski BMR, Smith EM, Meyer WJ et al: Corticotropin-releasing activity of monokines. Science 1985; 230:1035–1037.
14. Besedovsky H, Del Rey A, Sorkin E , Dinarello CA: Immunoregulatory feedback between interleukin-1 and glucocorticoid hormones. Science 1986; 233:652–654.
15. Cannon JG, Tompkins RG, Gelfand JA et al: Circulating interleukin-1 and tumor necrosis factor in septic shock and experimental endotoxin fever. J Infect Dis 1990; 161:79–84.

16. Marano MA, Fong Y, Moldawer LL et al: Serum cachectin/tumor necrosis factor in critically ill patients with burns correlates with infection and mortality. Surg Gynecol Obstet 1990; 170:32–38.
17. Jurney TH, Cockrell JL Jr, Lindberg JS et al: Spectrum of serum cortisol response to ACTH in ICU patients—correlation with degree of illness and mortality. Chest 1987; 92:292–295.
18. Werb MR, Zinman B, Teasdale SJ et al: Hormonal and metabolic responses during coronary artery bypass surgery: role of infused glucose. J Clin Endocrinol Metab 1989; 69:1010–1018.
19. Fisher CJ, Opal SM, Dhainaut JF et al: Influence of an anti-tumor necrosis factor monoclonal antibody on cytokine levels in patients with sepsis. Crit Care Med 1993; 21:318–327.
20. Fisher CJ, Slotman GJ, Opal SM, et al: Initial evaluation of human recombinant interleukin-1 receptor antagonist in the treatment of sepsis syndrome: a randomized, open-label, placebo-controlled, multicenter trial. Crit Care Med 1994; 22:12–21.
21. Blake MJ, Udelsman R, Feulner GJ et al: Stress-induced heat shock protein 70 expression in adrenal cortex: an ACTH sensitive, age-dependent response. Proc Natl Acad Sci, USA 1991; 88:9873–9877.
22. Reincke M, Allolio B, Wurth G, Winkelmann W: The hypothalamic-pituitary-adrenal axis in critical illness: response to dexamethasone and corticotropin releasing hormone. J Endocrinol Metab 1993; 77: 151–156.
23. Jarek MJ, Legare CJ, McDermott MT et al: Endocrine profiles for outcome prediction from the intensive care unit. Crit Care Med 1993; 21:543–550.
24. Salem M, Tainsh RE, Bromberg J et al: Perioperative glucocorticoid coverage: a reassessment 42 years after emergence of a problem. Ann Surg 1994; 219:416–425.
25. Udelsman R, Goldstein DS, Loriaux DL, Chrousos GP: Catecholamine-glucocorticoid interactions during surgical stress. J Surg Res 1987; 539–545.
26. Cupps TR, Gerrard TL, Falkoff RJ et al: Effects of in vitro corticosteroids on B cell activation, proliferation, and differentiation. J Clin Invest 1985; 75:754–761.
27. Schaffner A: Therapeutic concentrations of glucocorticoids suppress the antimicrobial activity of human macrophages without impairing their responsiveness to gamma interferon. J Clin Invest 1985; 76: 1755–1764.
28. Chernow B, Vernoski B, Zaloga GP et al: Dexamethasone causes less steroid-induced alkalemia than methylpredinisolone or hydrocortisone. Crit Care Med 1984; 12:384–386.
29. Salomäki TE, Leppäiluoto J, Laitinen JO et al: Epidural versus intravenous fentanyl for reducing hormonal, metabolic, and physiologic responses after thoracotomy. Anesthesiology 1993; 79:672–679.
30. Khosla S, Wolfson JS, Demerjian Z, Godine JE: Adrenal crisis in the setting of high-dose ketoconazole therapy. Arch Intern Med 1989; 149: 802–804.
31. Zaloga GP: Hormones: vasopressin, growth hormone, glucagon, somatostatin, prolactin, G-CSF, GM-CSF. In: Chernow B, ed: The pharmacologic approach to the critically ill patient, 3rd ed. Baltimore, Williams & Wilkins, 1994; pp. 700–714.
32. Villar J, Ribiero S, Mullen JB et al: Induction of the heat shock response reduces mortality rate and organ damage in a sepsis-induced acute lung injury model. Crit Care Med 1994; 22:914–921.

33. Ribiero S, Villar J, Downey GP et al: Sodium arsenite induces heat shock protein-72 expression in the lungs and protects rats against sepsis. Crit Care Med 1994; 22:922–929.
34. Buchman TG: Manipulation of stress gene expression: a novel therapy for the treatment of sepsis? Crit Care Med 1994; 22:901–902.
35. Parker LN, Levin ER, Lifrak ET: Evidence for adrenocortical adaptation to severe illness. J Clin Endocrinol Metab 1985; 60:947–952.
36. Spratt DI, Cox P, Orav J et al: Reproductive axis suppression in acute illness is related to disease severity. JPEN J Parenter Enteral Nutr 1993; 76:1548–1554.
37. Zaloga GP, Chernow B, Smallridge RC et al: A longitudinal evaluation of thyroid function in critically ill surgical patients. Ann Surg 1985; 201:456–464.
38. Burman K: Thyroid hormones. In: Chernow B, ed: The pharmacologic approach to the critically ill patient, 3rd ed. Baltimore, Williams & Wilkins, 1994; pp. 741–757.
39. Wilmore DW: Catabolic illness: strategies for enhancing recovery. N Engl J Med 1991; 325:695–702.
40. Ponting GA, Halliday D, Teale JD, Sim AJW: Postoperative positive nitrogen balance with intravenous hyponutrition and growth hormone. Lancet 1988; 1:438–439.
41. Chernow B, Zaloga GP, McFadden E et al: Hypocalcemia in critically ill patients. Crit Care Med 1982; 10:848–851.
42. Chernow B, Bamberger S, Stoiko M et al: Hypomagnesemia in postoperative intensive care patients. Chest 1989; 95:391–397.
43. Zaloga GP, Chernow B: Hypocalcemia in critical illness. JAMA 1986; 256:1924–1929.
44. Zaloga GP, Chernow B: The multifactorial basis for hypocalcemia during sepsis: studies on the PTH-vitamin D axis. Ann Intern Med 1987; 107:36–41.
45. The Diabetes Control and Complications Trial Research Group: The effect of intensive treatment of diabetes on the development and progression of long-term complications in insulin-dependent diabetes mellitus. N Engl J Med 1993; 329:977–986.
46. Giroir BP: Mediators of septic shock: new approaches for interrupting the endogenous inflammatory cascade. Crit Care Med 1993; 21:780–789.

CHAPTER 4

Pain Management and Sedation in the Intensive Care Unit

Philip G. Boysen
William S. Blau

Case Report

A 79-year-old female patient returned to the intensive care unit (ICU) following surgery for removal of renal cell carcinoma. The location of the patient's left kidney required that the incision be carried into the left chest. The extensive procedure resulted in a blood loss of 3 L, which was replaced with both autologous and homologous blood and 8 L of Ringer's lactate and normal saline. Prior to the procedure, an epidural catheter had been threaded into the L8-L9 interspace. Because of the extent of the procedure, the large blood loss and fluid replacement, the late hour of the day, and the patient's age, it was elected to keep the patient intubated and mechanically ventilated overnight. The epidural catheter was utilized for pain relief. The patient received an infusion of fentanyl, 5 μg/ml, combined with a 1/16% bupivicaine solution at a rate of 6 ml/hr. This rendered adequate pain relief.

Approximately 3 hours after her arrival in the ICU, the patient was awake and somewhat agitated. The agitation appeared related to the presence of the endotracheal tube. The chest film then revealed evidence of fluid overload, and diuresis was begun. However, the patient required 60% oxygen and a positive end-expiratory pressure (PEEP) of 10 cm H_2O to maintain a PaO_2 of 78 mm Hg and 94% saturation. It was not believed safe to remove the endotracheal tube and to discontinue mechanical ventilation. Sedation, in addition to analgesia, was considered. The patient was initially given a bolus of 1 mg of midazolam and then started on an infusion of 1.5 mg/hr. This appeared to calm her. She was still arousable to stimuli.

By morning, the patient had diuresed 2 L of fluid. The F_{IO_2} was 0.4, and the PaO_2 was 94 mm Hg on 5 cm/H_2O PEEP. Midazolam was discontinued, and the patient was extubated 80 minutes later. She made an uneventful recovery and was discharged with the epidural catheter still in place for pain relief.

The treatment of pain in any clinical setting presents a real challenge.[1] Treatment of pain and anxiety in the critically ill patient includes its own set of problems. Not only are these patients more acutely ill, but often the severity of their illness far exceeds that of patients encountered in other clinical environments. Many such patients require mechanical ventilation, and the required transtracheal tube leaves them unable to speak or communicate adequately. The confusion and agitation, often a part of illness, result in the need for restraints. While perhaps clinically indicated and necessary for a patient's well-being, restraints often further complicate the patient's reaction to the clinical situation and environment. We often fail to recognize the undertreatment of pain and anxiety in any hospital setting, and specifically the ICU, until the patient can be interviewed subsequently as to the course, conduct, and reactions to the acute illness.[2–4] Unfortunately, it then becomes all too clear how inadequate our treatments often were.

• *Anxiety and pain in the ICU can contribute to agitation and can result in a significant increase in metabolic demands.*

Inadequate treatment of pain, suffering, and anxiety causes adverse physiologic sequelae. Frequently, the patient's metabolic rate increases. Such a response utilizes valuable energy substrates otherwise destined for nutrition and reparative processes.[5] Alterations in blood pressure and heart rate in response to pain may be obscured, since such changes may be due to other physiologic consequences of the illness. Stress alone can increase blood coagulability and water retention, presumably by secretion of antidiuretic hormone (ADH), as well as breakdown and interference with tissue reparative processes and immune function.[6,7] The autonomic hyperreactivity and stress placed on the cardiac and pulmonary systems may be further detrimental to the patient's outcome, especially in the presence of underlying chronic disease.[8] Following injury or surgical procedures, pain and agitation can delay the return of normal bowel function and can contribute to a prolongation of the illness. Last, increased awareness of chronic pain syndrome and difficulties in developing adequate treatment have become better recognized.[9,10] The cumulative evidence suggests that pain management, especially with neuraxial local anesthetics and opioids, can modify these physiologic responses.[7,8,11–17]

The Agency for Healthcare Policy and Research (AHCPR) published clinical practice guidelines for acute pain management in 1992. These guidelines were intended to provide a logical sequence for assessment and management of acute pain. The Joint Commission for Accreditation of Healthcare Organizations, the United

States Department of Health and Human Services, and the Society of Critical Care Medicine have begun to include pain control criteria as part of their patient recommendations and guidelines. The spectrum of available methodology and agents to treat pain syndromes has dramatically increased in the last 10 years. Many patients now have increased awareness of the various treatment methods. This awareness has changed their expectations as well as their interactions with their physicians. Even some trauma patients are able to communicate with their surgeons and anesthesiologists during the preoperative assessment. A spectrum of the pain control options available can often be reviewed at such a time. This can provide coordination of the preoperative assessment, intraoperative management, and eventual postoperative delivery of a therapeutic regimen. Care can be tailored to the individual patient's needs. Clearly, this has become one of the more satisfying aspects of practice in the critical care environment. The ability to support vital organ function and at the same time relieve pain and suffering requires a degree of clinical acumen and expertise that serves as part of the bedrock of a critical care practice. This chapter reviews current methodologies of particular interest to the ICU-oriented clinician and provides a strategy for a multifaceted approach to the relief of pain and anxiety.

- *When possible, pain management should be discussed in advance with patients. Many patients are aware of some of the newer techniques available.*

PAIN RELIEF

Nociception

Nociception refers to the global realization and response to a variety of noxious stimuli, which include pain.[18] Nociception represents culmination of a step-wise process that follows an irritant or painful stimulus. This stimulus causes transduction of the signal that is then secondarily transmitted along a nerve network. Modulation of the signal occurs at the spinal cord level. Following modulation, the signal moves in a rostral or cephalic direction. Arrival of the signal at the brain stem signals perception of the noxious stimulus as pain. All this elicits a rapid response. The systematic approach to transduction, transmission, modulation, and perception of pain allows us to identify sites at which to interrupt the nociceptive response. For the critically ill patient, pain control and treatment can be aimed at any or all of these sites. This approach can be termed "balanced analgesia"(Fig. 4–1). Ultimately, the goal is to alter the patient's pain perception in order to minimize or eliminate any response to noxious stimulation.

- *Pain modulation can involve several steps along the anatomic route from stimulation at the peripheral site to brain perception.*

In the periphery, transduction of a noxious stimulus into an electrical signal can be inhibited by nonsteriodal anti-inflammatory drugs (NSAIDs), which decrease levels of inflammatory mediators generated at the site of tissue injury.[77] Following transduction, the transmission or passage of the signal from the nociceptor to the central nervous system by primary afferent nerve fibers can be reduced or blocked by field blocks, regional anesthesia, cryoanalgesia,[19] or interpleural anesthetics.[20] Several methods can modify or

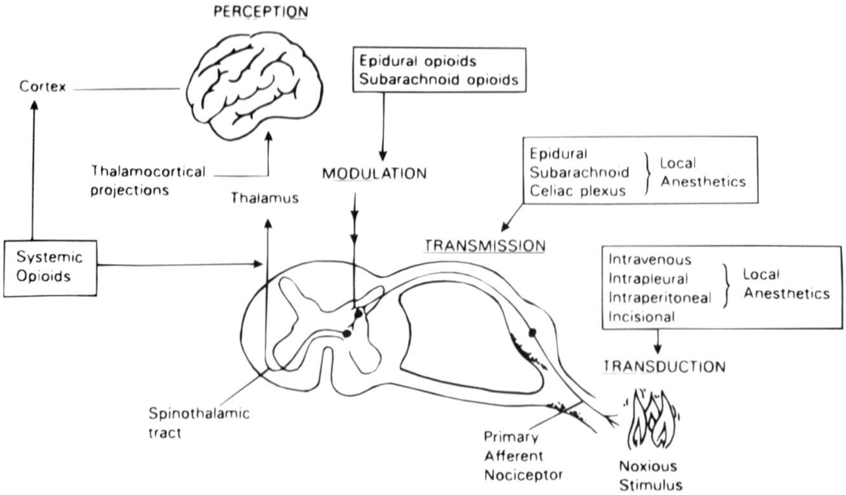

Figure 4–1.
Sites of interruption of the nociceptive response to achieve "balanced analgesia." (Modified from Ferrante FM, VadeBoncouer TR: Epidural analgesia with combinations of local anesthetics and opioids. In: Ferrante FM, VadeBoncouer TR, eds: Postoperative pain management. New York, Churchill-Livingstone, 1992.)

interrupt the signal at the spinal cord level. These include intrathecal injection or epidural anesthesia/analgesia with local anesthetics or narcotics.

The use of techniques such as transcutaneous electrical nerve stimulation (TENS) and spinal injection of opioids to modify the processing of nociceptive information at the spinal cord or higher central nervous system levels is derived from the gate-control theory of pain transmission.[21] Nociceptive impulses, which travel from the periphery in Aδ or C nerve fibers, result in the release of substance P and other neurotransmitters that excite the first central transmitting cells in the dorsal horn of the spinal cord. Non-nociceptive input from larger, myelinated nerve fibers tends to prevent opening of the "gate" for further transmission of nociceptive input and to stimulate enkephalinergic interneurons. Descending inhibitory tracts also stimulate these same interneurons, which then block the release of substance P. This process implies a delicate balance of the neural, neurohormonal, and neuroendocrine aspects of the network (Fig. 4–2).

The neuroendocrine response to surgical stress, trauma, and painful stimuli disrupts the steady state and overwhelms the system. Changes in body mass and tissue reserve, and the patient's immune status, may all be modulated by this response. Myocardial oxygen demand, respiratory muscle function, and other factors may aggravate or further stimulate the neuroendocrine response. An increased tendency to blood coagulation and thromboembolism can result, with consequent formation of pharmacologic foci within the thrombus and ultimately release of many more mediators.

• *Pain can increase myocardial oxygen demands and can interfere with normal respiratory muscle function. Pain may also increase coagulation.*

Many of these hormones and mediators are now undergoing investigation to determine their effect on the stress response.[5,6] The inflammatory response, for example, involves not only substance P

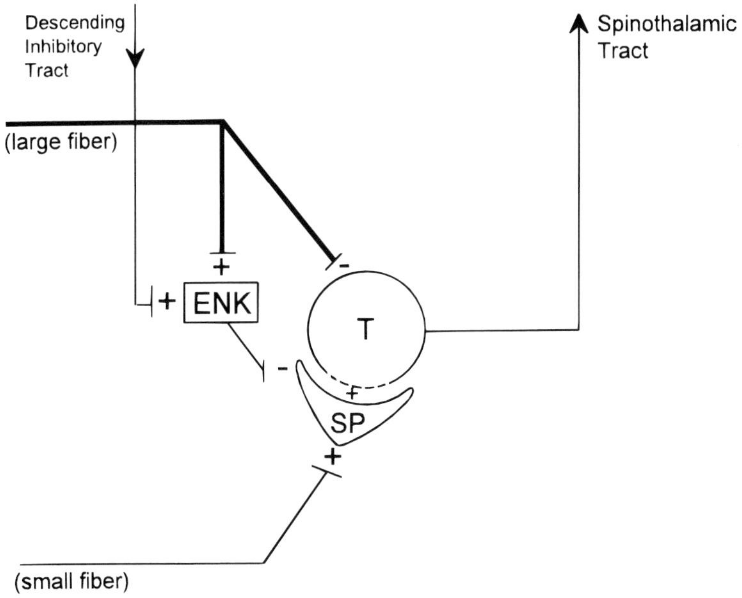

Figure 4–2.
Modification of the gate control theory. Impulses through the small fiber release substance P (SP), which excites the first central transmission cells (T). Large fiber impulses inhibit the opening of the "gate" and stimulate an enkephalinergic interneuron (ENK). The descending inhibitory tract also stimulates the enkephalinergic interneuron, which blocks the release of substance P. Fibers from the dorsal horn form the spinothalamic tract (ST).

and tissue necrosis factor (TNF), but also interleukin-1 (IL1). Modulation of the release or activity of these substances will soon be possible. At the level of the hypothalamus, corticotropin-releasing hormone, and ADH are secreted as part of the pain response. They impede tissue repair and cause water retention. The pituitary may release corticotropin (ACTH) and a series of beta endorphins.[22] The adrenal response to pain and includes the release of cortisol from cortex and the secretion of catecholamines and probably leu-enkephalins and met-enkephalins.

Pain Assessment

Communication problems can make assessment of pain difficult. Visual signals, as well as written messages for the patient who is lucid enough to categorize his or her nociceptive state, can overcome such obstacles. A visual pain scale can include a work analysis of simple descriptive intensities, a numeric intensity scale from no pain to the worst possible pain, or a simple visual analog scale. The acutely ill patient, unable to phonate, can simply point to the scale and characterize the pain level and response (Fig. 4–3).

- *Visual analog scales can help patients to communicate their pain level.*

Importantly, responses to the visual stimulus not only should be part of the initial assessment, but also should be repeated following initiation of therapy and should be charted on the flow sheet along with other vital signs and trended data. Even in patients capable of

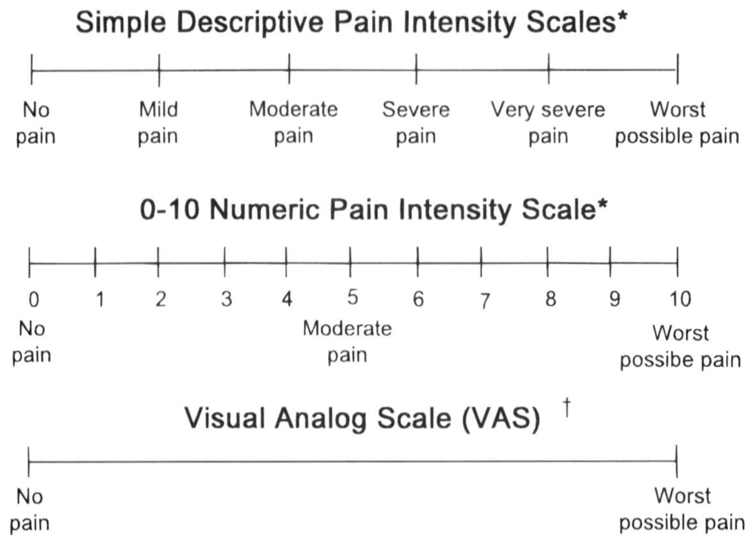

Figure 4–3.
Scales by which to measure pain that do not require the patient to speak. [*]If used as a graphic rating scale, a 10-cm baseline is recommended;[†] a 10-cm baseline is recommended for VAS scales. (From Agency for Healthcare Policy and Research (AHCPR): Acute pain management guideline and from acute pain management: operative or medical procedures and trauma. Clinical practice guidelines. Rockville, MD, Agency for Healthcare Policy and Research, Public Health Service, US Dept of Health and Human Services, AHCPR Publication No. 92–0032, February 1992.)

verbal communication, the visual analog scale or pain intensity scale can be helpful to initiate a response to therapeutic intervention and continually trend and analyze feedback data from the patient.

Systemic Techniques

The most common therapy for acute pain utilizes intravenous administration of opioid agonists. The opioid receptor characteristics include multiple sites and function. These receptors are variously occupied and activated by different agents (Table 4–1). Commonly used opioids for the critically ill are morphine, meperidine, fentanyl, sufentanil, and shorter-acting agents such as alfentanil. Table 4–2 includes a comparative analysis of these different agents. Systemic opioid analgesia has most often been administered intermittently, either intramuscularly or, preferably, intravenously on an as-needed (PRN) schedule. This cost-effective and easy-to-administer approach often results in inadequate pain relief for most acutely ill patients. This problem can be traced to the pharmacokinetic variability of these drugs among patients and the particular characteristics of the agent administered. In order to maintain blood levels within the therapeutic range, the dose should be of a specific strength and interval so that levels are obviously neither toxic nor subtherapeutic. An inadequate dose or a prolonged dosage interval may cause the patient to experience acute pain, and large narcotic

Table 4–1.
Opioid Receptor Sites and Function are Occupied by Agonists/Antagonists

Site	Effect	Agonist	Antagonist
Mu-1	Supraspinal analgesia	Beta endorphin Meptazinol Morphine	Naloxone Pentazocine Nalbuphine
Mu-2	Hypoventilation Bradycardia Physical dependence Euphoria Ileus	Meperidine Fentanyl Sufentanil Alfentanil	
Delta	Modulate mu receptor activity	Leu-enkephalin	Naloxone Met-enkephalin
Kappa	Analgesia Sedation Hypoventilation(?) Miosis	Dynorphin Pentazocine Butorphanol Nalbuphine Buprenorphine Nalorphine	Naloxone
Sigma	Dysphoria Hypertonia Tachycardia Tachypnea Mydriasis	Pentazocine(?) Ketamine(?)	Naloxone

doses may then be necessary to bring the pain response back under control. Larger doses or more frequent intervals, however, can exceed the therapeutic range necessary to achieve pain control and can result in toxic side effects, such as respiratory depression. If it were not for the variation among individuals, administration of the necessary dose at intervals that approximate the beta elimination half-life of the drug would almost always result in an appropriate response.

For this reason, regimens were devised to halve the dose and give the drug twice as frequently (Fig. 4–4). A logical next step would be a continuous infusion to maintain therapeutic blood levels

Table 4–2.
Pharmacokinetics of the Most Widely Used Opioid Agonists and the Antagonist Naloxone

Opioid	pK	Protein Binding (%)	Volume of Distribution ($L \cdot kg^{-1}$)	Clearance ($ml \cdot kg^{-1} \cdot min^{-1}$)	Elimination Half-Time (min)
Morphine	7.93	26–36	3.2–3.4	15–23	114
Meperidine	8.5	64–82	2.8–4.2	10–17	180–264
Fentanyl	8.43	79–87	3.2–5.9	11–21	185–219
Sufentanil	8.01	92.5	2.86	13	148–164
Alfentanil	6.5	89–92	0.5–1	5–7.9	70–98
Naloxone			1.8	30	60–90

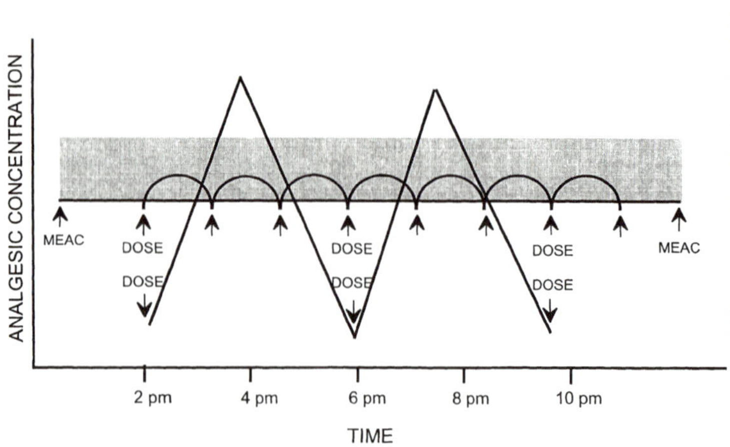

Figure 4–4.
Dosing intervals in relation to maintenance of therapeutic blood levels for analgesia or anxiolysis.

(Table 4–3). Unfortunately, variations in the drug pharmacokinetics also interfere with this strategy. Such methodology presumes that the drug infusion rate equals its clearance rate. If the infusion rate exceeds the clearance, then accumulation begins. If the infusion rate does not match the clearance, blood levels fall to subtherapeutic ranges. For this reason, intravenous techniques were further refined into patient-controlled analgesia (PCA).[23,24]

This PCA method of stress-response alteration relies on the model of nociception. The PCA paradigm extends one step beyond a continuous infusion. In addition to maintenance of drug plasma concentrations in the therapeutic range, continuous infusion of many drugs can cause downregulation of receptor sites and an alteration in the activity of the drug simply because of maintenance of constant plasma concentrations. PCA can close the loop between the model of nociception and drug administration.[25,26] When the first aura of pain begins to appear and before pain is well established, the patient can administer a small intravenous dose, fixed in amount, and at designated intervals (Table 4–4). There is little tendency for oversedation or depressive narcosis. Should either occur, the patient would not be awake enough to be able to attempt a redose. If desired, a slow concurrent infusion of the drug can be

• *To be most effective, patients should initiate the PCA pump at the first perception of pain. A continuous or basal infusion of an agent can aid patients who do not use a PCA pump to its full potential.*

Table 4–3.
Continuous Intravenous Opioid Infusion

	Beta Elimination Half-time β (hr)	Load Dose	Maintenance Dose (hr)
Morphine	3–6	5–10 mg	1–3 mg
Fentanyl	3–5	100–200 μg	30–150 μg
Sufentanil	3–5	10–20 μg	4–15 μg

Table 4–4.
Intravenous Patient-Controlled Analgesia

Drug	Load Dose	Maintenance Dose	Lockout (min)	Basal Rate (rate/hr)
Morphine	0.05–0.10 mg/kg	0.5–3.0 mg	6–8	0.5–2.0 mg
Meperidine	0.5–1.0 mg/kg	5–30 mg	6–8	5–20 mg
Hydromorphone	0.01–0.02 mg/kg	0.1–0.5 mg	6–8	0.1–0.3 mg
Fentanyl	0.5–1.0 μg/kg	15–75 μg	4–6	15–60 μg
Sufentanil	0.07–0.10 μg/kg	2–10 μg	4–6	2–8 μg

used and the PCA-designated dose self-administered to "top-off" the effect.[27] Almost any opioid agonist can be used effectively in a PCA system.[28] The variability of individual response to pain, trauma, mediator release, and altered pharmacokinetics makes the PCA system a viable option for the cooperative, critically ill patient.[29,30]

There is a general belief that smaller and less frequent dosing of narcotics is efficacious if it prevents the original nociceptive response. In the vernacular, "you can't get behind pain." Once full-blown nociception is established, it will require more narcotic to achieve satisfactory pain control than if smaller doses of the drug had been used to interrupt the initial pain response. This phenomenon has been termed central hypersensitization or "wind-up."[31,32] When this occurs, peripheral and central sensitization develops as an initial response following expansion of receptive fields in the dorsal horn. The dorsal horn wind-up causes further neuronal discharge, which amplifies the response.[33,34] The entire response represents an early protective mechanism. Avoidance of this series of events allows smoother pain control and lower overall doses. Wall's theory of the prevention of postoperative pain indicates that surgical trauma also creates a barrage of nociceptive transmissions. This, in turn, induces electrophysiologic and morphologic changes within the spinal cord.[35] Unfortunately, the sequelae of these alterations may long outlast the initial noxious stimulus. This situation absolutely characterizes the problem faced by many clinicians when treating a critically ill patient.

- *Undesirable responses to pain such as tachycardia are not necessarily reduced even though pain may ultimately be controlled.*

The enhancement of nociceptive transmission and the afferent barrage also introduced other pain-management concepts. Preemptive analgesia holds that inhibition of cord neuroblastic changes long outlasts the initial neural blockade.[36] This is a reverse of the Wall theory of system activation. For many patients, the surgical incision or initial trauma represents the priming mechanism that initiates pain response.

Neuraxial Opioids and Local Anesthetics

At the level of the spinal cord, neuraxial opioids modulate the transmission of pain stimuli.[37] Intrathecal and epidural routes of administration of opioid agonists take advantage of these receptor sites in the dorsal horn of the spinal cord.[38,39] The first narcotic employed, morphine sulfate, can be placed into the intrathecal or epidural space and then readministered through an indwelling catheter.[40–43] The technique now includes many other opioid agonists.

Morphine, hydromorphone, and hydrophilic opioids, based on their pharmacokinetics, maximize the therapeutic response. They have a slow onset, but long duration, combined with a high degree of cerebral spinal fluid (CSF) solubility. While a single dose has a prolonged effect, the duration of action remains unpredictable. Side effects commonly develop and include respiratory depression, as discussed later in this chapter. The hydrophilic nature of the drug causes considerable spread. One result is thoracic analgesia obtained via lumbar administration of the drug.

The properties of the lipophilic opioids, fentanyl and sufentanil, include low CSF solubility and spread and rapid onset of analgesia. These drugs also have a short duration of action. Single-dose administration results in a brief response, and lumbar administration provides poor thoracic analgesia. We prefer thoracic placement of the epidural catheter when we use these agents. This minimizes side effects. Their short duration of action makes these drugs particularly amenable to continuous infusion (Table 4–5). This technique can be combined with a PCA pump to deliver patient-controlled epidural analgesia (PCEA) (Table 4–5).[44]

- *The short duration of action of fentanyl makes it an ideal drug to use for a continuous infusion in the epidural space.*

- *Opioids combined with local anesthetics reduce the overall narcotic requirements.*

Simultaneous administration of opioids and local anesthetics can moderate the pain response and possibly enhance mediator release blockade. This is particularly true with continuous infusion and works in most, but not all, clinical situations.[45–47] Many different combinations have been devised (Table 4–6).[48–50] The final choice often depends on local preference.

Epidural analgesia can cause significant side effects.[51] Urinary retention and pruritus are common. Respiratory depression, while rare, more often develops with hydrophilic agents, such as mor-

Table 4–5.
Patient-Controlled Epidural Analgesia: Recommended Concentration-Dosing Protocols

	Bolus Load (ml)	Dose (ml)	Onset (min)	Basal Rate (ml/h)
Fentanyl 2 μg/ml Bupivacaine 0.125%	4–12	2–4	10	2–8
Fentanyl 5 μg/ml Bupivacaine 0.0625%	6–12	2–6	10	2–8
Fentanyl 10 μg/ml Bupivacaine 0.05%	5–10	2–5	10	2–5
Fentanyl 10 μg/ml Bupivacaine 0.025%	5–10	2–5	10	2–5
Sufentanil 2 μg/ml Bupivacaine 0.0625%	4–10	2–4	10	2–4
Morphine 0.1 mg/ml	10–20	0.5–2.0	20	0–4

Table 4–6.
Continuous Epidural Infusion Analgesia

Drug	Concentration	Infusion Rate (ml/h)
Fentanyl Bupivacaine	2 μg/ml 0.125%	4–20
Fentanyl Bupivacaine	5 μg/ml 0.0625%	4–15
Sufentanil Bupivacaine	1 μg/ml 0.125%	4–8
Sufentanil Bupivacaine	2 μg/ml 0.0625%	4–8
Morphine Bupivacaine	0.05 mg/ml 0.125%	4–8
Morphine Bupivacaine	0.1 mg/ml 0.0625%	2–8
Morphine	0.1 mg/ml	2–8

phine. The actual incidence is less than 1%.[52] Respiratory depression associated with epidural narcotics has a biphasic time course—at 2 and 8 hours after dosing. However, late respiratory depression has also been documented.[53] Simultaneous administration of intravenous narcotics can be particularly dangerous.[54] In an ICU, patients may receive mechanical ventilation, and most have an indwelling urinary catheter. Therefore, the complications are often not as serious. For example, pruritus is not a frequent complaint of the critically ill.

- *Fentanyl used in continuous infusions of less than 1 μg/kg/hr rarely causes respiratory depression in a critically ill patient.*

The immediate complications of catheter placement or from the initial drug dose can also be significant.[55] The most important immediate complication involves intrathecal or intravascular drug administration. Since spread of the epidural block depends on the volume of the agent rather than on baricity, intrathecal placement of a large volume of agent results in "total" spinal autonomic collapse and apnea. Recent data, however, suggest that small doses of intrathecal morphine can provide effective pain relief.[56] Similarly, an initial intravascular injection rapidly results in toxic local anesthetic levels.

- *Epidural catheters should be aspirated from time to time to make sure the tip has not migrated into either the CSF or a blood vessel.*

Other Regional Analgesic Techniques

Peripheral or autonomic nerve block therapies are not currently widely used as part of ICU pain management.[57,58] Intercostal nerve blocks are efficacious for the treatment of thoracic pain following chest trauma, thoracotomy, or cholecystectomy.[59–62] Utilization of a catheter permits redosage or continuous infusion.[63] Other specific nerve blocks can be maintained by intermittent or continuous dosing. These include sciatic,[64] femoral,[65] or interscalene[66] approaches. A psoas compartment block provides immediate and prolonged relief.[67]

Interpleural analgesia, when it works, provides effective pain relief. However, it usually requires that 20 to 25 ml 0.5% bupivi-

Table 4–7.
Dosages of Nonsteroidal Anti-inflammatory Agents

Ibuprofen (Motrin)	400 mg PO q4–6h
Naproxen (Naprosyn)	500 mg PO initially, then 250 mg PO q6–8h
Indomethacin (Indocin)	25–50 mg PO q8h
Ketorolac (Toradol)	30–60 mg IM Loading dose 30 mg q6h IM 10 mg q6h PO

caine be injected into the thorax and the patient positioned so that the drug accumulates in the paravertebral gutter for 20 to 30 minutes. If a chest tube has been placed, suction on the tube can result in "spotty" analgesia.[68,69]

The three major sympathetic blocks, celiac, stellate ganglion, and lumbar, may be performed in critically ill patients and can forestall chronic pain syndrome. Lumbar sympathetic blocks are particularly useful for one-sided lower extremity pain and trauma.[70–72] Stellate ganglion blocks may ameliorate upper extremity pain.[73]

Nonsteroidal Anti-Inflammatory Drugs (NSAIDS)

NSAIDs have been underutilized for general pain management. NSAIDs are effective alone for mild-to-moderate pain and can serve as adjuncts to opioids or regional anesthetic techniques.[74] They not only enhance the effect but reduce the required dosage of these other agents.[75] While most NSAIDs are only available in an oral dosing form, ketorolac can be administered both orally and parenterally. Ketorolac provides pain relief to a degree similar to narcotics[76,77] (Table 4–7). Ketorolac can interfere with platelet adhesiveness, which can potentially lead to clotting abnormalities.

• *The NSAIDs can provide adequate pain relief but may interfere with platelet function.*

SEDATION

In critically ill patients, pain alone may not be an issue. Instead, the anxiety of acute illness, combined with tracheal intubation, mechanical ventilation, and immobilization, can overwhelm the patient. Like pain, anxiety is often undertreated.[78] The patient with problems such as acute or chronic respiratory failure due to chronic obstructive pulmonary disease (COPD), or hypoxemic respiratory failure secondary to near-drowning or aspiration, may be agitated, uncooperative, and frightened. Other causes of agitation in the postoperative or posttraumatic period include head injury or anoxic damage as well as withdrawal from alcohol or other agents. Patients who receive long-term benzodiazepine therapy may also exhibit withdrawal signs. On occasion, patients may have an idiosyncratic reaction to a narcotic or other drug and may become acutely agitated. Obviously, treatable causes of agitation such as hypoxia and electrolyte disturbances must first be corrected. Although opioid

• *Before sedatives are instituted, the clinician must be sure that other correctable causes of agitation are not present. Examples include undetected hypoxemia or untreated pain.*

agonists provide some degree of sedation as well as analgesia, these effects are secondary. Sedation or, more appropriately, anxiolysis should be considered as a separate therapeutic goal. In fact, sedatives have a variety of other desirable effects, such as amnesia and seizure prophylaxis. Even after very high-dose narcotics (e.g., 50 to 100 μg/kg of fentanyl) for cardiac surgery, some patients recall their operations. A surprising number of patients can repeat conversations and relate anxious intraoperative moments.

Sedation and anxiolysis are, in fact, distinct pharmacologic results. Conscious sedation implies that the patient appears awake and is somnolent, but will respond to verbal stimulation. However, such patients are often sluggish and have slurred speech. Anxiety relief may occur at lower doses. The patient is awake, responsive to the environment with eyes open, and appropriately communicative. He or she appears unthreatened by the immediate environment and events. Anxiolysis can also be effected by a cognitive-behavioral and nonpharmacologic approach.[79–81]

Assessment

Anxiety assessment has been suggested as a parallel analysis to analgesic assessment. A visual analog scale or a verbal scheme (i.e., no worries, intense worries, on a scale of 1 to 10) can provide insight into the patient's mental condition. Postsurgical or posttraumatic interviews help increase clinical acumen as both patient and clinician quietly reflect on previous experience. As for clinical signs, unfortunately, tachycardia and hypertension can indicate either pain or anxiety. Other nonspecific signs may be failure to cooperate and confused or slurred speech.

When sedative agents are prescribed, individual nurses and physicians seem to have their own idea of the appropriate end point. However, such subjectivity provides an elusive goal. Each unit should probably consider adoption of a set of objective criteria to identify end points of therapy. This can prevent the highly variable sedation levels often a result of the bedside nurse and time of day.

- *An objective end point should be utilized when ordering sedation therapy.*

Choice of Agents

For critically ill patients, benzodiazepines have become the agents of choice to achieve sedation and anxiolysis. These drugs are often combined with opioid agonists. Diazepam, lorazepam, and midazolam have been and continue to be useful. Each has some advantages and disadvantages (Table 4–8).[82] The lipid solubility and widespread distribution of diazepam produce a long elimination half-life, and its active metabolites can further prolong the clinical effect (Fig. 4–5).[83] Lorazepam, also lipid soluble, has a long duration of action and provides intense amnesia. Midazolam's water solubility and shorter half-life make it popular for continuous infusion.[84] However, continued infusion has demonstrated increased dosing requirements. Reports have indicated that even small dosages can cause profound respiratory depression in the elderly.[85] The pharma-

- *The ability to use midazolam as a continuous infusion makes it the ideal benzodiazepine.*

Table 4–8.
Comparative Pharmacokinetics of the Benzodiazepines

	Equivalent Dose ($mg \cdot kg^{-1}$)	Volume of Distribution ($L \cdot kg^{-1}$)	Protein Binding (%)	Clearance ($ml \cdot kg^{-1} \cdot min^{-1}$)	Elimination Half-Time (h)
Diazepam	0.3–0.5	1–1.5	96–98	0.2–0.5	21–37
Midazolam	0.15–0.3	1–1.5	96–98	6–8	1–4
Lorazepam	0.05	0.8–1.3	96–98	0.7–1	10–20

cokinetic differences among these drugs are listed in Table 4–8. Various sedative-analgesic combinations have also been proposed.[86]

Benzodiazepines

Benzodiazepine receptors are multiple and modulate four separate pharmacologic effects. Facilitation of the action of gamma-aminobutyric acid (GABA)—an inhibitory transmitter—results in sedation and muscle relaxation. Interactions with separate sites on the receptor cause amnesia and suppress seizure activity (Fig. 4–6).[87] When given alone, these agents are remarkably free of side effects other than respiratory depression. When combined with narcotics, hypotension may be severe.

Routes of benzodiazepine administration depend on the particular agent. As mentioned, midazolam can be continuously infused. Diazepam and lorazepam do not readily lend themselves to a continuous infusion because of their high degree of lipid solubility and long half-life. However, such a strategy can be successfully employed with close monitoring.

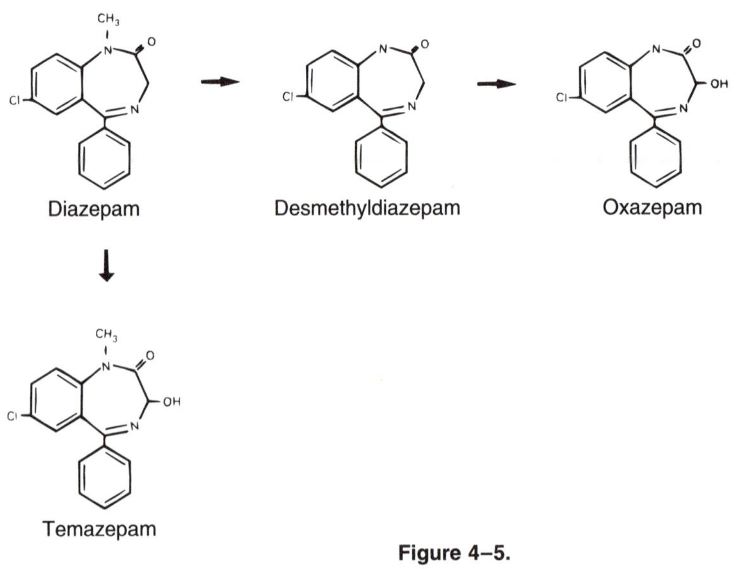

Figure 4–5.
The active metabolites of diazepam.

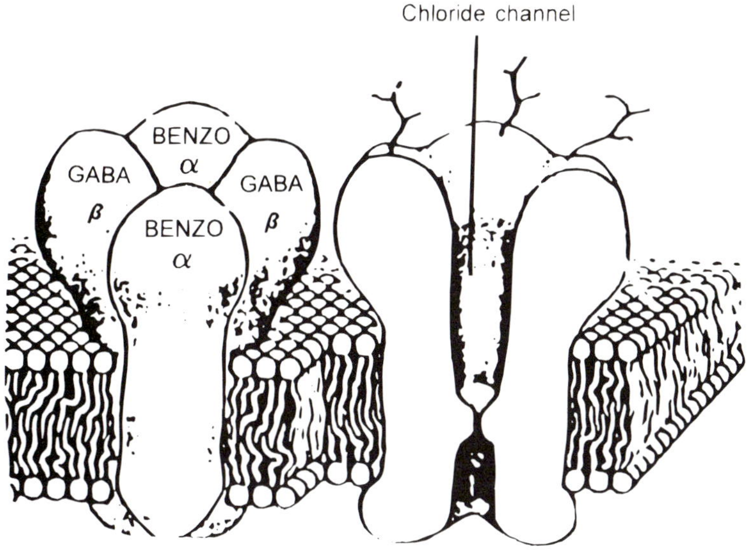

Figure 4–6.
The model of the benzodiazepine receptor. The drug attaches to the alpha site and facilitates the action of the inhibitory neurotransmitter GABA. (From Mohler H, Richards JG: The benzodiazepine receptor: a pharmacologic control elements of brain function. Eur J Anesthesiol 1988; 2:15–24.)

A particularly intriguing dosing protocol, called patient-controlled anxiolysis, has emerged.[88,89] It espouses the same principle as PCA therapy. The clinician controls the dose and the time interval. Within these limits, the patient can control the frequency of drug administration. The psychologic impact of autonomy and control helps to provide anxiolysis at lower drug doses. This method also minimizes the tendency to overmedicate, with possible respiratory depression. The noncontinuous infusion helps to avoid tolerance or tachyphylaxis.

A new agent has been developed to "reverse" the benzodiazepine effect.[90] Flumazenil, with a structure somewhat similar to that of midazolam, can occupy but not activate the receptor site. While the use of reversal agents has increased, it is probable that reversal of amnesic effects occurs with very small doses.[91] Clinical indications for benzodiazepine reversal include drug overdosage or induced cardiovascular instability. The half-life of flumazenil is usually less than that of the benzodiazepine, so effective use will require multiple flumazenil doses or a continuous infusion.

- *Flumazenil can reverse the effects of benzodiazepines, but its effects may not outlast the duration of action of the benzodiazepine.*

Propofol

Propofol, originally an anesthetic induction agent, has become an effective sedative for critically ill patients. The agent undergoes rapid redistribution to fat stores, and the liver rapidly conjugates the drug.[92,93] This permits easy titration to the desired effect. Furthermore, the drug's effects dissipate within 15 minutes of discontinuation.[94] The agent has minimal cardiovascular effects. Some degree of hypotension may develop in the volume-depleted patient.

- *Propofol is a mild vasodilator.*

Propofol can minimally reduce intracranial pressure.[95] However, more importantly, its short duration of action can make it useful in the management of the agitated brain-injured patient. Once the drug has been discontinued, the patient can be at baseline within 15 minutes and ready for a neurologic evaluation. The drug has clearly made it easier to manage the agitated patient but still permit ongoing evaluation of neurologic status.

• Calories from propofol should be counted when measuring the patient's caloric intake.

Propofol is prepared in a 10% fat emulsion. Therefore, its caloric content of 1 kcal/ml must be taken into account. Tolerance does not usually develop. It has no direct analgesic properties, but it does provide amnesia for recent events.

In summary, treatment of pain and anxiety in the critically ill patient provides both challenges and rewards. Analgesia and sedation are important methods to help maintain the patient's vital signs within appropriate ranges and to reduce overall metabolic demands. Both therapies should be part of the standard regimen in the care of critically ill postoperative patients.

REFERENCES

1. Fields HL: Pain. New York, McGraw-Hill, 1987.
2. Parker MO: Perceptions of a critically ill patient experiencing therapeutic paralysis. Crit Care Med 1984; 12:69–71.
3. Jones J, Hoggart B, Withey J et al: What the patient says: a study of reactions to an intensive care unit. Intensive Care Med 1979; 5:89.
4. Loper KA, Butler S, Nessly M et al: Terror in the ICU: paralyzed with pain. Anesth Analg 1989: 68:51.
5. Wilmore DW: Catabolic illness: strategies for enhancing recovery. N Engl J Med 1991; 325:695–702.
6. Kehlet H: The stress response to surgery: release mechanisms and the modifying effect of pain relief. Acta Chir Scand Suppl 1989; 550: 22–28.
7. Kehlet H: Surgical stress: the role of pain and analgesia. Br J Anaesth 1989; 63:189–195.
8. Rutberg H, Hakanson E, Anderberg B et al: Effects of the extradural administration of morphine, or bupivacaine, on the endocrine response to upper abdominal surgery. Br J Anaesth 1984; 56:233–238.
9. Muse M: Stress-related, posttraumatic chronic pain syndrome: criteria for diagnosis, and preliminary report on prevalence. Pain 1985; 23: 295.
10. Merskey H: Classification of chronic pain: description of chronic pain syndromes and definition of pain terms. Pain 1986; 3(Suppl):S1-S225.
11. Moller IW, Dinesen K, Sondergard S et al: Effect of patient-controlled analgesia on plasma catecholamine, cortisol and glucose concentrations after cholecystectomy. Br J Anaesth 1988; 61:160–4.
12. Bormann B, Weidler B, Dennhardt R et al: Influence of epidural fentanyl on stress-induced elevation of plasma vasopressin (ADH) after surgery. Anesth Analg 1983; 62:727–732.
13. Kehlet H: Modification of responses to surgery by neural blockade: clinical implications. In: Cousins MJ, Bridenbaugh PO, eds: Neural blockade in clinical anesthesia and management of pain, 2nd ed. Philadelphia, JB Lippincott, 1988; pp. 145–188.

14. Scott NB, Mogensen T, Bigler D et al: Continuous thoracic extradural 0.5% bupivacaine with or without morphine: effect on quality of blockade, lung function and the surgical stress response. Br J Anaesth 1988; 62:253–257.
15. Murray MJ, Offord KP, Yaksh TL: Physiologic and plasma hormone correlates of survival in endotoxic dogs: effects of opiate antagonists. Crit Care Med 1989; 17:39.
16. Rawal N, Tandon B: Epidural and intrathecal morphine in intensive care units. Intensive Care Med 1985;:129.
17. Nimmo WS, Duthie DJR: Pain relief after surgery. Anaesth Intensive Care 1987; 15:68.
18. Katz N, Ferrante FM: Nociception. In: Ferrante FM, Vadeboncouer TR, eds: Postoperative pain management. New York, Churchill-Livingstone, 1992.
19. Maiwand MO, Makey AR, Rees A: Cryanalgesia after thoracotomy: improvement of technique and review of 600 cases. J Thorac Cardiovasc Surg 1986; 92:291.
20. Kvalheim L, Reiestad F: Intrapleural catheter in the management of postoperative pain. Anesthesiology 1984; 61:A231.
21. Wall PD, The prevention of postoperative pain (editorial). Pain 1988; 33:289–290.
22. McSermott WV: Endorphins, I presume. Lancet 1980; 2:1353.
23. Ferrante FM, Orav EJ, Rocco AG et al: A statistical model for pain in patient-controlled analgesia and conventional intramuscular opioid regimens. Anesth Analg 1988; 67:457–461.
24. Forrest WH, Smethurst PWR, Kienitz ME: Self-administration of intravenous analgesics. Anesthesiology 1970; 33:363–365.
25. Sechzer PH: Objective measurement of pain. Anesthesiology 1968; 29: 209–210.
26. Sechzer PH: Studies in pain with the analgesic-demand system. Anesth Analg 1971; 50:1–10.
27. Owen H, Szeley SM, Plummer JL et al: Variables of patient-controlled analgesia. 2. Concurrent infusions. Anaesthesia 1989; 44:11–13.
28. Scott JC, Ponganis KV, Stanski DR: EEG quantitation of narcotic effect: the comparative pharmacodynamics of fentanyl and alfentanil. Anesthesiology 1985; 62:234–241.
29. Pasternak G: Multiple morphine and enkephaline receptors and the relief of pain. JAMA 1988; 259:1362–1367.
30. Jacobs JR, Watkins WD: Pharmacokinetics in multiple organ failure. Crit Care 1988; 9:163–176.
31. Woolf CJ: Evidence for a central component of post-injury hypersensitivity. Nature 1983; 306:686–688.
32. Coderre TJ, Melzack R: Cutaneous hyperalgesia: contributions of the peripheral and central nervous systems to the increase in sensitivity after injury. Brain Res 1987; 404:95–106.
33. Cook AJ, Woolf CJ, Wall PD, McMahon SB: Dynamic receptive field plasticity in the rat spinal cord dorsal horn following C-primary afferent input. Nature 1987; 325:151–153.
34. Sugimoto T, Takemura M, Sakai A, Ishimaru M: Rapid transneuronal destruction following peripheral nerve transection in the medullary dorsal horn is enhanced by strychnine, picrotoxin and bicuculline. Pain 1987; 30:385–393.
35. Wall PD, Woolf CJ: The brief and prolonged facilitatory effects of unmyelinated influenced by peripheral nerve section. Neuroscience 1986; 17:1199–1205.

36. Katz J, Kavanagh BP, Sandler AN et al: Preemptive analgesia: clinical evidence of neuroplasticity contributing to postoperative pain. Anesthesiology 1992; 77:439–446.
37. Snyder SH: Opiate receptors and internal opiates. Sci Am 1977; 236: 44–56.
38. Cousins MJ, Mather LE, Glynn CJ et al: Selective spinal analgesia. Lancet 1979; 1:1141–1142.
39. Cousins MJ, Mather LE: Intrathecal and epidural administration of opioids. Anesthesiology 1984; 61:276–310.
40. Nordberg G, Hedner T, Mellsrtand T et al: Pharmacokinetic aspects of epidural morphine analgesia. Anesthesiology 1983; 58:545–551.
41. Behar M, Olshwang D, Magora F, Davidson JT: Epidural morphine in the treatment of pain. Lancet 1979; 1:527–529.
42. Lanz E, Theiss D, Riess W et al: Epidural morphine for postoperative analgesia: a double-blind study. Anesth Analg 1982; 61:236–240.
43. Bromage PR, Camporesi E, Chestnut D: Epidural narcotics for postoperative analgesia. Anesth Analg 1980; 59:473–480.
44. Lysak SZ, Eisenach JC, Dobson CE: Patient controlled epidural analgesia (PCEA) during labor: a comparison of three solutions with continuous epidural infusion (CEI) control. Anesthesiology 1988; 69:A690.
45. Rauck R, Knarr D, Denson D et al: Comparison of the efficacy of epidural morphine given by intermittent injection or continuous infusion for the management of postoperative pain. Anesthesiology 1986; 65:A201.
46. Fischer RL, Lubenow TR, Liceaga A et al: Comparison of continuous epidural infusion of fentanyl-bupivacaine and morphine-bupivacaine in management of postoperative pain. Anesth Analg 1988; 67: 559–563.
47. Badner NH, Reimer EJ, Komar WE, Moote CA: Low-dose bupivacaine does not improve postoperative epidural fentanyal analgesia in orthopedic patients. Anesth Analg 1991; 72:337–341.
48. Ferrante FM, VadeBoncouer TR: Epidural analgesia with combinations of local anesthetics and opioids. In: Ferrante FM, VadeBoncouer TR, eds. Postoperative pain management. New York, Churchill-Livingstone, 1992.
49. Lee A, Simpson D, Whitfield A, Scott DB: Postoperative analgesia by continuous extradural infusion of bupivacaine and diamorphine. Br J Anaesth 1988; 60:845–850.
50. Dahl JB, Rosenberg J, Hansen BL, et al: Differential analgesic effects of low-dose epidural morphine and morphine-bupivacaine at rest and during mobilization after major abdominal surgery. Anesth Analg 1992; 74:362–365.
51. Gustafsson LL, Schlidt B, Jacobson K: Adverse effects of extradural and intrathecal opiates: report of a nationwide survey in Sweden. Br J Anaesth 1982; 54:479–485.
52. McCaughey W, Grahan JL: The respiratory depression of epidural morphine: time course and effect of posture. Anaesthesia 1982; 37: 990–995.
53. Robson JA, Brodsky JB: Latent dural puncture after lumber epidural block. Anesth Analg 1977; 56:725–735.
54. Gustafsson LL, Fechting B, Klingstedt C: Late respiratory depression after concomitant use of morphine epidurally and parenterally. Lancet 1981; 1:892–893.
55. Bromage PR: The price of intraspinal narcotic analgesia: Basic constraints. Anesth Analg 1981; 60:461–463.

56. Neustein SM, Cohen E: Intrathecal morphine during thoracotomy. Part II: effect on postoperative meperidine requirements and pulmonary function tests. J Cardiothorac Vasc Anesth 1993; 7:157–159.
57. Raja SN, Meyer RA, Campbell JN: Peripheral mechanisms of somatic pain. Anesthesiology 1988; 68:571–590.
58. Murphy TM. Nerve blocks. In: Miller RD, ed: Anesthesia, 2nd ed. New York, Churchill-Livingstone, 1986; pp. 1024–1034.
59. Nunn JF, Slavin G: Posterior intercostal nerve block for pain relief after thoracotomy. Br J Anaesth 1980; 52:253–260.
60. Bridenbaugh PO, Dupen SL, Moore DC et al: Postoperative intercostal nerve block analgesia versus narcotic analgesia. Anesth Analg 1973; 52:81–85.
61. Bridenbaugh PO: Intercostal nerve blockade for evaluation of local anesthetic agents. Br J Anaesth 1975; 47:306–308.
62. Moore DC, Bush WH, Scurlock JE: Intercostal nerve block: a roentgenographic anatomic study of technique and absorption in humans. Anesth Analg 1980; 59:815–825.
63. Murphy DF: Continuous intercostal nerve blockade for pain relief following cholecystectomy. Br J Anaesth 1983; 55:521–524.
64. Smith BE, Fischer HB, Scott PV: Continuous sciatic nerve block. Anaesthesia 1984; 39:155–157.
65. Rosenblatt RM: Continuous femoral anesthesia for lower extremity surgery. Anesth Analg 1980; 59:631–632.
66. Rosenblatt RM, Cress JC: Modified Seldinger technique for continuous interscalene brachial plexus block. Reg Anesth 1981; 6:82–84.
67. Chayen D, Nathan H, Chayen M: The psoas compartment block. Anesthesiology 1976; 45:95–99.
68. Haak-van der L, vanKleef JW, Burm AGL et al: Preoperative interpleural administration of sufentanil or bupivicaine reduces intraoperative intravenous sufentanil requirements during thoracotomy. J Cardiothorac Vasc Anesth 1993; 7:526–528.
69. Ferrante FM, Chan VWS, Arthur CR et al: Interpleural analgesia after thoracotomy. Anesth Analg 1991; 72:105–109.
70. Winnie AP, Ramanurthy S, Durrani Z: The inguinal paravascular technic of lumbar plexus anesthesia: the "3-in-1 block." Anesth Analg 1973; 52:989–996.
71. Parkinson SK, Mueller JB, Little WL et al: Extent of blockade with various approaches to the lumbar plexus. Anesth Analg 1989; 68: 243–248.
72. Lofstrom B: Lumbar sympathetic block. In: Ericksson E, ed: Illustrated handbook in local anesthesia. Philadelphia, WB Saunders, 1980; pp. 144–148.
73. Lofstrom B: Stellate ganglion block. In: Ericksson E, ed: Illustrated handbook in local anesthesia. Philidelphia, WB Saunders, 1980; pp. 141–143.
74. Gillies GW, Kenny GN, Bullingham RE et al: The morphine sparing effect of ketorolac tromethamine. Anaesthesia 1987; 42:727–731.
75. Ziel R, Krupp P: Significance of membrane-stabilizing effect of nonnarcotic analgesics. In: Bonica JJ, Albe-Fessard D, ed: Advances in pain research and therapy, vol 1. New York, Raven, 1976; pp. 517–521.
76. O'Hara DA, Fragen RJ, Kinzer M et al: Ketorolac tromethamine as compared with morphine sulfate for treatment of postoperative pain. Clin Pharmacol Ther 1987; 41:556–561.
77. Dahl JB, Kehlet H: Non-steroid anti-inflammatory drugs: rational for use in severe postoperative pain. Br J Anaesth 1991; 66:703–712.

78. Oden RV: Acute postoperative pain incidence, severity, and the etiology of inadequate treatment. Anesthesiol Clin North Am 1989; 7:1–15
79. Tan SY: Cognitive and cognitive-behavioral methods of pain control: a selective review. Pain 1982; 12:201.
80. Clum GA, Luscomb RL, Scott L: Relaxation training and cognitive redirection strategies in the treatment of acute pain. Pain 1982; 12: 175.
81. Rooney SM, Jain S, Goldiner PL: Effect of transcutaneous nerve stimulation on postoperative pain after thoractomy. Anesth Analg 1983; 62: 1010.
82. Wood JH: Use and abuse of benzodiazepines. JAMA 1989; 16: 3476–3479.
83. Freeman JW, Hopkinson RB: Therapeutic progress in intensive care sedation and analgesia. Part II: drug selection. J Clin Pharmacol Ther 1988; 13:41–51.
84. Behn M et al: Continuous midazolam infusion for sedation of respirator patients. Anaesthesist 1987; 65:228–232.
85. Berggren L, Erikson I, Mollenholt P et al: Changes in respiratory pattern after repeated doses of diazepam and midazolam in healthy subjects. Acta Anaesthesiol Scand 1987; 31:381–386.
86. Adams HA: Sedative-analgesic medicaton in intensive care patients needing ventilator treatment. Anaesthesist 1988; 7:268–276.
87. Mohler H, Richards JG: The benzodiazepine receptor: a pharmacologic control elements of brain function. Eur J Anesthesiol 1988; 2:15–24.
88. Loper AK, Ready LB, Brody M: Patient-controlled anxiolysis with midazolam. Anesth Analg 1988; 67:1118–1119.
89. Loper KA, Ready LB: Patient controlled anxiolysis with midazolam (letter). Crit Care Med 1989; 17:200–201.
90. Forster A, Rouiller M, Morel D et al: Double-blind study evaluating a specific benzodiazepine antagonist. Anesthesiology 1983; 59:A375.
91. Ghoneium MM, Block RK, Sumping ST, et al: The interaction of midazolam and flumazenil on human memory. Anesthesiology 1993; 79: A361.
92. Somons PJ, Cockshott ID, Douglas EJ et al: Blood concentrations, metabolism and elimination after subanesthetic, intravenous doses of ^{14}C propofol ("Diprivan") to male volunteers. Postgrad Med J 1985; 61(Suppl 3):64.
93. White PF: Propofol: pharmacokinetics and pharmacodynamics. Semin Anesth 1988; 7(Suppl 1):4–20.
94. Roekaerts PMHJ, Huygen FJPM, deLange S: Infusion of propofol versus midazolam in the intensive care unit following coronary artery surgery. J Cardiothorac Vasc Anesth 1993; 7:142–147.
95. Ping ADM, Lelausque JN, Chetanneau A et al: Effects of propofol on cerebral hemodynamics and metabolism in patients with brain trauma. Anesthesiology 1990; 73:404–409.

CHAPTER 5

Acute Electrolyte Imbalances in the Critically Ill Postoperative Patient

Andrea Gabrielli
A. Joseph Layon

Case Report

Mrs. H. was a 73-year-old female patient. Three days before her admission to the intensive care unit (ICU), she had a left femoral-tibial bypass graft. The patient had a history of congestive heart failure, and therapy had included digitalis. She weighed 55 kg.

Admission to the ICU took place because of a deterioration in mental status and symptoms suggestive of heart failure, including rales, shortness of breath, and a respiratory rate of 30/min. The patient had not made any urine over the 6 hours prior to ICU admission. Intravenous fluids included D5 0.25 normal saline at 85 ml/hr.

On admission to the ICU, the patient was responsive only to painful stimuli. Vital signs were: blood pressure, 116/92 mm Hg; pulse, 116/min; respiratory rate, 32/min; temperature, 38°C. Laboratory data revealed: sodium, 122 mEq/L; potassium, 6.1 mEq/L; glucose, 228 mg/dl.

Pulmonary artery catheterization revealed a wedge pressure of 24 mm Hg. Following 40 mg of furosemide, the patient began a brisk urine output over the next 3 hours. The wedge pressure decreased to 18 mm Hg. Cardiac output increased from 2.8 to 4.1 L/min. Fluid therapy was changed to normal saline at 75 ml/hr. Because of the high-peaked T waves on the electrocardiogram (ECG) at the time of ICU admission, the patient also received

50 g of glucose and 10 U of intravenous insulin. Four hours later, the patient's serum potassium concentration was 4.7 mEq/L.

The following day, intravenous hyperalimentation was initiated. The patient was scheduled to receive 1.5 L/day of D25 solution, which would also provide 1.25 g/kg/day of amino acids. Eighteen hours later, the patient's blood glucose level was 483 mg/dl, and her inorganic phosphorus level had decreased to 1.7 mEq/L. Continuous insulin infusion was initiated, and phosphate was given in the form of sodium phosphate to correct the deficiency.

The outcome of resuscitation in the patient who has undergone surgery or who has suffered traumatic or thermal injury or, for that matter, any kind of hemodynamic instability is clearly related to thorough knowledge of the normal physiology of fluid and electrolytes. In particular, the immediate postoperative period is characterized by dramatic movement of fluid and essential mono- and divalent essential ions in different body compartments. Therefore, any reasonable interpretation of postoperative fluid and electrolyte derangements requires an understanding of these various compartments.

BODY AND FLUID COMPARTMENTS

Total body water (TBW) averages 60% of body weight in men and 50% on average in women, with a variation of approximately 10% in the thin or obese individual. In the "ideal" 70-kg man, TBW is 42 L; the intracellular compartment contains 66% of this (28 L), and the extracellular fluid compartment (ECF) contains 34% (14 L). The ECF (20% of body weight, or 34% of the TBW) is composed of intravascular (3.5 L) and interstitial (10.5 L) subcompartments.

• *Free water distributes throughout the total body water compartment, which equals 60% of body weight. One liter of isosmotic saline solution increases the intravascular compartment by 20 to 30% following redistribution which may take up to 1 hour.*

When "free" (nonosmotically active) water is added to any compartment, an even distribution through the TBW occurs. Following equilibration, which takes approximately 30 minutes, 1 L of free water (5% dextrose in water = D5W) contributes less than 100 ml to the intravascular space. In contrast, after rapid infusion of 1 L of isosmotic normal saline solution (0.9% saline solution), the intravascular compartment increases by 300 ml, or 200 ml more than results from the same volume infusion of D5W. Since all fluids are a combination of free water and isotonic solution (for example, 1000 ml of 0.45% saline = 500 ml of 0.9% saline + 500 ml of free water), it is possible to predict the relative distribution for any standard intravenous solution.

The distribution of colloid solution in human body compartments is somewhat more complicated. With these solutions, the volume increase of the intravascular compartment after fluid challenge depends on both the fluid's oncotic activity and its tonicity, as well as on the integrity of the capillary membrane.

SURGICAL TRAUMA: HISTORICAL REVIEW

Several studies have attempted to identify the redistribution pathway of fluids in postsurgical patients. In 1931, Blalock used a dog model to identify and quantify the redistribution of plasma volume into traumatized tissue and the peritoneal cavity following surgery.[1] Thirty-five years later, Shires and associates, using ^{35}S-labeled sodium sulfate in 18 human patients with hemorrhagic shock, found a large discrepancy between the measured blood loss and the apparent decrease of sodium sulfate at equilibrium.[2] This volume was not lost from the body, but rather had become "nonfunctional" and was redistributed into an area in which the sulfate no longer equilibrated with the ECF; this was termed "third space" fluid. That portion of ECF into which sulfate rapidly equilibrated was termed "functional extracellular fluid volume" (FEFV). The same investigators noted that the decrease of FEFV, as well as sodium and water retention, was more severe after "major" abdominal surgery than after "minor" orthopedic surgery.

Several mechanisms have been proposed to describe this normal homeostatic mechanism. Both 17-hydroxycorticosteroids and aldosterone were found to be elevated in the immediate postoperative period.[3] However, case studies in adrenalectomized patients showed the same degree of sodium and water retention postoperatively as patients with intact adrenal glands.[4] Increased levels of antidiuretic hormone (ADH) associated with low serum osmolarity (as low as 255 mOsm/L) and high urine osmolarity (as high as 900 mOsm/L)[5] have been found for about 5 postoperative days. This response cannot be seen as "inappropriate" considering the attempt to restore the ECF volume. Again, sodium and water retention could not be attributed to ADH in groups of hypophysectomized patients with decreased urine flow rate but without a corresponding increase in urine osmolarity.[6] Atrial natriuretic factor seems to play a role in the correction of ECF volume deficit, although the full significance of this mechanism has not yet been completely elucidated.[7] It is likely that each of these has a part in postoperative fluid retention.

- *Retention of sodium and water in the postoperative period is principally due to antidiuretic hormone as well as to atrial natriuretic factor.*

The final effect of FEFV loss is net sodium retention. This is not a problem as long as isotonic fluids are used to replete the FEFV. However, when free water (D5W) is inappropriately used, water intoxication may occur. The risk of using hypotonic solutions to expand the FEFV includes the onset of the water intoxication syndrome, accompanied by the development of hyponatremia, impaired renal function, CNS deterioration, and cardiovascular collapse.[8] Perhaps the first description of this phenomenon was by Schroeder, who in 1949 described postsurgical patients with oliguria who were not responsive to large infusions of D5W. These patients demonstrated an elevated blood urea nitrogen (BUN) and urea clearance less than 10% of normal; hyponatremia was accompanied by progressive anuria and CNS deterioration.[9] Stokes and co-workers studied D5W-induced salt depletion in dogs and in human patients.[10] These investigators found, in spite of severe hyponatremia and consequent hypo-osmolarity, a high urine osmolarity compared

- *Replacement of the functional extracellular fluid volume should be accomplished with an isotonic rather than a hypotonic solution. Hypotonic solutions contribute to hyponatremia and possible water intoxication.*

with that of plasma, along with a reduction of glomerular filtration rate (GFR) of up to 80%. Treatment with hypertonic saline restored the GFR and caused excretion of a large volume of hypotonic urine.

In critically ill patients, the handling of free water may be severely impaired due to precarious renal blood flow (RBF). Furthermore, in postsurgical patients, anesthetics act directly by depressing renal function or indirectly by producing changes in cardiovascular function and neuroendocrine activity. Barbiturates and inhalational anesthetics tend to decrease RBF and GFR in a reversible fashion. Along with a drop in blood pressure and cardiac output, opioids tend to reduce the GFR independent of RBF. This follows release of ADH in the presence of painful stimulation. While ketamine and the benzodiazepines have not been clearly defined in this regard, the neuromuscular blocking agents seem not to influence the GFR and RBF significantly. Spinal and epidural anesthetic techniques may decrease RBF and GFR resulting from relative central hypovolemia caused by peripheral pooling. Positive pressure ventilation, positive end-expiratory pressure, and their net negative effect on preload have also been associated with reduced urine flow, creatinine clearance, and urinary sodium excretion.[11,12]

• *Factors that depress renal function in postsurgical patients include barbiturates, inhalational anesthetics, hypotension, and opioids. Spinal and epidural anesthetics as well as positive-pressure ventilation all decrease renal blood flow.*

Postsurgical patients often demonstrate a limited urinary dilution capability, frequently in the range of 1.2 to 1.6 ml/mOsm solute, rather than 10 ml/mOsm in the nonstressed patient.[13] This may be exacerbated by hyponatremia resulting from the use of hypo-osmotic solutions in the perioperative period. If an isotonic intravenous solution is utilized during surgery, and D5W is used thereafter, the amount of sodium excreted into the urine in the immediate postoperative period will appear to follow a biphasic pattern, increasing in the first 5 hours (perhaps because of a large intraoperative sodium load) and thereafter progressively diminishing, with a net positive free water balance over the first 24 hours. The highest urinary concentration achieved was just below 700 mOsm/L.[14] In anesthetized dogs, excessive utilization of D5W may be responsible for the metabolic acidosis seen secondary to a decrease in the amount of sodium reaching the acidifying mechanism of the distal nephron.[15] Since acidification of urine depends on the distal tubular exchange of sodium for hydrogen ion, hyponatremic animals given only D5W are pointedly unable to do this. Finally, excess use of free water in the perioperative period and consequent hyponatremia can cause severe cardiovascular depression and hypotension both related to decreased FEFV. This can be reversed by hypertonic sodium solution.[16]

The immediate postoperative period includes a redistribution of fluid and electrolytes from the intravascular/interstitial space to nonfunctional ECF, the so-called "third" space. Sodium and water retention in the first 24 hours postoperatively may be considered a natural compensatory mechanism to maintain the intravascular volume. This mechanism is partially impaired by the negative effect of the anesthetic, surgical trauma, and mechanical ventilation. These factors directly impair renal and cardiovascular function or exert their effects through the neuroendocrine axis. Proper fluid and elec-

• *Replacement of fluid lost from the nonfunctional extracellular space requires use of isotonic or hypertonic solutions.*

trolyte management is therefore essential to provide volume sufficient to replace the sequestered ECF, plus an additional amount of water and solute for insensible loss and optimal renal function. In general, we should limit the intake of free water in the perioperative period and should provide balanced or physiologic electrolyte solutions, such as normal saline or lactated Ringer's solutions. Careful use of hypertonic solution (3% sodium chloride, for example) may also be considered, to limit the total amount of fluid necessary to maintain intravascular volume.

SODIUM

Sodium is the dominant cation of the ECF; the normal concentration ranges between 135 and 145 mEq/L. The sodium concentration is a reflection of the ECF tonicity. Because tonicity may vary independent of ECF volume, hyponatremia and hypernatremia may occur with increased, decreased, or normal ECF volume. For these reasons, in the acute postoperative period the volume must be assessed separately from tonicity.[17] Sodium, like glucose, is an effective osmole because gradients can cause free water to shift across the cell membrane. Under normal conditions, sodium serves as the major determinant of the effective plasma osmolarity, which can be calculated using the following formula:

- *Sodium serves as the principal determinant of osmolarity.*

$$\text{Effective Osmolarity} = \text{Plasma Na}^+ \text{ (mEq/L)} \times 2 + \frac{\text{Glucose (mg/dl)}}{18} + \frac{\text{BUN (mg/dl)}}{2.8} \quad (1)$$

If the presence of other effective osmoles is suspected, the total osmolarity should be measured. Other osmoles could include mannitol, methanol, ethanol, ethylene glycol, and isopropyl alcohol.[19] The difference between measured and calculated osmolarity represents the osmolar gap.

Hyponatremia

Physiology

Hyponatremia is defined as a serum sodium concentration less than 135 mEq/L and is one of the most common electrolyte disorders in the postoperative critically ill patient. Three variants of hyponatremia are described: isotonic, hypertonic, and hypotonic.

Isotonic Hyponatremia. Aside from laboratory error, common diseases characterized by hyperlipemia (familial lipoprotein lipase deficiency, diabetes mellitus, oral contraceptive use) and hyperproteinemia (multiple myeloma, angioimmunoblastic lymphadenopathy) may create a spurious reduction in serum sodium concentration (pseudohyponatremia)[17–19] with a normal measured osmolarity. This phenomenon develops because of reduced water in plasma secondary to the increase in lipids or protein. Isotonic hyponatremia is thus characterized by a spurious decrease in serum sodium with a normal measured osmolarity. The erroneous value can be corrected utilizing a different technique for measuring the electrolyte, such as an ion-selective electrode or preanalysis ultracentrifugation of the sample.[20]

Hypertonic Hyponatremia. The presence of hyperglycemia has also been associated with pseudohyponatremia. Practically:

For each 100 mg/dl rise in plasma glucose concentration above 100 mg/dl, sodium is decreased approximately 1.6 mEq/L (2)

• Hyperglycemia contributes to hyponatremia. Correction should include continuous or intermittent insulin infusion.

High-dose mannitol infusions administered for head injury or renal failure cause the same situation. Free water redistributes from the intracellular to the extracellular space. This particular situation is associated with high osmolar state ($>$ 290 mOsm/kg H_2O) and generally, profound intracellular dehydration.[21] Hypertonic hyponatremia is characterized by a decrease in the serum sodium and a serum osmolarity greater than 290 mOsm/kg H_2O. Therapy includes correction of hyperglycemia with insulin and replacement of free water. Insulin should be administered by either continuous or intermittent intravenous infusion. Usually, if the patient's glucose concentration is greater than 350 mg/dl, continuous infusion will be required. Serum glucose should be monitored hourly.

Once spurious causes of hyponatremia have been ruled out, a rational approach to further evaluation depends on an accurate assessment of the total body salt and water content. This requires knowledge. In critically ill patients, the use of hypotonic solutions during surgery, as well as in the presence of reduced renal perfusion, contributes to impaired free water excretion and hyponatremia. The physiologic response to hyponatremia, suppression of ADH, is appropriately blunted in patients inadequately resuscitated or in those with diminished intravascular volume, including congestive heart failure (CHF) and cirrhosis.[22,23]

Hypotonic Hyponatremia. This complex form of hyponatremia is associated with three subtypes (hypervolemic, isovolemic, and hypovolemic). It is characterized by a decreased serum sodium and a serum osmolarity less than 270 mOsm/kg H_2O. Differentiation is made by assessment of ECF volume (Table 5–1).

Increased Total Body Salt and Water Content (Hypervolemic Hyponatremia)

Pathophysiology. This involves four relatively common clinical situations: cirrhosis, CHF, renal failure (acute and chronic), and the nephrotic syndrome. The decreased effective intravascular volume is associated with an increased extracellular interstitial fluid and, clinically, an edematous state. The urine sodium concentration is usually low, below 10 to 15 mEq/L, with urine osmolarity ranging between 350 and 400 mOsm/kg H_2O. However, in these patients, the ability to concentrate urine is lost in very advanced disease or during acute hypoperfusion of the kidneys, as during the postoperative period and critical illness. Treatment is directed at improving

Table 5–1.
Hypotonic Hyponatremia

Diagnosis
- ↓ P_{Na+}, plasma osmolality < 270 mOsm/kg H_2O
- Differentiate type by assessment of ECF volume

Causes
- Hypovolemic
  - Extrarenal
    - GI loss: vomiting, diarrhea
    - Burns
    - Third space (e.g., pancreatitis)
  - Renal
    - Diuretics
    - Adrenal failure
    - Renal parenchymal disease
- Hypervolemic
  - Advanced renal disease
    - Acute renal failure
    - Chronic renal insufficiency
  - Edematous states
    - Congestive heart failure
    - Cirrhosis of the liver
    - Nephrotic syndrome
    - Severe hypoproteinemia, second-degree nutritional/GI disease
- Isovolemic
  - Stress
  - Adrenal insufficiency
  - Hypothyroidism
  - Drugs
  - K^+ depletion/diuretic use
  - Psychogenic polydipsia
  - Syndrome of inappropriate antidiuretic hormone secretion

Management
- Hypovolemic: isotonic saline
- Hypervolemic/isovolemic: restrict free H_2O
- Manage underlying disorders

Complications
- CNS: seizures, coma, death, residual effects
- Decompensation of underlying disorders

(From Layon AJ, Bernards WC, Kirby R: Fluids and electrolytes in the critically ill. In: Civetta JM, Taylor RW, Kirby RR, eds: Critical care, 2nd ed. Philadelphia, JB Lippincott, 1992; pp. 457–480.)

renal perfusion, obtained by optimization of cardiac output and reduction of afterload in patients with CHF and renal failure, and by the use of colloid plasma expanders in patients with cirrhosis and nephrotic syndrome. Free water restriction may be required in more chronic situations.

A special category of perioperative hyponatremia with increased water content is part of the transurethral resection of the prostate (TURP) syndrome.[24] The pathophysiology of acute hyponatremia in these patients is related to use of hypotonic solutions that are absorbed via the periprostatic venous bed. The rate of absorption is related to the height of the irrigating solution container (usually significant if it is more than 60 cm above the site of the operation).

- *Following a TURP, hyponatremia develops rapidly. The likelihood of seizures depends on the rapidity of change as well as the final value.*

In these patients, the volume of hypotonic fluid absorbed may be calculated as follows:

$$\text{Volume absorbed} = \left(\frac{\text{Preop Na}^+}{\text{Postop Na}^+} \times \text{ECF}\right) - \text{ECF} \qquad (3)$$

where *ECF* is calculated as approximately 0.2 times body weight. An awake patient and the use of a regional anesthetic technique instead of general anesthesia allow better assessment of the neurologic deficits secondary to acute brain edema resulting from an acute decrease in serum sodium to or below 125 mEq/L, as well as their prompt correction.

Immediate Therapy. Treatment includes use of loop diuretics (furosemide, 20 to 40 mg IV every 2 to 4 hours). Osmotic diuretics should generally be avoided as initial therapy, considering possible fluid overload, but they may be used after loop diuretics initiate significant urine flow greater than or equal to 2 ml/kg/hr. This management, along with the use of a 0.9% saline solution, should be titrated to raise the serum sodium at a rate of 1 mEq/L/hr. The use of hypertonic saline solutions should generally be reserved for patients with severe neurologic impairment, in whom a faster elevation of serum sodium (up to 2 mEq/L/hr) is recommended. The serum sodium is corrected to about 125 mEq/L rapidly; thereafter, normal homeostatic mechanisms can usually be allowed to complete the correction.

Normal Total Body Salt and Water Content (Isovolemia)

Pathophysiology. These involve all clinical situations associated with the syndrome of inappropriate ADH secretion (Table 5–2), as well as stress and drug-related hyponatremia. In the former patients,

Table 5–2.
Chronic Disorders Leading to the Syndrome of Inappropriate Antidiuretic Hormone Secretion (SIADH)

Pulmonary disorders
Bronchogenic carcinoma
Acute or chronic infection (especially tuberculosis)
Central nervous system disorders
Tuberculous meningitis
Other bacterial/viral CNS infections
Head trauma
Subarachnoid hemorrhage
Guillian-Barré syndrome
Acute intermittent porphyria
Endocrine disorders
Adrenal insufficiency
Hypothyroidism

(From Cooke CR, Turin MD, Walker WG: The syndrome of inappropriate antidiuretic hormone secretion (SIADH): pathophysiologic mechanisms in solute and volume regulation. Medicine 1979; 58:240–251.)

the excess of ADH enhances the reabsorption of free water from the collecting ducts, thus expanding the ECF. The temporary expansion of intravascular volume results in increased renal perfusion and GFR with decreased proximal tubular reabsorption and enhanced distal sodium delivery. The combination of high circulating ADH levels and normal distal sodium delivery creates inappropriately concentrated urine. The net effect is a urine osmolarity higher than the serum value or, viewed slightly differently, the inability to elaborate maximally diluted urine (i.e., less than 100 mOsm/kg). Reduced aldosterone secretion in these patients, in the face of sodium restriction when water intake is not limited, is related to the euvolemic state and is promptly reversed when fluid is restricted.

A special category of isovolemic hyponatremia is seen in the immediate postoperative period in patients who are resuscitated with hypotonic solution. A low output of urine of relatively low osmolarity (379 ± 31 mOsm/kg H_2O) can be seen as result of a net sodium retention and impaired renal function.[25] In these patients, postoperative hyponatremia is a combined result of the nonosmotic release of ADH and the utilization of hypotonic intravenous fluids.

Immediate Therapy. Immediate therapy is carried out as described for hypervolemic hyponatremia. Additionally, free water restriction may be required in a long-term setting.

Decreased Total Body Salt and Water Content (Hypovolemia)

Pathophysiology. Critically ill patients may present on an emergency basis with severe sodium and water deficits secondary to renal and extrarenal losses. Diuretics are a very common cause of hyponatremia.[26] Among these drugs, the carbonic anhydrase inhibitor acetazolamide decreases sodium reabsorption via inhibition of HCO_3^- absorption. Thiazides, such as hydrochlorothiazide, affect the sodium and chloride transport mechanism in the thick ascending limb of the loop of Henle. Loop diuretics, such as furosemide, also prevent reabsorption of sodium and chloride in the thick ascending loop of Henle and decrease the interstitial tonicity necessary for the production of hypertonic urine in the ADH-stimulated collecting tubule; the result is isosthenuria. Potassium-sparing diuretics, such as spironolactone, also restrict sodium entry in the collecting tubule. Finally, osmotic diuretics, such as mannitol, affect all levels of the glomerulus, resulting in fluid loss secondary to an osmotic gradient.

• *Most diuretics, including the loop variety, as well as thiazides, ultimately result in hyponatremia because of excess sodium loss.*

Other causes of renal sodium losses include acute adrenal insufficiency, related to deficits of both mineralocorticoids, which increase renal sodium excretion, and glucocorticoids, which decrease suppression of ADH release in response to hypotonicity.[18] Occasionally, acute renal disease, such as postobstructive tubulointerstitial nephropathy, may be associated with sodium wasting and ECF contraction. A salt-wasting syndrome has been described in patients affected by subarachnoid hemorrhage secondary to elevated levels of an atrial natriuretic factor (ANF)-like protein and relatively diminished vasopressin concentration. The presence of an ANF-like

• *Significant sodium may be lost following head injury. This is the so-called salt-wasting syndrome.*

substance was recently identified in the hypothalamus.[27] In this syndrome, urine sodium may be as high as 200 mEq/L and is associated with hypovolemia.

Nonrenal sources of sodium and water losses in the postoperative patient include prolonged vomiting, diarrhea, an acute abdomen with third-space fluid losses, and extensive thermal, chemical, or electrical burns. Compared to the group with renal losses, these patients show a low urine sodium concentration in an attempt to minimize the effect of extrarenal sodium and water losses.

A recent management review classifies as acute hyponatremia any clinical situation associated with decrease of serum sodium of more than 0.5 mEq/L/hr to a level less than or equal to 120 mEq/L.[28] In these cases, the only compensatory mechanism after the first 24 hours is loss of sodium, potassium, chloride, and water from the brain cells and loss of interstitial fluid by bulk flow into the CSF. Experimental animal data suggest that brain edema is a consequence of a plasma to brain osmotic gradient secondary to overly rapid correction of acute hyponatremia.[29] Many causes of acute hyponatremia have been recorded in postoperative critically ill patients.[30] These include the administration of hypotonic fluid to patients with impaired inability to excrete H_2O (elderly women are particularly susceptible to this complication), the TURP syndrome, and inappropriate exogenous administration of ADH in neurosurgical patients or oxytocin in obstetric patients.

With respect to chronic hyponatremia, there is some disagreement regarding medical therapy.[31] Although it is not always possible to differentiate acute from chronic hyponatremia in the critically ill postoperative patient, especially if the patient presents to the hospital on an emergency basis, we can generally assume that a clinical history longer than 2 to 3 days makes chronic hyponatremia more likely. Chronic brain cell adaptation of hyponatremia includes extracellular shift of potassium, chloride, and water, as well as severe loss of organic osmoles in the form of amino acids.[30]

- *Rapid correction of hyponatremia may lead to paralysis, dysarthria, or cardiac arrhythmias.*

Thus, in patients with the chronic disorder, rapid correction of hyponatremia may produce a paradoxic acute intracellular brain shrinkage, comparable to that seen in acute severe hypernatremia. A very serious neurologic complication related to rapid correction of severe chronic hyponatremia is central pontine myelinolysis.[32] This syndrome involves a rapidly evolving para- or quadriparesis, dysarthria, dysphagia, and hemodynamic instability. Severe diffuse, demyelinating lesions, resembling acute hypoxic damage, have been found in hyponatremic patients with a history of alcoholism, malnutrition, and hepatic cirrhosis.[32] The variability of results in neurologic outcome after correction of chronic hyponatremia seems related to three major factors: (1) a clear definition of chronic versus acute hyponatremia does not clearly exist, and on occasion the data do not permit such differentiation; (2) individual, and probably gender-related, variability likely affects the effectiveness of brain cell compensatory mechanisms; and (3) preexisting clinical conditions may influence the outcome of treatment.

Immediate Therapy. Severe symptomatic hyponatremia is a life-threatening condition associated with a mortality that may reach as high as 50% if the sodium concentration is reduced to less than 120 mEq/L in fewer than 24 hours.[31] Symptoms, related to cerebral edema and brain stem herniation,[33] include progressive weakness, lethargy with progressive headache, and obtundation culminating in generalized seizures, coma, and ultimately death. Characteristic ECG changes have also been detected and include a decrease in the height of the P wave and increased QRS voltage.[34] In critically ill postoperative patients, the early symptoms may not necessarily be detected. *Acute hyponatremia* may be corrected at a rate of 1 mEq/L/hr to a maximum of 2 mEq/L/hr, to prevent severe mortality and morbidity.[31] The amount of sodium necessary to reach a desired level is calculated as follows:

• Correction of hyponatremia should begin at sodium levels of 120 mEq/L or higher. Solutions include normal hypotonic saline.

$$\text{Na}^+ \text{ requirement (mEq/L)} = \text{TBW} \times (\text{desired serum Na}^+ - \text{actual serum Na}^+) \quad (4)$$

In *chronic hyponatremia* the best neurologic outcome seems to be obtained when correction is carried out slowly, at a rate less than 0.5 mEq/L/hr. In both cases, the addition of furosemide (usually 20 to 40 mg IV) repeated at 2- to 4-hour intervals or an osmotic diuretic agent such as mannitol (0.5 mg/kg) may be used with either 0.9 or 3% saline solutions to replete the vascular volume. Volume should be titrated, based on the rate of free water excretion and the intravascular volume status. The target value of this therapy should be a sodium concentration of about 125 mEq/L; once this value is achieved, we allow evaporative and urinary losses to restore the sodium level to normal over several days.

Hypernatremia

Hypernatremia is defined as an increase of sodium concentration above 145 mEq/L. A serum sodium concentration above 160 mEq/L implies severe dehydration or solute gain. Hypertonic states cause intracellular dehydration. Hypernatremia represents a common cause of hyperosmolarity. The body's principal defense against hypernatremia due to free water loss is ADH release and subsequent renal free water retention. This mechanism increases the urine osmolarity to as high as 800 to 1200 mOsm/kg H_2O and significantly decreases the urine volume.

Causes

Hypernatremia in a critically ill patient is caused by either free water loss or solute gain. The extracellular volume may be normal, decreased, or increased, depending on the pathogenesis of the hypernatremia. Frequently, hypernatremia develops secondary to hypertonic fluid infusions as part of the patient's intravenous therapy. It has become popular to use concentrated saline solutions of 1.5 to 3%. Such therapy usually results in less overall volume being infused. Hypernatremia can develop secondary to either large volumes or rapid infusion rates.

• Today, a common cause of hypernatremia is the use of hypertonic saline solutions.

Table 5–3.
Causes of Diabetes Insipidus (DI)

Acquired neurogenic DI
Head trauma
Postsurgical
Meningoencephalitis
Vascular injury
Postanoxia/ischemia injury
Acquired nephrogenic DI
Pyelonephritis
Postobstructive uropathy
Metabolic abnormalities
Hypokalemia
Hypercalcemia
Drug-induced
Amphotericin B
Lithium chloride
Secondary DI
Excessive intravenous fluid loading

(From Hall J, Robertson GP: Diabetes Insipidus. Probl Crit Care 1990; 4:346.)

Diabetes insipidus (DI) characteristically has large free water losses. Urine volume usually exceeds 3 ml/kg/hr. Urine specific gravity varies between 1.000 and 1.003. Urine sodium concentrations rarely exceeds 15 mEq/L. Brain trauma secondary to closed head injury or elective surgery for removal of a craniopharyngioma is the most common cause (Table 5–3). Symptoms usually begin within 12 hours of surgery or as brain swelling increases.

Burn patients can readily develop hypernatremia. The cause is the large free water losses from the burn site. The greater the burn, the higher the likelihood of such an occurrence.

Salt added to enteral feeding formulas can cause hypernatremia. Similarly, any medication in a salt base such as ticarcillin can increase serum sodium values.

Duration of the deficit depends on the amount of suprasellar damage; healing usually occurs in 2 days to a few weeks. Return of normal function is probably due to release of ADH from higher levels of the hypothalamopituitary tract when lower portions are destroyed.[35] The diagnosis of postoperative DI depends on demonstration of hypotonic (< 250 mOsm/kg H_2O), polyuria (> 2 ml/kg/hr), together with an increase in plasma osmolarity (> 300 mOsm/kg H_2O). Other causes such as gastroenteritis, glycosuria, mannitol administration, or renal failure should be excluded.

Treatment

Failure to treat hypernatremia can cause significant brain water shifts. Obviously, lost free water as from DI or burns must be replaced. Since sodium and water equilibrate through all compartments, the volume of distribution is TBW, which is 60% of body weight. If the current sodium concentration and weight are known, the amount of water to reach a new lower concentration can be easily calculated.

• Correction of hypernatremia should take into account that salt distributes across total body water, which comprises 60% of body weight.

$$\text{Water deficit (L)} = [0.6 \times \text{body weight (kg)}] \times [\text{known Na conc (mEq/L)} - \text{desired Na conc (mEq/L)}] \quad (5)$$

DI can be treated by replacement of varing fractions of free water lost, usually 0.5 to 0.75 ml for every 1 ml of urine. Replacement on an ml-per-ml basis only continues to increase urine output. Replacement fluid can be D5W or 0.25 normal saline. Large volumes of D5W can cause hyperglycemia, hence the use of 0.25 normal saline. If urine volumes continue to exceed 250 to 300 ml/hr, pitressin or DDAVP can reduce volume and simplify management. Pitressin (5 units IV) provides shorter term therapy than DDAVP (5 units IV) and should probably be used first. If the problem is not self-limiting, then DDAVP can be given.

Patients who have undergone surgery for craniopharyngioma are often awake enough to take oral fluids to replace lost free fluids. Again, care should be maintained to prevent hyperglycemia.

Serum sodium should probably be followed every 4 to 6 hours. If levels exceed 155 mEq/L, a bolus infusion of 500 to 1000 ml of free water or 0.25 normal saline may be needed.

POTASSIUM

Total body potassium in a 70-kg adult averages 3500 mEq (50 mEq/kg), only 70 mEq of which is in the ECF, with a normal concentration of 3.5 to 5 mEq/L. Therefore, small changes in serum concentration represent large changes in total body composition. Potassium is important for generation of transmembrane potential. The intracellular fluid (ICF)/ECF gradient is normally maintained by the sodium-potassium-adenosine triphosphatase (ATPase) pump, which moves potassium into the cells and sodium out.

Potassium homeostasis is regulated by both renal and extrarenal mechanisms. In general, chronic potassium balance is regulated by the kidneys, while acute potassium balance is determined by both renal and extrarenal mechanisms.[36] During the first 4 to 6 hours following an acute potassium load, about 50% is excreted by the kidneys. Of the remaining 50%, 80% is transferred into the cells and 20% is distributed into the ECF. The intracellular uptake of potassium is regulated by several mechanisms. Insulin enhances muscle and splanchnic potassium transport. Catecholamines and adrenergic-type drugs, such as the beta_2 agonist bronchodilators, lower plasma potassium concentration via the beta_2 receptor and are antagonized in this action by beta_2 blocker agents.[37] Aldosterone, in addition to its well-known kaliuretic action, increases potassium excretion in sweat and salivary glands. Further, aldosterone shares with glucocorticoids the role of enhancing potassium secre-

• The principal determinants of potassium distribution are insulin and the acid-base status of the patient.

tion by gut epithelial cells. Extracellular pH affects potassium distribution. Acidosis leads to potassium extravasation from cells. The converse also holds.[38] As a general rule, a decrease of 0.1 pH units increases the plasma potassium by 0.5 mEq/L. Severe hyperkalemia, if present, may also develop secondary to the combination of renal dysfunction and protein catabolism (starvation).[39]

The renal tubules control long-term homeostasis of potassium. Potassium is freely filtered by the glomeruli; 70% is reabsorbed along with water and sodium in the proximal tubule and with sodium and chloride at the level of the thick ascending limb of the Henle's loop. Active secretion of potassium into the distal tubule and collecting ducts occurs under the influence of aldosterone; this agent augments sodium reabsorption at the expense of potassium. Potassium excretion is affected by the rate of tubular flow; the higher the renal flow rate, the greater the loss of potassium. Potassium secretion is decreased during acidosis as hydrogen is lost in its place from the renal tubule. The reverse occurs during alkalosis.

Hypokalemia

Pathophysiology

• *For critically ill patients, hypokalemia exists at values less than 4.5 mEq/L.*

In the critically ill patient, hypokalemia should be defined as a value less than 4.5 mEq/L. Such levels tend to potentiate cardiac arrhythmias, particularly when hypothermia exists or the patient is on digitalis therapy. There are three basic mechanisms by which hypokalemia occurs. The first mechanism is *intracellular shift.* The "stressed" critically ill postoperative patient may present with high insulin and epinephrine levels, both of which contribute to intracellular potassium shift.[40] In patients receiving $beta_2$ or alpha-adrenergic antagonists, this response may be attenuated,[41] although there is some controversy.[42] An iatrogenic hypokalemia may be related to too rapid a correction of hyperglycemia in the setting of diabetic ketoacidosis. Finally, hypothermia, even in a patient with mild metabolic acidosis, induces intracellular shift of potassium.[43]

The second mechanism is *reduced intake.* In severe starvation, or immediately after starting parenteral nutrition, the potassium supply may not be adequate. Even these patients cannot reduce urinary potassium losses below 10 mEq/L. The third mechanism is *increased loss.* Pharmacologic influences such as diuretic therapy,[44] magnesium deficiency, and glucocorticoid excess may result in severe potassium depletion. Long-term diuretic therapy can cause profound, unexpectedly severe total body potassium deficits.

• *Patients receiving long-term diuretic therapy may have significantly reduced total body potassium values despite a normal serum potassium level.*

Upper gastrointestinal losses may cause hypokalemia on the basis of three different mechanisms: (1) loss of potassium from the gastrointestinal tract; (2) metabolic alkalosis, secondary to chloride losses, resulting in a hydrogen ion for potassium exchange in the kidney; and (3) hypovolemia and hyperaldosteronism in which correction of hypovolemia acutely improves renal blood flow, enhancing kaliuresis.

Immediate Therapy

There are conflicting recommendations on the use of potassium to correct hypokalemia. In a critically ill patient, hypokalemia is generally corrected with intravenous therapy. Potassium chloride can be safely infused at rates of 20 to 30 mEq/hr via central vein.[45] Serum hypokalemia (< 2.2 mEq/L) coupled with life-threatening arrhythmias may require bolus administration of potassium chloride. Usually, this is done at a rate of 1 mEq every 2 to 3 minutes up to a total of 5 mEq. This should be followed by the continuous infusion described.

- *Potassium should not be infused at rates greater than 20 to 30 mEq/hr via a central vein.*

Two other electrolyte abnormalities frequently associated with hypokalemia are hypophosphatemia and hypomagnesemia. In particular, magnesium replenishment limits renal potassium wasting and is a cofactor of sodium-potassium transport.[46] Therefore, assessment of these two electrolytes is recommended in patients with acute or severe hypokalemia. Both phosphorus and magnesium are discussed later in this chapter.

Hyperkalemia

Hyperkalemia means a serum potassium level that is greater than 5.5 mEq/L. Factitious hyperkalemia may be caused by hemolysis secondary to prolonged tourniquet time or lysis of leukocytes (when more than 50,000 cells/μL are present[47]) or platelets (when more than 600,000 cells/μL are present); the plasma potassium level is normal in these patients.[48] True hyperkalemia is secondary to increased potassium input, redistribution of potassium between intracellular and extracellular compartments, and/or impaired renal potassium excretion.[47]

- *Hyperkalemia is defined as serum levels greater than 5.5 mEq/L.*

Pathophysiology

With regard to *increased input,* an important cause of iatrogenic hyperkalemia is intravenous potassium infusion at rates of more than 40 mEq/hr. More commonly, however, critically ill patients may present with high levels of potassium secondary to *shift from the intracellular to the extracellular compartment.* The most acute and severe shift results from acute metabolic acidosis. The ability of ECF to act as a buffer because of extracellular bicarbonate concentration, rather than the arterial pH per se, appears to govern this redistribution of potassium. This helps to explain why the ratio of increase in serum potassium to decrease in pH is inconstant, between 0.5 and 1.3 mEq/L per 0.1 unit of fall of arterial pH. This rise tends to be higher later in the course of acute acidosis, when the ECF's ability to buffer is at its nadir. Conversely, respiratory acidosis from elevated CO_2 results in a less marked elevation in serum potassium.[49]

Other causes of an acute rise in ECF potassium include diabetes in combination with hypoaldosteronism, massive cardiac glycoside

Table 5–4.
Etiologies of Drug-Induced Hyperkalemia

Increased K^+ input
KCl supplements/salt substitutes
Potassium penicillin
Transfusion of stored blood
Oxprenolol
Altered compartment distribution
Beta blockers/alpha agonists
Succinylcholine
Hypertonic solutions
Arginine
Digoxin
Barbiturates/heroin/phencyclidine/amphetamines
Decreased K^+ output
K^+-sparing drugs
Angiotensin-converting enzyme inhibitors
Cyclosporine
Nonsteroidal anti-inflammatory agents
Heparin

(From Layon AJ, Bernards WC, Kirby R: Fluids and electrolytes in the critically ill. In: Civetta JM, Taylor RW, Kirby RR, eds: Critical care, 2nd ed. Philadelphia, JB Lippincott, 1992; pp. 457–480.)

overdose, the use of succinylcholine in patients with burn injury or upper motor neuron lesions, and acute adrenal failure.[50,51] Additionally, an acutely ischemic limb may be associated with rhabdomyolysis and hyperkalemia. This situation becomes clinically significant in severe renal dysfunction, such as in the case of acute renal failure secondary to myoglobinuria.[52]

• *Severe limb ischemia can cause hyperkalemia.*

Finally, although patients with chronic renal failure are able to maintain potassium homeostasis until the GFR approximates 10 ml/min, in critically ill patients, an increase in potassium intake or release may result in hyperkalemia sooner and with a higher GFR (*decreased output*). Many commonly used drugs have been associated with hyperkalemia in selected settings (Table 5–4).[51] Drugs that affect renal potassium excretion may impair the GFR directly, or they may interfere with the renin-angiotensin-aldosterone system.

Hyperkalemia produces symptoms very similar to those of hypokalemia. High potassium concentrations may depolarize the cell membrane and may reduce conduction velocity. Systemic manifestations include muscle weakness and decreased deep tendon reflexes. The effects of hyperkalemia on electrical impulse formation and conduction in the heart overshadow all others in clinical importance.[53] Hyperkalemic ECG findings usually appear when the concentration of serum potassium is around 6 mEq/L (peaked T waves, widening of QRS complex) and progress to a continuous sine-wave appearance. Low serum sodium and calcium and high serum magnesium concentrations lower the threshold for malignant cardiac dysrhythmia in the setting of hyperkalemia.

• *High-peaked T waves appear when serum potassium exceeds 6 mEq/L.*

Immediate Therapy

Any potassium level above 5.5 mEq/L, coupled with ECG changes or a value greater than 7 mEq/L, requires emergency therapy. The cardiac effects of hyperkalemia can be minimized by a rapid intravenous infusion of 10% calcium chloride solution (1 g Ca^{2+}/10 ml). Furthermore, 50 to 100 ml of 7.5% sodium bicarbonate solution or 100 to 200 ml of 5% sodium chloride, both intravenously administered, will temporarily depress the membrane threshold potential. This treatment should be followed by intravenous glucose/insulin solution to facilitate intracellular potassium shift. The solution we commonly use is 10% dextrose in water mixed with 10 U regular insulin/100 g of dextrose. This solution is very effective in lowering the serum potassium concentration within 30 minutes of infusion initiation. As a bridge therapy before instituting dialysis, gastrointestinal resins, such as sodium polystyrene sulfonate (Kayexalate) can subacutely control elevated potassium levels, once more rapidly acting therapy has been initiated. The dose for this agent is 20 to 30 g by mouth or nasogastric tube in 50 ml 70% sorbitol every 4 hours, or 50 to 100 g in 200 ml water by retention enema.[54] For serum potassium levels less than about 6 mEq/L, usually all that is required is to restrict the potassium intake and to liberalize sodium intake.

• Measures to reduce an elevated serum potassium level rapidly include calcium chloride, sodium bicarbonate, and glucose-insulin infusions.

CALCIUM

Calcium, the most abundant electrolyte in the human body, is found in a concentration of 15 to 20 g/kg of body weight (99% skeletal, 1% soft tissue, and ECF). Total plasma calcium level varies between 8.5 and 10 mg/dl and circulates in the blood in three major forms: (1) a *protein-bound* form (normally 4.0 to 4.5 mg/dl); (2) a *chelated or nonionized* form (0.5 to 1.0 mg/dl); (3) and an *ionized* form (4.2 to 4.8 mg/dl or 2.1 to 2.4 mEq/L).

Calcium homeostasis comes under the control of several hormones.[55] Parathyroid hormone (PTH), secreted by the parathyroid gland in response to low ionized calcium and magnesium, raises the calcium level. It further stimulates osteoclast activity, which enhances intestinal calcium absorption. Calcitonin counteracts the action of the PTH at the level of the skeleton. Vitamin D enhances intestinal and renal tubular absorption of calcium.

Functions ascribed to calcium include excitation-contraction coupling, hormonal and neurotransmitter secretion, cell division, cell motility, enzyme activity, and blood coagulation. In the heart, calcium contributes to the plateau phase of the cardiac action potential and is responsible for spontaneous depolarization.

At the ultrastructural level, cytoplasmic calcium increases as a specific intracellular response to electrical or chemical stimuli. In other words, calcium serves as a "second messenger" analogous to cyclic adenosine monophosphate (cAMP).[56] The serum ionized fraction, thought to be the physiologically active component, is af-

• *Ionized calcium levels are more important in the critically ill patient than are total calcium values.*

fected by a variety of factors in critically ill patients, independent of the total calcium level. Therefore, in these patients, direct measurement of ionized serum calcium is recommended. Free fatty acids increase ionized calcium binding to albumin, resulting in an ionized fraction that is as much as 10 times lower than the normal level. This is relatively common in critically ill patients.[57]

Hypocalcemia

Pathophysiology

Hypocalcemia occurs in 15 to 50% of critically ill patients. Serum ionized calcium values are less than 2 mEq/L (4 mg/dl or 1 mM/L). The causes of hypocalcemia can be grouped into four general categories (Table 5–5).

Impaired PTH secretion is the most common cause of surgically induced hypocalcemia and develops in 13 to 30% of patients who undergo parathyroid surgery[58] or extensive neck dissections. Hypocalcemia becomes evident on postoperative day 1 or 2 and lasts up to 5 days, provided the parathyroid gland damage is not permanent.

More commonly, acute hypocalcemia may be the result of a circulating chelator such as phosphate. This anion, commonly ele-

Table 5–5.
Causes of Hypocalcemia

- Impaired parathyroid hormone secretion or action
  - Primary parathyroid gland dysfunction
  - Secondary parathyroid gland dysfunction
    - Neck surgery/trauma
    - Infiltrative disease
    - Burns
    - Sepsis
    - Hungry bone syndrome
- Chelation/precipitation
  - Elevated phosphate
  - Citrate/EDTA/EGTA
  - Pancreatitis
  - Fat embolism
  - Rhabdomyolysis
  - Protamine
  - Radiographic contrast dye
  - Ethylene glycol intoxication
  - Sodium sulfate
  - Sodium fluoride
- Vitamin D deficiency
  - Malabsorption (of any cause)
  - Liver failure
  - Renal failure
  - Poor dietary intake
  - Hypomagnesemia
- Decreased bone turnover
  - Hypothyroidism
  - Toxic shock syndrome
  - Drugs (see Table 5–6)

Table 5–6.
Drugs Causing Hypocalcemia

Altered metabolism of 25-OH-Vitamin D
Anticonvulsants (phenytoin)
Ethanol
Glutethimide
Hypomagnesemia
Altering bone turnover
Phosphate-containing antacids
Mithramycin
Calcitonin
Citrate/EDTA/EGTA
Loop diuretics (furosemide, bumetanide)
Radiographic contrast dyes
Sodium sulfate
Sodium fluoride
Ethylene glycol (via oxalate production)
Cis-platinum
Protamine
Gallium
Diphosphonates

(Data from Wilson RF, Binkley LE, Sabo FM, et al: Electrolyte and acid-base changes with massive blood transfusions. Am Surg 1992; 9:535–544; and Zaloga GP: Calcium disorders. Probl Crit Care 1990; 4:382–401.)

vated in trauma, rhabdomyolysis, hyperpyrexia, and renal failure, may cause soft tissue calcium precipitation.[59] Severe pancreatitis and citrate from rapid blood infusion (> 60 ml/kg/hr) have also been implicated as causes of hypocalcemia.[60] Sepsis has been identified as a major contributor to hypocalcemia in the critically ill, on a multifactorial basis.[61,62]

Vitamin D deficiency occurs from malabsorption, liver, or renal failure. It can cause hypocalcemia in critically ill patients, but it is rarely responsible for acute hypocalcemia.

Decreased bone turnover is caused by multiple drugs (Table 5–6), as well as by calcitonin release after thyroidectomy and in toxic shock syndrome.[63] No matter the etiology of the hypocalcemia, a normal serum potassium level, through potentiation of PTH and vitamin action, is a marker of a good response to calcium therapy. If hypomagnesemia is present, magnesium as the chloride salt, rather than as the sulfate salt, should be administered, because the latter may combine with calcium and may worsen coexisting hypocalcemia.[64]

The clinical signs of hypocalcemia relate to the severity and the rapidity of the decrease in calcium level.[65] Although it is a hallmark of hypocalcemia, tetany rarely develops in critically ill postoperative patients. Paresthesias, muscle spasms, and laryngospasm may develop. However, in this population, hypotension and/or low cardiac output are more likely. In the heart, decreased ionized calcium inhibits relaxation and may reduce contractility to the point of hypotension, ventricular arrhythmias, or refractory heart failure. A charac-

• *Hypocalcemia causes hypotension and/or low cardiac output.*

teristic prolongation of the ST segment may lead to an increased QT interval on the ECG.[66]

Immediate Therapy

Hypocalcemia in critically ill patients requires therapy directed both at symptoms and at the underlying cause. Evaluation of hypocalcemia should include acid-base status, albumin level, and electrolytes such as phosphorus and magnesium. Injudicious use of calcium in patients with tissue hypoxia and septic shock can cause clinical deterioration, probably related to generalized enzyme activation and free radical production.[67] While a mild degree of ionized hypocalcemia (> 1.8 mEq/L) does not usually require any specific treatment, we most often treat patients with this or lower values with 1 g of calcium chloride. This is three times the amount of ionized calcium found in gluconate.

Acute symptomatic hypocalcemia, which presents with laryngospasm, hypotension, and/or ventricular arrhythmias, requires immediate treatment. One to two grams of calcium chloride should be given immediately over 2 to 4 minutes via a central line. If hypomagnesemia is a possibility, in absence of renal failure, we and others[66] recommend the empiric administration of 1 to 2 g of magnesium to potentiate the action of calcium.

- *Acute hypocalcemia requires immediate therapy with 1 to 2 g calcium chloride.*

If symptomatic hypocalcemia persists, such as following parathyroid surgery, a slow central infusion of calcium is indicated over 4 to 6 hours (10 to 15 mg/kg). The calcium level is usually monitored every 1 to 4 hours. Calcium augments the effect of digitalis and may precipitate digitalis toxicity. Other adverse effects include hypertension, nausea and vomiting, skin flushing, and bradycardia. Chronic hypocalcemia is rarely an ICU emergency and is usually related to hypoparathyroidism or vitamin deficiency. In these cases, therapy may be individualized based on the patient's blood and urine calcium levels.

Hypercalcemia

Pathophysiology

The most common causes of hypercalcemia in the critically ill are malignant neoplasia and primary hyperparathyroidism (Table 5–7). This includes single adenomas (80%), diffuse hyperplasia (15%), and multiple endocrine neoplasms. Malignant diseases associated with hypercalcemia include bronchogenic carcinoma, breast cancer, multiple myeloma, lymphoma, and renal cell carcinoma.[55] These tumors cause elevations in serum calcium due to direct tumor osteolysis or tumor-produced humoral substances, such as parathroid hormone-related peptide, which stimulate bone reabsorption.[66] The humoral substances are also responsible for the stimulation of renal adenylate cyclase, which causes inhibition of phosphate reabsorption[56] and production of prostaglandins. The prostaglandins induce leukocyte production of osteoclast activating factor.[68]

Table 5–7.
Causes of Hypercalcemia

Malignant diseases
Hyperparathyroidism
Primary
Secondary
Multiple endocrine neoplasia syndrome
Immobilization
Pheochromocytoma
Granulomatous disease
Tuberculosis
Sarcoid
Fungus (coccidioidomycosis, histoplasmosis)
Lymphoproliferative disorders
Exogenous vitamin D
Vitamin A intoxication
Exogenous calcium
Hyperthyroidism
Addison's disease
Thiazide diuretics/lithium (decreased excretion)
Theophylline (increased PTH secretion)

(From Zaloga GP: Calcium disorders. Probl Crit Care 1990; 4:382–401.)

Less common causes of acute hypercalcemia include prolonged immobilization, as a result of increased bone reabsorption exceeding urinary excretion and PTH suppression. From 10 to 20% of patients with hyperthyroidism experience direct effects of thyroid hormone on bone reabsorption.[69,70] In patients with pheochromocytoma, hypercalcemia may be due to catecholamine effects on bone or PTH secretion. Elevated calcium levels may develop during the recovery phase of acute renal failure and postrenal transplantation because of secondary hyperparathyroidism.[71] Finally, the thiazide group of diuretics enhances distal tubular reabsorption of calcium and can result in hypercalcemia.[55]

Immediate Therapy

Hypercalcemia is defined as an ionized serum calcium level greater than 2.6 mEq/L (5.2 mg/dl or 1.3 mM/L). The decision to treat hypercalcemia relates to the level of serum calcium and the presence of clinical manifestations.[72] Immediate treatment becomes necessary if the total serum calcium level exceeds 14 mg/dl (> 3.5 mM/L). This value must be adjusted for the serum albumin value or for an ionized calcium level greater than 6 mg/dl (> 1.5 mM/L or > 3 mEq/L).

Symptoms of hypercalcemia involve a variety of organs. Although ECG changes, such as shortening of the QT interval and flattening and inversion of T waves, are common, they do not correlate with the degree of hypercalcemia.[73] However, malignant ven-

• *During hypercalcemia, electrocardiographic changes do not correlate with the degree of hypercalcemia.*

tricular arrhythmias and enhanced sensitivity to the digitalis glycosides can be noted. Central nervous system symptoms include progressive obtundation and coma. Dehydration aggravates these symptoms. Gastrointestinal symptoms, such as nausea, vomiting, and constipation, as well as renal dysfunction, also occur.

The therapy of hypercalcemia has four basic goals: (1) to correct dehydration; (2) to enhance renal excretion of calcium; (3) to inhibit accelerated bone reabsorption; and (4) to treat the underlying disorder.

The expansion of intravascular volume to increase calciuresis requires an isotonic salt solution such as 0.9% saline with volume based on the patient's baseline cardiovascular status. Loop diuretics inhibit calcium reabsorption in the ascending limb of the loop of Henle.

Long-term therapy utilizes biphosphonates (etidronate, pamidronate, or clodronate) to bind to hydroxyapatite in bone and to inhibit the dissolution of crystals. The dosage of etidronate is 7.5 mg/kg intravenously over 4 hours every day for 3 to 7 days; the effect is seen within 2 days and is maximized at about 7 days. Therapy is safe, with only mild and reversible increases in phosphate and creatinine concentrations. Short-term use does not impair bone formation, although long-term use can result in osteomalacia. Mithramycin, in a dosage of 25 μg/kg over 4 to 6 hours, inhibits RNA synthesis in osteoclasts. This drug has potentially toxic effects on liver, kidney, and bone marrow, However, side effects are not usually seen at this dosage unless more than three to four doses are given. The agent may be repeated several times at 1- to 2-day intervals. Calcitonin, at a dose of 4 MRC U/kg every 12 hours, inhibits bone reabsorption and increases renal calcium excretion. Maximal urinary calcium excretion is reached within 12 to 24 hours. However, this agent may not work in 25% of patients. Glucocorticoids, such as hydrocortisone, 3 mg/kg/day for 3 to 5 days, inhibit the growth of neoplastic lymphoid tissue in hematologic malignancy and also inhibit active intestinal absorption of calcium both directly and likely by a reduction in the level of 1,25-$(OH)_2$-vitamin D. Intravenous phosphate dramatically binds intravenous calcium, but it may create precipitates in the blood vessels and soft tissues. This agent has only limited use.

MAGNESIUM

Magnesium is the second most important intracellular cation in the body. It activates many enzyme systems, including phosphatases, transphosphorylases, pyrophosphatases, carboxylases, hexokinases, and adenylacetylase.[74] Hence, magnesium physiology and pharmacology involve numerous body systems such as the central nervous, musculoskeletal, and cardiovascular systems.[75]

• *Magnesium levels affect both the central nervous system and the cardiovascular system.*

Much of the body's magnesium is found in the bone (about 60%), with the rest principally located in soft tissue, primarily muscle. Less than 1% is distributed in the plasma, reaching a total concentration of 1.7 to 2.4 mg/dl (1.4 to 2.0 mEq/L). Magnesium circulates in the plasma in three forms: (1) a protein-bound fraction (30%); (2) a chelated fraction (15%); and (3) an ionized fraction (55%), although the ionized form is not routinely measured by most laboratories. The ionized fraction is responsible for the cation's physiologic action. The small intestine takes up the daily dietary magnesium intake of 25 to 30 mEq. Stool and kidney excretion and renal tubular reabsorption maintain magnesium homeostasis. Magnesium blood levels regulate excretion and reabsorption. ECF expansion, hypercalcemia, loop and osmotic diuretics, phosphate depletion, metabolic acidosis, and protein and alcohol intake all stimulate renal excretion.

Hypomagnesemia

Pathophysiology

Hypomagnesemia results from inadequate intake, impaired absorption, or excessive losses. Low renal magnesium excretion (less than 1 to 2 mEq/day) suggests a nonrenal cause of hypomagnesemia. Such patients, challenged with an intravenous magnesium sulfate load of 75 g over 12 hours, retain more than 25 to 50% of the ion administered.[76] Inadequate intake results from starvation or incorrect parenteral nutrition. This situation creates an acute intracellular shift of magnesium associated with the administration of glucose and amino acids or insulin treatment of hyperglycemic patients.[77] Inflammatory bowel disease decreases gut absorption. Pancreatic and biliary diseases are associated with malabsorption.[76] Esophageal surgery seems to be associated with a magnesium deficiency, probably secondary to severe malnutrition.

Diuretics, aminoglycoside antibiotics, amphotericin B, *cis*-platinum, cardiac glycosides, acute ethanol intoxication, and rapid replacement of potassium all alter renal magnesium conservation.[46,77]

Hypomagnesemia commonly develops in the postoperative critically ill patient.[78] Although no correlation between the severity score and the degree of hypoproteinemia and postoperative serum magnesium has been found, patients with severe hypomagnesemia (serum $Mg^{2+} \leq 1$ mEq/dl) have a higher mortality rate than those with higher magnesium levels.[78] The presence of hypokalemia, hypophosphatemia, hyponatremia, and hypocalcemia may help to predict hypomagnesemia.[79]

The clinical consequences of hypomagnesemia involve the cardiovascular system as well as the central and peripheral nervous systems. Magnesium produces significant cardiovascular effects because of its influence on intracellular transfer of sodium and potassium via ATPase. Hypomagnesemia allows intracellular concentrations of potassium and sodium to decrease and increase, respectively, leading to unstable function of the Purkinje system.[80] Changes on the ECG may vary from slight to marked widening of the QRS interval to peaked T waves or ST depression, simulating ischemia. Magnesium sulfate has been effectively used to treat refractory ventricular tachycardia (including torsades de pointes) and fibrillation.[77]

• *Magnesium sulfate is effective in the treatment of ventricular tachycardia including torsades de pointes and ventricular fibrillation.*

Neurotoxic effects of hypomagnesemia include increased neuromuscular activity from tetany and psychiatric disturbances including acute delirium and convulsions. Often, hypocalcemia is present at the same time, secondary to hypomagnesemia-induced resistance to action of PTH or failure to synthesize the hormone.[81]

Immediate Therapy

• *The usual dose for replacement magnesium therapy is 2 g of magnesium sulfate.*

Except in life-threatening cardiac dysrhythmias, preeclampsia, eclampsia, or seizures, magnesium replacement may be administered slowly—1 to 3 g (8 to 24 mEq) magnesium sulfate over 30 minutes intravenously every 4 to 6 hours until the serum level normalizes. In emergency situations, however, 1 to 2 g (8 to 16 mEq) magnesium sulfate may be administered intravenously over 2 to 4 minutes; thereafter, an infusion of 1 to 2 g/hr for several hours may be instituted in patients with normal renal function.[82]

Hypermagnesemia

Pathophysiology

Hypermagnesemia is defined as a serum magnesium concentration above 3 mg/dl (2.4 mEq/L, 1.2 mM/L). Above 4 mEq/L, symptoms of lethargy and loss of deep tendon reflexes develop. Most cases of hypermagnesemia result from the administration of magnesium-containing antacids, laxatives, and enemas or from nutritional products in patients with renal disease. Hypermagnesemia can occur following intravenous magnesium therapy in patients with premature labor or preeclampsia or eclampsia.

• *Hypermagnesemia causes central nervous depression and interferes with peripheral nerve impulse transmission. Magnesium reduces the amount of available acetylcholine at the neuromuscular junction.*

The clinical effects of hypermagnesemia relate to actions of magnesium on the peripheral and central nervous systems, the circulation, uterine contractility, and the blood flow of the mother and fetus.[75] Change in membrane transport, as well as central nervous system depression, has been noted when magnesium salt is applied directly to nervous tissue in vitro;[82–83] it also potentiates the effect of local anesthetic-induced nerve block.[84] Although there is currently no clear evidence that magnesium crosses the blood-brain barrier, studies in patients with eclampsia have indicated that, when magnesium is injected parenterally, the electrolyte acts as a neuronal depressant.[85] Some of the changes, however, such as decreased reflexes, may be explained on the basis of action on the neuromuscular end plate. Magnesium decreases both liberation of acetylcholine at the neuromuscular junction and the sensitivity of the motor end plate to the neurotransmitter. This potentiates the actions of both nondepolarizing and depolarizing neuromuscular blocking agents. This action is antagonized by anticholinesterase agents, as well as by calcium.

Magnesium produces significant vasodilation while maintaining contractile forces of the myocardium. However, serum concentrations above 5 to 7 mEq/L are associated with cardiac toxicity. High levels of magnesium in obstetric patients have reduced the frequency and amplitude of uterine contractions, with a concomitant increase in uterine arterial blood flow.[86]

Immediate Therapy

Definitive therapy to lower serum magnesium level consists of discontinuation of all exogenous magnesium. More acute therapy includes 0.9% saline (500 to 1000 ml) and loop diuretics (10 to 40 mg of furosemide IV) to enhance renal excretion. Calcium, an antagonist of magnesium action, may be administered intravenously in a dose of 500 to 1000 mg as the chloride salt. In patients with renal failure, magnesium may be removed by dialysis. Neuromuscular and cardiac toxicity can be transiently antagonized by intravenous calcium at a dose of 500 to 1000 mg of calcium chloride over 5 minutes.

- *Therapy for hypermagnesemia includes calcium chloride and/or renal dialysis.*

PHOSPHORUS

The body contains between 500 and 800 g (11 to 14 g/kg lean tissue) of phosphorus, with 80% in bone, 9% in skeletal muscle, and the rest distributed in the soft tissues. Less than 2% of the anion is distributed in the extracellular fluid. Intracellular concentrations of phosphorus approximate 100 mEq/L.[87] Phosphorus is required for protein, fat, and carbohydrate metabolism. It provides the source of high-energy bonds in tri- and dinucleotides in the mitochondrial respiratory chain and in synthesis of nucleic acids.[88] Since phosphorus is an intracellular ion, serum levels may not always reflect the status of intracellular stores. The average daily intake of phosphorus is 800 to 1000 mg; the normal total serum phosphorus level in adults is 2.5 to 4.5 mg/dl. The kidney primarily controls blood phosphorus concentration.[89] Levels can vary as much as 50% during the day. Renal excretion maintains circulating levels. PTH, vitamin D, calcitonin, and glucocorticoids reduce renal phosphate reabsorption and cause phosphaturia. Other causes of phosphaturia include glucagon, vasopressin, acetylcholine, prostaglandin, acidosis, volume expansion, saline, diuretics, magnesium, and potassium depletion. Growth hormone, thyroxine, and hypophosphatemia increase, and hyperphosphatemia suppresses, renal phosphate reabsorption.[89] Finally, acid-base alterations influence the serum phosphorus level.[90] Respiratory alkalosis increases the intracellular pH and activates phosphofructokinase. This requires an intracellular phosphorus shift. Metabolic alkalosis causes an intracellular phosphate shift, but it also increases renal phosphate excretion because of expanded extracellular fluid (e.g., infusion of bicarbonate). Urinary phosphate assists in the differentiation of the two clinical situations. Acid-base alterations are also influenced by hypophosphatemia. For example, mild metabolic acidosis can develop because of renal bicarbonate wasting, decreased excretion of titratable acids, and decreased ammoniagenesis. The abnormalities are buffered by release of alkali from bone, hence the usually mild nature of the aberrations.[90–93]

Hypophosphatemia

Pathophysiology

Hypophosphatemia is defined as a blood phosphorus concentration below 2.5 mg/dl, but a value less than or equal to 1 mg/dl may be life-threatening. Three primary mechanisms are at work in this process: (1) intracellular shift of phosphate; (2) increased renal loss of phosphate; and (3) decreased gastrointestinal absorption of phosphate. Transcellular shifts of phosphorus can result from carbohydrate loading, total parenteral nutrition (the refeeding syndrome), or rapid correction of diabetic ketoacidosis. High catecholamine levels and glucagon secretion—often seen in acutely stressed, postoperative, burn, or trauma patients—also contribute to acute hypophosphatemia because of intracellular shift and urinary excretion, respectively.[88,94]

• *Carbohydrate loading shifts phosphorus intracellularly, causing hypophosphatemia.*

Respiratory alkalosis and hypophosphatemia, as discussed earlier, have been associated with induced hyperventilation in neurotrauma patients[95] and in salicylate poisoning. Increased renal losses of phosphorus are also found in patients with renal tubular dysfunction, hyperparathyroidism, hypomagnesemia, hypokalemia, hyperthermia, and diuretic use.

Reduced gastrointestinal absorption of phosphorus occurs in malabsorption states, emesis, and prolonged gastric suctioning (resulting in decreased intake), diarrhea, and phosphate binding resins. A frequently seen clinical situation in critically ill patients admitted to the hospital is the combination of an intravenous infusion of dextrose-containing solutions and the administration of oral phosphate-binding antacids such as aluminum or magnesium hydroxide. Again, the presence of low urinary phosphate (< 100 mg/day) allows one to discriminate gastrointestinal from renal losses.[88] While hypophosphatemia at values greater than 1 mg/dl is seen in approximately 30% of postsurgical patients,[96] significant morbidity and mortality have been associated with severely depressed phosphate levels (< 1 mg/dl) in critically ill patients.[95,97] Patients with severely low phosphate levels may complain of muscle weakness, or tremor, and they may have respiratory distress secondary to decreased diaphragmatic contractility. Although reversible with intravenous phosphate, this level of hypophosphatemia may contribute to failure to wean the patient from the mechanical ventilator.[98–100]

In long-term alcohol abusers, and in diabetics during recovery from ketoacidosis, rhabdomyolysis due to decreased phosphate levels has been noted. In most cases, it has been mild and asymptomatic.[101] Defective adenosine triphosphate (ATP) synthesis contributes to skeletal muscle dysfunction.[100] The intracellular myocyte composition changes include increased intracellular sodium and water, and decreased magnesium and potassium.[101]

Severe hypophosphatemia does not affect myocardial performance.[102] The major cardiovascular abnormality is labile blood pressure associated with postural hypotension in awake patients.[103,104] Central nervous system symptoms correlate with the severity of the hypophosphatemia. They range from irritability to psychotic or confusional states[105] to seizures and coma.[106] Peripheral neuropathy may be present as well.[107]

• *Hypophosphatemia causes central nervous system depression or confusion and occasionally seizures.*

Immediate Therapy

Treatment of hypophosphatemia involves, first of all, correction of the underlying causes of phosphorus depletion. Severe or symptomatic hypophosphatemia requires treatment with intravenous phosphate. An intravenous infusion of 7.5 to 15 mg/kg (0.25 to 0.5 mM/kg) sodium or potassium phosphate over 4 hours has been shown to be safe in patients with serum phosphate levels in the range of 0.5 to 1 mg/dl.[107] Significant changes in the mean serum calcium, potassium, and magnesium concentrations are not seen at these or lesser (0.1 mM/kg) doses.[108,109] Treatment risks include hyperphosphatemia, hypocalcemia, hyperkalemia (with potassium phosphate), hypomagnesemia, hyperosmolarity, and metastatic calcification if preexisting hypercalcemia is present. These electrolytes require close following during phosphate infusion.

Hyperphosphatemia

Pathophysiology

Hyperphosphatemia is present if the serum phosphorus concentration exceeds 4.5 mg/dl. The critically ill patient is most apt to be seen with this problem in the setting of renal dysfunction or a drug-induced reduction of the renal excretion of phosphorus.[94] In renal failure, the level of phosphate remains within a normal range until the GFR falls below 20 to 25 ml/min. Hyperphosphatemia, as well as renal failure, impairs the conversion of 25-OH-vitamin D to 1, 25-$(OH)_2$-vitamin D, contributing to hypocalcemia and secondary hyperparathyroidism. Two more basic mechanisms for hyperphosphatemia include increased phosphate or vitamin D uptake (e.g., ingestion of laxatives, enemas, or vitamin D), and, more commonly in the ICU, increased extracellular shift (e.g., acidosis, chemotherapy and tumor lysis, malignant hyperthermia, hemolysis, and rhabdomyolysis). Accurate history and measurement of the GFR and urinary phosphate excretion help to determine the cause of the hyperphosphatemia. Clinical features of hyperphosphatemia reflect hypocalcemia and ectopic calcification when the calcium-phosphate product exceeds 75 mg/dl (normal, 30 to 40 mg/dl).

Immediate Therapy

Treatment consists, first, of correction of the underlying cause. Dietary phosphate and other exogenous sources should be restricted. Phosphorus may be removed via oral phosphate binders, such as aluminum hydroxide. Severe states of hyperphosphatemia or symptomatic patients, such as those with soft tissue calcifications, should be treated with intravenous saline and loop diuretics; acetazolamide in a dose of 500 mg every 6 hours prevents proximal tubular reabsorption of phosphate. If renal function is compromised, peritoneal dialysis or hemodialysis may be used to eliminate the phosphate. The possibility of acute hypocalcemia should be anticipated and careful monitoring of this electrolyte implemented.

REFERENCES

1. Blalock A: Trauma to the intestines: the importance of the local loss of fluid in the production of low pressure. Arch Surg 1931; 22:314–324.
2. Shires T, Williams J, Brown F: Acute change in extracellular fluids associated with major surgical procedures. Ann Surg 1961; 154: 803–810.
3. Moore FD, Steenburg RW, Ball MR, et al: Studies in surgical endocrinology: the urinary excretion of 17-hydroxycorticoids and associated metabolic changes, in cases of soft tissue trauma of varying severity and in bone trauma. Ann Surg 1955; 141:145–174.
4. Robson JS, Horn DB, Dudley HA, Stewart CP: Metabolic response to adrenalectomy. Lancet 1955; 2:325–326.
5. Hayes MA, Williamson RJ, Heidenreich WF: Endocrine mechanisms involved in water and sodium metabolism during operation and convalescence. Surgery 1957; 41:353–386.
6. Hayes MA, Coller FA: The neuroendocrine control of water and electrolyte excretion during surgical anesthesia. Surg Gynecol Obstet 1952; 95:142–149.
7. Layon AJ, Bernards WC, Kirby R: Fluids and electrolytes in the critically ill. In: Civetta JM, Taylor RW, Kirby RR, eds: Critical care, 2nd ed. Philadelphia, JB Lippincott, 1992; pp. 457–480.
8. Bartholomew LG, Scholz DA: Reversible postoperative neurological symptoms: report of five cases secondary to water intoxication and sodium depletion. JAMA 1956; 162:22–26.
9. Schroeder HA: Renal failure associated with low extracellular sodium chloride: the low salt syndrome. JAMA 1949; 141:117–124.
10. Stokes JM, Bernard HR, Balfour J: Effects of experimental electrolyte depletion upon renal water and solute excretion. Arch Surg 1962; 85:540–548.
11. Payen DM, Farge D, Beloucif S et al: No involvement of antidiuretic hormone in acute antidiuresis during PEEP ventilation in humans. Anesthesiology 1987; 66:17–23.
12. Qvist J, Pontoppidan H, Wilson RS et al: Hemodynamic responses to mechanical ventilation with PEEP: the effect of hypervolemia. Anesthesiology 1975; 42:45–55.
13. Hayes MA, Goldenberg IS: Renal effects of anesthesia and operation mediated by endocrines. Anesthesiology 1963; 24:487–499.
14. Kapadia CR, Chan STF, Johnson AW et al: The hourly pattern of urine solute and electrolyte excretion following standard surgical trauma. Br J Surg 1983; 70:286–289.
15. Hutchin P, McLaughlin JS, Hayes MA: Renal response to acidosis during anesthesia and operation. Ann Surg 1961; 154:161–180.
16. Smith LL, Moore FD: Refractory hypotension in man: is this irreversible shock? N Engl J Med 1962; 267:733–742.

17. Defronzo RA, Thier SO: Pathophysiologic approach to hyponatremia. Arch Intern Med 1980; 140:897–902.
18. Goldberg M: Hyponatremia. Med Clin North Am 1981; 65:251–269.
19. Colbert N, Andrieu JM: Hyponatremia associated with angioimmunoblastic lymphadenopathy. Acta Haematol 1983; 70:389–391.
20. Jamieson MJ: Hyponatremia. Br Med J 1985; 290:1723–1728.
21. Aviram A, Pfau A, Czaczkes JW, Ullman TD: Hyperosmolarity with hyponatremia, caused by inappropriate administration of mannitol. Am J Med 1967; 42:648–650.
22. Levine TB, Franciosa JA, Vrobel T, Cohn JN: Hyponatremia as a marker for high renin heart failure. Br Heart J 1982; 47:161–166.
23. Schrier RW: Pathogenesis of sodium and water retention in high-output and low-output cardiac failure, nephrotic syndrome, cirrhosis, and pregnancy. N Engl J Med 1988; 319:1127–1134.
24. Azar I: Transurethral prostatectomy syndrome. In: Refresher courses in anesthesiology, vol. 17. Philadelphia, JB Lippincott, 1989; pp. 1–15.
25. Chung H-M, Kluge R, Schrier RW, Anderson RJ: Postoperative hyponatremia: a prospective study. Arch Intern Med 1986; 146:333–336.
26. Laski ME: Diuretics: mechanism of action and therapy. Semin Nephrol 1986; 6:210–223.
27. Wijdicks EFM, Ropper AH, Hunnicutt EJ et al: Atrial natriuretic factor and salt wasting after aneurysmal subarachnoid hemorrhage. Stroke 1991; 22:1519–1524.
28. Cluitmans FHM, Meinders AE: Management of severe hyponatremia: rapid or slow correction? Am J Med 1990; 88:161–166.
29. Sterns HR, Thomas DJ, Herndon RM: Brain dehydration and neurological deterioration after rapid correction of hyponatremia. Kidney Int 1989; 35:69–75.
30. Stern RH: The management of symptomatic hyponatremia. Semin Nephrol 1990; 10:503–514.
31. Narins RG: Therapy of hyponatremia; does haste make waste? N Engl J Med 1986; 314:1573–1575.
32. Tien R, Arieff AI, Kucharczyk W et al: Hyponatremic encephalopathy: is central pontine myelinolysis a component? Am J Med 1992; 92:513–522.
33. Feig PU, McCurdy DK: The hypertonic state. N Engl J Med 1977; 297:1444–1454.
34. Gibson TC, Sugioka K, Sugioka M: The effect of acute alterations in blood sodium on the electrocardiogram. J Electrocardiol 1974; 7: 127–136.
35. Leaf A: Neurogenic diabetes insipidus. Kidney Int 1979; 15:572–580.
36. Bia MJ, DeFronzo RA: Extrarenal potassium homeostasis. Am J Physiol 1981; 240:F257-F268.
37. Todd EP, Vick RL: Kalemotropic effect of epinephrine: analysis with adrenergic agonists and antagonists. Am J Physiol 1971; 220: 1964–1969.
38. Alexander EA, Perrone RD: Regulation of extrarenal potassium balance. In: Maxwell MH, Kleeman CR, Narins RG, eds: Clinical disorders of fluid and electrolyte metabolism, 4th ed. New York, McGraw-Hill, 1987; pp. 105–117.
39. Fulop M: Hyperkalemia in diabetic ketoacidosis. Am J Med Sci 1990; 299:164–169.
40. Brown MJ, Brown BC, Murphy MB: Hypokalemia from $beta_2$-receptor stimulation by circulating epinephrine. N Engl J Med 1983; 309: 1414–1419.

41. Williams ME, Gervino EV, Rosa RM et al: Catecholamine modulation of rapid potassium shifts during exercise. N Engl J Med 1985; 312:823–827.
42. Minaker KL, Rowe JW: Potassium homeostasis during hyperinsulinemia: effect of insulin level, ß-blockade, and age. Am J Physiol 1982; 242:E373-E377.
43. Sprung J, Cheng EY, Gamulin S et al: The effect of acute hypothermia and serum potassium concentration on potassium cardiotoxicity in anesthetized rats. Acta Anesthesiol Scand 1992; 36:825–830.
44. Freis ED, Papademetriou V: How dangerous are diuretics? Drugs 1985; 30:469–474.
45. Kruse JA, Carlson RW: Rapid correction of hypokalemia using concentrated intravenous potassium chloride infusions. Arch Intern Med 1990; 150:613–617.
46. Dyckner T: Relation of cardiovascular disease to potassium and magnesium deficiencies. Am J Cardiol 1990; 65:44K-46K.
47. Oster JR, Perez GO, Gastro A, Vaamonde CA: Plasma potassium response to acute metabolic acidosis induced by mineral and nonmineral acids. Miner Electrolyte Metab 1980; 14:28–36.
48. Miller CE, Remenchik AP: Problems involved in accurately measuring the K content of the human body. Ann NY Acad Sci 1963; 110: 175–188.
49. Scribner BH, Fremont-Smith K, Burnell JM: The effect of acute respiratory acidosis on the internal equilibrium of potassium. N Engl J Med 1955; 34:1276–1285.
50. Sterns RH, Cox M, Feig PU, Singer I: Internal potassium balance and the control of plasma potassium concentration. Medicine 1981; 60: 339–354.
51. Ponce SP, Jennings AE, Madias NE, Harrington JT: Drug-induced hyperkalemia. Medicine 1985; 64:357–370.
52. Celoria G, Zarfos K, Berman J: Effects of acute lower limb ischemia on femoral venous efflux. J Vasc Dis 1990; 6:439–444.
53. Goodyer AVN, Goodkind MJ, Stanley EJ: The effects of abnormal concentrations of the serum electrolytes on left ventricular function. Am Heart J 1964; 67:779–791.
54. Zaloga GP, Chernow B: Life-threatening electrolyte and metabolic abnormalities. In: Parrillo JE, ed: Current therapy in critical care medicine. Toronto, BC Decker, 1987; pp. 245–257.
55. Zaloga GP, Chernow B, Cook D et al: Assessment of calcium homeostasis in the critically ill surgical patient. Ann Surg 1985; 202: 587–594.
56. Landers DF, Becker GL, Wong KC: Calcium, calmodulin, and anesthesiology. Anesth Analg 1989; 69:100–112.
57. Zaloga GP, Willey S, Tomasic P, Chernow B: Free fatty acids after calcium binding: a cause for misinterpretation of serum calcium values and hypocalcemia in critical illness. J Endocrinol Metab 1987; 64:1010–1014.
58. Kale N, Basaklar AC, Somnez K et al: Hungry bone syndrome in a child following parathyroid surgery. J Pediatr Surg 1992; 27: 1502–1503.
59. Zaloga GP, Chernow B: Hypocalcemia in critical illness (letter). JAMA 1987; 257:626.
60. Wilson RF, Binkley LE, Sabo FM et al: Electrolyte and acid-base changes with massive blood transfusions. Am Surg 1992; 9:535–544.

61. Burchard KW, Simms HH, Robinson A et al: Hypocalcemia during sepsis: relationship to resuscitation and hemodynamics. Arch Surg 1992; 127:265–272.
62. Zaloga GP, Chernow B: The multifactorial basis for hypocalcemia during sepsis: studies of the parathyroid hormone-vitamin D axis. Ann Intern Med 1987; 107:36–41.
63. Zaloga GP: Calcium disorders. In: Zaloga GP, ed: Endocrine emergencies. Problems in critical care, vol 4. Philadelphia, JB Lippincott, 1990; pp. 382–401.
64. Eisenbud E, LoBue CC: Hypocalcemia after therapeutic use of magnesium sulfate. Arch Intern Med 1976; 136:688–691.
65. Ginsburg R, Esserman LJ, Bristow MR: Myocardial performance and extracellular ionized calcium in a severely failing human heart. Ann Intern Med 1983; 98:603–606.
66. Agus ZS, Wasserstein A, Goldfarb S: Disorders of calcium and magnesium homeostasis. Am J Med 1982; 72:473–487.
67. Zaloga GP, Sager A, Prielipp R, Ward K: Low dose calcium administration increase mortality during septic peritonitis (abstract). Crit Care Med 1990; 18:S209.
68. Shaw JW, Oldham SB, Rosoff L et al: Urinary cyclic AMP analyzed as a function of the serum calcium and parathyroid hormone in the differential diagnosis of hypercalcemia. J Clin Invest 1977; 59:14–21.
69. Bergstrom WH: Hypercalciuria and hypercalcemia complicating immobilization. Am J Dis Child 1978; 132:553–554.
70. Gordon DL, Suvanich S, Erviti V et al: The serum calcium level and its significance in hyperthyroidism: a prospective study. Am J Med Sci 1974; 268:31–36.
71. Kukreja SC, Hargis GK, Rosenthal IM, Williams GA: Pheochromocytoma causing excessive parathyroid hormone production and hypercalcemia. Ann Intern Med 1973; 79:838–840.
72. Bilezikian JP: Management of acute hypercalcemia. N Engl J Med 1992; 326:1196–1203.
73. Ellman H, Dembin H, Seriff N: The rarity of shortening of the Q-T interval in patients with hypercalcemia. Crit Care Med 1982; 10: 320–322.
74. Quamme GA, Dirks JH, Maxwell MH et al: Magnesium metabolism. In: Maxwell MH, Kleeman CR, Narins RG, eds: Clinical disorders of fluid and electrolyte metabolism, 4th ed. New York, McGraw-Hill, 1987; pp. 297–316.
75. Aldrete JA: Magnesium physiology and pharmacology in anesthesia. Anesthesiol Rev 1987; 14:33–39.
76. Berkelhammer C, Bear RA: A clinical approach to common electrolyte problems: hypomagnesemia. Can Med Assoc J 1985; 132:360–368.
77. Zaloga GP, Roberts JE: Magnesium disorders. In: Zaloga GP, ed: Endocrine emergencies. Problems in critical care, vol 4. Philadelphia, JB Lippincott, 1990; pp. 425–436.
78. Chernow B, Bamberger S, Stoiko M et al: Hypomagnesemia in patients in postoperative intensive care. Chest 1989; 95:391–397.
79. Whang R, Oei TO, Aikawa JK et al: Predictors of clinical hypomagnesemia: hypokalemia, hypophosphatemia, hyponatremia, and hypocalcemia. Arch Intern Med 1984; 144:1794–1796.
80. Paddle BM, Haugaard N: Role of magnesium in effects of epinephrine on heart contraction and metabolism. Am J Physiol 1971; 221: 1178–1184.
81. Flink EB: Magnesium deficiency: etiology and clinical spectrum. Acta Med Scand 1981; 647(Suppl):125–137.

82. Libet B, Gerard RW: Control of the potential rhythm of the isolated frog brain. J Neurophysiol 1930; 2:153–169.
83. Zaloga GP: Electrolyte disorders. In: Civetta JM, Taylor RW, Kirby RR, eds. Critical care, 2nd ed. Philadelphia, JB Lippincott, 1992; p. 499.
84. Akutagawa T, Saito H, Katz JD, Kitahata LM: Magnesium ion enhances lidocaine induced nerve block (abstract). Anesthesiology 1980; 53:525.
85. Pritchard JA, Cunningham FG, Pritchard SA: The Parkland Memorial Hospital protocol for treatment of eclampsia: evaluation of 245 cases. Am J Obstet Gynecol 1984; 148:951–963.
86. Stallworth JC, Yeh S-Y, Petrie RH: The effect of magnesium sulfate on fetal heart rate variability and uterine activity. Am J Obstet Gynecol 1981; 140:702–706.
87. Janson C, Birnbaum G, Baker FJ: Hypophosphatemia. Ann Emerg Med 1983; 12:107–116.
88. Zaloga GP: Phosphate disorders. In: Zaloga GP, ed: Endocrine emergencies. Problems in critical care, vol 4. Philadelphia, JB Lippincott, 1990; pp. 416–424.
89. Lee DBN, Kurokawa K: Physiology of phosphorus metabolism. In: Maxwell MH, Kleeman CR, Narins RG, eds: Clinical disorders of fluid and electrolyte metabolism, 4th ed. New York, McGraw-Hill, 1987; pp. 245–295.
90. Stoff JS: Phosphate homeostasis and hypophosphatemia. Am J Med 1982; 72:489–494.
91. O'Donovan DJ, Lotspeich WD: Activation of kidney mitochondrial glutaminase by inorganic phosphate and organic acids. Nature 1966; 212:930–932.
92. Dominguez JH, Gray RW, Lemann J: Dietary phosphate deprivation in women and men: effect on mineral and acid balances, parathyroid hormone, and the metabolism of 25-OH-vitamin D. J Clin Endocrinol Metab 1976; 43:1056–1068.
93. Knochel JP: Hypophosphatemia. West J Med 1981; 134:15–16.
94. Swaminathan R, Bradley P, Morgan DB, Hill GL: Hypophosphatemia in surgical patients. Surg Gynecol Obstet 1979; 148:448–454.
95. Knochel JP: The pathophysiology and clinical characteristics of severe hypophosphatemia. Arch Intern Med 1977; 137:203–220.
96. Aubier M, Murciano D, Lecocgic Y et al: Effect of hypophosphatemia on diaphragmatic contractility in patients with acute respiratory failure. N Engl J Med 1985; 313:420–424.
97. Agusti AGN, Torres A, Estopa R, Agusti-Vidal A: Hypophosphatemia as a cause of failed weaning: the importance of metabolic factors. Crit Care Med 1984; 12:142–143.
98. Fisher J, Magid N, Kallman C et al: Respiratory illness and hypophosphatemia. Chest 1983; 83:504–508.
99. Knochel JP, Barcenas C, Cotton JR et al: Hypophosphatemia and rhabdomyolysis. J Clin Invest 1978; 62:1240–1246.
100. Hettleman BD, Sabina RL, Drezner MK et al: Defective adenosine triphosphate synthesis: an explanation for skeletal muscle dysfunction in phosphate-deficient mice. J Clin Invest 1983; 72:582–589.
101. Montanari A, Borghi L, Curti A et al: Skeletal muscle cell abnormalities in acute hypophosphatemia during total parenteral nutrition. Miner Electrolyte Metab 1984; 10:52–57.
102. Rasmussen A, Buus S, Hessov I: Postoperative myocardial performance during glucose-induced hypophosphatemia. Acta Chir Scand 1985; 151:13–15.

103. Nanji AA, Freeman HJ: Postural hypotension and labile blood pressure associated with severe hypophosphatemia. Int J Cardiol 1984; 5:379–381.
104. Saglikes Y, Massry SG, Iseki K et al: Effect of phosphate depletion on blood pressure and vascular reactivity to norepinephrine and angiotensin II in the rat. Am J Physiol 1985; 248:F93-F99.
105. Nanji AA: The psychiatric aspect of hypophosphatemia. Can J Psychiatry 1984; 29:599–600.
106. Silvis SE, Pargas PD: Paresthesias, weakness, seizures, and hypophosphatemia in patients receiving hyperalimentation. Gastroenterology 1972; 62:513–520.
107. Yagnik P, Singh N, Burns R: Peripheral neuropathy with hypophosphatemia in a patient receiving intravenous hyperalimentation. South Med J 1985; 78:1381–1384.
108. Zaloga GP, Chernow B: Divalent ions: calcium, magnesium, and phosphorus. In: Chernow B, ed: Essentials of critical care pharmacology. Baltimore, Williams & Wilkins, 1989; pp. 348–381.
109. Gadisseux P, Sica DA, Ward JD, Becker DP: Severe hypophosphatemia after head injury. Neurosurgery 1985; 17:35–39.

CHAPTER 6

Fluid Therapy in the Early Postoperative Period

Loren D. Nelson

Case Report

The patient was a 48-year-old 80-kg white man admitted to the intensive care unit (ICU) following operative debridement for necrotic pancreatitis. In addition, drains were placed and packing was left in situ. The patient was kept intubated and was brought to the ICU. During the operation, he had received 6 L Ringer's lactate and 3 units of packed red cells. He made 80 ml of urine during the 3-hour case.

In the ICU, the patient initially had the following vital signs: blood pressure, 90/60 mm Hg; and pulse, 130/min. Pulmonary artery catheterization was carried out, and the results were as follows: pulmonary artery pressure (PAP), 20/12 mm Hg; wedge pressure, 8 mm Hg; and central venous pressure (CVP), 6 mm Hg. Initial cardiac outputs averaged 4.5 L/min. Urine output was 10 ml over the first hour.

Mechanical ventilator support included: positive end-expiratory pressure (PEEP), 10 cm H_2O; pressure support, 15 cm H_2O; FIO_2, 0.4; and intermittent mandatory ventilation, 8/min. Blood gas values were: PO_2, 111 mm Hg; PCO_2, 41 mm Hg; and pH 7.35. Laboratory data included: hematocrit/hemoglobin, 27/9.3; sodium, 137 mEq/L; potassium, 3.0 mEq/L; chloride, 99 mEq/L; and bicarbonate, 20 mEq/L. The patient was given 2 L of normal saline over the next 1.5 hours. This raised the cardiac output to 4.8 L as the wedge pressure increased to 10 mm Hg. The patient began to develop peripheral edema. Therefore, the remainder of resuscitation was then carried out with another 750 ml of plasma protein fraction (Plasmanate) and 2 units of packed red cells. The clinicians believed that both these components were more likely to remain in the intravascular space. In addition, 3% saline was started at an infusion rate of 60 ml/hr.

By the next day, the patient's values were: cardiac output, 6.9 L/min; PAP, 38/20 mm Hg; wedge pressure, 16 mm Hg; CVP, 12 mm Hg; and heart rate, 107/min. Positive fluid balance was 5.8 L. Blood gases were essentially unchanged on the same ventilator settings: PO_2, 103 mm Hg; PCO_2, 40 mm Hg; and pH 7.34 mm Hg.

Appropriate management of fluid administration is an essential element in the care of all patients undergoing surgical procedures. Fluid management has been traditionally, but arbitrarily, divided into three phases: preoperative, intraoperative, and postoperative. This chapter will review principles of fluid therapy in the early postoperative period.

THE RESUSCITATION CONTINUUM

Although perioperative fluid management has often been described as having three discrete phases,[1] in fact, it is a continuum. Each phase may dramatically alter the fluid management necessary in subsequent phases. For example, the patient who is profoundly dehydrated from preoperative vomiting who does not have adequate preoperative volume resuscitation can be anticipated to have a greater than normal intraoperative fluid requirement. Similarly, the patient with prolonged preoperative shock may receive satisfactory preoperative volume resuscitation but may have increased intraoperative fluid requirements because of high insensible losses that occur as the sequelae of shock.

Postoperative fluid management is affected even more dramatically by intraoperative events. Most patients undergoing surgical procedures who are well resuscitated intraoperatively require only a reasonable amount of maintenance fluid in the early postoperative period. Patients who experience intraoperative dehydration, hypovolemia, or shock may experience massive volume changes in the early postoperative period. The loss of normal homeostatic mechanisms caused by anesthesia seems to amplify the magnitude of postoperative fluid shifts.

Perioperative volume resuscitation is a continuum with each phase of resuscitation being highly dependent upon the previous phase.

NORMAL DISTRIBUTION OF FLUID AND ELECTROLYTES

In the uninjured patient there is a reasonably consistent distribution of the total body water into three primary compartments. Normally,

Table 6–1.
Normal Distribution of Total Body Water*

Space of Distribution	Lean Body Mass (%)	Total Body Water (%)	Volume in 70-kg Person
Total Body	60	100	42L
Intracellular	40	66	28L
Interstitial	15	25	10.5L
Intravascular	5	8	3.5L

* The distribution of water by percentage in each body fluid compartment and estimated volume of each compartment in a 70-kg person.

(Data modified from Demling RH, Wilson RF: Fluids, electrolytes, and acid-base balance: terminology. In: Demling RH, Wilson RF, eds: Decision making in surgical critical care. Philadelphia, BC Decker, 1988; pp. 127–132.)

total body water accounts for approximately 60% of the lean body mass of an adult (Table 6–1). This water is divided into intracellular and extracellular components. The intracellular component accounts for approximately two thirds or 40% of lean body mass. The extracellular component accounts for the other third or 20% of lean body mass. This is divided further into interstitial and intravascular components. Three quarters of the extracellular fluid or 15% of lean body mass is in the interstitial space, and one quarter of extracellular water or 5% of lean body mass is in the intravascular space.[2–4] While these rules can generally be applied to healthy adults, they cannot be applied to critically ill patients with shock or sepsis.

- *The usual distribution of fluid into various compartments may vary considerably in critically ill patients.*

There are dramatic alterations in the distribution of total body water in patients in significant catabolic states.[4] There is an overall increase in total body water with a large fraction of the increase in the interstitial space (Table 6–2). There is often depletion of the intravascular space and, occasionally, depletion or excess intracellular water. The actual alteration in the distribution of total body water primarily depends on the patient's underlying condition. Prolonged shock and sepsis are associated with the largest increases in interstitial fluid.

- *Sepsis and shock significantly increase the interstitial fluid compartment.*

Table 6–2.
Body Composition Changes During Catabolic States*

Component	Normal (%)	Catabolic (%)
Body weight (kg)	70.4	58.9
Extracellular water (L)	25.6 (36)	31.9 (54)
Body cell mass (kg)	24.7 (35)	14.7 (25)
Body fat (kg)	20.1 (29)	12.3 (21)

* The changes in body composition associated with severe catabolic states. Body weight decreases due to decreases in body cell mass and fat even though extracellular water increases both in absolute amount and percentage of total weight.

(Data modified from Wilmore DW: Homostasis: bodily changes in trauma and surgery. In: Sabiston DC, ed: Textbook of surgery: the biological basis of modern surgical practice. Philadelphia, WB Saunders, 1986; pp. 23–37; and Shizgal HM: Body composition. In: Fischer JE, ed: Surgical nutrition. Boston, Little, Brown, 1983; pp. 1–17.)

Table 6–3.
Normal Electrolyte Distribution*

Solute	Concentration (mEq/L) Plasma	Interstitial	Intracellular	Total Amount	Extracellular (%)	Intracellular (%)	Bone (%)	Exchangeable
Sodium	144	137	10	67	50	10	40	41
Potassium	4	4	140	58	2	94	4	44
Chloride	107	113	4	42	60	15	25	30
Bicarbonate	27	28	10	—	50	50	—	10–12
Magnesium	1.5	1.4	31	32	1	50	49	—
Calcium	2.5	2.4	0	940	<1	<1	99	—

* The normal distribution of most common electrolytes. The concentration in each body fluid compartment is shown in the first three columns. The total amount of each electrolyte (mEq/kg) is shown in column 4. The percentages of total electrolyte in extracellular and intracellular fluid and bone are shown in columns 5 to 7. The amount of freely exchangeable electrolyte (mEq/kg) is shown in column 8.

(Data modified from Goodenough RD, Burke JF: Fluid, electrolyte, and acid-base homeostasis in surgery. In: Burke JF, ed: Surgical physiology. Philadelphia, WB Saunders, 1983; pp. 35–50; and Demling RH, Wilson RF: Fluids, electrolytes, and acid-base balance: terminology. In: Demling RH, Wilson RF, eds: Decision making in surgical critical cases. Philadelphia, BC Decker, 1988; pp. 127–132.)

• *Interstitial fluid accumulation following shock results from altered permeability, not from the fluid volume administered.*

This has significant implications for the treatment of the highly stressed patient. Fluid therapy in critical illness must be directed toward appropriate fluid volume and electrolytes to meet the increased requirements of the interstitial space (Table 6–3). The alteration in membrane permeability causes an increase in the interstitial fluid volume and accounts for a significant amount of postresuscitation edema. It must be emphasized that postresuscitation edema develops because of permeability changes and not fluid administration. However, the fluid administration, which maintains an adequate circulatory volume, clearly contributes to interstitial and intracellular fluid increases and the resultant edema.

POSTOPERATIVE FLUID LOSSES

Postoperative fluid losses can be divided into three general categories: insensible, measurable, and "third space." Insensible fluid losses occur by evaporation or excretion from the lungs and skin. Measurable losses include those from the urinary tract, gastrointestinal (GI) tract, or through other tubes and drains. These measurable losses are quantifiable and analyzable in terms of their protein and electrolyte composition. The most difficult type of fluid shift to estimate takes place in the "third space" (body cavities, interstitial spaces, and intracellular spaces).

Insensible Postoperative Fluid Losses

Insensible fluid losses are the unmeasureable losses from the patient to the environment. The volume of insensible loss depends on a large number of factors related to both the patient and the environment. Normal insensible fluid losses for the average 70-kg individual range between 600 and 1200 ml per day.[5] However, they may vary greatly depending on conditions (Table 6–4).

Table 6–4.
Electrolyte and Water Composition of Secretions

Site	Volume (ml/d)	Na (mEq/L)	K (mEq/L)	Cl (mEq/L)	HCO^3 (mEq/L)
Urine	800–1500	10–80‡	90%*	97%*	—
Feces	0–250	0–20‡	10%*	3%*	—
Sweat	0–1000	10–60‡	0–5%*	0–10%*	—
Pulmonary	600–900	—	—	—	—
Salivary‡	500–2000	2–10	20–30	8–18	30
Gastric†	100–4000	9–116	0–32	8–154	—
Duodenal†	100–2000	140	5	80	—
Ileal†	100–9000	80–150	2–8	43–137	30
Colonic†	—	60	30	40	—
Pancreatic†	100–800	113–185	3–7	54–95	115
Biliary†	50–800	131–164	3–12	89–180	35

* Values listed are the percentage of total daily excretion from each site.

† Values listed are the ranges of volumes or concentrations of each solute present in each body fluid.

‡ Values listed are the sodium losses per day (mEq/day) from each site.

(Data modified from Shires GT, Canizaro PC: Fluid and electrolyte management of the surgical patient. In: Sabiston DC, ed: Textbook of Surgery: the biological basis of modern surgical practice. Philadelphia, WB Saunders, 1986; pp. 64–86.)

Normally, about half of the insensible fluid loss in a healthy individual occurs through the lungs. Estimated evaporative losses of free water from the lungs range from 0 to 8 ml/kg/day or about 400 to 500 ml/day.[5] Lung evaporative losses depend on the patient's exhaled minute ventilation, the patient's temperature, the room temperature, the relative humidity, and the relative hydration state of the patient. Losses tremendously increase in the highly catabolic, febrile patient with high minute ventilation. Lung evaporative losses from patients who require mechanical ventilation or humidified, closed breathing circuits may be negligible. In some circumstances, patients may gain water from the mechanical ventilator circuit.

Insensible losses from the skin also depend on the patient and on environmental factors. The presence or absence of fever and the general hydration state of the patient affect normal skin evaporative losses. The integrity of the skin directly controls evaporative cutaneous losses. Fluid losses through injured skin contribute to electrolyte and protein losses in patients with cutaneous burns.

Insensible losses may also occur from other open wounds related to surgical procedures or trauma. These open wounds may also contribute to the loss of electrolytes and protein. Normal minimal fluid and electrolyte losses and ranges of normal losses are easily estimated (Table 6–5). The volume of fluid lost via insensible routes may be staggering in patients with shock or sepsis who have severe capillary permeability defects.

Measurable Postoperative Fluid Losses

Measurable postoperative fluid losses occur from the urinary tract, the GI tract, and from other tubes and drains placed in body cavities,

Table 6–5.
Normal Adult Water and Electrolyte Requirements*

Component	Minimal Needs	Usual Needs
Sodium	0.3	0.7–3.6
Potassium	0.3–0.5	0.7–2.1
Calcium	0.2	0.4–1.1
Magnesium	0.2–0.4	0.3–0.7
Chloride	0.3	0.7–3.6
Water	870	1500

* The normal adult electrolyte requirements. Values for electrolytes are in mEq/kg/d and for water are in ml/m^2.

(Data modified from Goodenough RD, Burke JF: Fluid, electrolyte, and acid-base homeostasis in surgery. In: Burke JF, ed: Surgical physiology. Philadelphia, WB Saunders, 1983; pp. 35–50.)

hollow viscera, and various ducts. The measurable postoperative fluid losses are usually the easiest to manage since they are clearly quantifiable and the composition of the fluid losses can be accurately measured.

Postoperative urinary losses are primarily dependent upon the patient's solute load, intravascular volume status, and overall renal function. The normal solute load that must be excreted by the kidneys of a healthy 70-kg individual equals about 600 mOsm/day. This means that, in the presence of normal renal function, in which the kidney can concentrate 600 to 1200 mOsm/L of urine, the minimal obligatory urine output is about 500 to 1000 ml/day. Severely catabolic postoperative patients may have a much greater solute load presented to the kidneys. Kidneys that have sustained an injury from shock, sepsis, nephrotoxins, or diuretics may be unable to concentrate urine. In the absence of unusual solute, 0.5 ml/kg/hr is considered adequate.

- *A catabolic patient may have a significant increase in solute load to the kidneys and therefore greater fluid loss.*

In critically ill postoperative patients, solute loads may be increased in sepsis, after trauma, and in other catabolic states, and with osmotic loads from hyperglycemia, intravenous contrast administration, or osmotic diuretics. Catabolic states may interfere with the kidney's ability to concentrate urine to the normal maximum values, and the presence of increased solute loads necessitate higher urinary outputs. One solute load often overlooked is the sodium load that occurs following large volume crystalloid resuscitation in preoperative or intraoperative periods. A large volume crystalloid resuscitation may double the patient's total body sodium, causing an obligatory high solute volume (sodium) loss from the kidneys.

- *Large volume crystalloid resuscitation may ultimately result in large volume urinary outputs with high sodium losses.*

Acute or chronic endocrine abnormalities may dramatically alter urinary composition and volume. Aldosterone secretion is mediated by changes in the renin-angiotensin system. This is the hormone primarily responsible for the balance between sodium and potassium excretion by the kidneys.[4] Many postoperative states are associated with high renin formation and therefore with secondary hyperaldosteronism. In the presence of high levels of aldosterone, there is retention of sodium and high losses of urinary potassium. This at least partially explains the high incidence of postoperative hypokalemia.

Antidiuretic hormone (ADH) is secreted from the anterior pituitary and is primarily responsible for the control of water reabsorption from the distal tubule.[4] ADH secretion normally increases following trauma or major surgery. This increase in ADH causes retention of free water often in excess of the increased sodium retention due to aldosterone. This results in the dilutional hyponatremia so commonly seen in postoperative patients.

- *Appropriate antidiuretic hormone release following surgery or trauma results in an increase in free water accumulation and relative hyponatremia.*

Lack of ADH impairs free water reabsorption and results in hyperosmolar states caused by hypernatremia. Reduced ADH levels cause diabetes insipidus, a common clinical condition in patients with severe brain injury. It results in an inappropriately high urine output and free water loss.

The GI tract is the second major source of measurable postoperative fluid losses. The proximal GI tract acts as the secretory portion and the more distal GI tract the absorptive portion. Secretions from the proximal GI tract include saliva (up to 1000 ml/day), gastric (up to 1000 ml/day), and biliary/pancreatic (up to 1000 ml/day). A large volume of proximal secretions into the GI tract is normally reabsorbed in the distal small bowel (small amount) and colon (nearly all). This results in fluid loss from normal stool output of only about 100 ml/day. Obstruction of the proximal small bowel may cause upper GI tract fluid losses, which approach 3000 ml/day. Loss of distal tract absorption properties may result in stool losses of similar magnitude. The electrolyte composition of the fluid from each segment of the GI tract varies and may be estimated from standard tables or measured directly from the collected fluid (see Table 6–4). Assessment of the volume and composition of the fluid losses helps to optimize postoperative fluid management.

The third source of measurable losses includes that from tubes and drains that may be placed in body cavities, ducts, or soft tissues. Fluid losses from these spaces are often high in protein and usually have an electrolyte composition similar to that of serum.

Third-Space Postoperative Fluid Losses

By far the most complex and confusing perioperative fluid losses are the so called "third-space" fluid losses. Traditionally, the first resuscitation space has been considered to be the intravascular volume. It is difficult to know what the "second space" was meant to describe, but most likely it relates to the intracellular space. The "third space" refers to fluid present in the interstitial space and intracavitary areas such as the pleural and peritoneal cavities. In actuality there is a flux of fluid that occurs between these spaces and a dynamic equilibrium defined by the Starling equation.[6,7]

- *The "third space" refers to the interstitial space.*

The Starling equation quantitates the flux of fluid across membranes:

$$Q_f = K_f[(p_{mv} - p_{pmv}) - \delta(\pi_{mv} - \pi_{pmv})]$$

Table 6–6.
Classification of Hypovolemic Shock*

	Class I	Class II	Class III	Class IV
Blood loss	<750 ml	750–1500 ml	1500–2000 ml	>2000 ml
Blood volume	<15%	15–30%	30–40%	>40%
Heart rate	<100	>100	>120	>140
Blood pressure	normal	normal	normal to ↓	decreased
Urine output	>30 ml/hr	20–30 ml/hr	5–15 ml/hr	nil

* Initial presentation in unresuscitated shock.

Modified from Committee on Trauma, American College of Surgeons: Advanced trauma life support course: instructor manual. (Chicago American College of Surgeons, 1984; p. 185.)

It is clear from the Starling equation that fluid flux is governed by hydrostatic (p) and oncotic (π) pressure gradients across the membrane in question. The relative importance of these gradients is modified by the filtration factor (K_f) and the reflection coefficient (δ). The membrane in question determines the filtration factor. The reflection coefficient is also determined by the membrane characteristics, but, more importantly, by acute pathophysiologic changes within the patient. The reflection coefficient is often (mistakenly) assumed to be near 1.0. This would mean that oncotic pressure differences between the microvascular space (mv) and the perimicrovascular (pmv, interstitial) space have the same effect on fluid flux as the hydrostatic pressure gradient across the membrane. This assumption has not been borne out by scientific evidence. In fact, the reflection coefficient for the lung approximates 0.8 in normal conditions[6,8] and may fall to extremely low levels (0.1 to 0.3) in conditions associated with permeability pulmonary edema (i.e., acute respiratory distress syndrome).

Postoperative third-space fluid losses that follow uncomplicated elective surgical procedures are often quite minimal. When surgical procedures are complicated by large amounts of tissue injury (related either to dissection or direct trauma) fluid losses may increase dramatically. Third-space fluid losses are also increased in conditions of shock or sepsis (Table 6–6).

Shock and sepsis may dramatically increase third-space fluid losses by direct alteration of the reflection coefficient. This removes the beneficial effects of the normal oncotic pressure gradient, which tends to return fluid from the interstitium to the microvascular spaces. In addition, acute alternation of the reflection coefficient results in large molecules (such as albumin) that normally contribute to serum oncotic pressures, freely entering the interstitial space and contributing to additional third-space losses.

SELECTION OF POSTOPERATIVE FLUID REPLACEMENT

Two basic "rules" govern fluid management in virtually all patients. The first and most important rule is: "replace to the intravascular space what is lost from the intravascular space." If a patient bleeds

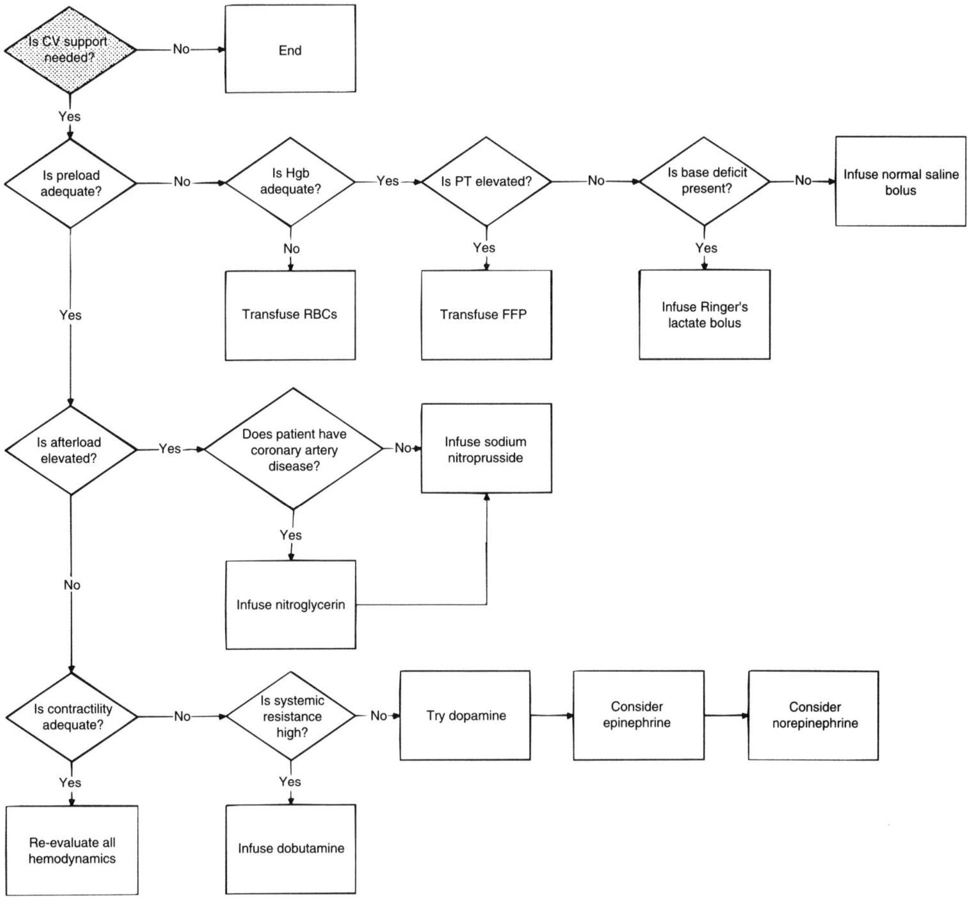

Figure 6–1.
An algorithm for the support of oxygen transport and stroke volume in critically ill patients with a pulmonary artery catheter in place. If cardiovascular (CV) support is needed, as determined by oxygen transport variables, preload is augmented, afterload reduced, and contractility enhanced. Preload augmentation is part of the postoperative fluid management in many critically ill surgical patients. Hgb, Hemoglobin concentration; PT, prothrombin time; RBCs, red blood cells; FFP, fresh frozen plasma.

and loses red blood cells and plasma, appropriate volume replacement must include red blood cells and plasma. If a patient loses fluid into the interstitial space, the resuscitation fluid management must include crystalloid solutions that approximate the electrolyte composition of interstitial fluid (Fig. 6–1).

A second general rule that can be applied to most patients in the perioperative period directs replacement of fluids with the assumption that homeostasis is more easily restored in an "economy of abundance." The vast majority of surgical patients can handle overreplacement of estimated fluids, and a brisk diuresis develops as the patient begins to mobilize fluid. Underresuscitation may result in prolongation of a hypoperfused state and lead to shock, worsened organ system dysfunction, or organ system failure. Even greater volumes of fluid may be required at a later period of time. Early fluid resuscitation may minimize the sequelae of prolonged hypovolemia and actually decrease the total volume of fluid required by the patient. The "economy of abundance" should not imply that patients be fluid overloaded. Rather, fluid resuscitation of patients should be tailored to their precise needs with the understanding that

- *In most patients, "over resuscitation" compared with "under resuscitation" results in fewer complications.*

underresuscitation is probably more detrimental in the long term than overresuscitation.

The next consideration in the selection of perioperative fluid replacement is the relative priority of different types of fluid (Fig. 6–1). Clearly, the bleeding patient needs blood more than crystalloid. A patient with a significant coagulopathy may need fresh frozen plasma more than albumin and the patient with thrombocytopenia may need platelets more than plasma.

Red Blood Cells

Restoration of red cell mass is vitally important in a patient with significant hemorrhage. The transfusion of red blood cells not only restores intravascular volume and peripheral perfusion, but also reestablishes oxygen-carrying capacity. Red blood cells improve oxygen delivery more than any other fluid.[9] Red cells provide a significant intravascular space to the interstitium. Red cells have an advantage over other oncotic agents in that they aid in maintenance of a favorable oncotic effect even in the presence of an extremely low reflection coefficient that would otherwise allow albumin and other large molecules to leak into the interstitium.

The transfusion of red blood cells has risks. The first is an immunologically mediated reaction to the red blood cells, plasma proteins, or potential allergens present in the blood. Modern blood banking techniques have reduced the incidence of major transfusion reactions to well within a clinically acceptable range. Major hemolytic reactions to transfused blood are almost unheard of today and are virtually always related to personnel and clerical errors.[10] Minor allergen-related reactions still occur and are usually manifested by fever and/or a rash beginning shortly after the administration of the blood. Very rarely, the allergic reaction may precipitate bronchospasm or even laryngospasm, which requires aggressive medical treatment. Much more commonly, however, the reaction terminates upon discontinuance of the blood product administration. Occasionally the administration of an antihistamine with or without an antipyretic may become necessary.

The other major concern that follows the transfusion of blood and blood products is the spread of transfusion-associated diseases.[11,12] Improved screening of blood and blood donors has decreased the incidence of hepatitis B virus transmission in blood products. In the 1980s, hepatitis C became a larger problem. At this time, improved screening techniques have significantly decreased the incidence of hepatitis C transmission resulting from transfusion of blood products.[13]

Also in the 1980s, the relationship between human immune deficiency virus (HIV) and transfusion of blood and blood products became painfully clear. Without question, there was a period in the mid-1980s during which blood and blood products donated by HIV-positive individuals were present in the world's blood pool. As increased awareness of HIV risk factors and better screening techniques for donated blood and blood donors became available, the risk of HIV transmission decreased dramatically. In the mid-1990s, the estimated risk of disease transmission from transfused blood is less than 0.1% per unit of blood products transfused.

• Better screening tests for blood transfusion have reduced the incidence of AIDS to less than 0.1% and the incidence of hepatitis C to 1 to 3%.

Programs that employ the directed donation of blood have not significantly reduced the incidence of blood-related infection problems. Autotransfusion and the preoperative banked autologous blood have eliminated this risk in patients who undergo elective surgical procedures.[14]

Another concern raised in the late 1980s and early 1990s was the potential immunosuppression that develops in patients who are transfused with significant amounts of blood. Data in regard to the immunosuppressive effects of transfusion are extremely difficult to interpret and often conflict.[15–22] Patients who receive significant amounts of blood exhibit a reduced immune response. They demonstrate increased tolerance to transplantation of solid organs.[23] Patients who receive significant volumes of blood may become immunosuppressed. As such, they may have an increased risk for recurrence of certain tumors, most notably those in the head and neck and in the colon.[24] However, it is not entirely clear whether the tumor recurrence relates to a larger initial tumor load, thus necessitating a greater magnitude of surgery and increased risk of bleeding and thus transfusion. Moreover, shock may predispose patients to a depressed immunologic response.[18]

• Red blood cell transfusion can increase tolerance to organ transplantation.

Patients who manifest significant signs of impaired oxygen transport related to a decrease in intravascular volume and compounded by a decreased oxygen-carrying capacity should receive red blood cells. This will improve total body oxygen delivery.[25–28] Concerns of infection or immunosuppression should be of secondary importance compared to the patient's immediate resuscitative needs.

• One unit of transfused blood roughly equals 1 L of increased cardiac output.

Fresh Frozen Plasma

Indications for fresh frozen plasma in postoperative patients are relatively clear.[28] Patients with a significant coagulopathy manifested by prolonged prothrombin time and who are either bleeding or at significant risk for bleeding should receive fresh frozen plasma. Fresh frozen plasma should not be used for restoration of intravascular volume if patients have no evidence of coagulopathy or active bleeding. Fresh frozen plasma may be used to reverse the effects of warfarin (Coumadin) and related anticoagulants in patients who are bleeding or who require emergency surgical procedures. The effects of these anticoagulants may also be reversed by parenteral administration of vitamin K when intravascular volume, active bleeding, and the need for reanticoagulation are not significant clinical concerns.

• Fresh frozen plasma should be used to correct coagulation defects, not for volume replacement.

Administration of fresh frozen plasma to patients at risk for large volume blood losses who have been transfused with packed red cells (rather than whole blood) may be prudent.[29–33] However, dilutional coagulopathies from large volume transfusions rarely result from the loss of clotting factors in patients who do not have significant liver disease. Bleeding related to massive transfusion is much more commonly associated with a dilutional thrombocytopenia or hypothermia.[34,35]

Other Blood Products

Other blood products occasionally need to be transfused in the patient who has received large volumes of red cells because of persistent bleeding or hemorrhagic shock. The most common blood product is platelets for treatment of persistent bleeding in patients with dilutional thrombocytopenia or acquired platelet dysfunction.[30,36] The indications for platelet transfusion generally are not based solely upon the total platelet count.[34] However, some guidelines are available. Spontaneous onset of bleeding is extremely uncommon in adult patients with functional platelets whose counts exceed 20,000/mm^3. Patients at high risk for bleeding complications probably should be transfused platelets to keep the total platelet count greater than 50,000/mm^3. Patients with active bleeding who require continued transfusion probably should receive platelets to maintain the total platelet count greater than 100,000/mm^3.[37]

• *In actively bleeding patients, the platelet count should be kept above 100,000 mm^3.*

Once the clinical indication for platelet transfusion has been identified, the dose of platelets should be tailored to the patient's size. Generally, 1 unit of platelets is transfused for ever 10 kg of body weight. This dose of platelets should raise the total platelet count by approximately 50,000/mm^3. An increase of less than 50,000 with this dose implies ongoing platelet sequestration or consumption. The transfusion may be repeated as necessary, depending on the patient's bleeding status and platelet count.

Assessment of platelet dysfunction in surgical patients is often difficult, and precise tests for platelet function are often available only in specialized laboratories. When there is no evidence of significant coagulopathy (i.e., prothrombin time and partial thromboplastin times are normal) and the total platelet count is greater than 100,000/mm^3, the bleeding time may be a useful test to assess the adequacy of platelet function. In the absence of other coagulopathies and a normal platelet count, a bleeding time in excess of 9 minutes may be suggestive of platelet dysfunction. A bleeding time of less than 6 minutes rules out significant coagulopathy or platelet dysfunction in most patients.

• *Bleeding time can provide significant information on the adequacy of platelet function.*

Cryoprecipitate is occasionally indicated in the patient who is bleeding or is at great risk for bleeding from factor VIII deficiency or decreased fibrinogen. Cryoprecipitate contains more factor VIII on a volume basis than does fresh frozen plasma. Cryoprecipitate is also the most concentrated source for fibrinogen for patients who have a consumptive coagulopathy, who have not responded to fresh frozen plasma, and who have hypofibrinogenemia. Since it is a pooled unit, cryoprecipitate carries a higher infection risk than a unit of fresh frozen plasma. This must be balanced against the clinical situation. The dose of cryoprecipitate is usually 10 units.

• *Cryoprecipitate, on a volume basis, contains a greater amount of factor VIII than does fresh frozen plasma. However, the risks of hepatitis and AIDS are significantly increased with this agent.*

Albumin and Other Colloids

The administration of albumin and other colloid solutions as part of the postoperative fluid management can still generate controversy.[38–40] The two points on which nearly all agree are: (1) colloids are significantly more expensive than crystalloids; and (2) colloids are more efficient in acutely increasing intravascular volume.[41,42] The areas that remain questionable include: (1) Do colloids improve outcome? (2) Do colloids worsen organ system dysfunction? (3) Do colloids achieve their physiologic intent?

- *Colloids require less volume to restore intravascular volume than do crystalloids. However, outcome may favor crystalloids.*

Numerous clinical and basic studies have demonstrated that colloid administration is approximately threefold more efficient in the restoration of intravascular volume than crystalloid administration. This means that resuscitation with colloid can be accomplished with one third the volume necessary with crystalloids. The increased efficiency of colloid to raise intravascular volume carries a risk of intravascular overload and hydrostatic pulmonary edema.[43–46] The implication for resuscitation of hypovolemic shock following surgery is that careful clinical monitoring must be performed to prevent intravascular fluid overload.

Colloid solutions that are typically available in the United States today include concentrated (25%) albumin solution, 5% albumin or purified protein fraction solutions, colloid starch suspensions, and dextrans.[47] The adverse effects on platelet aggregation and the potential for allergic reactions preclude dextrans as a perioperative intravascular volume expander. The remainder of this section will deal with albumin and starch-containing solutions.

A number of prospective randomized clinical trials have compared a pure crystalloid volume resuscitation with combined crystalloid and colloid resuscitation in both surgical and nonsurgical patients. There are reported advantages and disadvantages of each resuscitation regimen. Some differences reflect patient selection and others the physiologic end points selected or the type of fluid administered.[48] One of the more interesting overviews in regard to the use of colloid solutions for fluid management was performed by Velanovich.[49] This was a meta-analysis of prospective randomized trials with specific resuscitation end points and outcome. Crystalloid and crystalloid-colloid regimens were compared. The most striking feature seemed to be an outcome (i.e., mortality) advantage of pure crystalloid solutions in surgical patients and an outcome advantage of mixed crystalloid-colloid resuscitations in medical patients (Fig. 6–2). The differences were statistically significant although the clinical implications of the meta-analysis are not entirely clear.

It is easy to understand the observed outcome advantage of colloid over crystalloid since colloid more efficiently expands the intravascular volume.[50] However, it is unclear whether colloids are worth the great increase in patient cost incurred by their use. Colloids are approximately 15- to 60-fold more expensive than crystalloids on a volume basis. When the efficiency factor is included, colloids will still cost 5 to 15 times as much as crystalloids used to similar resuscitation end points.

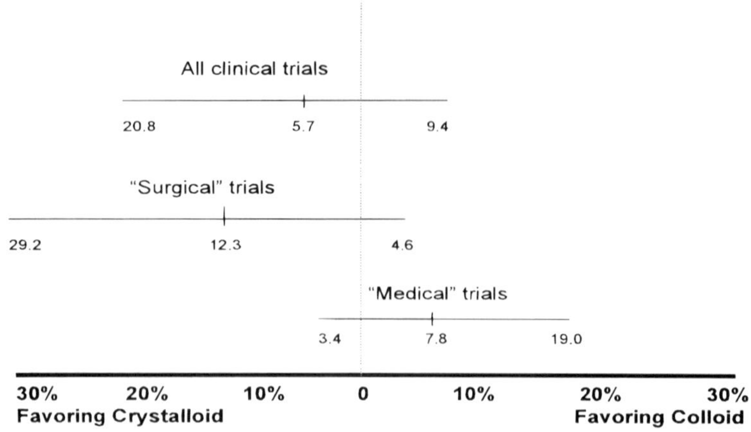

Figure 6–2.
Meta-analysis allows the pooling of data from several similar studies to compare defined outcomes between patients resuscitated with pure crystalloid and those receiving crystalloid and colloid. The chart displays the average and range of mortality advantages of two resuscitation regimens. The data show a slight outcome (mortality) advantage (5.7%) of crystalloid over colloid resuscitation for all studies. Patients with trauma and "surgical" diseases showed an advantage with crystalloid (12.3%), but "medical" patients showed an outcome advantage with colloid (7.8%). (Modified from Velanovich V: Cystalloid versus colloid fluid resuscitation: a meta-analysis of mortality. Surgery 1989; 105:65–71.)

- *Some studies suggest that albumin administration may interfere with some organ function including the lung.*

Albumin may have detrimental effects on end-organ function. Several studies have demonstrated an impairment in coagulation following colloid administration.[51–54] Additional studies have shown rather unequivocal evidence that albumin administration impairs renal function[55,56] and the kidney's ability to excrete sodium. Other studies have demonstrated a possible adverse effect on myocardial contractility[57,58] and vasodilation[59] using commercially prepared albumin solutions. Finally, a number of studies suggest that pulmonary function is more severely compromised following albumin resuscitation versus a pure crystalloid resuscitation.[43,44,46,60–63] There appears a propensity to develop hydrostatic pulmonary edema from overresuscitation when albumin solutions are used. The second pulmonary problem encountered with colloids involves patients with permeability defects in the lung microvasculature. Increased colloid oncotic pressures may potentially develop in the lung interstitium as colloid leaks through the endothelium.[64] The presence of colloid in the pulmonary interstitium or alveoli may theoretically pull more fluid into these spaces and prolong the need for mechanical ventilation.

The starch-derived colloids, such as hydroxyethyl starch, may have a slight cost advantage over albumin-containing solutions. Additionally, starch-derived colloids eliminate concern for administration of blood-derived products. The starch-derived colloids seem to be equally efficacious when compared with albumin solutions in their ability to reach similar physiologic resuscitation end points.[65] Unfortunately, starch-derived colloid solutions share the high cost and lack of demonstrable improvement in patient outcome seen with other colloid solutions.

Finally, some data indicate that starch-containing solutions may interfere with the body's reticuloendothelial system, particularly the Kupffer cells of the liver. Because of minor effects on coagulation, theoretic limits to the volume of starch solution administration have been suggested.[41] Generally, these limits are somewhere between 1 and 2 L per day.

The most clear-cut guide to the use of colloid solutions would seem to be the first rule of volume resuscitation: to replace to the intravascular space what is lost from the intravascular space. When patients have high albumin and protein losses due to reaccumulation of ascites, pleural effusions, or extrinsic losses from burns and other soft tissue injuries, it would seem appropriate to replace these albumin losses with albumin solutions. It would also seem prudent to replace albumin in patients who have marked impairment of hepatic albumin synthesis. However, in the vast majority of postoperative patients colloid-containing solutions have little or no role, are quite costly, and show no benefit in improving patient outcome.

Crystalloid Solutions

Sodium-containing crystalloid solutions are the mainstay of perioperative fluid management. These solutions may be tailored to meet precise electrolyte and volume requirements in a variety of clinical situations and may be used to meet insensible fluid losses, measurable fluid losses, and the third-space fluid losses acquired by critically ill surgical patients.

Normal postoperative maintenance fluid requirements are usually met by the administration of a solution approximating half normal saline and supplemented as needed with a potassium-containing electrolyte solution. A maintenance fluid administration rate of approximately 1 ml/kg/hr will generally meet insensible fluid losses and minimal obligatory urinary fluid losses in patients whose clinical situation is uncomplicated. Additional maintenance fluid is often added to meet the requirement of an "economy of abundance," with the assumption that normal kidneys will eliminate excess sodium and water. Thus, a total maintenance fluid administration volume for a patient without extraordinary fluid losses may approximate 1.25 to 2.0 ml/kg/hr of half normal saline with supplemental potassium as needed. Five percent dextrose added to this routine maintenance will maintain the solution isotonic.

Additional postoperative fluid is needed to meet specific measurable fluid losses. In particular, extreme losses of fluid from the GI tract deplete or lower optimal intravascular volume. These losses should be replaced. Since the electrolyte composition of GI secretions varies with location, the electrolyte constitution of specific replacement fluids should be tailored to that which is lost (see Table 6–4). When small to moderate GI losses occur, the electrolyte com-

- *Large gastrointestinal tract fluid losses may require specific electrolyte correction. Ordinarily large gastric losses result in a hypochloremic alkalosis.*

position of the replacement fluid can be based on the known usual composition of that fluid. Daily monitoring of serum electrolyte concentrations may help in the day-to-day modification of maintenance and replacement fluids. When patients have extraordinarily high GI losses, it may be prudent to measure the electrolyte composition of these losses, to better tailor the specific replacement fluids.

The choice of fluids for the postoperative resuscitation of the hemodynamically unstable patient is difficult. As indicated previously, fluid losses from the interstitium of patients who have sustained prolonged shock or sepsis are unpredictable and are difficult to estimate. There is building evidence that electrolyte composition of resuscitation fluid for the patients in shock should serve to normalize the electrolyte composition of the interstitial space.

The initial studies that demonstrated the improved efficacy of crystalloid resuscitation for hypovolemic shock were performed by Shires and associates in the 1960s.[66,67] These carefully controlled animal and clinical studies demonstrated an improvement in outcome when resuscitation was continued to normalize not only the intravascular volume, but also the interstitial volume. When animals were resuscitated after a period of hemorrhagic shock with all their shed blood, the mortality was 80%. When the animals were resuscitated with all their shed blood plus a volume of plasma estimated to normalize the intravascular volume, the mortality remained at 70%. Only when the animals were given their shed blood plus a volume of balanced salt solution with the approximate composition of interstitial fluid to a volume that normalized *interstitial* volume did mortality dramatically fall to 30%. These results led Shires and others to advocate shock resuscitation with a combination of the estimated blood volume which had been lost plus balanced salt solution to normalize hemodynamics.[67–71]

It is clear that resuscitation of hypovolemic shock which includes restoration of interstitial volume is of great importance in critically ill postoperative patients (Fig. 6–3). It has become apparent that restoration of the interstitial sodium concentration may be of greater importance. Studies that have used hypertonic saline have demonstrated that smaller resuscitation volumes can achieve reach similar physiologic end points.[72–75] The advantage of hypertonic solutions over isotonic solutions is the reduced volume requirement.[76,77] Generally, when solutions that contain approximately twice the sodium concentration of normal saline are used, half the usual volume is required to reach the same physiologic end point. Hypertonic salt solutions can reduce postresuscitation edema. Hypertonic solutions have been used for resuscitation of major burns,[76,77] severe closed head injuries,[78–81] and hypovolemic shock.[82] Although these solutions are clearly associated with a lower resuscitation volume load, the effect on patient outcome and mortality has yet to be delineated.[83,84] In general, hypertonic saline solutions should be infused at a rate less than 100 ml/hr. This will avoid hypernatremia of greater than 160 mEq/L. Standard hypertonic saline solutions can result in hyperchloremia and metabolic acidosis. Substitution of acetate for chloride by the addition of 100 to 200 mEq of sodium acetate to a liter of normal saline can accomplish this end.

• *Hypertonic saline for fluid resuscitation can result in less overall volume administered. However, it can cause hyperchloremic acidosis.*

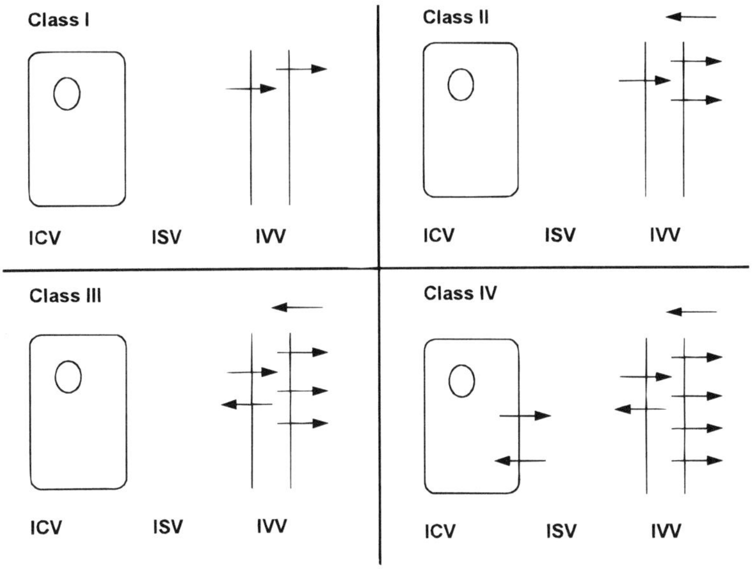

Figure 6–3.
Fluid flux in patients with hemorrhagic shock. In class I shock, fluid leaving the intravascular volume (IVV) is replaced by interstitial fluid by the process known as "plasma refill". In class II shock, more volume is lost from the intravascular space, and plasma refill continues from the interstitial volume (ISV). At this time, intravenous fluid is usually given to supplement the intravascular volume. In class III shock, the capillary membrane integrity is being lost, and fluid begins to leak freely between the IVV and the ISV; edema begins to appear. In class IV shock, the cell membrane integrity is lost, allowing flux of fluid between the intracellular space (ICV), the interstitium, and intravascular space.

ASSESSMENT OF VOLUME REQUIREMENTS

The nature of postoperative fluid losses must be determined. As indicated earlier, insensible losses are generally easy to estimate and may be replaced primarily with free water and a very small amount of sodium. Measurable losses can be calculated, and when the electrolyte composition of the fluid loss is in question, it can be measured directly. The most difficult assessment of fluid is estimation of third-space losses caused by direct injury, shock, or sepsis.

Three general means have been used to assess the adequacy of circulating volume and the adequacy of resuscitation following trauma or major surgical procedures: (1) general end-organ perfusion; (2) hemodynamic monitoring; and (3) oxygen transport monitoring.[85]

General End-Organ Perfusion

In the vast majority of surgical patients, the only necessary assessment of intravascular volume is the state of end-organ perfusion. These include brain, skin, and kidneys. Evaluation of these systems and measurement of vital signs and response to fluid challenges serve as adequate indicators of circulating volume in more than 90% of surgical patients.

Completely normal mental status indicates maintenance of cerebral perfusion. Unfortunately, in most surgical patients mental status is difficult to assess because of residual effects of anesthetics, narcotics, sedatives, and other drugs. In addition, cerebral perfusion can be well maintained into the later stages of hypovolemic shock. Since most of the body's compensatory mechanisms are aimed at cerebral perfusion preservation central nervous system function does not change until the advanced stages of shock.

Cutaneous perfusion can also assess the adequacy of circulatory volume. A patient with warm skin and good distal capillary refill generally has an adequate circulating volume. However, states associated with vasoderegulation such as sepsis, spinal cord injury, and regional anesthetics often cause a significant maldistribution of blood flow that favors skin perfusion at the expense of more vital organs. In these patients, warm skin may actually imply a worsening in their vasoregulatory state. Furthermore, patients with acute and chronic vascular disease may show markedly impaired cutaneous perfusion when central perfusion is, in fact, totally adequate.

Urine output and renal function are probably the most important clinical indicators of the adequacy of circulating volume. Patients who have normal vital signs and adequate urine output are generally well perfused. A number of factors may pathologically increase urine output even during conditions of relative intravascular volume depletion.

One of the most common causes of inappropriately high urinary output in postoperative patients is the presence of an osmotic diuresis. This osmotic diuresis may be initiated by hyperglycemia and glucosuria, intravenous contrast for radiographic procedures, or an osmotic diuretic such as mannitol. In addition, large amounts of sodium associated with volume resuscitation can induce diuresis. Alcohol intoxication may also present a slight increase in osmotic load. Alcohol can also inhibit secretion of ADH.

A period of shock, which causes significant renal tubule injury, but then is partially resuscitated, may be associated with an nonoliguric form of acute renal insufficiency.[86] In this situation, the renal tubules cannot concentrate urine, and they put out a high urine volume in spite of continued intravascular volume depletion. Postobstructive diuresis following decompression of a previously distended urinary tract can cause diuresis.

Prior administration of diuretic agents may also significantly increase urinary output, at least transiently, even with a depleted intravascular volume. Drugs such as dopamine, which has a direct diuretic and naturetic effect, may also increase urinary output in spite of reduced circulating volume. Vasopressors or inotropes can contract the vascular bed and can thereby initially create the impression of adequate hemodynamics and renal perfusion in spite of intravascular volume depletion. When attempts are made to decrease the infusion of the vasopressor, significant hemodynamic deterioration will develop.

Hemodynamic Measurements in the Assessment of Intravascular Volume

Traditional vital signs are essential in the assessment of circulating volume. Heart rate, blood pressure, and the response of these variables to a change in body position are part of the routine assessment in nearly all surgical patients. In the absence of significant underlying heart disease and medications that alter normal cardiovascular reflexes, a normal blood pressure and a slow heart rate generally imply an adequate circulatory volume. In the presence of significant cardiac disease or medications affecting the autonomic nervous system and normal cardiovascular reflexes, the interpretation of pulse and blood pressure must be done with caution.

Tachycardia is a relatively sensitive but extremely nonspecific response (Table 6–6). Tachycardia usually occurs with intravascular volume depletion and shock but also may be caused by pain, anxiety, agitation, fever, hypoxemia, hypercarbia, acidemia, and a variety of other abnormalities often seen in critically ill postoperative patients. The presence of tachycardia therefore should be a red flag that alerts the health care team to look further into the causes.

Blood pressure is of such fundamental importance that many of the body's autonomic responses are geared specifically to its maintenance. Baroreceptors present in the carotid sinus and aortic arch trigger reflexes to induce vasoconstriction, tachycardia, and increased myocardial contractility. These persist until volume depletion becomes so severe that the homeostatic mechanisms fail. A delay in therapy until blood pressure decreases and indicates intravascular volume depletion can result in significant delays in appropriate treatment and may compromise the patient's outcome.

• *During hypovolemic states, blood pressure may remain normal until intravascular volume has been depleted by 20 to 25%.*

Because of the problems associated with the assessment of general perfusion status, end-organ function, and traditional vital signs, clinicians have searched for other means to detect hypovolemia at an early point in time. The so-called "tilt test" can, in some patients, demonstrate the inability to compensate fully for decreased circulating volume. In the absence of medications that impair autonomic nervous system function and hemodynamic response to stress, head elevation of a hypovolemic patient will usually induce tachycardia and perhaps lower blood pressure. Generally, this is an indication of marginal or compromised circulating intravascular volume.

In spite of all of the noninvasive assessment means available to the clinician, a small number of postoperative patients will need invasive hemodynamic monitoring to better assess their intravascular volume status and the adequacy of perfusion.[85,87,88] Complete hemodynamic monitoring may also be necessary to guide fluid administration in patients with complex postoperative courses and multiple organ system dysfunction or failure. In the 1990s, complete hemodynamic monitoring implies placement of a flow-directed pulmonary artery catheter capable of measurement of intravascular pressures and cardiac output.[89] One of the most difficult issues associated with pulmonary artery catheterization concerns determination of the adequacy and appropriateness of the measured values in an individual patient. Hemodynamic monitoring should provide a data base that will provide the clinician information necessary to optimize the delivery of oxygen and other substrates that meet the requirements of metabolically active tissues.

• *Rather than a specific cardiac output level, patients should be manipulated to a cardiac output which meets metabolic demands.*

Cardiac output, determined by the heart rate and stroke volume, depends on the interactions among preload, afterload, and contractility. There are no normal values for cardiac output and only wide ranges of normal cardiac indices adjusted for the body surface area of the patient. Since blood pressure is relatively constant in most healthy patients, metabolic demands determined by tissue mass necessitate variations in cardiac output according to the patient's size. Since there are no normal values for cardiac output, all of the variables used to assess normal hemodynamics must be based on cardiac index and, therefore, the size of the patient.

Cardiac preload remains the single most important determinant of stroke volume index. Fiber length of the cardiac myofibrils at end-diastole defines preload. The fiber length directly relates to the end-diastolic volume, which may be used as an indicator of ventricular preload. For the many years that the flow-directed pulmonary artery catheter has been available, clinicians have often assumed that ventricular compliance is relatively fixed and, therefore, end-diastolic pressures, to some degree, reflect preload. Commonly, the pulmonary artery occlusion pressure (PAOP) has been used as an indication of left ventricular end-diastolic pressure. This assumption requires a properly positioned catheter, carefully transduced measurements, and no significant mitral valve disease. A patient who has an inadequate cardiac index and a low PAOP is generally believed to have intravascular volume depletion. A volume challenge may be given with the intent of improved cardiac index secondary to a raised ventricular end-diastolic volume (see Fig. 6–1). This assumption is generally valid as long as PAOP is low.

Elevations in PAOP follow an absolute increase in circulating volume, a decrease in left ventricular function, or an increase in intrathoracic pressure secondary to positive pressure mechanical ventilation. Therefore, a low PAOP in a patient with inadequate cardiac output can generally be assumed to be an indicator of volume depletion, and a volume challenge may be safely applied. Patients with a high PAOP are much more difficult, since a high PAOP is not necessarily associated with an increased or even adequate ventricular end-diastolic volume. A high PAOP will only reflect intravascular volume overload if intrapleural pressures and left ventricular function are normal.

• *New pulmonary artery catheters that permit calculation of end-diastolic volume provide a better aid to fluid resuscitation than does the use of pulmonary capillary occlusion pressure.*

Because of the difficulties involved in interpretation of pressure measurements as an indicator of preload, new technology has become available to assess ventricular end-diastolic volume. This technology uses a thermodilution technique.[90] This indirect measurement of end-diastolic volume seems to be a better indicator of both preload and preload-recruitable increases in cardiac output in response to fluid challenge.[91–93]

Ventricular afterload assessment presents equal difficulties. Afterload is generally defined as the impedance to ejection from the left ventricle.[94,95] Determinants of ventricular afterload include aortic valve resistance, left ventricular compliance, aortic compliance, systemic vascular resistance, and the mass and viscosity of the blood. The most easily assessed and treatable variable is systemic vascular resistance. Since this value requires the cardiac output values, it must be indexed to body surface area in order to be interpreted. While there are many determinants of systemic vascular resistance index, isolated intravascular volume depletion in the absence of confounding medications and other pathophysiologic states (i.e., sepsis) is usually associated with an increase in systemic vascular resistance index.[96]

Oxygen Transport as an Assessment of Intravascular Volume Adequacy

Since the early 1980s, the adequacy of cardiac output has generally been defined in terms of oxygen transport variables. These include the delivery of oxygen from the left ventricle, the uptake of oxygen by the peripheral tissues, and the ratio of these two variables, the oxygen utilization coefficient. Intravascular volume depletion usually results in a compromise in oxygen delivery to the tissue. Severe reductions in oxygen delivery may result in flow-limited oxygen consumption, which, when unchecked, may result in anaerobic metabolism, further shock, and death of the patient.[97,98]

The addition of mixed venous oximetry to the flow-directed pulmonary artery catheter has allowed on-line assessment of these oxygen transport indices.[99] A decrease in mixed venous oxygen saturation acts as a sensitive but nonspecific indicator of global oxygen transport imbalance. A decrease in mixed venous oxygen saturation indicates an increase in the oxygen utilization coefficient (oxygen extraction ratio), which means that a greater fraction of delivered oxygen has been consumed. Mixed venous oxygen saturation is also used in the calculation of the arterial-venous oxygen content difference (Ca-vDO_2). This indicates the adequacy of cardiac output to meet tissue oxygen consumption. An increase in Ca-vDO_2 indicates greater extraction of oxygen by the tissue to maintain the necessary oxygen consumption (Fig. 6–4). When hemodynamic measurements indicate that reduced preload may be at least partially responsible for an impairment in oxygen transport, a volume challenge intended to optimize preload, thus improving cardiac output and oxygen delivery, seems warranted.[85,100,101]

- *A decrease in mixed venous oxygen saturation usually indicates inadequate oxygen delivery.*

Treatment with preload augmentation to reach an optimal oxygen-delivery value or to achieve a level of oxygen consumption that is independent of delivery may prove to be a desirable therapeutic end point.[102,103] This is most efficiently achieved by transfusing red blood cells, which increase oxygen-carrying capacity. When hemoglobin concentration has been optimized, other fluids may be used.

Lactic acidosis represents the final indicator of inadequate oxygen transport. This marks the onset of anaerobic metabolism. The demand for oxygen at the tissue level has exceeded the actual use of oxygen by the tissue (Fig. 6–4). The clearance of lactate and the

- *Development of lactic acidosis usually indicates that all compensatory systems to meet oxygen demands have been exhausted.*

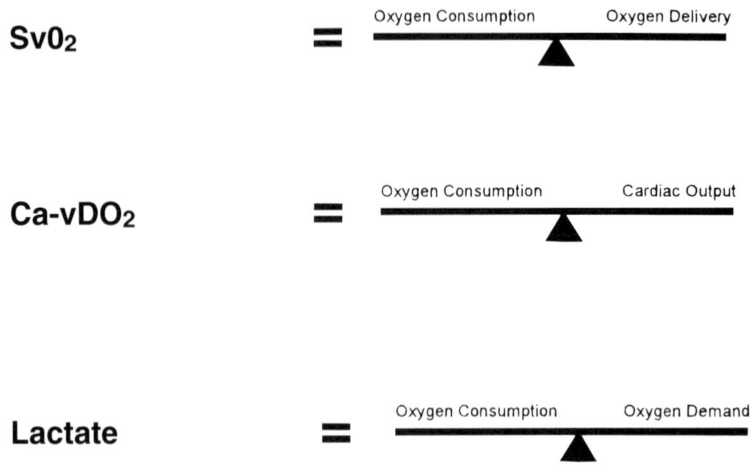

Figure 6–4.
The three critical balances. Three oxygen transport balances are often assessed in critically ill postoperative patients. Each of the balances assess the relationship between oxygen consumption and other variables. The balance between oxygen consumption and oxygen delivery is assessed by measuring the mixed venous oxygen saturation (SvO_2) or the oxygen utilization coefficient (extraction ratio, VO_2/DO_2). The balance between oxygen consumption and cardiac output is determined by the Fick equation to be equal to the arterial-venous oxygen content difference, $Ca\text{-}vDO_2$. The balance between oxygen demand (the volume needed to function aerobically) and oxygen consumption (the volume actually used) is reflected by the arterial lactate level. When oxygen demand exceeds oxygen consumption, excess lactate appears.

accompanying metabolic acidosis generally indicates an improvement in oxygen transport balance.[104,105] The fluid challenge may be an important diagnostic and therapeutic maneuver in patients with lactic acidosis unexplained by other reasons.[106]

CLINICAL RECOMMENDATIONS

Knowledge of normal fluid and electrolyte physiology and of normal fluid losses aids the clinician in the selection of postoperative fluid management. Knowledge of the electrolyte composition of extraordinary fluid losses helps greatly in the replacement of the lost electrolytes. Assessment of third-space fluid losses in critically ill patients presents a difficult problem. These fluid losses must be replaced with a balanced electrolyte solution that approximates the normal electrolyte concentration of interstitial fluid. The volume required to meet the interstitial space requirements can be difficult to estimate or to assess. The clinician should maintain an adequate circulating blood volume and oxygen transport balance in order to optimize organ perfusion. Resuscitation from shock and maintenance of good end-organ function will restore the integrity of the capillary membranes. The excess interstitial fluid will be reabsorbed by the lymphatic system and returned to the intravascular space. The resultant increase in intravascular volume will be followed by postresuscitation diuresis, which will occur over the next 48 to 72 hours.

The priorities for postoperative fluid management continue to be: (1) replacement of red cell mass; (2) replacement of coagulation factors in the patient at high risk of bleeding; (3) replacement of intravascular volume; and (4) maintenance of adequate interstitial volume. A physiologic approach to fluid replacement, based on a careful assessment of fluid needs determined by the patient and goal-directed administration of fluids to predetermined physiologic values, is effective in reducing postoperative organ system dysfunction and failure.

REFERENCES

1. Gold MS: Perioperative fluid management. Crit Care Clin 1992; 8: 409–421.
2. Goodenough RD, Burke JF: Fluid, electrolyte, and acid-base homeostasis in surgery. In: Burke JF, ed: Surgical physiology. Philadelphia, WB Saunders, 1983; pp. 35–50.
3. Layon AJ, Bernards WC, Kirby RR: Fluids and electrolytes in the critically ill. In: Civetta JM, Taylor RW, Kirby RR, eds: Critical care. Philadelphia, JB Lippincott, 1992; pp. 457–480.
4. Shizgal, HM: Body composition. In: Fischer JE ed: Surgical nutrition. Boston, Little, Brown, 1983; pp. 1–17.
5. Wilmore DW: Homeostasis: bodily changes in trauma and surgery. In: Sabiston DC, ed: Textbook of surgery: the biological basis of modern surgical practice. Philadelphia, WB Saunders, 1986; pp. 23–37.
6. Civetta JM: A new look at the Starling equation. Crit Care Med 1979; 7:84.
7. Peters RM, Hargens AR: Protein vs electrolytes and all of the Starling forces. Arch Surg 1981; 116:1293–1298.
8. Taylor AE: Capillary fluid filtration: Starling forces and lymph flow. Circ Res 1981; 49:557–575.
9. Czer LSC, Shoemaker WC: Optimal hematocrit value in critically ill postoperative patients. Surg Gynecol Obstet 1978; 147:363.
10. Myhre B: Fatalities from blood transfusion. JAMA 1980; 244: 1333–1335.
11. Aach RD, Kahn RA: Post-transfusion hepatitis: current perspectives. Ann Intern Med 1980; 92:539.
12. Miller RD: Medical intelligence: complications of massive blood transfusions. Anesthesiology 1973; 39:82–93.
13. Gitnick G: Non-A, non-B hepatitis: etiology and clinical course. Annu Rev Med 1984; 35:265.
14. Glover JL, Broadie TA: Autotransfusion in trauma. Crit Care Q 1983; 6:33–43.
15. Agarwal N, Murphy JG, Cayten CG, Stahl WM: Blood transfusion increases the risk of infection after trauma. Arch Surg 1993; 128: 171–177.
16. Alexander JW: Transfusion-induced immunomodulation and infection. Transfusion 1991; 31:195–196.
17. Chaudry IH, Ayala A, Ertel W, Stephan R: Hemorrhage and resuscitation: immunological aspects. Am J Physiol Soc 1990; 259:R663-R678.

18. Cue JI, Peyton JC, Malangoni MA: Does blood transfusion or hemorrhagic shock induce immunosuppression? J Trauma 1992; 32: 613–617.
19. Edna TH, Bjerkeset T: Association between blood transfusion and infection in injured patients. J Trauma 1992; 33:659–661.
20. Graves TA, Cioffi WG, et all: Relationship of transfusion and infection in a burn population. J Trauma 1989; 29:948–954.
21. Mezrow CK, Bergstein I, Tartter PI: Postoperative infections following autologous and homologous blood transfusions. Transfusion 1992; 32:27–30.
22. Rosemurgery AS, Hart MB, Murphy CG et al: Infection after injury. Am Surg 1992; 58:104–107.
23. Opelz G, Sengar DPS, Mickey MR, Terasaki P: Effect of blood transfusions on subsequent kidney transplants. Transplant Proc 1973; 5: 253–259.
24. Wu HS, Little AG: Perioperative blood transfusions and cancer recurrence. J Clin Oncol 1988; 6:1348–1354.
25. Fortune JB, Feustel PJ, Saifi J et al: Influence of hematocrit on cardiopulmonary function after acute hemorrhage. J Trauma 1987; 27: 243–249.
26. Phillips TF, Soulier G, Wilson RF: Outcome of massive transfusion exceeding two blood volumes in trauma and emergency surgery. J Trauma 1987; 27:903–910.
27. Watkins GM, Glover JL, Greenburg AG, Friedman BA: Panel: "Present use of blood and blood products." J Trauma 1981; 21: 1005–1012.
28. Wilson RF: Complications of massive transfusions. Surg Rounds 1981; 8:47–54.
29. Heimbach DM: Hemostasis in massively transfused trauma patients. In: Fresh frozen plasma: indicators and risks. Bethesda, MD, National Institutes of Health Consensus Development Conference, 1984; pp. 38–39.
30. Counts RB, Haisch C, Simon TL et al: Hemostasis in massively transfused trauma patients. Ann Surg 1979; 7:91–98.
31. Harrigan C, Lucas CE, Ledgerwood AM et al: Serial changes in primary hemostasis after massive transfusion. Surgery 1985; 98: 836–843.
32. Hewson JR, Neame PB, Kumar N et al: Coagulopathy related to dilution and hypotension during massive transfusion. Crit Care Med 1985; 13:387–391.
33. Martin DJ, Lucas CE, Ledgerwood AM et al: Fresh frozen plasma supplement to massive red blood cess transfusion. Ann Surg 1985; 202:505–510.
34. Reed RL II, Ciavarella D et al: Prophylactic platelet administration during massive transfusion. Ann Surg 1986; 203:40–48.
35. Valeri CR, Feingold H et al: Hypothermia-induced reversible platelet dysfunction. Ann Surg 1987; 205:175–181.
36. Collins JA: Problems associated with the massive transfusion of stored blood. Surgery 1974; 75:274.
37. Yeston NS, Niehoff JM, Dennis RC: Transfusion therapy. In: Civetta JM, Taylor RW, Kirby RR, eds: Critical care, 2nd ed. Philadelphia, JB Lippincott, 1992; pp. 427–443.
38. Bisonni RS, Holtgrave DR, Lawler R et al: Colloids versus crystalloids in fluid resuscitation: an analysis of randomized controlled trials. J Fam Pract 1991; 32:387.

39. D'Angio R, Orlando R: Fluid resuscitation: colloid versus crystalloid. Conn Med 1986; 50:689–691.
40. Rackow EC, Falk JL, Fein IA: Fluid resuscitation in circulatory shock. Crit Care Med 1983; 11:839.
41. Rackow EC, Falk JL, Fein IA et al: Fluid resuscitation in circulatory shock: a comparison of the cardiorespiratory effects of albumin, hetastarch and saline solutions in patients with hypovolemic and septic shock. Crit Care Med 1983; 11:839–850.
42. Stahl WM: Crystalloid versus colloid resuscitation. Trauma Q 1985; 5:15–23.
43. Lucas CE, Ledgerwood AM, Higgins RE et al: Impaired pulmonary function after albumin resuscitation from shock. J Trauma 1980; 20: 446.
44. Metildi LA, Shackford SR, Virgilio RW et al: Crystalloid versus colloid in fluid resuscitation of patients with severe pulmonary insufficiency. Surg Gynecol Obstet 1984; 158:207.
45. Schaeffer RC, Reniewicz RA, Chilton SM et al: Effects of colloid or crystalloid solutions on edemagenesis in normal and thrombomicroembolized lungs. Crit Care Med 1987; 15:1110–1115.
46. Virgilio RW, Rice CL, Smith DE et al: Crystalloid vs. colloid resuscitation: is one better? Surgery 1979; 85:129.
47. Dawidson I, Eriksson B: Statistical evaluation of plasma substitutes based on 10 variables. Crit Care Med 1982; 10:653–657.
48. Vincent JL: Plugging the leaks: new insight into synthetic colloids. Crit Care Med 1991; 19:316.
49. Velanovich V: Crystalloid versus colloid fluid resuscitation: a meta-analysis of mortality. Surgery 1989; 105:65–71.
50. Lucas CE, Bouwman DL, Ledgerwood AM, Higgins R: Differential serum protein changes following supplemental albumin resuscitation for hypovolemic shock. J Trauma 1980; 20:47.
51. Cogbill TH, Moore EE, Dunn EL et al: Coagulation changes after albumin resuscitation. Crit Care Med 1981; 9:22.
52. Johnson SD, Lucas CE, Gerrick SJ et al: Altered coagulation after albumin supplements for treatment of oligemic shock. Arch Surg 1979; 114:379–383.
53. Lucas CE, Ledgerwood AM, Mammon EF: Altered coagulation protein content after varied resuscitation regimens. J Trauma 1982; 22: 1.
54. Lucas CE, Ledgerwood A, Mammon EF: Altered coagulation after albumin resuscitation. Ann Surg 1982; 196:198–202.
55. Lucas CE, Weaver D, Higgins RF et al: Effects of albumin versus non-albumin resuscitation on plasma volume and renal excretory function. J Trauma 1978; 18:564.
56. Siegel DC, Cochin A, Geocaris T et al: Effects of saline and colloid resuscitation on renal function. Ann Surg 1973; 177:51–57.
57. Dahn MS, Lucas CE, Ledgerwood AM et al: Negative inotropic effect of albumin resuscitation for shock. Surgery 1979; 86:235.
58. Kovalik SG, Ledgerwood AM, Lucas CE et al: The cardiac effect of altered calcium homeostasis after albumin resuscitation. J Trauma 1981; 21:275.
59. Bland JHL, Laver MB, Lowenstein E: Vasodilator effect of commercial 5% plasma protein fraction solutions. JAMA 1973; 224–1721.
60. Gallagher TJ, Banner MJ, Barnes PA: Large volume crystalloid resuscitation does not increase extravascular lung water. Anesth Analg 1985; 64:323.

61. Holcroft JW, Trunkey DD: Pulmonary extravasation of albumin during and after hemorrhagic shock in baboons. J Surg Res 1975; 18: 91.
62. Holcroft JW, Trunkey DD: Extravascular lung water following hemorrhagic shock in the baboon: comparison between resuscitation with Ringer's lactate and plasmanate. Ann Surg 1974; 180:408–417.
63. Weaver DW, Ledgerwood AM, Lucas CE et al: Pulmonary effects of albumin resuscitation for severe hypovolemic shock. Arch Surg 1978; 113:387.
64. Moss GS: An argument in favor of electrolyte solution for early resuscitation. Surg Clin North Am 11972; 52:3.
65. Gold MS, Russo J, Tissot M et al: Comparison of hetastarch to albumin for perioperative bleeding in patients undergoing abdominal aortic aneurysm repair: a prospective, randomized study. Ann Surg 1990; 211:482.
66. Shires GT, Carrico CT, Cohn D: The role of extracellular fluid in shock. Int Anaesth Clin 1964; 2:435.
67. Shires T, Cohn D, Carrico J et al: Fluid therapy in hemorrhagic shock. Arch Surg 1964; 88:688.
68. Canizaro PC, Prager MD, Shires GT: The infusion of Ringer's lactate solution during shock. Am J Surg 1971; 122:494.
69. Carrico CJ, Canizaro PC, Shires T: Fluid resuscitation following injury: rationale for the use of balanced salt solutions. Crit Care Med 1976; 4:46–54.
70. Gann DS, Carlson DE, Byrnes GJ et al: Role of solute in the early restitution of blood volume after hemorrhage. Surgery 1983; 94:439.
71. Shires GT, Cunningham JN, Baker CRF et al: Alterations in cellular membrance function during hemorrhagic shock in primates. Ann Surg 1972; 176:288.
72. Auler JOC, Pereira MHC, Gomide-Araral RV et al: Hemodynamic effects of hypertonic sodium chloride during surgical treatment of aortic aneurysms. Surgery 1987; 101:594.
73. Bauer M, Marzi I, Ziegenfu BT et al: Comparative effects of crystalloid and small volume hypertonic hyperoncotic fluid resuscitation on hepatic microcirculation after hemorrhagic shock. Circ Shock 1993; 40:187–193.
74. Cone JB, Wallace BH, Caldwell FT Jr et al: Beneficial effects of a hypertonic solution for resuscitation in the presence of acute hemorrhage. Am J Surg 1987; 154:585.
75. Gross D, Landau EH, Klin B et al: Treatment of uncontrolled hemorrhagic shock with hypertonic saline solution. Surg Gynecol Obstet 1990; 170:106.
76. Monafo WW, Halverson JD, Schechtman K: The role of concentrated sodium solutions in the resuscitation of patients with severe burns. Surgery 1984; 95:129.
77. Moylan JA, Reckler JM, Mason AD: Resuscitation with hypertonic lactate saline in thermal injury. Am J Surg 1973; 125:580.
78. Freshman SP, Battistella FD, Matteucci M et al: Hypertonic saline (7.5%) versus mannitol: a comparison for treatment of acute head injuries. J Trauma 1993; 35:344–348.
79. Prough DS, Johnson JC, Poole GV et al: Effects on intracranial pressure of resuscitation from hemorrhagic shock with hypertonic saline versus lactated Ringer's solution. Crit Care Med 1985; 13:407.
80. Sutin KM, Ruskin KJ, Kaufman BS: Intravenous fluid therapy in neurologic injury. Crit Care Clin 1992; 8:367–408.

81. Todd MH, Tommasino C, Moore S: Cerebral effects of isovolemic hemodilution with a hypertonic saline solution. J Neurosurg 1985; 63:944.
82. Peters RM, Shackford SR, Hogan JS et al: Comparison of isotonic and hypertonic fluids in resuscitation from hypovolemic shock. Surg Gynecol Obstet 1986; 163:219.
83. Vassar MJ, Fischer RP, O'Brien PE et al: A multicenter trial for resuscitation of injured patients with 7.5% sodium chloride. Arch Surg 1993; 128:1003–1013.
84. Vassar MJ, Perry CA, Holcroft JW: Prehospital resuscitation of hypotensive trauma patients with 7.5% NaCl versus 7.5% NaCl with added dextran: A controlled trial. J Trauma 1993; 34:622–633.
85. Domsky MF, Wilson RF: Hemodynamic resuscitation. Crit Care Clin 1993; 10:715–726.
86. Baxter CR, Zedlitz WH, Shires GT: High-output acute renal failure complicating traumatic injury. J Trauma 1964; 4:467.
87. Imm A, Carlson RW: Fluid resuscitation in circulatory shock. Crit Care Clin 1993; 9:313–333.
88. Booth FVMcL: Fluid resuscitation of the critically ill: monitoring in resuscitation. Crit Care Clin 1992; 8:455.
89. Shoemaker WC, Appel PL, Kram HB et al: Prospective trial of supranormal values of survivors as therapeutic goals in high-risk surgical patients. Chest 1988; 94:1176–1186.
90. Reuse C, Vincent JL, Pinsky MR: Measurements of right ventricular volumes during fluid challenge. Chest 1990; 98:1450.
91. Cheatham ML, Chang MC, Eddy VA et al: Right ventricular end-diastolic volume index and pulmonary artery occlusion. Chest 1993; 104:78S.
92. Diebel LN, Wilson RF, Taggett MG et al: End-diastolic volume: a better indicator of preload in the critically ill. Arch Surg 1992; 127:817.
93. Eddy VA, Chang MC, Cheatham MLL et al: Reevaluation of the bedside approach to preload assessment. Chest 1993; 104:73S.
94. Lappas DG, Fahmy NR: The heart. In: Burke JF, ed: Surgical physiology. Philadelphia, WB Saunders, 1983; pp. 476–496.
95. Nelson LD: Continuous venous oximetry in surgical patients. Ann Surg 1986; 203:329.
96. Mellander S, Johannson B: Control of resistance, exchange, and capacitance functions in the peripheral circulation. Pharmacol Rev 1968; 20:117.
97. Hankeln K, Radel C, Becz M et al: Comparison of hydroxy-ethyl starch and lactated Ringer's solution on hemodynamics and oxygen transport in critically ill patients in prospective crossover studies. Crit Care Med 1989; 17:133.
98. Haupt MT, Gilbert EM, Carlson RW: Fluid loading increases oxygen consumption in septic patients with lactic acidosis. Am Rev Respir Dis 1985; 131:912.
99. Nelson LD: Continuous venous oximetry in surgical patients. Ann Surg 1986; 203:329.
100. Barone JE, Snyder AB: Treatment strategies in shock: use of oxygen transport measurements. Heart Lung 1991; 20:81.
101. Komatsu T, Shibutani K, Okamoto K et al: Critical level of oxygen delivery after cardiopulmonary bypass. Crit Care Med 1987; 15:194.
102. Shoemaker WC: A new approach to physiology, monitoring, and therapy of shock states. World J Surg 1987; 11:133.

103. Yu M, Levy MM, Smith P et al: Effect of maximizing oxygen delivery on morbidity and mortality rates in critically ill patients: a prospective randomized, controlled trial. Crit Care Med 1993; 21:830–838.
104. Kasnitz P, Druger GL, Yorra F, Simmons DH: Mixed venous oxygen tension and hyperlactatemia: survival in severe cardiopulmonary disease. JAMA 1976; 236:570–574.
105. Rutherford EJ, Morris JA, Reed GW et al: Base deficit stratifies mortality and determines therapy. J Trauma 1992; 33:417–423.
106. Falk JL, Rackow EC, Leavy J et al: Delayed lactate clearance in patients surviving circulatory shock. Acute Care 1985; 11:212.

CHAPTER 7

Electrocardiographic Monitoring in Critical Care

Mark L. Franklin
Jeffrey S. Vender

Case Report

A 56-year-old male patient underwent operative removal of a rectal tumor. It required partial resection of the sacrum. The 4-hour procedure resulted in an extensive blood loss requiring 6 units of packed red blood cells as well as fresh frozen plasma and platelets. The patient also received 9 L of Ringer's lactate solution.

The previous history included a myocardial infarction 3 years earlier. He had a left bundle branch block. Therapy included oral nitrates.

On arrival in the intensive care unit (ICU), the patient's temperature was 34.1°C. His initial potassium concentration was 3.8 mEq/L. Although the patient's vital signs were stable, the monitor demonstrated premature ventricular contractions (PVCs).

Initial resuscitation included a warming blanket as well as warming of all intravenous fluids. Over the next 3 hours, 60 mEq/L of potassium chloride were infused in an attempt to raise the potassium value to above 4.5 mEq/L. The patient's heart rate was 48/min. In view of the PVCs, he was given 0.2 mg of atropine. The heart rate increased to 68/min, with a decrease in the number of PVCs.

Over the first 3 hours, the urine output averaged 20 ml/hr. This was in spite of fluid maintenance of 150 ml/hr and an additional 2 L of normal saline by bolus administration. Vital signs included: blood pressure, 116/84 mm Hg; pulse, 88/min; and central venous pressure, 12 mm Hg. Since the patient had not yet responded to fluids, it was elected to place a pulmonary artery catheter. In view of the patient's left bundle branch block, an external pacer was first applied and set to a rate of 90/min. It was then elected to insert a pulmonary artery catheter with a pacing port. After the catheter was successfully placed, the wire was advanced into the right ventricle. After capture was obtained, the pacer was set at a rate of 70/min.

In today's modern ICU, the most ubiquitous monitor is the electrocardiograph (ECG). The majority of patients admitted to an ICU have either cardiovascular instability or problems that affect that stability. The ECG provides a noninvasive, real-time, reproducible, validated assessment of cardiac function. It can be used to detect rhythm disturbances, myocardial ischemia, and electrolyte changes.

PRINCIPLES OF ECG MONITORING

Basic Electrophysiology

Within the heart, a well-described electrical conduction system initiates and conducts impulses that result in organized myocardial contraction.[1] Normally, the sinoatrial (SA) node spontaneously depolarizes to initiate an electrical impulse. The SA node lies in the right atrium at the junction of the superior vena cava and the right atrial appendage. The generated impulse spreads out over both atria and to the atrioventricular (AV) node. At the AV node, a brief delay ensues before the impulse continues down through the bundle of His, and on to the right and left bundles and the Purkinje branches. The QRS portion of the ECG results from conduction through the ventricles. The electrical transmission through the His bundle occurs very rapidly and does not produce externally detectable electrical activity. The T wave represents repolarization of the ventricles. Table 7–1 provides a description of the cardiac waves, segments,

Table 7–1.
Electrocardiographic Findings

- Heart rate and rhythm
- Waves and morphology
    - P wave: artrial impulse conduction
    - QRS complex
        1. Q wave: initial negative deflection before the R wave
        2. R wave: positive deflection
        3. S wave: negative deflection after the R wave
    - T wave: ventricular repolarization
    - U wave: ventricular repolarization
- Segments and intervals
    - PR interval: conduction to AV node and His-Purkinje system
    - ST segment: isoelectric period before ventricular repolarization
        - J point: junction of the QRS and ST segment
    - QT interval

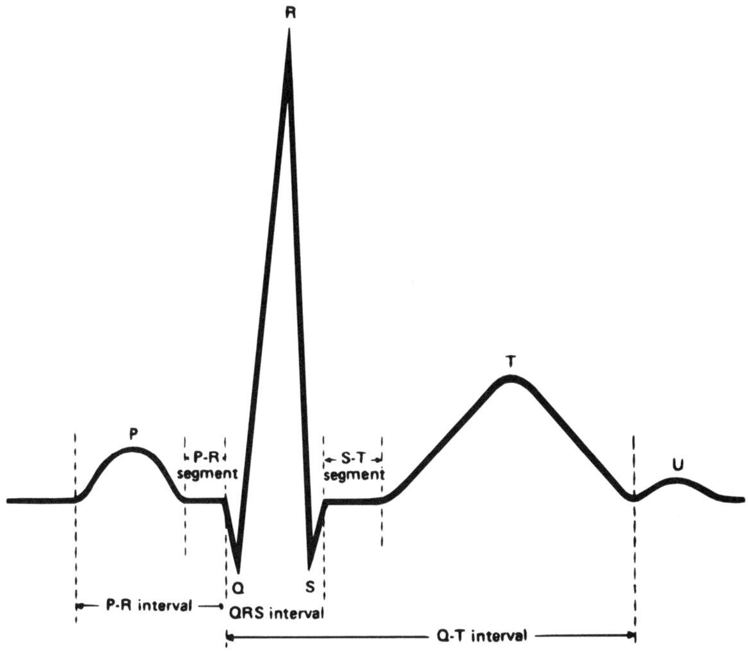

Figure 7–1.
A normal ECG trace. The various waves, segments, and intervals are identified. See text for greater detail. (From Chung EK: Principles of cardiac arrhythmias, 3rd ed. Baltimore, Williams & Wilkins, 1983.)

and intervals of a normal ECG. Repolarization of the atria is hidden in the QRS complex.

Electrocardiographic recording of the foregoing activity describes a characteristic pattern (Fig. 7–1). Firing of the SA node produces the P wave on the ECG trace, and atrial contraction follows. Passage of the electrical impulse through the AV node and the His/Purkinje system produces myocardial contraction of the ventricles. This activity can be divided into four phases: the septal vector, the apicoanterior vector, the left ventricular vector, and the basal vector. Each vector separately contributes to the QRS complex. The ST segment, T wave, and U wave all reflect ventricular repolarization.[2] The ST segment, the area from the conclusion of the QRS complex to the T wave, is normally isoelectric (without any slope). ST-segment depression or elevation may reflect ischemia. T-wave inversion also signals myocardial damage secondary to ischemia (see the discussion of ischemia later in this chapter). Table 7–2 indicates the normal duration of ECG waves.

Impulses are generated by spontaneous depolarization of the just described specialized neural tissue within the endocardium (Figs. 7–2 and 7–3). Myocardial tissue usually maintains a resting potential at −80 to −90 mV with a sodium-potassium-adenosine triphosphatase (ATPase) pump. Certain cells (the AV and SA nodes) have a slightly higher resting potential. These cells can undergo spontaneous depolarization and can initiate a cardiac cycle. Attainment of a threshold potential results in a formation of an action

- *The SA node normally controls heart rate due to its normal intrinsic rate of 60 to 100/min. The AV node and His bundle can serve as secondary pacemakers.*

Table 7–2.
Normal Duration of ECG Waves

Wave	Duration
P wave	<0.11 sec (and amplitude <2.5 mm)
PR interval	(isoelectric) 0.12–0.20 sec
QRS	<0.12 sec
	longer duration indicates abnormal ventricular conduction
ST segment	if not isoelectric may indicate ischemia
QT interval	less than half the preceding RR interval
T wave	<5 mm in standard leads
	<10 mm in precordial leads

potential. The SA node normally fires at a rate of 60 to 100/min. Other neural tissue can also display spontaneous depolarization. However, the slower rise in phase 4 results in a slower rate and maintains the SA node as the primary heart pacemaker. The AV node usually fires at a rate of 45 to 50/min, and the His bundle and Purkinje fibers fire at a rate of 30 to 40/min.

Lead Systems

Various lead configurations allow the measurement of a potential difference (Fig. 7–4). The standard bipolar leads are the three limb leads (left arm, left leg, and right arm). A triangle (Einthoven's) forms among the leads conventionally termed I, II, and III. Connection of the bipolar leads causes a central terminal point at zero potential. Different leads can be formed as each of the limb leads

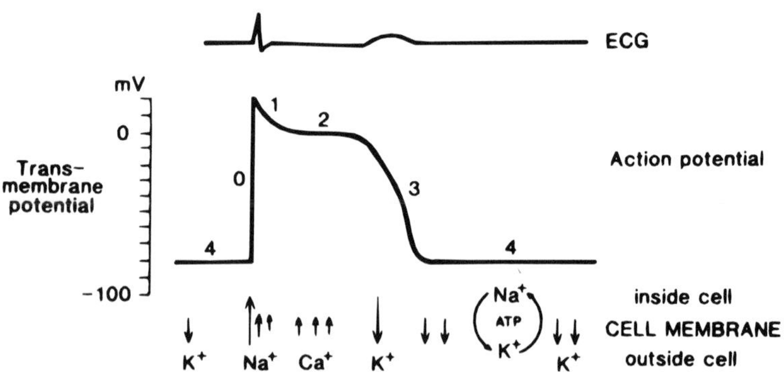

Figure 7–2.
The cardiac action potentials. As fast gating channels open, sodium (Na) rapidly crosses the cell membrane (phase 0). Phase 2 represents the isoelectric ST segment, when the cell is refractory. During repolarization (phase 3), potassium (K) rapidly exits the cell and restores a negative potential. This corresponds to the ECG T wave. During the isoelectric phase 4, the Na-K-adenosine triphosphatase (ATPase) pump exchanges Na out of the cell and K into the cell. (From Textbook of advanced cardiac life support, 4th ed. New York, American Heart Association, 1994. Reproduced with permission. Copyright American Heart Association.)

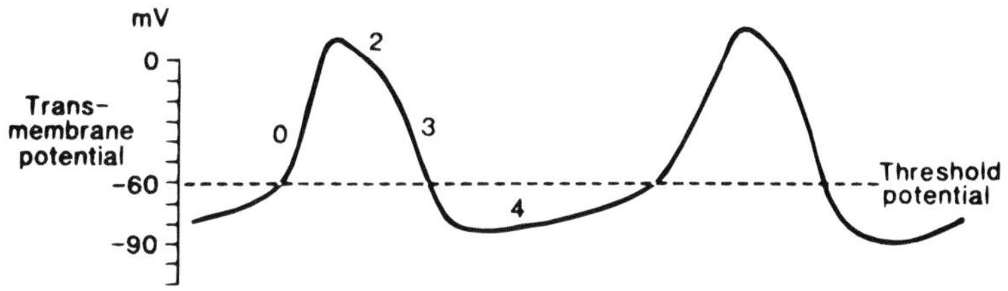

Figure 7–3.
Action potential of pacemaker cardiac cells. Note that during phase 4 the cell becomes progressively less negative until a threshold is reached. Once this threshold is reached, the cell depolarizes. (From Textbook of advanced cardiac life support, 4th ed. New York, American Heart Association, 1994. Reproduced with permission. Copyright American Heart Association.)

becomes active with a potential measured between the central zero point and a limb lead. These are termed the unipolar augmented leads, aVR, aVL, and aVF.

Precordial leads provide further information about the heart. Use of the standard bipolar leads to create a zero potential permits a potential to be measured between the central zero and six precordial positions. The nomenclature (V_1 to V_6) of the six precordial leads refers to the location on the chest wall.

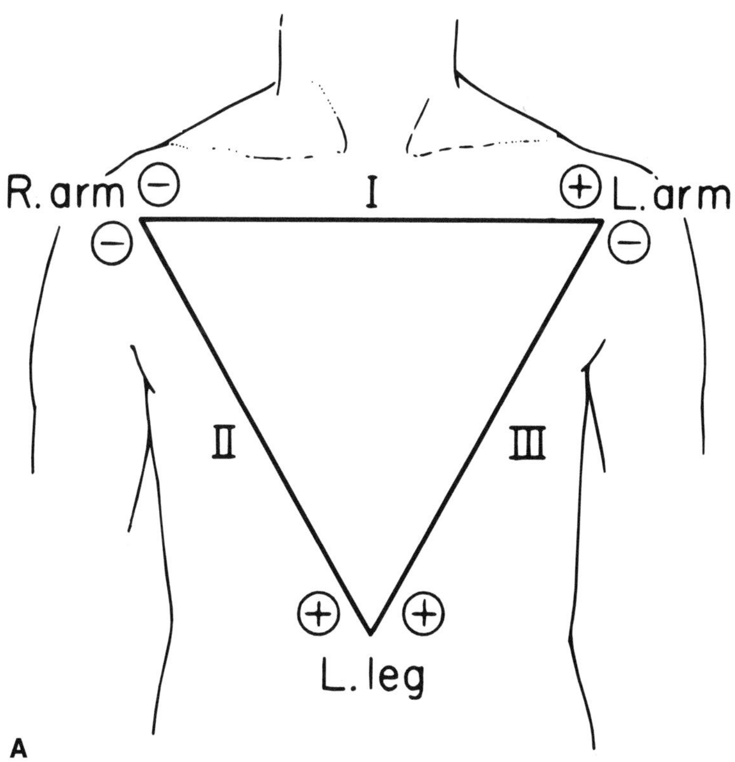

A

Figure 7–4.
ECG lead configurations. A, The bipolar leads (I, II, and III) and the augmented cardiac leads. The augmented cardiac leads (aVR, aVL, and aVF) are created by the potential between each limb lead and a central zero point. (*continued*)

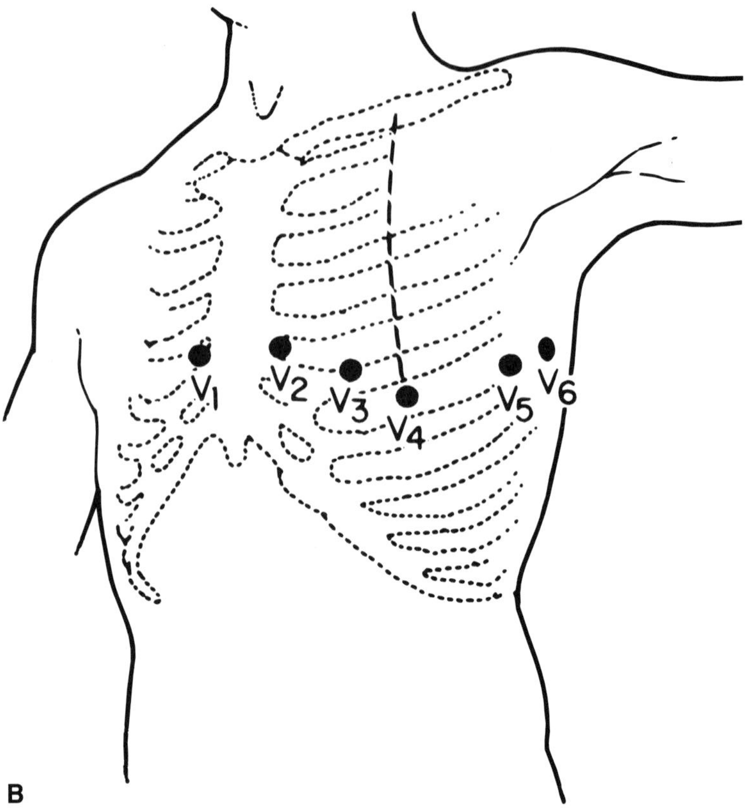

B

Figure 7–4. *(continued).*
B, The precordial leads. These also form from a potential recorded between a central zero point and the chest lead placement. (From Thys DM: The normal ECG. In: Thys DM, Kaplan JA, ed: The ECG in anesthesia and critical care. New York, Churchill Livingstone, 1987.)

Commonly used monitoring systems consist of either three or five electrode leads. The three-lead placement in the conventional locations of left arm, right arm, left leg (LA, RA, and LL) produces leads I, II, III, aVR, aVL, and aVF. Modification of the lead configuration may increase the ability to detect ischemia or arrhythmias. Modification of bipolar leads is designated with the negative lead as central (C) and its position at the left arm.[3] The positive electrode is designated at its precordial position.

The central subclavicular lead (CS_5) results from the placement of the RA electrode under the right clavicle and the LA at V_5. Selection of lead II provides a modified V_5 and can aid in detection of anterior wall ischemia. The modified central lead 1 (MCL_1) is created by the placement of the left arm electrode under the clavicle and the left leg at V_1 (right fourth intercostal space) while recording lead III. It is advantageous in the detection of arrhythmias and conduction blocks.

• *The modified V_5 lead requires that the right arm electrode be placed under the right clavicle and the left arm electrode at the V_5 position.*

With a five-lead system, all six standard bipolar leads can be recorded as well as a unipolar lead. Many monitors allow for the continuous monitoring of two or more leads. The larger P-wave

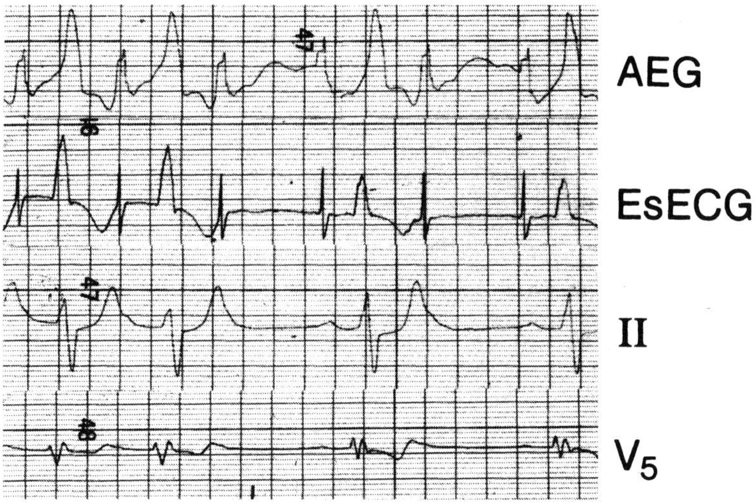

Figure 7–5.
Esophageal and intracardiac leads. Note the increased amplitudes of the P wave recorded from the intracardiac (AEG) and esophageal (Es) waves. These are due to increased proximity to that chamber. In this circumstance, the diagnosis of second degree heart block type II becomes apparent. (From Kates RA, Zaidan JR, Kaplan JA et al: Esophageal lead for intraoperative electrocardiographic monitoring. Anesth Analg 1982; 61:781.)

deflection on lead II best monitors rhythm disturbances. Although any precordial lead can be utilized, V_5 is commonly chosen to monitor for ischemia. The sensitivity of V_5 ischemia detection approximates 75%, while that of V_4 averages about 61%. The combination increases the sensitivity to 90%. On the contrary, lead II detects only 33% of ischemic events. The combination of lead II and lead V_5 increases sensitivity to 80%, while the combination of leads II, V_4, and V_5 raises it further to 98%.[4]

• Standard lead II monitors rhythm disturbances. V_5 is best for ischemia detection.

Invasive leads, such as intracardiac, esophageal, and tracheal, also offer an advantage of proximity to the heart and can provide a greater deflection in the ECG trace. Esophageal leads, due to their proximity to the atria, provide a relatively large P wave. Intracardiac leads produce the greater deflection within any chamber (Fig. 7–5). Intracardiac leads have been used in the placement of central venous lines. Esophageal and intracardiac leads help distinguish atrial from ventricular dysrhythmias.[5,6] A pulmonary artery catheter with pacing electrodes can also provide large deflections and improve the diagnosis of arrhythmias and conduction problems. Because of less electrical interference and production of a more stable signal, intracardiac leads can be used to trigger intra-aortic balloon pump counterpulsation.[7]

• Atrial and ventricular dysrhythmias can sometimes be diagnosed with the use of an intracardiac or esophageal lead.

Monitoring and Recording

In order to best examine the heart, the ECG trace must truly reflect its electrical activity. This is no small feat since the measured potential equals only about 1 mV. An ECG monitor permits the detection, amplification, display, and recording of this small electrical potential of the heart.[8] Signal interference can provide misleading information. It is important to check other leads in order to ensure that information from a single lead is accurate. Silver chloride electrodes with an adhesive surface are attached the skin. To record the best signal, good skin contact is essential. Accurate lead placement becomes important for interpretation of the traces. Muscle contraction produces electrical activity that may interfere with the cardiac signal. Changes in body position alter the relative position of the heart in the thorax. The resultant altered axis may produce misleading information. The respiratory cycle changes thoracic impedance, which will change the recorded electrical potential.

ISCHEMIA

Due to the prevalence of coronary artery disease, detection of perioperative myocardial ischemia significantly contributes to decreased cardiac morbidity.[9] Monitoring and treatment of ischemia have been shown to decrease morbidity.[10] ECG monitoring allows for detection of dysrhythmias and ischemia. Newer microprocessor and computer technology can provide automated analysis of ST segments. Concievably, this may further decrease morbidity. Ischemia monitoring in the postoperative period has taken on a new significance with the recognition of an increased number of adverse cardiac events in that period.[11] Although the focus of ischemia detection is ST-segment depression, dysrhythmias may also herald ischemia.

Many currently available monitors provide for display and recording of two or more ECG leads. Most frequently, leads II and V_5 are chosen. Rhythm disturbances can be easily determined with lead II because of the large P-wave deflection. The distribution of ST-segment depression correlates well with the specific ischemic area. Since ST-segment changes that denote ischemia occur laterally, monitoring leads V_4 and V_5 will detect 90% of ischemic episodes. Significant ST-segment depression and, to a lesser degree, elevation provide evidence of ischemia.[4] ST-segment depression is considered significant when it is greater than 0.1 mV (one small box of standard chart paper).[12] Because each lead best reflects a portion of myocardium, the ECG can localize the ischemic areas. The precordial leads relay information from the right, septal, anterior, and lateral myocardium utilizing leads V_1 through V_6, respectively. Leads II, III, and aVF provide information on the inferior myocardium.

• *Significant ST depression is a change of 0.1 mV from baseline. Precordial leads can differentiate right, septal, anterior, and lateral wall ischemia.*

The ECG demonstrates changes in ST segments and T waves during ischemia. ST-segment depression and, to a lesser degree, elevation are highly suggestive of myocardial ischemia. Automated ST-segment analysis determines the depression or elevation from a isoelectric baseline (Fig. 7–6). The isoelectric baseline represents an average of a number of morphologically identical beats, determined from the PR interval. A template for each lead of the normal trace is stored in memory. From this template, the ST-segment change

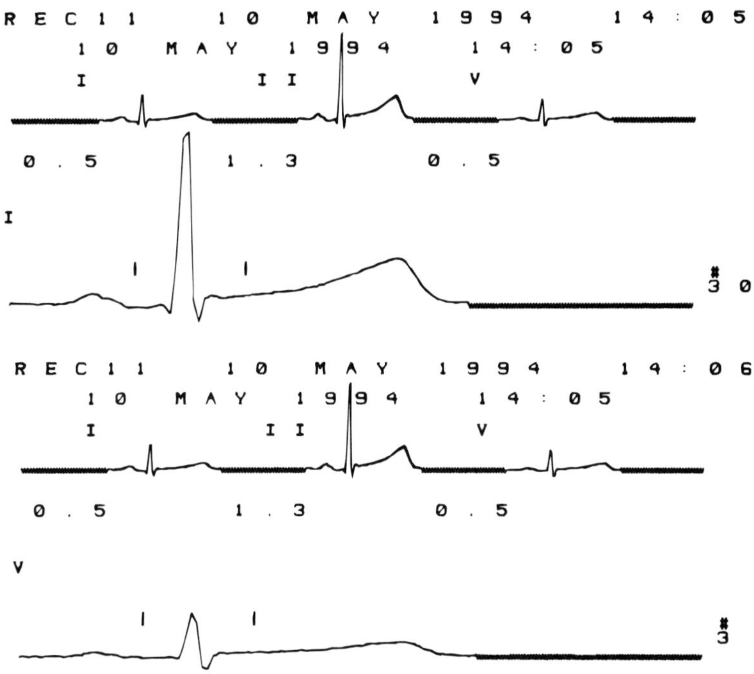

Figure 7–6.
An example of automated ST segment monitoring. Three different leads (I, II, and V) are continuously monitored. The first and third traces show an average ECG trace with an illustration of the magnitude of ST-segment change for the isoelectric interval. The dark horizontal bars in the second and fourth trace indicate the isoelectric interval between the P wave and the QRS complex. This is compared with the ST segment.

can be determined. Motion artifacts, premature beats, and other rhythm changes are excluded, since they are usually not of similar morphology. Additionally, this information can be stored and used to trend changes in ST segments. Electronic alarms can warn when the ST-segment deviation exceeds preset thresholds. Although each manufacturer produces a slightly different product and software, all these devices essentially operate in a similar manner.[12]

Although these changes suggest ischemia, other nonischemic events can produce the same type of changes. Hypothermia, hypoglycemia, hyperkalemia, alkalosis, and changes in electrical axis (changes in position) all may mimic ischemia.

ECG INTERPRETATION

A systemically guided approach to ECG interpretation is essential to minimize errors and improve diagnostics. A good approach has been offered by Kaplan and requires answers to six very important questions:[13] (1) What is the heart rate? (2) Is the rhythm regular? (3) Does a P wave precede every QRS complex? (4) Is the QRS complex normal? (5) Is the disturbance dangerous? (6) Is therapy required?

MECHANISMS OF DYSRHYTHMIAS

Dysrhythmias are any change in ECG recording outside of a normal sinus rhythm. They may result from abnormal spontaneous impulse initiation, abnormal impulse conduction, or both.[14] Automaticity or the spontaneous depolarization in phase 4 of the action potential results in an initiation of an ECG cycle. As described previously, under normal circumstances, the cells of the SA node, the AV node, and the His-Purkinje system normally maintain automaticity. Other cells do not ordinarily possess this ability. Disease processes may allow spontaneous depolarization and initiation of abnormal impulses. These alterations in automaticity may result in dysrhythmias.[15]

- *Abnormal impulse generations or conductions can result in arrhythmias.*

Impulse conduction abnormalities may also result in dysrhythmias. When areas of cardiac tissue are diseased, conduction of impulses may be inhibited or exaggerated. This allows an impulse to reenter the conduction pathway (Fig. 7–7). This circus conduction continues through or around diseased tissue to initiate another apparent impulse. Reentrant dysrhythmias may also result from a decrease in impulse conduction through an area. Instead, retrograde conduction occurs through the diseased area and reexcites a recently depolarized area (Fig. 7–7).[12]

- *Reentry conduction phenomena develop as a result of a diseased area that inhibits or exaggerates impulse conduction. This permits retrograde conduction and can reexcite a depolarized area.*

Triggered automaticity refers to electrically active cells that, with one or more afterdepolarizations, can trigger an impulse.[16] Afterdepolarizations occur during the relative refractory period and may be additive. A delay in repolarization can also result in an afterpotential. If sufficient afterpotentials exist, the threshold to trigger an action potential can be reached.

- *Delayed repolarization can cause afterpotentials, which, in sufficient number, can trigger an action potential.*

Dysrhythmias prevent achievement of optimal cardiac performance. Cardiac output and subsequently blood pressure may fall. Additionally, changes in rhythm may herald other problems, such as hypoxemia, hypercarbia, acidosis, ischemia, electrolyte disturbances, and the like.

Disturbances in cardiac rhythm can sometimes be unnoticed by the patient. The more common presenting symptoms include palpitations, tachycardia, lightheadedness, nausea, and other constitu-

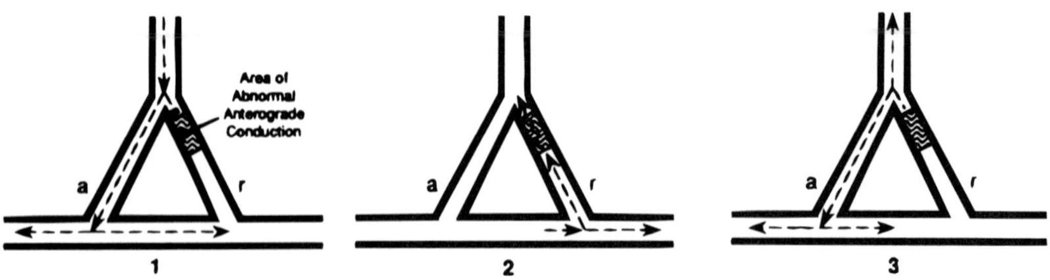

Figure 7–7.
Mechanisms of reentry arrhythmias. In 1, as the impulse travels down one path (a), its normal conduction is blocked through the abnormal fibers (r). However, in 2, retrograde impulse conduction occurs through the abnormal retrograde pathway and spreads out over the rest of the myocardium. In 3, the anterograde (a) path has recovered sufficiently that the retrograde conducted impulse will continue through the anterograde path and complete the circuit. (From Springman SR, Atlee JL: The etiology of intraoperative arrhythmias. Anesthesiol Clin North Am 1989; 7:2.)

tional symptoms. Due to the decrease in cardiac output, fainting, hypotension, and cardiac arrest can occur.

SUPRAVENTRICULAR DYSRHYTHMIAS

Sinus Bradycardia

Sinus bradycardia appears as a normal ECG with a rate less than 60/min. This may be an entirely normal finding, due to decreased cardiac demands. Inferior wall ischemia, hypoxia, increased vagal tone, and drugs (narcotics) may also cause bradycardia. A high spinal block or injury may result in bradycardia due to inhibition of the cardioaccelerator nerves. Table 7–3 lists common causes of sinus bradycardia.

- *Inferior wall ischemia can cause sinus bradycardia.*

Bradycardia is usually asymptomatic. However, if the rate falls below 40/min, blood pressure may also decrease, usually because of the reduced cardiac output. The decision to treat bradycardia should be based on evidence of decreased perfusion. Therapy should eliminate the inciting cause. Vagolytic agents (atropine and glycopyrrolate), beta agonists (isoproterenol, ephedrine, and epinephrine), and pacing are all accepted therapy for refractory bradycardia.

- *Bradycardia should not be treated unless it reduces perfusion.*

Sinus Tachycardia

Sinus tachycardia represents the most common dysrhythmia in the perioperative period. Normal P waves are followed by a narrow QRS complex at a rate greater than 100/min. Higher rates are normal in infants and children. Causes include increased sympathetic activity (stress, hypoxia, hypercarbia, acidosis, hypovolemia, pain, drug effects, fever, congestive heart failure, etc.) on the SA node. Table 7–4 lists common causes of sinus tachycardia. Therapy primarily involves correction of the underlying problem. Heart rate increases are associated with increased myocardial oxygen demand and may be detrimental in patients with ischemic heart disease. The decision to use beta blockade to slow the heart rate must be clear. The decision to pharmacologically (beta blockade) slow the heart rate should be carefully considered. The effect of a slower heart rate with a potential for decreased cardiac output must be balanced against ischemia attenuation.

- *Sinus tachycardia can cause myocardial ischemia. Heart rate should normally be maintained at less than 100/min.*

Table 7–3.
Common Causes of Sinus Bradycardia

Beta blockade
Hypoxemia
Narcotics
Hypothermia
Inferior myocardial ischemia
Increased vagal tone
Decreased cardiac demand

Table 7–4.
Common Causes of Sinus Tachycardia

Hypovolemia
Hypercarbia
Hypoxemia
Acidosis
Fever
Anxiety
Pain
Sympathomimetic agents
Congestive heart failure
Thyrotoxicosis
Increased metabolic demands

Sinus Dysrhythmia

Sinus dysrhythmia is characterized by varying heart rates with normal conduction and morphology. Commonly, the rate will increase during inspiration and slows with expiration. This asymptomatic rhythm more often occurs in children and young adults.

Atrial Flutter

• *Atrial flutter can develop secondary to pulmonary emboli, myocarditis, and ischemia. Cardioversion is reserved for patients in whom pharmacologic therapy has failed.*

Atrial flutter develops because of a rapid atrial discharge, usually at a rate of 300/min. The high rate usually results in atrioventricular (AV) block with a variable ventricular rate up to 150/min. The ECG trace has a "*saw tooth*" pattern of P waves with a normal QRS configuration (Fig. 7–8). Heart disease (usually left atrial enlargement) frequently coexists with this rhythm. Atrial flutter also develops with pulmonary emboli, valvular heart disease, hyperthyroidism, and myocarditis. Goals of therapy include restoration of normal sinus rhythm and/or slowed ventricular response rate. Synchronized cardioversion, initially at a low energy (50 to 100 J) should be undertaken in patients whose condition is unstable and in those who have failed other therapy.[17] Vagal maneuvers, beta blockade, calcium channel blockade, and digitalis are also commonly employed. Both chronic atrial flutter and fibrillation increase the risk of thrombus formation and embolization. These patients may require anticoagulation.

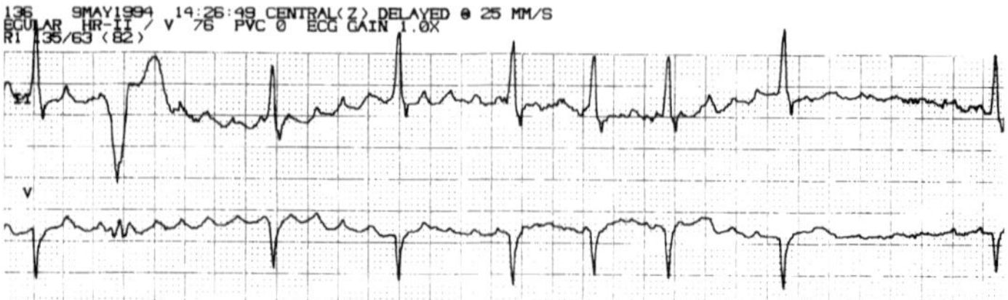

Figure 7–8.
Atrial flutter. Note the irregular "saw-tooth" pattern of the P waves.

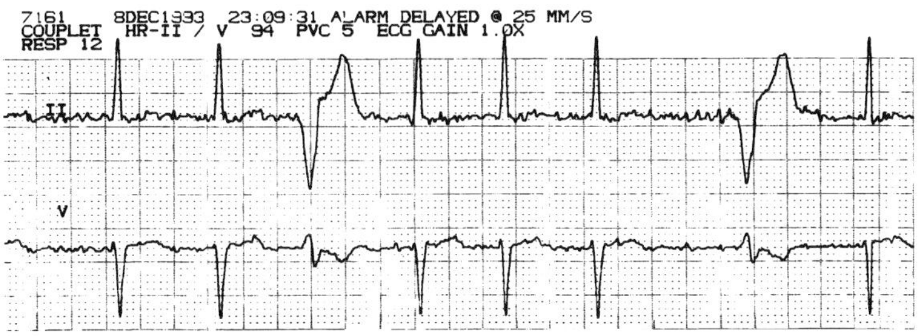

Figure 7–9.
Atrial fibrillation. The fine fibrillation at baseline is readily apparent. The ventricular rate is slow, with premature ventricular beats.

Atrial Fibrillation

Rapid and irregular discharge from an atrial focus without P waves characterizes atrial fibrillation. The ECG trace reveals a fine fibrillatory baseline with an *irregularly irregular* narrow QRS complex (Fig. 7–9). The QRS complex may be abnormal if there is aberrant ventricular conduction. The increased mortality compared with patients in sinus rhythm reflects the significance of this dysrhythmia.[18] Patients at risk to develop this rhythm are similar to those with atrial flutter. Increases in left atrial size, especially greater than 4.5 cm, enhance the likelihood of development of atrial fibrillation.[19] Cardiac output may be compromised, with decreased ventricular filling and the concomitantly decreased ventricular preload due to a lack of atrial systole.

• *Atrial fibrillation develops because of atrial enlargement or ischemia. Cardiac output may be compromised in patients who have limited left ventricular function.*

Therapy, as with atrial flutter, primarily involves restoration of sinus rhythm and/or control of the ventricular response rate. Cardioversion with or without pharmacotherapy will often be the therapy of choice for conversion to a sinus rhythm. The energy requirements are usually greater than for atrial flutter (> 200 J). As with atrial flutter, in conscious patients with atrial fibrillation, anesthesia should be considered during the actual cardioversion. Initial pharmacotherapy classically consists of digitalis preparations to slow conduction through the AV node. This requires a loading dose of the drug to achieve a therapeutic level. In acute situations, the total dose may be given in one or two divided doses over 2 hours. This dose is usually 1.0 to 1.5 mg. After the rate slows, patients often convert to sinus rhythm. If serum potassium levels fall below 4.5 mEq/L, atrial fibrillation may recur. Patients are also susceptible to digitalis toxicity when relative hypokalemia coexists. Other more rapid acting drugs include beta blockers and calcium channel blockers. These agents can effectively slow the ventricular rate. The most common beta blockers are esmolol and propranolol. Verapamil is currently the most useful calcium channel blocker. However, its vasodilatory properties can cause systemic hypotension.

• *Pharmacologic therapy for atrial flutter includes digitalis, beta blockade, and calcium channel blockers. Cardioversion is used for patients with hemodynamic compromise.*

Premature Atrial Beats

Premature atrial beats (PAB) are the result of an ectopic pacemaker focus in either atrium that spontaneously initiates a depolarization

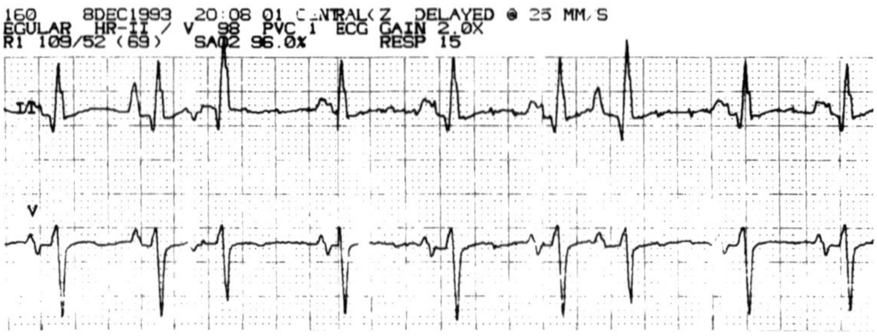

Figure 7–10.
Premature atrial beats. The third and seventh beats are premature atrial beats. Each QRS complex is preceded with a P wave. The morphology of the P waves varies. Also note the large biphasic P wave with normal sinus conducted beats.

(Fig. 7–10). The resultant P-wave morphology may be abnormal, and the PR interval may be longer or shorter than preceding beats. Depolarization includes the SA node. This resets the pacemaker so that the next cycle develops at its normal interval, i.e., no compensatory pause. Aberrant ventricular conduction causes abnormal QRS morphology. It can be difficult to differentiate from a premature ventricular beat (PVB). The presence of a compensatory pause is consistent with a PVB. The compensatory pause develops when the next beat occurs at a normal interval from the premature beat. Other factors consistent with PAB and that distinguish it from PVB include a P wave, a right bundle branch block pattern, and an rSR′ in V_1.

- *Premature atrial beats, unlike premature ventricular, beats do not have a compensatory pause.*

These abnormal depolarizations are of little clinical significance and rarely need therapy. Occasionally, frequent PABs lead to more serious supraventricular dysrhythmias. Therapy is similar to that of atrial flutter and atrial fibrillation.

Supraventricular Tachycardia

Repeated episodes of rapid, supraventricular, premature complexes that originate from an atrial site characterize supraventricular tachycardia (SVT) (Fig. 7–11). This classification includes tachydysrhyth-

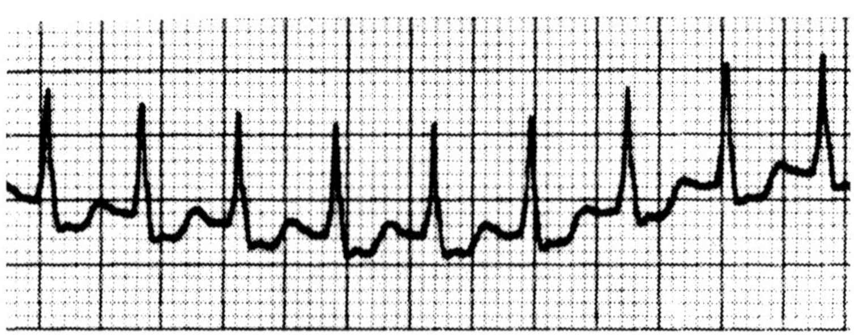

Figure 7–11.
Supraventricular tachycardia (SVT). Note the narrow QRS complex without clearly discernible P waves. The origin of the impulse is above the AV node. Other SVTs may have different morphology with aberrant conduction. (From Dimich I, Pratilas V, Thys DM; Dysrhythmias. In: Thys DM, Kaplan JA, ed: The ECG in anesthesia and critical care. New York, Churchill Livingstone, 1987.)

mias that develop at or above the AV node. Unless the source involves multiple atrial foci, the rhythm is usually regular. The QRS complex may be either narrow or wide, depending on the conduction through the AV node and His-Purkinje system. Often, it is difficult to distinguish an SVT rhythm with aberrant ventricular conduction from ventricular tachycardia. Intracardiac or esophageal leads can help to make this distinction. These rhythms develop in patients with systemic illnesses, pulmonary disease, digitalis toxicity, and hyperthyroidism.[20]

A slowed heart rate allows longer filling times and increases cardiac output. Carotid sinus massage or pharmacologic elevation of blood pressure (phenylephrine) may reflexly increase vagal tone. Calcium channel blockers and beta blockers have also been used successfully. The use of adenosine (6 mg) to break this reentrant tachycardia has become the pharmacotherapy of choice. Adenosine, due to its very short half-life, produces fewer hemodynamic side effects.[21] If the tachycardia is not due to reentry, adenosine will not convert the rhythm, but will slow AV conduction to allow diagnosis.[22] If these efforts fail or if the patient remains or becomes unstable, synchronized cardioversion at low energy (100 J) can be used.

• *Supraventricular tachycardia is regular in appearance and may have a narrowed or widened QRS complex. Adenosine can sometimes interrupt ventricular tachycardia. However, it aids more in diagnosis rather than in treatment.*

VENTRICULAR DYSRHYTHMIAS

Junctional Rhythm

When the junction of the atrium and the ventricle produces a spontaneous depolarization, a junctional rhythm results. Spontaneous depolarization occurs in the area surrounding the AV node. However, the AV node usually does not initiate impulse generation. The ECG trace demonstrates a narrow QRS complex with abnormal or absent P waves (Fig. 7–12). The P wave may be located before, after, or hidden within the QRS complex, depending on the location of the impulse origination. The rate can be quite variable. Decreases in cardiac output and blood pressure will develop due to the lack of atrial augmentation of ventricular filling.

A patient in stable condition usually requires no therapy. In the

• *A junctional rhythm has a narrow QRS complex with abnormal or absent P waves. Premature ventricular beats occur at an ectopic focus below the AV node. There is no P wave, and a compensatory pause follows.*

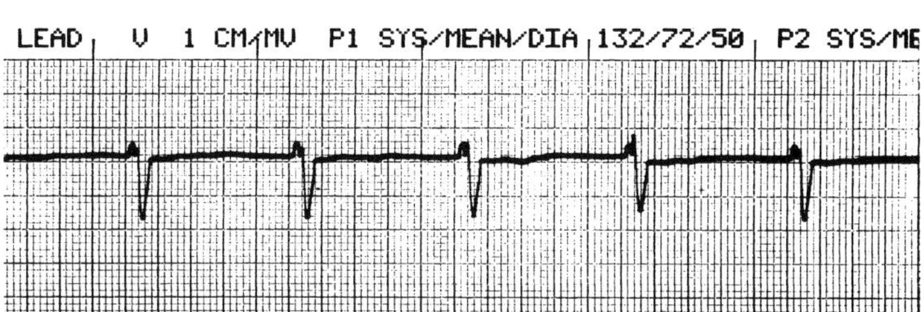

Figure 7–12.
Junctional rhythm. The P wave occurs shortly before each QRS complex and is almost hidden in it. Although the rate is slow, the normal blood pressure verifies the stability of this rhythm disturbance.

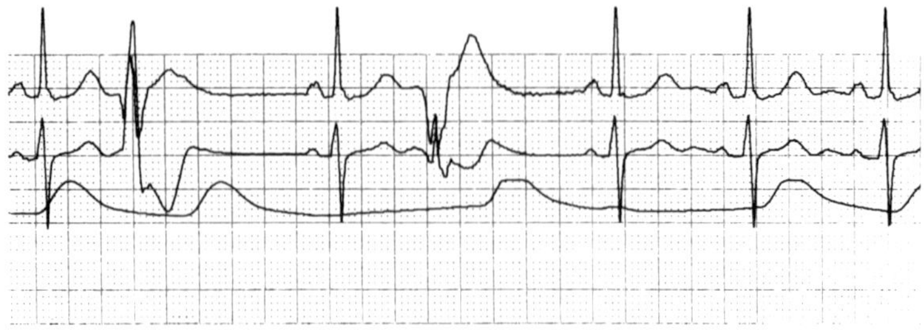

Figure 7–13.
Premature ventricular beats. The second and forth beats are premature. They have a different morphology and emanate from different foci.

presence of hypotension and decreased perfusion, the therapeutic goal becomes increased SA node output. Beta agonists, atropine, and pacing at a higher rate can successfully restore perfusion.

Premature Ventricular Beats

An ectopic focus below the AV node initiates this impulse. The impulse then spreads through the myocardium and produces a PVB. This results either from increased automaticity or from reentrant mechanisms. Depending on the location of origin of the impulse generation, the morphology varies. Each beat will not have a prior P wave. The QRS complex is wide, with an abnormal T wave that has the opposite vector (Fig. 7–13). A compensatory pause usually follows. The depolarization of the SA node resets it so that the next impulse occurs at the appropriate interval. Frequently, PVBs occur cyclically, such as in bigeminy or trigeminy.

- *Ischemia, hypercarbia, and acidosis can all cause premature ventricular beats.*

There are many causes of this rhythm disturbance, some benign and others more significant. Direct myocardial stimulation may produce PVBs. Myocardial ischemia, hypercarbia, and acidosis are all common inciting events. Table 7–5 lists common causes of PVBs. Drugs commonly associated with ventricular irritability include inhalational anesthetics, sympathomimetics, and aminophylline. This rhythm can degenerate into ventricular fibrillation.

Therapy primarily involves relief of the inciting event. Acute

Table 7–5.
Causes of Premature Ventricular Beats

Hypoxia
Acidosis
Hypercarbia
Myocardial stimulation
Myocardial ischemia
Sympathomimetic agents
Aminophylline
Inhalational anesthetics
Pancuronium

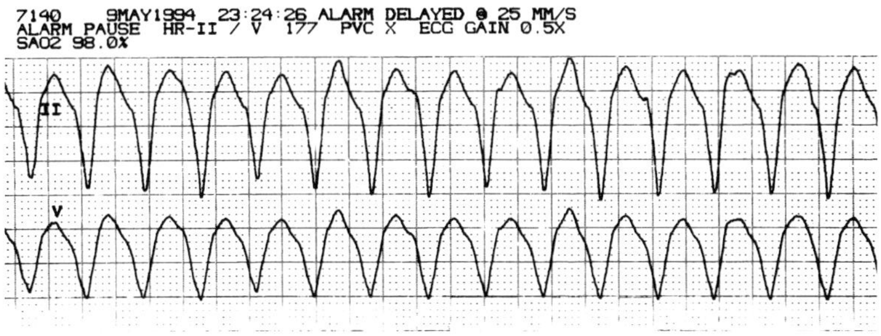

Figure 7–14.
Ventricular tachycardia. The QRS complex is widened, with abnormal T waves. The ventricular rate approximates 150 beats/min. There are no apparent P waves.

intravenous antiarrhythmic agents (lidocaine, procainamide, and bretylium) are more commonly utilized in the critical care environment. Quinidine, amiodarone, and disopyramide are oral agents that have been successfully used to treat ventricular ectopy. Correction of any ischemia remains essential. In addition, hypokalemia should be corrected to values above 4.5 mEq/L.

• *Lidocaine provides the most effective therapy for temporary inhibition of premature ventricular beats.*

Ventricular Tachycardia

Ventricular tachycardia represents a potentially life-threatening dysrhythmia. It is defined as four or greater consecutive PVBs (Fig. 7–14). There are no P waves. Although usually regular, the QRS complex can exhibit an irregular and widened complex with a rate of 70 to 250/min. Typical rates average 150/min. It is at times difficult to distinguish ventricular tachycardia from SVT with aberrant conduction. An invasive lead such as an esophageal or intracardiac lead can help detect the difference. AV dissociation, left axis deviation, and a compensatory pause all suggest ventricular tachycardia.[23]

• *Ventricular tachycardia may be regular or irregular and has a wide QRS complex. Rates average 150/min.*

Ventricular tachycardia requires immediate therapy to prevent its degeneration into ventricular fibrillation. Therapy can be divided into two modes, depending on hemodynamic stability. If the patient maintains adequate blood pressure and cerebral perfusion, pharmacologic therapy can be tried initially. Agents include lidocaine, procainamide, and bretylium. Often, the last two drugs are not immediately available. Failure of these agents to convert the dysrhythmia should be rapidly followed by synchronized electrocardioversion (200 to 360 J). In patients in unstable condition, electrocardioversion (sequentially from 200 to 360 J) should be the primary therapy. If the initial cardioversion fails, an intravenous antiarrhythmic agent can be used in conjunction with another attempt at cardioversion.[17]

• *If ventricular tachycardia does not respond immediately to lidocaine, synchronized cardioversion will be required.*

Ventricular Fibrillation

Ventricular fibrillation represents discoordinate electrical activity of the ventricle (Fig. 7–15). The ECG shows either a fine or a coarse fibrillatory wave. There is no organization that allows for muscle

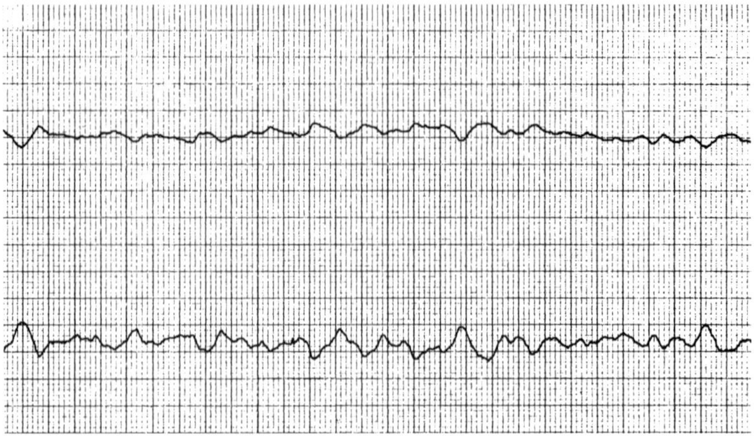

Figure 7–15.
Ventricular fibrillation. The two traces, leads II and V, come from the same patient. The entire trace is chaotic, without organized electrical activity. This rhythm is incompatible with effective myocardial contraction and must be rectified.

• *Definitive therapy for ventricular fibrillation is immediate defibrillation.*

contraction. Therapy consists of immediate electrocardioversion (360 J). The earlier defibrillation can be initiated, the greater the chance of success. If initial attempts at cardioversion fail, an intravenous antiarrhythmic agent can be given along with further attempts at cardioversion. Epinephrine should also be used. However, in general, pharmacologic attempts at conversion routinely fail.

Torsades de Pointes

Torsades de pointes is a polymorphic ventricular tachycardia with a variable morphology.[24] Characteristically, the QRS complex changes in amplitude from an isoelectric baseline (Fig. 7–16). It commonly occurs in patients with a prolonged QT interval. Causes

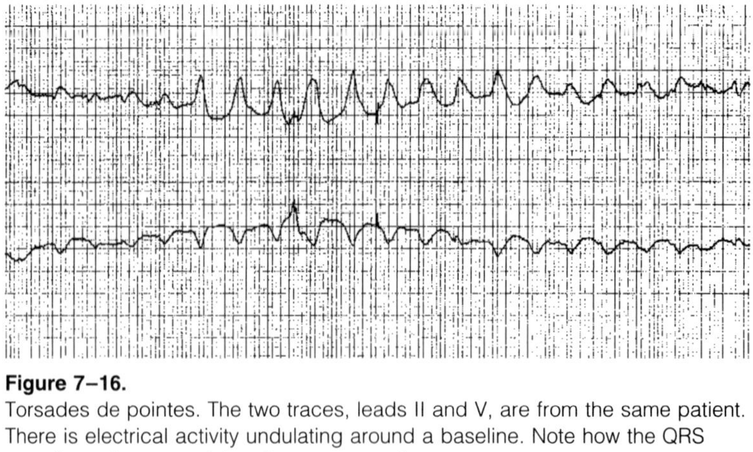

Figure 7–16.
Torsades de pointes. The two traces, leads II and V, are from the same patient. There is electrical activity undulating around a baseline. Note how the QRS complex enlarges and then becomes smaller.

of the prolonged QT include electrolyte abnormalities (hypomagnesemia and hypokalemia), myocarditis, congenital abnormalities, and drugs. Quinidine, phenothiazines, disopyramide, and beta blockers have been implicated as causal agents of this rhythm.

• Hypomagnesemia and hypokalemia are common causes of torsades de pointes.

This dysrhythmia does not readily respond to therapy. Management involves attempts to correct the underlying problem and to decrease the QT interval. Antiarrhythmic agents, such as quinidine, that can exacerbate the rhythm must be avoided.[25] Many clinicians consider overdrive pacing the therapy of choice. Sympathomimetic therapy to increase heart rate and decrease the QT interval may be useful.[24]

• Quinidine should be avoided in torsades de pointes. Overdrive pacing can be the most effective therapy.

Asystole

Asystole means lack of any cardiac electrical activity. Therapy consists of cardiopulmonary resuscitation (CPR), intracardiac epinephrine, isoproterenol, atropine, and pacing. If these modalities fail, cardioversion may be attempted. At times, a fine ventricular tachycardia may be mistaken for asystole.

Pulseless Electrical Activity

This rhythm was previously known as electromechanical dissociation. The designation has been changed to include disturbances that demonstrate electrical activity but without production of a pulse. Recent ECG evidence has noted myocardial contraction but of insufficient force to eject any blood. Common causes are listed in Table 7–6. Therapy should be directed at correction of the underlying problem. In addition to CPR, intracardiac epinephrine and atropine may increase cardiac output.

• Electromechanical dissociation still has cardiac contraction but with inadequate force. Intracardiac epinephrine may correct the situation.

Table 7–6.
Causes of Pulseless Electrical Activity

Hypoxia
Hypovolemia
Hypothermia
Acidosis
Cardiac tamponade
Tension pneumothorax
Myocardial infarction
Pulmonary embolus
Drug overdose
Hyperkalemia

(Adapted from Emergency Cardiac Care Committee and Subcommittees, American Heart Association: Guidelines for cardiopulmonary resuscitation and emergency cardiac care. III: Adult ACLS. JAMA 1992; 268:2199.)

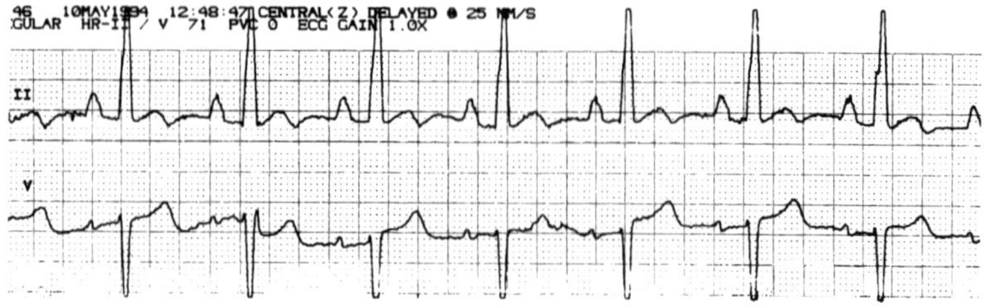

Figure 7–17.
First degree heart block. The PR interval is greater than 0.20 seconds. In addition, the P waves are large and biphasic in lead V.

CONDUCTION BLOCKADE

Optimal cardiac function depends on the coordinated and sequential contraction of the atria followed by the ventricles. Any defect in conduction immediately causes cardiovascular compromise. Some conduction abnormalities are asymptomatic. Conduction blocks can be divided into those at the level of the AV node and those in the His-Purkinje system.

Atrioventricular Conduction Blocks

First degree AV block results from delayed but normal conduction of the impulse through the AV node (Fig. 7–17). The ECG has a normal P wave and QRS complex, but the PR interval exceeds 20 msec. The blockade does not necessarily have to be in the AV node but can also occur in the distal conduction system.[26] This change can occur in normal, healthy patients, especially those with bradycardia. First degree AV block is a benign rhythm change and does not require therapy.

• *A Mobitz type I block results from ischemia in the distribution in the right coronary artery. It does not require therapy. A type II block has a normal PR interval. Therapy should be directed to increase rate.*

Second degree AV block has two types, based on ECG differences. Mobitz type I block has a progressively longer PR interval, until a P wave does not conduct (Fig. 7–18). This is the Wenckebach phenomenon. Mobitz type II block has a normal PR interval with occasional lack of conduction of P waves (Fig. 7–19). Although type I block may occur in healthy patients, it more commonly develops in those with an underlying disease process. AV node ischemia (usually

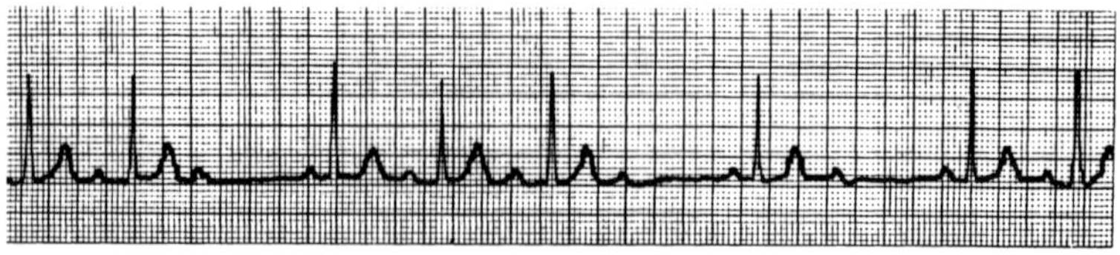

Figure 7–18.
Second degree heart block, type I. The progressively increased PR intervals have a pause in ventricular conduction. Atrial and ventricular conduction varies. (From Textbook of advanced cardiac life support, 4th ed. New York, American Heart Association, 1994. Reproduced with permission. Copyright American Heart Association.)

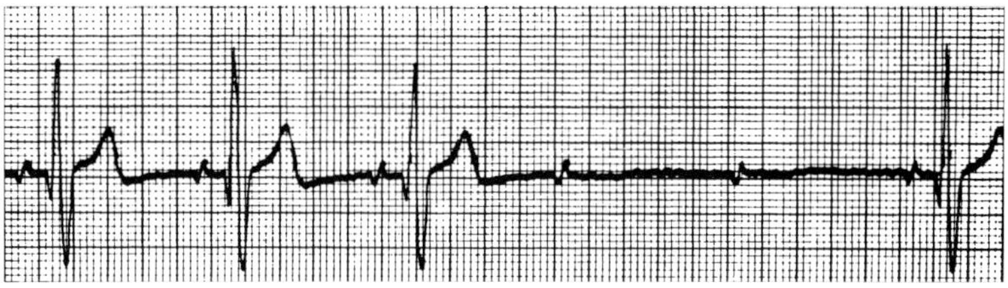

Figure 7–19.
Second degree heart block, type II. P waves are conducted in the first three beats followed by nonconducted P waves. The last beat shows a normally conducted sinus beat. (From Textbook of advanced cardiac life support, 4th ed. New York, American Heart Association, 1994. Reproduced with permission. Copyright American Heart Association.)

of the right coronary artery) may produce these blocks. Type I block remains asymptomatic and usually does not require therapy. However, an underlying cause should be sought and treated. Type II block may reduce cardiac output. Directed therapy includes an increased ventricular rate by pacing, atropine, or epinephrine.

Third degree AV block means the lack of conduction between the atria and the ventricles (Fig. 7–20). This condition has also been referred to as AV dissociation. The ECG has P waves but without conduction to the ventricles. The ventricles instead respond at their own intrinsic rate. Therefore, the QRS appears as a wide complex, like a PVB. Complete heart block can result from multiple disease processes, but most commonly it is due to ischemia. With total disruption of AV conduction and the usual slow ventricular response rate of the ventricle, cardiac output can be significantly reduced. Primary therapy involves increasing the heart rate. Acutely, intravenous agents such as atropine or epinephrine may help. A pacemaker remains the therapy of choice. Initially, an external pacemaker may be used. However, a transvenous pacemaker is usually required for long-term therapy.

• *Treatment of third degree AV block is a transvenous pacemaker.*

Bundle Branch Blocks

Right bundle branch block results from delayed conduction through the right His bundle. A normal P wave conducts to an abnormal QRS complex. The QRS morphology demonstrates an rSR′ configuration (Fig. 7–21). This represents the initial depolarization of the septum, followed by the left and finally the right ventricle. The QRS complex is also prolonged, with a duration greater than 0.12 second.

• *A primary cause of right bundle branch block is ischemia and pulmonary hypertension.*

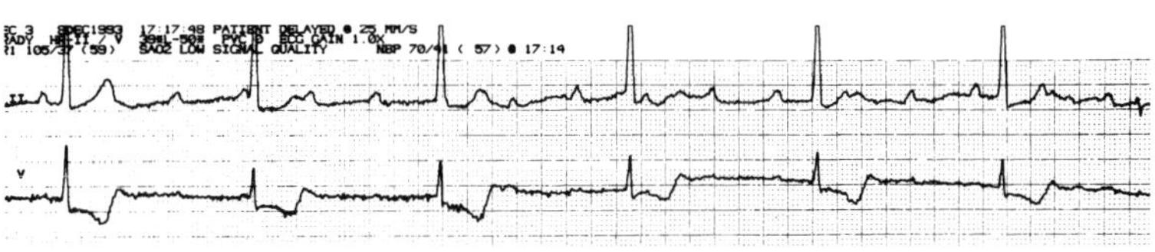

Figure 7–20.
Third degree heart block, also known as complete heart block and AV dissociation. There is no conduction of the P wave and no QRS complex.

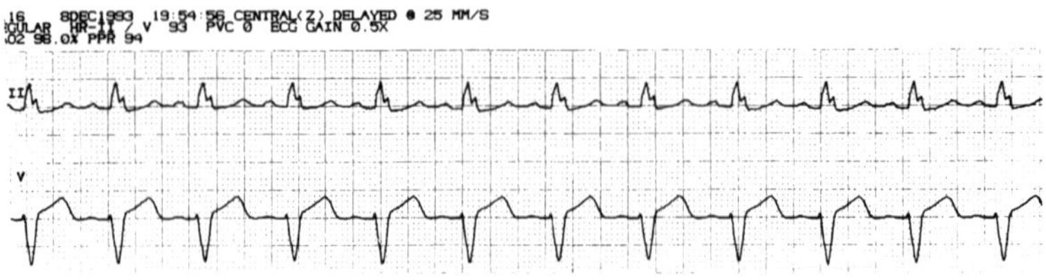

Figure 7–21.
Right bundle branch block.

Repolarization abnormalities may also be present. Causes of right bundle branch block include pulmonary disease (pulmonary hypertension and cor pulmonale), systemic hypertension, congenital heart defects, ischemia, and cardiomyopathies.

Left bundle branch block, like RBBB, also causes a conduction delay through the left ventricle. The septum and right ventricle depolarize first followed by the left ventricle (Fig. 7–22). The left ventricle depolarizes from the impulse through the right ventricle. The QRS duration is prolonged for more than 0.12 second. Septal depolarization causes a small r wave, followed by a large s wave due to right ventricle depolarization. A sloping r wave develops as the left ventricle depolarizes. The T wave is usually abnormal and inverted. This makes the diagnosis of ischemia and left ventricular hypertrophy (LVH) more difficult. The presence of left bundle branch block almost always indicates a disease process. Common causes include ischemia, prior infarction, hypertension, congestive heart failure, drug effects, or congenital defects.

• *Left bundle branch block principally results from ischemia or a prior infarction.*

The left bundle branch has two fascicles, the anterior and posterior, either of which may develop a conduction block. A *left anterior hemiblock* produces an initial r wave in the inferior leads (II, III, and aVF) and a q wave in the lateral leads (I, aVL, and V_5 to V_6) because of the initial posterior depolarization. There is a terminal s wave inferiorly and an r wave laterally as the anterior left ventricle depolarizes. Left axis deviation also appears. *Left posterior hemiblock* produces right axis deviation with initial negative deflections inferiorly, positive deflections laterally, and terminal deflections the opposite. The QRS duration is normal in both blocks; as long as one fascicle remains functional, the QRS duration appears normal. Calcific degeneration and ischemia to the conduction system are

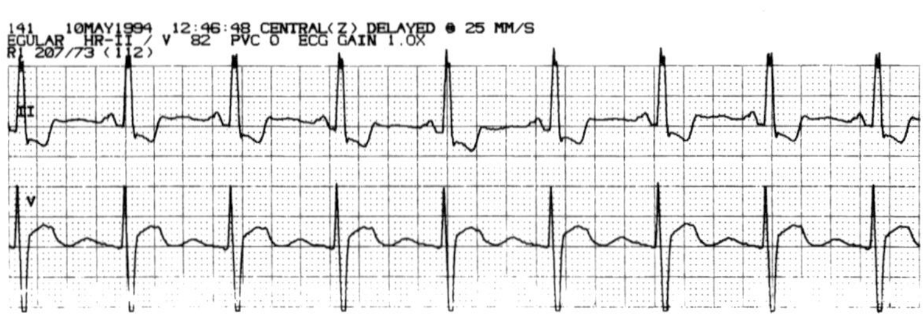

Figure 7–22.
Left bundle branch block.

commonly the problem. Usually, these rhythm disturbances are asymptomatic. However, they can progress to complete heart block. Therapy includes an increased heart rate either by pacing or by the administration of chronotropic agents. *Bifascicular block* occurs when a right bundle branch block exists along with either hemiblock. This increases the likelihood of development of complete heart block. Again, therapy consists of chronotropic agents and pacing.

• *Primary therapy for left anterior or posterior hemiblock is pacing.*

Ten percent of patients develop an acute right heart block during pulmonary artery catheterization. Therefore, catheter placement in a patient with a left bundle branch block could concievably lead to full heart block. Prior to placement of a pulmonary artery catheter, we place an external pacemaker on the patient. We then insert a catheter with a port for the pacing wire.

ELECTROLYTE EFFECTS ON THE ECG

The flux of ions across cardiac cells controls automaticity and contraction. Therefore, changes in electrolyte concentration have well-characterized effects on the ECG.

Potassium

Hyperkalemia classically produces large, peaked T waves (Fig. 7–23). As potassium rises above 6.5 to 7.0 mEq/L, the QRS complex beomes prolonged. With higher levels, the QRS complex becomes even wider and dysmorphic. Eventually, ventricular asystole or fibrillation occurs. Insulin (10 U) and glucose (50 g) infusions acutely lower potassium by driving it into cells. In addition, alkalemia induced with bicarbonate therapy or hyperventilation has the same effect.

Hypokalemia produces T-wave flattening. As the T wave becomes less prominent, a U wave becomes more apparent.[27] Hypokalemia increases the susceptibility of the heart to dysrhythmia. In postoperative patients, this will likely occur at serum potassium values less than 4.5 mEq/L. Chronic hypokalemia is well tolerated, but acute potassium decreases are more likely to result in dysrhyth-

• *Hypokalemia with values less than 4.5 mEq/L causes ventricular arrhythmias.*

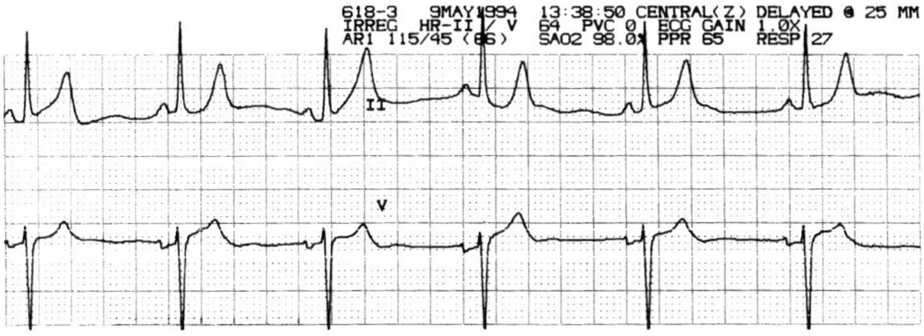

Figure 7–23.
Large T waves in a patient with elevated potassium. The potassium was only slightly increased at 5.3 mEq/dl.

mias. Hypokalemia increases the toxic effects of digitalis on the heart. Potassium chloride increases potassium values to acceptable ranges. The usual dose consists of 20 mEq/hr, for a total of 40 to 60 mEq over 3 hours. The values should then be rechecked.

Calcium

Changes in calcium concentrations affect the ST segment and QT interval. Hypocalcemia prolongs the ST segment and the QT interval.[28] Hypercalcemia has the opposite effect, a short QT interval. Hypercalcemia can also result in extrasystoles.

Magnesium

- *Hypomagnesemia causes ventricular dysrhythmias.*

Hypomagnesemia can result in low voltage of the P wave and the QRS complex. With very low concentrations for a protracted period of time, the PR interval may become prolonged and the QRS complex may widen. Normally, magnesium stabilizes myocardial membranes. Hypomagnesemia may predispose the patient to dysrhythmias. On the other hand, magnesium has a stabilizing effect on myocardial membranes. Therefore, magnesium infusions have been used to treat supraventricular and ventricular dysrhythmias. Hypermagnesemia has no notable effects on the ECG.

REFERENCES

1. Titus JL: Normal anatomy of the human cardiac conduction system. Anesth Analg 1973; 52:508.
2. Thys DM: The normal ECG. In: Thys DM, Kaplan JA, eds: The ECG in anesthesia and critical care. New York, Churchill Livingstone, 1987; pp. 1–15.
3. Griffin RM, Kaplan JA: ECG lead systems. In Thys DM, Kaplan JA, eds: The ECG in anesthesia and critical care.: New York, Churchill Livingstone, 1987; pp. 17–30.
4. London MJ, Hollenberg M, Wong MG et al: Intraoperative myocardial ischemia: localization by continuous 12 lead electrocardiography. Anesthesiology 1988; 69:232–241.
5. Kates RA, Zaidan JR, Kaplan JA: Esophageal lead for intraoperative electrocardiographic monitoring. Anesth Analg 1982; 61:781.
6. Donovan KD, Power BM, Hockings BE et al: Usefulness of atrial electrograms recorded via central venous catheters in the diagnosis of complex cardiac arrhythmias. Crit Care Med 1993; 21:532–537.
7. Lichtenthal PR: Multipurpose pulmonary artery catheter. Ann Thorac Surg 1983; 36:493.
8. Weinfurt PT: Electrocardiographic monitoring: an overview. J Clin Monit 1990; 6:132.
9. Mangano DT: Perioperative cardiac morbidity. Anesthesiology 1990; 72:153–184.
10. Rao TLK, Jacobs KH, El-Etr AA: Reinfarction following anesthesia in patients with myocardial infarction. Anesthesiology 1983; 59:499.
11. Mangano D, Browner W, Hollenberg M et al: Association of periopera-

tive myocardial ischemia with cardiac morbidity and mortality in men undergoing noncardiac surgery. N Engl J Med 1990; 323:1781–1788.

12. Muller JG, Barash PG: Automated ST-segment monitoring. Int Anesthesiol Clin 1993; 31:45–55.
13. Kaplan JA: Electrocardiographic monitoring. In: Kaplan JA, ed: Cardiac anesthesia. Orlando, FL, Grune & Stratton, 1979; p. 117.
14. Hoffman BF, Cranefield PF: The physiologic basis of cardiac arrhythmias. Am J Med 1964; 37:670.
15. Cranefield PF, Wit AL, Hoffman BF: Genesis of cardiac arrhythmias. Circulation 1973; 47:190.
16. Cranefield PF: Action potentials, afterpotentials, and arrhythmias. Circ Res 1977; 41:415.
17. Emergency Cardiac Care Committee and Subcommittees, American Heart Association: Guidelines for cardiopulmonary resuscitation and emergency cardiac care. III: Adult ACLS. JAMA 1992; 268:2199.
18. Gajowski J, Singer RB: Mortality in an insured population with atrial fibrillation. JAMA 1981; 245:1540.
19. Henry WL, Morganroth J, Pearlman AS et al: Relation between echocardiography determined left atrial size and atrial fibrillation. Circulation 1976; 53:273.
20. Jones RM, Broadbent MP, Adams AB: Anaesthetic considerations in patients with paroxysmal supraventricular tachycardia. Anaesthesia 1984; 39:307.
21. Camm AJ, Garratt CJ: Adenosine and supraventricular tachycardia. N Engl J Med 1991; 325:1621–1629.
22. DiMarco JP, Sellers TD, Lerman BB et al: Diagnostic and therapeutic use of adenosine in patients with supraventricular tachyarrhythmias. J Am Coll Cardiol 1985; 6:417–425.
23. Zipes DP, Fish C: Premature AV junctional contractions. Ann Intern Med 1971; 128:663.
24. Vukmir RB: Torsades de pointes: a review. Am J Emerg Med 1991; 9:250–255.
25. Kossman CE: Torsades de pointes: an addition to the nosography of ventricular tachycardia. Am J Cardiol 1978; 42:1054–1058.
26. Goldman MJ: Principles in clinical electrocardiography, 10th ed. East Norwalk, CT, Appleton & Lange, 1979.
27. Surawicz B: Relationship between electrocardiogram and electrolytes. Am Heart J 1967; 73:814.
28. Scheidegger D, Drop LJ: The relationship between duration of QT interval and plasma ionized calcium concentration. Anesthesiology 1979; 51:143.

CHAPTER 8

Myocardial Ischemia and Infarction in the Postoperative Setting of Noncardiac Surgery

Carl J. Pepine

Case Report

The patient was a 54-year-old man scheduled for an aortofemoral graft the following morning. He had a history of a myocardial infarction 3 years before. The patient reported two to three episodes of angina per week. It had always responded to nitroglycerin therapy. He had a history of hypertension currently treated with enalapril, 10 mg/day.

The examination revealed an obese male with: blood pressure, 160/86 mm Hg; regular pulse, 84/min; and respiratory rate, 16/min. The preoperative evaluation included an electrocardiogram (ECG) that demonstrated nonspecific ST-T-wave changes.

The surgeons wished to place the patient in the intensive care unit (ICU) preoperatively for invasive monitoring with a pulmonary artery catheter. They also inquired as to the need for other specific evaluations to delineate further the risk for adverse outcomes in the patient.

Each year in the United States, more than 25 million patients undergo noncardiac surgery. About 3 million of these patients are estimated to have known or to be at high risk for coronary artery disease (CAD) and about 4 million are more than 65 years old.[1] About 50,000 of these patients develop a perioperative myocardial infarction (MI), and more than half of the annual 40,000 deaths

• *Each year in the United States, 1 million patients who undergo noncardiac surgery suffer death, myocardial infarction, or heart failure due to cardiac ischemia.*

that are associated with noncardiac surgery are related to CAD. Overall, it has been estimated that about 1 million patients undergoing noncardiac surgery will have a serious cardiac-related adverse outcome (e.g., death, MI, unstable angina, or heart failure) and the cost of this in-hospital perioperative morbidity exceeds $10 billion annually.[1,2] Most of these adverse outcomes are directly related to cardiac ischemia or ischemia-associated myocardial injury and its health care costs are enormous. Since studies have suggested that the detection of myocardial ischemia before or during surgery identifies a subset of patients at high risk for perioperative events, considerable effort and cost have been focused on the preoperative and perioperative evaluation and care of such patients.

The purpose of this chapter is multifold. First, I will review the terminology and current state of the clinical problem of myocardial ischemia and CAD. Second, I will outline the rationale for focus on perioperative ischemia detection. Third, I will suggest a management strategy that relates to prevention, detection, and intervention in patients with known or suspected ischemia. Finally, throughout this review, where data are available, I will attempt to describe the impact on adverse outcomes and costs that might be realized by such a strategy.

TERMINOLOGY AND MECHANISMS OF ISCHEMIA-RELATED PERIOPERATIVE CARDIAC MORBIDITY

Readers of this chapter may not be regularly involved in the management of patients with transient myocardial ischemia or ischemic injury. Therefore, as background information, a number of pertinent definitions and important advances in our understanding of this area are reviewed. Particular attention is given to the pathophysiology of myocardial ischemia and the clinical syndromes that comprise ischemia-related adverse outcomes occurring in the perioperative period.

Throughout this chapter, the term "myocardial ischemia" is used to describe a condition that exists when oxygen supply to functioning myocardium declines below levels required to meet myocardial oxygen demands. This oxygen supply-demand imbalance usually results from a decrease in coronary artery blood flow or an increase in cardiac mechanical activity (e.g., heart rate, ventricular volume, blood pressure, contractility). As a consequence, the metabolism of myocardial cells is impaired to a degree sufficient to result in mechanical and electrical cardiac dysfunction. Ischemia-related mechanical dysfunction may include various degrees of diastolic (relaxation) followed by systolic (contraction) impairment. Ischemia-related electrical dysfunction may include various abnormalities of repolarization (ECG ST-segment and/or T-wave changes) and automaticity (ventricular rhythm disturbances).

• *Ischemia-related myocardial dysfunction may first involve diastolic and then systolic abnormalities.*

It should be recognized that myocardial ischemia is a condition (myocellular hypoxia) not directly measured in the clinical setting but inferred from signals (electrical, mechanical, and perfusion) recorded from the heart. Taken individually, these signals are neither highly sensitive nor highly specific for myocardial ischemia. Accordingly, a combination of these signals, as well as their time course in a patient with clinical characteristics highly suggestive of CAD (e.g., age, chest pain), is needed in order to fully evaluate ischemia. It is also important to note that all myocardial ischemia is transient. When the supply or demand disturbance is brief (e.g., several minutes) the ischemia-related cardiac functional disturbance resolves completely. However, when the supply or demand disturbance is prolonged (e.g., > 30 to 40 minutes), ischemia is resolved either by permanent injury to the myocardial cells (infarction) or by downregulation of contractile function, so that a new equilibrium between supply and demand for oxygen is reached. This latter concept is termed "hibernating myocardium," and should myocardial oxygen demand increase (e.g., tachycardia, blood pressure rise, ventricular volume enlargement) or oxygen supply become further reduced (e.g., hypoxemia, anemia, hypotension), infarction may ensue.

- *The ECG is a poor indicator of myocardial cellular ischemia.*

In clinical terms, "coronary artery disease" refers to atherosclerotic narrowing of a major coronary artery or its branch(es) of sufficient severity to limit coronary blood flow under physiologic conditions (e.g., rest, exercise, or other stress such as noncardiac surgery), to result in myocardial ischemia. The size of the coronary atheroma at any site is not the only factor that determines coronary blood flow. A number of dynamic factors are also important and they include coronary endothelial dysfunction, platelet and white cell activation, and vascular smooth muscle contraction. The term used to describe all such factors is coronary heart disease (CHD) or ischemic heart disease. Thus, patients with CHD have a form of heart disease whose primary manifestations result from myocardial ischemia due to CAD and related factors. The clinical syndromes of CHD range from totally asymptomatic ischemia, symptomatic ischemia (angina and its equivalents), myocardial necrosis (acute MI), myocardial failure (congestive heart failure secondary to ischemia-related left ventricular dysfunction or postinfarction scarring), and sudden cardiac death (lethal ventricular arrhythmias such as ventricular tachycardia and ventricular fibrillation or bradyarrhythmias such as severe bradycardia and asystole).

- *Coronary artery disease represents not only narrowing, but also functional impairment secondary to endothelial changes, platelet and white cell activation, and smooth muscle contraction.*

The most prevalent form of myocardial ischemia that occurs in patients with CHD during daily life, including the perioperative period, is *asymptomatic or unrecognized ischemia*. The prevalence of daily life ischemia varies greatly and depends on the extent, severity, and complexity of CAD and to a lesser extent on other clinical findings (e.g., age, stable angina, unstable angina). The method used for detection is also important (e.g., ECG, perfusion, or wall motion abnormality) in terms of prevalence. Regardless of the method used for detection, the presence of daily life ischemia identifies a subset of patients at high risk for adverse outcomes when compared with comparable patients without daily life ischemia.

- *Much myocardial ischemia may be unrecognized because of lack of symptoms.*

A number of ischemia-related cardiac *adverse outcomes* may occur in patients with CAD who undergo noncardiac surgery. *Cardiac death* is usually due to ventricular tachyarrhythmias, asystole, or profound left ventricular failure. Acute myocardial infarction (AMI) refers to a process of profound, prolonged, or repeated episodes of ischemia of sufficient severity to result in injury to myocardial cells. In its early stage this injury has two components. One is permanent and due to myocellular necrosis and the other is, to various degrees, reversible and due to both myocellular and coronary microvascular dysfunction. The stress of surgery itself, accompanying hemodynamic changes, neurohormonal activation and cardiac size changes due to volume shifts all may provoke perioperative ischemic injury.

• *Perioperative myocardial infarction usually occurs within 48 hours of surgery.*

Perioperative MI is usually clinically silent (painless) and difficult to detect, and it may or may not be associated with ECG Q waves.[3] The non-Q-wave MI may be detected only by cardiac enzyme efflux or new left ventricular wall motion abnormalities. Non-Q-wave perioperative MI typically occurs in the early postoperative period (~ 48 hours), with a time course similar to that observed for most perioperative ischemia.[1] *Heart failure* and/or *pulmonary edema* commonly occur somewhat later in the period (> 48 hours) and are often related to volume shifts in cases with ischemia-related left ventricular dysfunction.

• *Perioperative myocardial infarction has approximately a 40% risk of early death. Patients who initially survive have a 60% risk of late death or severe disability.*

"Cardiac risk" refers to the probability of future CAD-related adverse outcomes such as death, MI, and heart failure. A number of clinical factors are associated with increased cardiac risk, and these are addressed in the section of this chapter on multifactorial indexes. Perioperative MI has a very high (~ 40%) risk for early death. Survivors of perioperative MI have a very high risk (~ 60%) for death and/or disability over the next 1 to 2 years.

ASSESSING PERIOPERATIVE CARDIAC RISK

• *The risk of perioperative myocardial infarction in patients without prior evidence of heart disease is 0.5% or less.*

Data from several large series of patients show that the risk of an adverse outcome such as perioperative MI may be as low as 0.5% in patients without prior evidence to suggest CHD. However, in patients with evidence of CHD (e.g., prior MI) the risk of perioperative infarction averages approximately 6%,[4] or about 30 times higher. This risk, however, is not uniformly distributed across all subsets of patients with CAD. For example, risk of perioperative MI is inversely related to the time interval between the prior MI and the noncardiac surgery. The risk of perioperative reinfarction may be as high as 30% in the first several weeks after an infarction but only 2 to 5% 6 months after an infarction.[4] Other clinical factors such as age, heart failure, and diabetes interact with the type of noncardiac surgery to further determine risk. Various clinical risk scales have been derived attempting to identify patients who are at high risk.

Multifactorial Clinical Risk Indexes

Goldman and co-workers were among the first to devise a multifactorial index attempting to predict risk of cardiac adverse outcomes in noncardiac surgery according to a weighted set of clinical variables.[5] These included: presence of an S_3 gallop; jugular venous distention; MI within 6 months; rhythm other than sinus, including atrial premature contractions; need for emergency surgery; more than 5 premature ventricular contractions (PVCs)/min at any time before surgery; need for intra-abdominal, thoracic, or aortic surgery; age greater than 70 years; significant aortic valve stenosis on examination; and poor general medical condition. Although the Goldman risk index has been validated by several studies,[6] it only allows separation of patients relative to highest and lowest cardiac risk groups.[7,8] In these studies, patients in high cardiac risk classes have approximately an 8-fold higher incidence of serious cardiac events and approximately a 20-fold higher perioperative death rate than patients who are in the lower cardiac risk groups. Approximately half of these deaths occur in class 4 (the sickest) patients.

The applicability of the Goldman index to patients undergoing vascular surgical procedures has been questioned.[8,9] Those questions relate to a much higher cardiac event rate observed in patients undergoing noncardiac vascular surgery than for other procedures. Even individuals with low risk scores may have a 5 to 10% incidence of cardiac events. When the patients have a high prevalence of clinically silent or unrecognized CAD, a very low risk group cannot be identified by bedside markers alone.[9] These findings are consistent with the well-known close association between the presence of CAD and peripheral vascular disease. Coronary angiography performed routinely before vascular surgery demonstrates that the majority of these patients have severe multivessel disease, and in some the CAD may even be inoperable. Importantly, about a quarter of such patients with no history of CHD have multivessel disease at angiography similar to those who have a history or symptoms suggesting CHD. Severe CAD has been found in 70 to 90% of patients undergoing abdominal aortic surgery, carotid surgery and iliac artery surgery. Furthermore, early and late survival after surgery is significantly influenced by the presence and severity of CAD. The Goldman cardiac index has no provision for CHD other than a history of MI within 6 months. Assessments for angina are absent, and no provision is made for ischemic responses that are observed on stress testing. Hence it is not surprising that this index underestimates perioperative risk in patients with high risk for but not clinically overt CAD. In addition, the assessments for left ventricular function are limited to only recognition of an S_3 gallop and jugular venous distention.

- *Patients who undergo vascular surgical procedures appear to have a higher complication rate than indicated by the Goldman index. This probably results from associated underlying coronary artery disease.*

Subsequently, Detsky and associates proposed a modified cardiac risk index for use in noncardiac surgery patients that accounts for the presence and severity of angina pectoris and adds a more precise description of clinical heart failure as recent or remote pulmonary edema (Table 8–1).[8–10] These workers also simplified the

Table 8–1.
Multifactorial Cardiac Risk Index of Detsky and Colleagues

Variable	Points
Coronary artery disease	
Myocardial infarction ≤6 mo	10
Myocardial infarction >6 mo	5
Angina (Canadian Cardiovascular Society class)	
Class III	10
Class IV	20
Unstable angina <6 mo	10
Alveolar pulmonary edema	
Within 1 week	10
Ever	5
Valvular disease	
Suspected critical aortic stenosis	20
Arrhythmia	
Rhythm other than sinus, with or without atrial ectopy	5
Presence of >5 VPC/min at any time	5
Poor general medical status	5
Age >70 years	5
Emergency surgical procedure	10

VPC, Ventricular premature contractions.
(Data from Detsky AS, Abrams HB, Forbath N, et al: Cardiac assessment for patients undergoing noncardiac surgery: a multifactorial clinical risk index. Arch Intern Med 1986; 146:2131.)

scoring system into multiples of five. Finally, because the type of surgery is not a patient characteristic, the Detsky approach considered the type of surgery in the pretest probability, rather than in the index itself, as with the Goldman index. Thus, for any operative procedure, patients at low (0 to 15 points), intermediate (16 to 30 points), and high (> 30 points) risk may be identified. In clinical practice, this modified risk index helps identify risk for cardiac adverse outcomes within broad classes, but the index has not been extensively validated outside Detsky's hospital. This is an important limitation because the pretest probabilities are likely to vary widely in different practice settings dependent on patient case mix and referral bias. Finally, the Detsky index has limited sensitivity in the patient without either severe angina or left ventricular dysfunction.

Because of this limitation, Eagle and colleagues[11,12] modified the Detsky index to include ^{201}thallium stress test results. These investigators identified five clinical factors and two dipyridamole-thallium test results that were independently predictive of perioperative adverse outcomes of major vascular surgery.[12] These factors were: age greater than 70 years; ECG Q waves; diabetes; history of ventricular arrhythmias; angina; redistribution thallium defect; and ischemic ECG changes during the dipyridamole-thallium test. When three or more of the clinical factors were present, the risk for adverse outcomes was so high that additional testing with thallium was not warranted. If no clinical factors were present, the risk was so low that additional testing with thallium stress testing was not of added value. Thus, additional testing with dipyridamole-thallium for risk stratification was useful only for patients who had one or two of the clinical risk factors. This group comprised about half of the patients in their cohort. A similar approach has been suggested by others.[10]

Synthesis. It is important to recognize that preoperative clinical cardiac risk indices are limited in the evidence collected about ischemia and left ventricular dysfunction. Only jugular venous distention, third heart sound, and pulmonary congestion are included in the Goldman index, and only severe angina and pulmonary edema are included in the Detsky index. It is clear that other, less subjective, estimates of potential for ischemia and cardiac dysfunction during stress that simulates the perioperative period remain important predictors of adverse outcomes. So an objective test for ischemia and cardiac dysfunction during stress is likely to be helpful. These clinical risk scales generally are most useful for patients with relatively unstable CAD syndromes and/or clinical manifestations of left ventricular dysfunction who will be identified as high risk. In addition, these clinical risk scales are useful for noncardiac surgery populations with a very low likelihood of CAD (e.g., nonvascular surgery, younger patients). In a population with a moderate or high likelihood of CAD, many mildly symptomatic or asymptomatic patients who may be at high risk for adverse outcomes will not be identified. For this reason additional testing evolved.

Noninvasive Stress Testing

Recognition of the foregoing limitations led to the application of a number of noninvasive stress tests to refine risk stratification before noncardiac surgery (Table 8–2). Exercise testing was the first to be evaluated, in the early 1980s.

Treadmill Exercise Testing

Exercise treadmill testing (ETT) with monitoring of the ECG is the standard clinical method to determine which patients with CAD are likely to have functionally important coronary artery stenoses and are therefore at risk for adverse outcome. Patients with ETT-induced ischemia are at some increased risk; however, the risk varies widely and a number of other ETT markers for subsequent high adverse outcome risk without noncardiac surgery have been identified (Table 8–2). Any patients with these findings on ETT warrant strong consideration for coronary angiography and revascularization, if possible, in an attempt to modify their high risk for adverse outcomes.

- *In many asymptomatic patients, indices such as the Goldman index may not select out patients at high risk for cardiac complications. Abnormal ETT usually requires consideration of coronary angiography and a possible coronary artery bypass procedure.*

A number of studies of patients scheduled for major noncardiac vascular surgical procedures have been done using ETT.[13–17] These studies included about 700 patients and employed a treadmill or bicycle or arm ergometry. The largest study was by Carliner and associates,[15] who prospectively tested 200 consecutive patients (mean age 59) scheduled for abdominal, thoracic, or vascular (34%) procedures. Thirty-three patients developed adverse outcomes: (3

Table 8–2.
Criteria to Identify High Risk of Adverse Outcomes in Patients with Angina Pectoris or Other Ischemic Syndromes

ETT criteria
Failure to complete 6.5 METs or attain heart rate ≥120 b/min
≥2 mm ST depression
Postexercise ST depression >6 min
ST depression in multiple ECG leads
SBP response flat or decrease >10 mmHg
ST elevation in leads without Q waves
Exercise-induced VT
ECHO/MUGA criteria
EF ≤35%
Exercise decrease EF ≥5%
Multiple new defects
New defects at work load
^{201}Thallium or Sestimibi scintigraphy criteria
New defect at low work load
Multiple defects
Increase in cardiac size with exercise
Increase in lung uptake of thallium with exercise
AECG criteria
Any ischemic ST shift lasting 1 min
Other criteria still evolving

AECG, ambulatory electrocardiographic monitoring; ECG, electrocardiogram; ECHO, echocardiography; EF, ejection fraction; ETT, exercise treadmill testing; MET = metabolic equivalent; MUGA, multiple gated image acquisition analysis; SBP, systolic blood pressure; VT, ventricular tachycardia.

deaths, 3 nonfatal MIs, and 27 cases of ischemia or injury). An abnormal resting ECG was a significant predictor of risk. Five of the 6 patients with serious outcomes (death or nonfatal MI) had a maximum exercise capacity of less than 5 metabolic equivalents (METs), and one had ST-segment depression suggesting ischemia. Most of the other studies also found that low exercise capacity either in terms of METs (< 5) or maximum heart rate achieved (< 85% of maximum predicted or < 100 beats/min) was a strong predictor of adverse outcome.[13,14,16,17] When evidence for ischemia coexisted with poor exercise capacity, the risk was very high.[13,14]

• *An ECG in a patient with bundle branch block or left ventricular hypertrophy may be uninterpretable for ischemia. Dipyridamole-thallium testing requires a variation of blood flow of 4:1 between ischemic and nonischemic areas to be of clinical usefulness.*

Synthesis. In general, ETT is one of the useful ways to assess cardiovascular functional capacity, and it provides valuable information about risk stratification. The ETT is cost effective, and in my opinion, it is underutilized for perioperative risk stratification. However, many patients who undergo noncardiac surgery have ECGs that are uninterpretable for ischemia (e.g., bundle branch block, left ventricular hypertrophy), and others are unable to exercise to a sufficient degree to be tested adequately. Hence other noninvasive stress tests are needed.

Radionuclide Perfusion Imaging

Dipyridamole-^{201}thallium myocardial imaging has been extensively evaluated as an adjunct to clinical risk stratification for noncardiac surgery.[10–12,18–26] An extensive review of this test is beyond the scope of this chapter, but some areas are important to help understand its use and results. Thallium uptake by the myocardium is largely blood flow dependent but many important coronary artery stenoses do not reduce blood flow at rest. So some form of stress is added during testing to increase blood flow. Since exercise tolerance is often limited in patients with peripheral vascular disease, dipyridamole or adenosine is used as pharmacologic stress. These agents are potent coronary arteriolar dilatators and increase blood flow to myocardial regions supplied by arteries without functionally important stenoses, but flow does not increase to regions supplied by arteries with severe stenosis. However, limitations with thallium energy and resolution require a difference in blood flow of about 4:1 in order to recognize a myocardial region with reduced perfusion. Furthermore, soft tissue attenuation of the isotope energy can lead to imaging artifacts. The need to withhold all adenosine-active agents (e.g., theophylline, caffeine) and the requirement for delayed imaging 4 to 24 hours later are important limitations, in addition to cost.

Over the past decade, considerable experience has been published on testing patients before vascular surgery. These data suggest that most adverse outcomes occur in the minority of patients with an abnormal thallium stress test. This experience is discussed in detail in two reviews.[3,10] These studies are limited by small sample size and low power to detect adverse outcomes, lack of a common protocol and definitions, and other methodologic problems such as bias related to failure to withhold test results from investigators. Their results generally support the notion that the presence of areas of malperfused myocardium detected using thallium stress testing before peripheral vascular surgery can predict an increased risk for adverse outcome. A review of some recent studies with this test should help the reader in selection of patients for thallium stress testing.

- *An abnormal dipyridamole-thallium stress test is usually highly predictive of risk in patients undergoing noncardiac surgical procedures.*

More recently, the utility of exercise thallium scintigraphy in combination with other clinical factors in predicting perioperative adverse outcomes in patients who undergo elective vascular surgery has been suggested, but this conclusion is not uniform. McFalls and co-workers studied a group of 116 men (mean age 67 years); 43% had a history of CAD, including angina pectoris in 22%, MI in 28%, and bypass surgery in 16%.[25] These patients had a total of 22 perioperative MIs (18.9%), including 2 cardiac deaths (1.7%). A significantly greater proportion ($p < 0.05$) of patients with, than without, perioperative adverse outcomes had a history of CAD (77% versus 35%), angina (59% versus 14%), prior MI (50% versus 22%), abnormal ECG (68% versus 40%), or abnormal exercise thallium test (75% versus 47%). The group with adverse outcomes also had a significantly lower ejection fraction (45% versus 55%, $p < 0.005$). Independent predictors of adverse outcome were angina and fixed thallium defects (presumably unrecognized infarction or viable ischemic myocardium) after exercise. The finding that a fixed thallium defect was the only exercise thallium result predictive of

- *Predictors of myocardial complications include a combination of an abnormal thallium stress test, coronary artery disease, angina, and prior myocardial infarction, all coupled with an abnormal ECG.*

adverse outcome is at variance with most previously reported results. McFalls and associates suggest that these fixed defects, on 3- to 4-hour redistribution imaging, may represent severe ischemia (e.g., hibernating myocardium), rather than old infarction. Particularly interesting is the failure of reversible defects to predict outcomes. Thus, the data suggest that a reversible thallium defect after exercise is not as good a marker of high risk for adverse outcomes as previously thought.

Brown and Rowen tested the hypothesis that risk of perioperative cardiac events is not simply determined by the presence of myocardium at risk, but is directly related to the extent of myocardium at risk as reflected in thallium imaging.[26] The study cohort consisted of 231 consecutive patients who had a preoperative dipyridamole thallium study and underwent noncardiac surgery. Patients with vascular reconstruction or bypass constituted the largest subgroup ($n = 140$). For thallium imaging data, each of 3 planar projections was divided into 3 segments (total 9 segments), and each segment was interpreted as either normal or showing a transient or fixed defect. Perioperative adverse outcomes occurred in 19 patients, including 5 with cardiac death, 7 with nonfatal MI, and 7 with unstable angina. For cardiac death or nonfatal MI, the only significant multivariate predictors were the number of myocardial segments with transient thallium defects ($p < 0.0005$) and a history of diabetes ($p < 0.05$). For all adverse cardiac outcomes, the only significant multivariate predictors were the number of myocardial segments with transient defects ($p < 0.0001$), diabetes ($p < 0.05$), and calcium antagonist use ($p < 0.05$). These workers concluded that the probability of adverse outcomes in patients undergoing noncardiac surgery is best predicted by the extent of myocardium at risk, as reflected on thallium imaging, and a history of diabetes.

• *The risk of perioperative myocardial events may be related to the amount of myocardium noted to be abnormal during thallium testing.*

Hendel and Whitfield, in the largest series to date, used dipyridamole thallium scanning in 360 patients before elective vascular surgery.[24] Survivors were followed for a mean of 31 months. In the 327 patients who underwent vascular surgery, operative death and nonfatal MI occurred in 4.9 and 6.7%, respectively. Adverse cardiac outcomes (nonfatal MI or cardiac death) occurred in 14.4% of patients with a transient thallium defect, as opposed to only 1% with a normal scan ($p < 0.001$). Logistic regression analysis revealed that the best predictor of perioperative adverse outcomes was the presence of a reversible thallium defect, which elevated the risk by 4.3-fold. Late cardiac events occurred in 53 (15.2%) surgical survivors or nonsurgically treated patients. Patients with a fixed perfusion abnormality had a 24% late event rate, compared with 4.9% in those with a normal thallium study ($p < 0.01$). Cox analysis demonstrated that a fixed thallium defect was the best predictor of late events and increased the relative risk by almost 5-fold. A history of heart failure was the only significant variable that contributed additional value to that of a fixed thallium defect alone. Life-table analysis confirmed the strong relationship of a fixed thallium defect to cardiac event-free survival ($p < 0.0001$).

• *This study revealed that a reversible thallium scannning defect was the best predictor of perioperative myocardial complications.*

Fleisher and associates described three patients who had postoperative MI with normal or fixed defects on preoperative dipyridamole thallium scans.[22] All were interpreted preoperatively as negative for cardiac ischemic risk. All patients had ambulatory ECG (AECG) monitoring beginning the evening before surgery and continuing through the first 2 postoperative days. Two of the patients demonstrated either preoperative or early postoperative ischemia on AECG, which suggested that the thallium test results were falsely negative. The third patient did not demonstrate AECG ischemia during a postoperative day, which may have indicated progression of the underlying CAD. The authors concluded that preoperative dipyridamole thallium imaging may result in false-negative scans in selected high-risk populations.

The utility of preoperative stress thallium scintigraphy was determined in 59 patients by Kazmers and associates.[23] These patients were thought to have been at increased cardiac risk before major vascular surgery. Forty-seven had oral dipyridamole, and 12 underwent exercise stress thallium testing. Thallium redistribution abnormalities were present in 61% (n = 36), fixed defects (e.g., infarction) were present in 59% (n = 35), and some combination of defects was present in 76% (n = 45). There were 6 perioperative adverse outcomes in 5 patients (8.5%), including 3 patients with congestive heart failure, 2 with ventricular arrhythmia, and 1 with MI. Adverse outcomes occurred in 8.3% (3/36) of those with redistribution defects and in 8.7% (2/23) of those without redistribution (relative risk = 0.95). Perioperative MI was present in 2.8% (1/36) with redistribution versus 0% (0/23) without. These authors concluded that the utility of thallium stress testing has not been clearly established for prediction of perioperative cardiac risk after major vascular surgery.

• *In this study, thallium stress testing was not predictive of later myocardial events.*

In another study, by Younis and colleagues, 131 patients with peripheral vascular disease who underwent intravenous dipyridamole thallium testing were screened to determine cardiac event rates over an average follow-up of 18 months.[21] Of these 131 patients, 111 subsequently had peripheral vascular surgery. The patients with abnormal thallium scans after dipyridamole had a significantly higher risk of death or MI, both in the perioperative phase (7% versus 0%; $p < 0.001$) and at late follow-up (17% versus 6%; $p < 0.01$). The risk of a cardiac adverse outcome was twofold greater when a reversible, compared with a fixed, thallium defect was present. Multivariate analysis selected the number of thallium segments with perfusion defects, prior history of angina, and chest pain during dipyridamole testing as perioperative predictors of adverse outcomes. A reversible thallium defect was the only predictor of death or nonfatal MI during late follow-up. These workers concluded that intravenous dipyridamole thallium scintigraphy is a useful noninvasive test for risk stratification of patients before peripheral vascular surgery and provides prognostic information for risk of adverse outcome during the 2-year period after the test.

• *This study found that a reversible thallium defect was the only predictor of adverse cardiac events.*

Synthesis. A reversible thallium defect is associated with a significantly increased perioperative adverse outcome risk. Whether preoperative coronary angiography and revascularization reduce this

• *Although the reversible thallium defect can predict adverse outcome, a large percentage of patients with the reversible defect undergo surgery without development of any specific complications.*

risk is unknown. There are a large number of patients with CAD and reversible thallium defects, however, who do not have postoperative adverse outcomes, and the dipyridamole thallium test is very costly and inconvenient.

Left Ventricular Function Testing

Left ventricular function testing is another method used for risk stratification of patients undergoing major vascular surgery. Radionuclide angiography was first studied in patients at rest and during exercise in an attempt to improve preoperative risk assessment.[27–33] In these studies of several hundred patients referred for vascular surgery, resting ejection fraction less than or equal to 35% was a significantly better indicator of perioperative risk than any clinical marker. However, in more recent studies poor resting ejection fraction during radionuclide angiography did not have a strong relationship with perioperative adverse outcomes.[30–33] Exercise radionuclide angiography was then used to measure ejection fraction and wall motion responses to stress. Again, data were not particularly sensitive predictors of perioperative adverse outcomes. However, exercise capacity is limited in many vascular surgery patients and nuclear studies may not be available in all hospitals and are relatively expensive. In addition, radionuclide angiography for wall motion analysis has considerable technical limitations.

• *Stress echocardiography is becoming an important predictor of adverse myocardial events.*

Accordingly, the applicability of echocardiography using pharmacologic stress in this setting has been evaluated. The stress echocardiographic study, in addition to its relatively low cost, provides data on both global and regional left ventricular function, as well as valve function and any intracardiac, pericardial abnormalities. The results are immediately available, and the test can be performed in an office or other ambulatory setting without exposing the patient to radiation. An additional visit for delayed imaging, as for stress thallium studies, is not required. However, about 15 to 20% of patients do not have acoustical windows to permit acquisition of an echo adequate for the quantification of segmental wall motion. Initial studies using either dipyridamole or dobutamine stress echocardiography showed promise.[34–38] These studies had relatively small sample sizes and used selected groups of patients. Adenosine, dipyridamole, and dobutamine have all been used as stress agents, and Martin and co-workers compared these stressors in a blind study of 40 patients.[39] Coronary angiography was used as a reference criterion for the presence of severe CAD. These investigators found that dobutamine stress echocardiography was significantly more sensitive than either adenosine or dipyridamole stress. However, the adenosine stress study was found to be significantly more specific for the prediction of severe CAD.

Two recent studies used larger consecutive groups of patients who were specifically scheduled for elective vascular surgery. These two studies make an important contribution, and their data are reviewed. Poldermans and associates studied dobutamine stress echocardiography in 136 consecutive patients scheduled for elective vascular surgery, and all underwent cardiac risk assessment based on Detsky's classification.[40] None underwent stress thallium studies, coronary angiography, or myocardial revascularization before surgery. The authors found that dobutamine, plus atropine if necessary to achieve 85% of the age-predicted maximum heart rate without signs or symptoms of ischemia, was well tolerated. Adequate images were obtained in 134 of the 136 patients, and only one important complication (ventricular fibrillation) occurred. Three tests were discontinued prematurely because of side effects. Data from 131 patients were analyzed for outcomes. Dobutamine stress echocardiography showed new or worsened wall motion abnormalities in 35 of 131 patients. In the postoperative period, 15 patients had adverse outcomes (5 died of MI, 9 had unstable angina, and 1 developed pulmonary edema). All patients with adverse outcomes had a positive dobutamine stress echocardiogram, and no adverse outcomes occurred in the patients with negative tests. By multivariate logistic regression analysis, only age greater than 70 years and new wall motion abnormalities on dobutamine stress echocardiography were significant predictors of perioperative cardiac adverse outcomes. These authors concluded that dobutamine stress echocardiography is feasible, safe, and useful for identifying patients at high or low risk for perioperative adverse outcomes associated with noncardiac surgery. Furthermore these investigators believed that the test yielded additional information beyond that provided by clinical variables in patients scheduled for noncardiovascular surgery.

- *Wall motion abnormalities detected by echocardiography during dobutamine-induced stress appear to be significant predictors of adverse myocardial events.*

In another study, Davila-Roman and co-workers performed dobutamine stress echocardiography in 98 consecutive patients scheduled to undergo aortic or peripheral vascular surgery.[41] Dobutamine was infused in graded fashion until the maximum predicted heart rate, based on age, was reached. Five patients had inconclusive studies based on inadequate heart rates and were excluded. The remaining 93 patients were divided into 2 groups: 70 patients exhibited a normal response to the dobutamine infusion with no new wall motion abnormalities, and 23 patients had an abnormal response characterized by the development of new or worsening wall motion abnormalities suggesting the presence of myocardial ischemia. Sixty-eight of the 70 patients with a negative study subsequently underwent vascular or aortic surgery without perioperative adverse outcomes. Nineteen of the 23 patients with a positive study underwent coronary angiography, and all had less than 50% narrowing of one or more major coronary arteries Thirteen of these patients underwent bypass grafting or angioplasty before peripheral vascular or aortic surgery, and all 13 had an uneventful perioperative period. Four of the 10 patients who had positive studies but did not undergo coronary revascularization had perioperative adverse outcomes (MI occurred in 2, an ischemic episode requiring urgent coronary bypass grafting in 1 and heart failure in another). Events occurred in 20% of those who had positive results and no events occurred in those who had negative results ($p = 0.003$). The authors concluded that positive and negative dobutamine echocardiographic study results are significant predictors of the presence or absence of perioperative adverse outcomes. Furthermore, they recommend that when a positive test result occurs coronary angiography and further medical and/or surgical intervention or both be considered. Since a negative test indicates a low likelihood of perioperative adverse outcomes and no additional measures are needed. During the long-term follow-up period, 2 patients who had negative studies and 3 of the 23 with positive studies (15%) developed a cardiac adverse outcome ($p = 0.038$). Thus, the authors further conclude that this test provides information relative to long-term follow-up.

Synthesis. Based on accumulated data with dobutamine stress echocardiography, it is reasonable to conclude that the test is relatively safe, it costs less than radionuclide tests, and it is useful to predict the risk for adverse outcomes in patients undergoing noncardiac surgery. The test has not been applied to large populations, however, and it yields an inadequate echo in at least 10 to 15% of patients. A negative response identifies patients who can undergo noncardiac, in particular vascular, surgery with minimal risk and hence deserve no additional cardiac evaluation or intervention. A negative test result also seems to indicate a relatively favorable long-term prognosis. A positive dobutamine echocardiographic stress test, on the other hand, implies a considerable increase in risk of both perioperative and long-term adverse outcomes. At this point in time it would seem that the positive test results identify a subgroup of patients who should be considered for preoperative coronary angiography and myocardial revascularization when feasible before the planned surgery.

• *A positive dobutamine echocardiographic stress test demonstrates considerable risk for surgery. These patients may require further study and possible coronary artery revascularization before the intended operative procedure.*

Continuous Electrocardiographic (ECG) Monitoring

More recently, detection of ischemia during daily life by continuous, high-quality, multilead ECG monitoring has been shown to be a predictor of high risk for adverse outcomes when applied to patients with CAD.[42] Studies that applied this technique perioperatively have identified those patients at risk for perioperative adverse outcomes among patients scheduled to undergo peripheral vascular surgery.

Raby and associates were the first to apply this technology to 176 patients undergoing peripheral vascular surgery.[43] Thirty-two had episodes of ischemic-type ST-segment depression, and 73 of the 75 episodes of ischemia were asymptomatic. Thirteen patients had major postoperative adverse outcomes, including 1 with a fatal MI, 3 with nonfatal infarctions, 4 with unstable angina, and 5 with ischemia-related pulmonary edema. Of the 32 patients with ischemic episodes, before operation, 12 had postoperative adverse outcomes. In the 144 patients who did not have preoperative ischemic episodes, only 1 postoperative adverse outcome occurred.

• *In this study, preoperative ischemic episodes were highly predictive of myocardial infarction or ischemia-related pulmonary edema. Patients without preoperative ischemic events were highly unlikely to have an adverse outcome.*

Ouyang and her associates assessed the significance of early postoperative ischemia in 24 patients with clinically stable CAD who were undergoing peripheral vascular surgery.[44] Continuous ECG monitoring was initiated 17 hours preoperatively (mean), intraoperatively, and postoperatively for another 29 hours. This was done using 2 dual-channel recorders to yield information from 4 ECG leads. Fifteen patients (63%) had early postoperative ischemic episodes, 3 also had preoperative ischemia, and 5 had intraoperative ischemia. Patient characteristics, perioperative antianginal medications, and postoperative episodes of hemodynamic instability were similar in patients with and without ischemic episodes. However, 8 of the 15 patients (53%) with ischemia had postoperative adverse outcomes (2 patients with MIs, 2 with new congestive heart failure, and 4 with new-onset rest angina). Only 1 of 9 patients (11%) without ischemic episodes (11%) had postoperative adverse outcomes. The authors concluded that preoperative and early postoperative ischemia is usually silent, occurs frequently after vascular surgery, and is highly associated with postoperative adverse outcomes.

• *In this study, patients with preoperative ischemic ECG changes were likely to have an adverse outcome.*

In the most definitive report to date, Mangano and colleagues studied 476 men with CAD (243) or high risk for CAD (231) who were undergoing elective noncardiac surgery.[45] Ischemia was assessed by continuous ECG monitoring beginning 2 days before surgery and continuing for 2 days postoperatively. Eighty-three patients (18%) had postoperative cardiac adverse outcomes in the hospital. Postoperative ischemia occurred in 41% and was associated with a 2.8-fold increase in risk of all adverse outcomes ($p < 0.0002$) and a 9.2-fold increase in risk of ischemic events ($p < 0.004$).

• *Preoperative ischemia in this study resulted in a high risk of ischemic events or adverse outcomes.*

More recently, Fleisher and colleagues studied 67 patients undergoing vascular surgery and 97 nonvascular surgical patients, all of whom were at increased risk for cardiac disease, to determine whether preoperative ischemia on AECG was predictive of postoperative ischemia-related adverse outcomes.[46] The presence of preoperative ischemia in the nonvascular and vascular surgical patients had similar predictive values for postoperative adverse outcomes (0.38 and 0.38, respectively). Perhaps more important, the absence of preoperative ischemia predicted an excellent outcome in patients undergoing nonvascular surgery (0.99). The absence of ischemia was a less robust predictor of excellent outcome in the vascular patients (0.86).

• *Patients without ischemia during preoperative ECG monitoring were highly unlikely to have an adverse cardiac event.*

Pasternack and associates used real-time ECG monitoring in 200 patients undergoing peripheral vascular surgery to try to better define those at high risk of perioperative MI.[47] The patients were divided into those undergoing abdominal aortic aneurysm or lower extremity revascularization procedures (group I, $n = 120$) and those undergoing carotid artery endarterectomy (group II, $n = 80$). Ischemia was detected during the preoperative, intraoperative, or postoperative period in 61% of group I and in 68% of group II patients. Six group I and 3 group II patients had a perioperative MI, with 2 cardiac deaths. In both groups I and II, a variety of parameters based on monitoring of ischemia were compared between the subgroups of patients who had MI and those who did not. The results show that in both groups there was a significantly ($p \leq 0.05$) greater total duration of perioperative ischemic time, total number of perioperative ischemic episodes, and total duration

• *In this study, patients who had a perioperative myocardial infaction had a significantly greater perioperative ischemic time, as well as total number of perioperative ischemic events.*

of perioperative ischemic time as a percentage of total monitoring time in patients who developed a perioperative MI compared with those who did not. Multivariate logistic regression analysis of preoperative characteristics in all 200 patients showed that the occurrence of preoperative ischemia and angina at rest were the only significant predictors of perioperative MI. The authors concluded that perioperative monitoring for myocardial ischemia might noninvasively identify those patients undergoing peripheral vascular surgery who are at increased risk for perioperative MI permitting implementation of timely preventive measures in selected patients.

• During carotid endarterectomy, ischemia that developed during declamping had a high correlation with an adverse myocardial event.

Perioperative myocardial ischemia was evaluated by Landesberg and Erel in 36 consecutive carotid endarterectomy procedures carried out in patients with a high (72.2%) prevalence of ischemic heart disease.[48] These procedures were performed in patients who were given a cervical plexus block plus a prophylactic intravenous nitroglycerin infusion. Myocardial ischemia, based on perioperative (48 hours) continuous ECG recordings, was correlated with preoperative cardiac status, perioperative continuous intra-arterial blood pressure measurements, and postoperative cardiac outcome. In 2 patients, ST-segment analysis was uninterpretable because of bundle branch blocks. Altogether, 64 episodes of ischemia were detected in 18 (53%) of the procedures. In 8 (24%) procedures, ischemia occurred either during carotid artery clamping at the time of the largest rise in blood pressure or within 2 hours of declamping, when blood pressure tended to decline. There were 4 (12%) postoperative adverse outcomes 3 MIs (1 Q wave and 2 non-Q wave) and 1 episode of unstable angina. All 4 patients with adverse outcomes had early ischemia either at the time of cross-clamping or soon after declamping of the carotid artery. All MIs developed following prolonged (> 10 hours) ischemia, starting with the first 20 hours after surgery. Thus, ischemia that occurred during carotid clamping or soon after declamping was associated with cardiac adverse outcomes (sensitivity 100% and specificity 87%).

• In this study, preoperative ECG monitoring was unable to predict patients who would develop perioperative myocardial ischemia.

Kirwin and colleagues used continuous AECG monitoring as a low-cost preoperative method for detecting myocardial ischemia in 96 patients, whose mean age was 73 years, who were undergoing peripheral vascular surgery (elective aortic (24) or infrainguinal (72) operations).[49] Risk factors included hypertension (71%), history of CAD (66%), smoking (61%), and diabetes mellitus (47%). Nine of 96 patients (9.4%) had a positive AECG for ischemia. Only 1 patient (11%) developed postoperative MI, and there were no deaths. The incidence of postoperative MI in the nonischemic group, however, was 16% (14/87), and the mortality in this group was 6.9% (6/87). New and malignant arrhythmias requiring medical intervention were observed in 7 patients (7.4%), 2 cases of ventricular tachycardia and 5 cases of atrial flutter or fibrillation. Contrary to previous reports, AECG for ischemia was not a significant predictor of postoperative MI or mortality in these patients. However, the authors continue to recommend preoperative AECG monitoring as a diagnostic tool for unsuspected malignant arrhythmias.

Landesberg and associates used continuous perioperative ECG

recording in 151 consecutive patients undergoing major vascular surgery to determine the characteristics of myocardial ischemia and its relation to adverse outcome.[50] A total of 13 (8.6%) patients had postoperative cardiac adverse outcomes (6 MIs, 2 unstable angina, and 5 congestive heart failure). There were 342 perioperative ischemic episodes shown by ST-segment depression, and 164 of these (48%) occurred postoperatively. Postoperative ischemic episodes were significantly longer than episodes before or during operations (3.2 versus 1.7 and 1.5 min/hr monitored, respectively, $p < 0.001$). Both Detsky's cardiac risk index and long-duration (> 2 hours) preoperative ischemia were predictive of postoperative cardiac adverse outcomes (odds ratios in univariate analysis 3.3, $p = 0.03$, and 7.2, $p = 0.009$, respectively). However, long-duration (> 2 hours) postoperative ischemia was the only factor significantly associated with cardiac morbidity in multivariate logistic regression analysis (odds ratio 21.7, $p = 0.001$). Long periods of ST-segment depression preceded most (84.6%) postoperative cardiac events, including MIs, and no cardiac event was preceded by ST-segment elevation. Five of the 6 postoperative MIs were non-Q-wave infarctions. The authors concluded that long-duration subendocardial ischemia, rather than acute coronary artery occlusion, may cause postoperative myocardial injury and complications.

• *In this study, only postoperative mild cardiac ischemia, which lasted longer than 2 hours, proved predictive of cardiac morbidity.*

In another study, by Seegobin and co-workers, which assessed early postoperative adverse outcomes in 50 patients with CAD undergoing major noncardiac surgery, the ECG was monitored continuously for 24 hours after the onset of anesthesia, using a frequency-modulated (FM) AECG monitor.[51] Concurrent automated blood pressure and pulse were measured noninvasively at 3-minute intervals during anesthesia and subsequently at 5-minute intervals. Thirty patients were monitored with 2-site ECG recordings, from modified leads V_1 and V_5 (group A). Twenty patients had 17-site ECG monitoring, multiplexing a 4 by 4 array of precordial electrodes onto a single channel of the FM recorder (group B). Tapes were analyzed for noise, supraventricular and ventricular dysrhythmias, runs of tachy- and bradycardias, and ST-segment changes. These data were correlated with serial standard 12-lead ECGs and CK-MB assay in the 72 hours after surgery. Seven tapes from group A could not be analyzed. Ischemic ECG changes (> 1.0-mm ST-segment depression) observed during monitoring from groups A (14/23) and B (14/20) correlated with serial 12-lead ECG and/or CK-MB changes. The majority of patients with ischemic ST-segment changes (19/28, 70%) occurred shortly after anesthesia. In 14 of 28 (50%) patients, the ischemic ST-segment change occurred during episodes of tachycardia and/or elevated blood pressure (> 20% above baseline). Nine patients (9/23) in group A had no ischemic ST-segment change; however, 6 had serial 12-lead ECG and/or CK-MB changes of ischemic injury. Six patients (6/20) in group B had no ischemic ST-segment changes, and none of these patients had any change in serial 12-lead ECGs or CK-MB assay. No patient complained of chest pain during monitoring. The authors concluded that continual monitoring of heart rate and blood pressure and accu-

• *In this study, 50% of patients who developed ischemic ST-segment changes did so during tachycardiac or hypertensive events.*

rate ST-segment monitoring are essential for early detection and treatment of perioperative myocardial ischemia. The multiple-lead precordial system was more sensitive than traditional 2-lead AECG monitoring in detecting myocardial ischemia.

Synthesis. The foregoing data support the hypothesis that identification of ischemic ST-segment changes in the perioperative period delineates a group of patients at relatively high risk for early post operative adverse outcomes. The postoperative events are often preceded by prolonged periods of ischemia in the early postoperative period. High-quality multilead ECG systems are essential, and digital ECG monitoring with real-time analysis seems promising, considering its very low cost and objective on-line processing. Studies are lacking to conclude that prompt recognition and treatment of perioperative ischemia detected by ECG are of benefit in terms of prevention or reduction of the severity of adverse outcomes.

• *Both ischemia in the preoperative period and prolonged early postoperative ischemia lead to a high incidence of adverse myocardial events.*

Combination Monitoring Studies

ECG and Transesophageal Echocardiography. Since left ventricular regional wall motion abnormalities (RWA) reflect systolic dysfunction and are a very early sign of ischemia, continuous transesophageal echocardiography (TEE) was evaluated as an adjunct to ECG monitoring in 51 patients undergoing abdominal aortic surgery who were studied by Koolen and co-workers.[52] Motion of the entire left ventricular wall (9 segments) was semiquantitatively evaluated 15 minutes before and after aortic cross-clamping and 3 hours after declamping. In addition, limb lead II of the ECG was simultaneously recorded. At baseline, RWA were present in 16 patients (31%). New or worsened RWA 15 minutes after aortic cross-clamping developed in 17 patients, of whom 11 had persistent RWA still present 3 hours after declamping. This disorder was associated in 7 patients with enzyme-documented MI. Only 1 patient with an infarct demonstrated ST-segment changes of more than 1 mm. Thus, a single-limb ECG lead is relatively insensitive for perioperative myocardial ischemia detection. Furthermore, new and/or worsened RWA after aortic cross-clamping, which persists until at least 3 hours after declamping, is, to a considerable degree, associated with perioperative MI.

• *TEE-demonstrated wall motion abnormalities that persist are associated with perioperative myocardial infarction.*

Eisenberg and associates examined whether routine use of TEE and ECG monitoring has incremental value in identification of patients at high risk for perioperative ischemia-related adverse outcomes. This information was compared with preoperative clinical data and intraoperative monitoring using continuous 2-lead bipolar ECG lead system.[53] A total of 332 men who underwent noncardiac surgery and were at high risk for CAD had TEE, 12-lead ECG, and 2-lead ECG performed continuously during noncardiac surgery (47% vascular, 53% nonvascular). Monitoring results were not available to anesthesiologists or surgeons, and the data were blindly analyzed after surgery. In a subset of 285 patients who were adequately studied by all 3 techniques, 111 patients (39%) were identified as having had intraoperative myocardial ischemia by one or more monitoring techniques. By univariate analysis, intraoperative

• *Routine use of TEE does not add much to the identification of patients at high risk for perioperative ischemia.*

ischemia was associated with all perioperative cardiac adverse outcomes. This included the ischemia-related outcomes of cardiac death, nonfatal MI and unstable angina, congestive heart failure, and ventricular tachycardia. However, when monitoring results for TEE and the 12-lead ECG were added to a multivariate model that included preoperative clinical data and continuous 2-lead ECG results, the incremental value of TEE was small (odds ratio 2.6; 95% confidence interval (CI), 1.2 to 5.7; $p = 0.02$). The 12-lead ECG was not significant (odds ratio, 1.5; 95% CI, 0.6 to 3.8). Furthermore, when the multivariate analysis was repeated with only ischemia-related outcomes, neither TEE nor the 12-lead ECG retained significant associations (odds ratio, 2.2; 95% CI, 0.5 to 9.4, and odds ratio, 1.1; 95% CI, 0.2 to 6.1, respectively). These workers concluded that, when compared with preoperative clinical data and intraoperative monitoring using 2-lead ECG system, routine monitoring for myocardial ischemia with TEE or 12-lead ECG during noncardiac surgery has little incremental clinical value for identification of patients at high risk for perioperative ischemic outcomes.

ECG and Myocardial Perfusion Imaging. In order to stratify cardiac risk in patients undergoing vascular surgery, McPhail and co-workers compared dipyridamole stress myocardial perfusion imaging using Cardiolite (a ^{99m}technetium agent) with AECG monitoring for ischemia.[54] One hundred patients (86 men, 14 women; mean age, 67 years) underwent outpatient 48-hour AECG monitoring and Cardiolite imaging before vascular surgery (70 abdominal aortic aneurysm repair, 21 aortobifemoral grafts, 9 femoropopliteal grafts). Ischemia on AECG was defined as one or more periods when the ST segment was depressed 1 mm or more and lasted 1 minute or longer. Myocardial perfusion imaging was carried out with high-dose (0.84 mg/kg) dipyridamole, Cardiolite, and planar imaging. Ischemia was defined as a segmental perfusion abnormality following dipyridamole and with improved perfusion on rest imaging. The AECG identified ischemia in 30 of 100 (30%) patients. Perioperative MI occurred in 9 patients, and 2 died. The diagnostic accuracy of the tests was similar, with a low positive predictive value of 15 to 20%, but an extremely high negative predictive value of 94 to 96%. The cardiac adverse outcome rate in patients with negative results of both tests was only 2 of 48 (4.2%), with only 1 test positive in 3 of 40 (7.5%) and both tests positive in 4 of 12 (33%). These authors suggested that a reasonable approach to preoperative risk stratification would be to obtain either an AECG or a Cardiolite scan initially.

Synthesis. From the foregoing, it seems that the detection of perioperative ischemia by AECG during noncardiac vascular surgery is as good as either TEE wall motion monitoring or perfusion imaging in terms of predicting adverse outcome. However, all three technologies are relatively new and have not been tested for this purpose in large prospective evaluations. Whether a management strategy guided by detection of ischemia can alter the risk or severity of ischemia-related adverse outcomes in these patients has not yet been specifically addressed.

Invasive Cardiac Studies

In some centers, coronary angiography for risk stratification before vascular surgery is routinely recommended in all patients with known or suspected CAD. The rationale given is that the majority of these cases have severe CAD, and angiography-driven revascularization should eliminate or significantly reduce the risk for adverse outcomes. This approach has several important problems. First, simple knowledge of the coronary anatomy does not reliably predict either the functional significance of a coronary stenosis or the outcome in a given individual. Hence, taken alone, these coronary angiographic findings have the potential to lead to inappropriate decisions. Second, routine coronary angiography is costly and provides entry to even more costly therapeutic procedures (coronary angioplasty, bypass surgery) that may be unnecessary. Coronary angiography done in 1000 consecutive patients scheduled for peripheral vascular surgery by Hertzer and associates found that 92% had CAD.[55] About one quarter of these patients had prophylactic coronary bypass surgery. Here the identification of coronary stenosis drives the subsequent management rather than an estimate of the likely consequences associated with such a stenosis in a given patient with distinct individual characteristics (age, gender, old MI, diabetes, poor functional capacity, large area of myocardium at risk). The latter characteristics all interact to determine a given patient's long-term outcome. Third, increasingly a routine angiography-driven approach is challenged by third-party payers or is simply not reimbursed. Clearly, a routine invasive approach cannot be justified in this era of health care reform. Fourth, there are no objective data from controlled trials to suggest that routine coronary angiography and subsequent revascularization are of benefit before vascular surgery.

• *Coronary artery stenosis noted by angiography may not predict outcome unless associated factors such as diabetes, age, or previous myocardial infarction are taken into consideration.*

Finally, and perhaps the strongest argument against a routine invasive approach, is that a careful clinical evaluation using selective noninvasive tests appropriately can correctly identify the overwhelming majority of patients that comprise the group at increased cardiac risk. From this position appropriate invasive procedures can then be scheduled for the small subset of patients truly in need of and most likely to benefit from these procedures.

Synthesis. While routine preoperative coronary angiography before such procedures as peripheral vascular surgery has been advocated, the costs, risks, and implications of this approach as a routine prohibit its general application. Furthermore, coronary angiography does not provide data on the functional significance of given coronary stenosis.

ANTI-ISCHEMIC TREATMENTS TO ALTER PERIOPERATIVE CARDIAC RISK

Once an optimal testing strategy is developed and validated in a large variety of patient subgroups with different noncardiac surgical procedures and different practice settings, the question of which treatment provides optimal reduction of adverse outcomes can be addressed. It seems logical that myocardial ischemia can be used as a surrogate for major ischemia-related adverse outcomes. This will facilitate the initial testing of various treatment strategies. Ultimately, formal large-scale clinical trials will be needed to determine whether a given perioperative treatment strategy alters major adverse outcomes such as death and MI.

At present, only very preliminary data on anti-ischemic treatments are available. One prospective randomized trial used a single oral dose of a beta blocker in 128 patients scheduled for abdominal or vascular surgery.[56] Patients were randomized to 4 treatment groups: no beta-blocker control group (n = 39); 100-mg labetalol group (n = 29); 50-mg atenolol group (n = 30); and 20-mg oxprenolol group (n = 30). These agents were all given 2 hours before anesthesia induction. Ischemia occurred in 28% of controls but in only 2% of beta-blocker-treated patients. Although this difference was impressive, a single oral dose of these agents does not provide adequate beta blockade of cardiovascular responses at 2 hours. Two other nonrandomized studies provide data to support a protective effect of beta blockade for perioperative ischemia.[57,58] Another study examined the effect of intravenous diltiazem or placebo in 30 patients with chronic stable angina during noncardiac surgery.[59] Eleven placebo-assigned and 6 diltiazem-assigned patients had ischemia, but this difference was not statistically significant. A total of 25 ischemic episodes were recorded in the 11 placebo patients, versus only 8 ischemic episodes in the 5 diltiazem-assigned patients ($p < 0.002$). Coriat and co-workers studied the effect of low- and high-dose nitroglycerin infusion in 45 patients with chronic stable angina who underwent abdominal or vascular surgery.[60] These investigators found that the patients assigned to the high-dose nitroglycerin group were less likely to have intraoperative ischemia compared with the low-dose group.

- *Beta-blocker therapy and nitroglycerin appear to reduce the incidence of perioperative myocardial infarction.*

Recently, a meta-analysis of 22 trials suggests that aspirin is associated with a reduction of approximately 20% in the risk of MI, stroke, or vascular death in patients with peripheral vascular disease.[61] The same report found a highly significant reduction in death or pulmonary embolism in 53 trials of patients who underwent various surgical procedures. So it seems that aspirin should be used.

Synthesis. Based on the foregoing limited data, it is very difficult to support the routine use of any specific anti-ischemic agent except aspirin. In terms of revascularization before noncardiac surgery, there are no data from controlled trials to address this form of treatment. Observational data from several sources that suggest that revascularization may be protective for ischemia-related adverse outcomes associated with noncardiac surgery must be considered in terms of the 1 to 2% additional mortality associated with coronary bypass. When this risk is considered, no mortality benefit of routine preoperative coronary bypass grafting can be demonstrated. For these reasons, in addition to the enormous costs involved, a strategy of routine invasive study followed by prophylactic revascularization for all patients with CAD who are to undergo noncardiac surgery cannot be endorsed at this time. It is very unlikely that any additional measures like coronary angiography and revascularization could significantly alter the adverse outcome rates seen in low-risk patients. Other patients, however, who have markers suggesting high risk, may benefit from additional measures.

STRATEGY FOR PERIOPERATIVE CARDIAC ASSESSMENT THAT FOCUSES ON MYOCARDIAL ISCHEMIA

From the foregoing, it seems clear that methodology exists to identify groups of patients scheduled to undergo noncardiac surgery who are at high and low risk for adverse cardiac outcomes. The exact specialized testing required and the best use of these data to guide perioperative care are not yet settled. Until there are more data from large clinical studies, this important issue cannot be advanced. In the meantime, I will outline some guidelines that seem appropriate from my clinical practice. In my view, the objectives of preoperative assessment should be to identify patients at high or low risk for ischemia-related cardiac events and to detect and modify factors known to be associated with increased perioperative risk.

The history and physical examination findings are very important in the initial assessment, and these findings should form the basis for any additional testing (see Table 8–1). The goal is to identify high-risk and low-risk patients and use the results to suggest which patients need more comprehensive perioperative management. For example, in high-risk cases (e.g., recent MI, unstable angina), one may recommend that the surgery not be performed at that time and/or that coronary angiography be done (Fig. 8–1). Specific medications (e.g., beta blockers, nitrates) or monitoring procedures (e.g., TEE, AECG) are likely to be helpful in high-risk patients. In certain high-risk patients, benefit may occur from myocardial revascularization, with either percutaneous transluminal coronary angioplasty or coronary artery bypass grafting, before noncardiac surgery. Patients identified as low risk are also benefitted because no further preoperative evaluation is required, and their noncardiac surgery will not delayed by costly additional testing or treatments. In general, from the cardiovascular standpoint, patients without prior MI, angina, diabetes, evidence of heart failure, abnormal resting ECG, or ventricular arrhythmia overall comprise a very low-risk group for ischemia-related complications with noncardiac surgery. If they will not undergo vascular surgery, no additional testing will be needed (Fig. 8–2). Some may elect to add an ETT. I would recommend this option for all patients scheduled to undergo vascular surgery who are asymptomatic from the cardiac standpoint.

• *Patients without any risk factors for coronary artery disease probably will need few additional screening tests before surgery.*

Regardless of perioperative risk assessment, careful periopera-

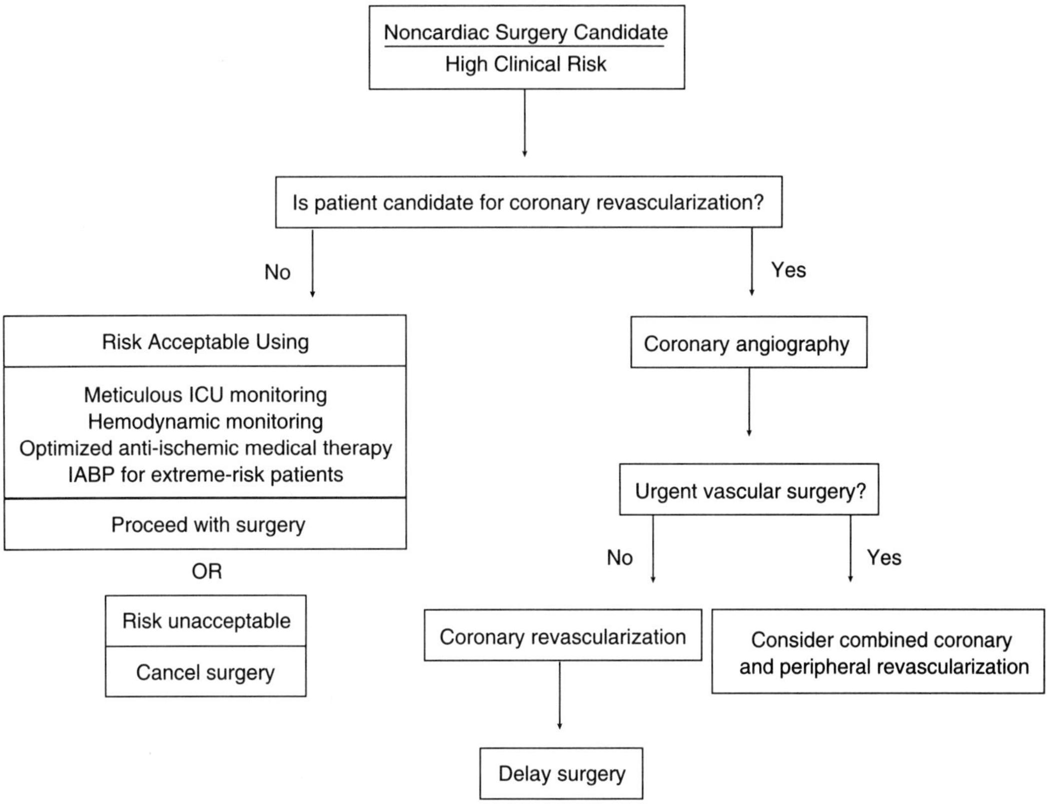

Figure 8–1.
Algorithm for preoperative management of the high-risk patient.

tive cardiac care can greatly minimize the severity and incidence of cardiac events. Cardiac medications including aspirin should be continued until the morning of surgery, when parenteral and intravenous medications can replace oral medications in the early postoperative period. This is particularly true with agents such as beta blockers and antihypertensive agents. With comprehensive perioperative invasive hemodynamic monitoring and oximetry, as well as high-quality multilead ECG monitoring, a significant decrease in perioperative ischemia can be achieved by early detection and attention to hemodynamic derangements before ischemia becomes manifest. In addition, intraoperative TEE can help monitor global and regional left ventricular function, particularly during aortic cross-clamping, which increases left ventricular afterload abruptly. This form of monitoring enables one to assess ischemia-related left ventricular dysfunction and to intervene early. Elective intra-aortic balloon pump support may be helpful in some high-risk patients, and preoperative revascularization may be useful in other patients. Despite these advances, it must be remembered that the mortality from a perioperative MI remains high. Approximately 40% of all perioperative infarctions will result in death. It has also been shown that 1- to 2-year outcomes of those who survive perioperative infarction are poor.[62] Consequently, any elective surgery must be deferred

- *When myocardial ischemia is noted perioperatively, steps should be taken immediately to correct the condition. These include heart rate and blood pressure reduction, as well as nitroglycerin therapy.*

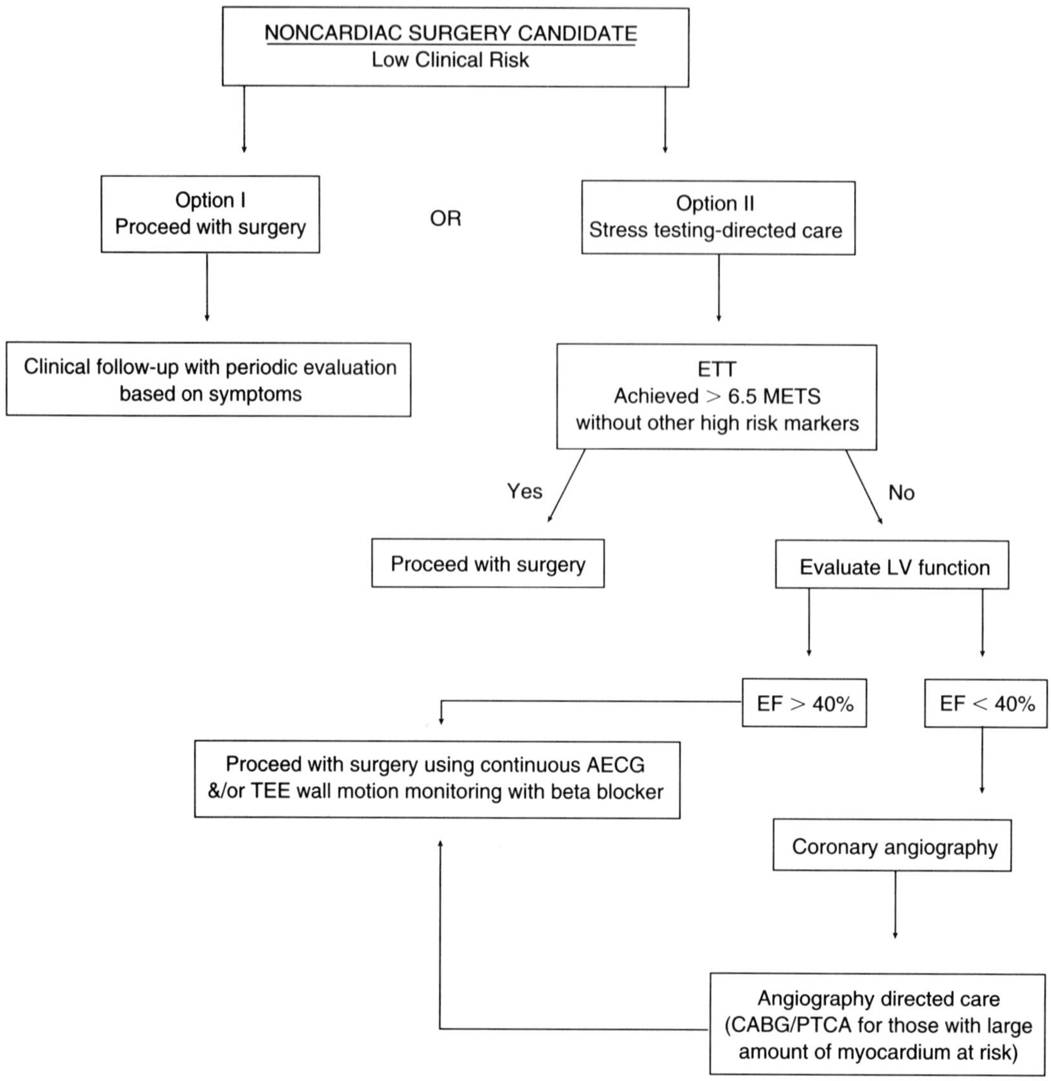

Figure 8–2.
Algorithm for preoperative management of the low-risk patient.

• *Patients at high risk for perioperative myocardial events and with known coronary artery disease may benefit from revascularization procedures before their specific surgical operation.*

until at least 6 months after a prior MI because of the high risk for recurrent MI. When surgery cannot be deferred, a possible combined procedure that includes both coronary revascularization and the emergency noncardiac surgery may minimize the risks.

The process of managing patients with known or suspect CAD who are to undergo elective vascular surgery requires ongoing risk stratification directed at identification of those at high risk for adverse outcomes. Considerable information for this process comes from the initial clinical assessment, which uses the multifactorial risk scores noted previously. In many cases, noninvasive stress testing provides a useful supplement to clinically based risk assessments (see Table 8–2). However, the reader should be aware that no prospective trial has provided data that compare patients randomly assigned to a conservative, clinically guided management strategy with those assigned to a more aggressive, ischemia-guided management strategy. Patients with severe angina (Canadian Cardiovascular Society class III, IV, or unstable), recent MI (< 6 months), heart failure, and resting ECG abnormalities of ischemia are at such high risk for adverse events that noninvasive risk stratification would not be likely to identify a subgroup with sufficiently low risk to justify any noninvasive test. Such high-risk patients are best managed with an early coronary angiogram and direct interventional strategy attempting to revascularize ischemic regions to reduce to risk for adverse events. Subgroups of high-risk patients will exist who are not willing to accept an interventional strategy as treatment for their CAD or have severe complicating illnesses or advanced age so that revascularization would not be an option. Another major group will be at such very low risk because they are unlikely to have CAD and heart failure (young patients, premenopausal women) after initial evaluation that the risk of adverse outcomes is so low that no abnormal test finding would prompt consideration for myocardial revascularization. I consider patients who do not clearly fall into one of the foregoing categories as reasonable candidates for risk stratification by noninvasive testing.

The goals of noninvasive testing are to estimate outcome and to use this information to help decide what additional tests and adjustments to therapy are required based on prognosis.

It is recommended that exercise or pharmacologic noninvasive stress testing should be an integral part of the evaluation of patients at high risk for CAD prior to elective noncardiac surgery even though they may not appear at risk for adverse outcomes based on clinical evaluation (Fig. 8–3). Those at high risk include men older than age 35 and postmenopausal women who have at least one other CAD risk factor such as smoking, hypertension, and hyperlipidemia or who have been scheduled for vascular surgery. The testing should include an evaluation for myocardial ischemia and an assessment of left ventricular function. The choice of test should be based on the patient's resting ECG, physical ability to perform exercise, and local expertise and technology available. In general, the exercise ECG should be considered for those who are physically able, provided their ECG is interpretable for ischemia (e.g., QRS duration $\leq$ 0.10 sec, resting ST-segment depression $\leq$ 0.5 mm, and R-wave amplitude $\geq$ 10 mm) in the absence of left ventricular hypertrophy and drugs that may affect ST segments. Clearly, patients with any of the foregoing, bundle branch block, or intraventricular conduction defects, or patients receiving digoxin therapy, should not undergo stress testing that uses the ECG signal for assessment of ischemia. Such patients are better served with an imaging modality to assess exercise-induced ischemia. For those who cannot exercise, a pharmacologic stress test with imaging (thallium, echocardiography) is the choice.

- *When feasible, the exercise ECG stress test may be the best screening tool to identify patients at risk for perioperative myocardial complications.*

In conclusion, advances in noncardiac surgical technology will encourage further use in wider groups of patients, many of whom will have CAD. In many such patients scheduled for noncardiac

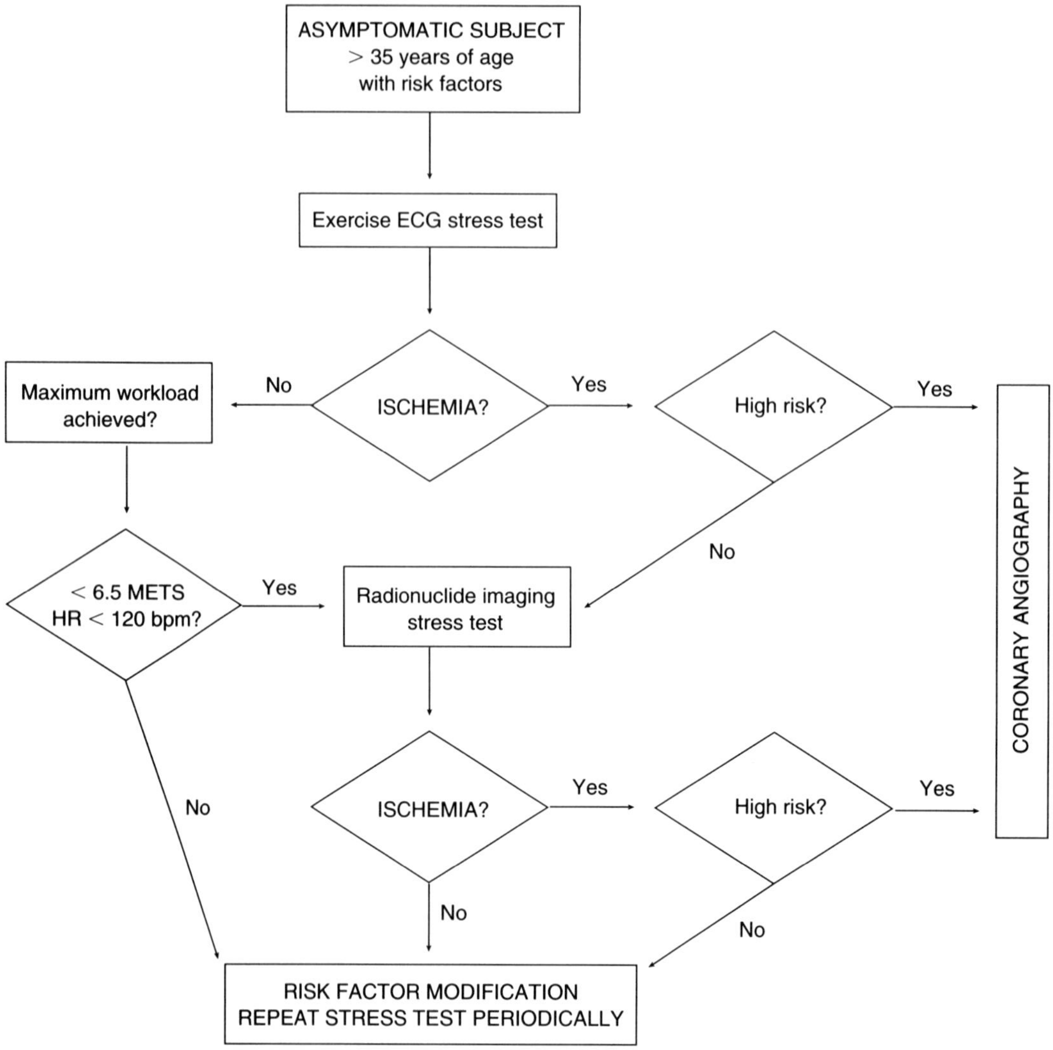

Figure 8–3.
Management of the asymptomatic patient.

surgery, adequate preoperative risk stratification can be done using simple clinical risk indices. In selected patients, additional noninvasive testing may be of benefit in identifying those at higher risk for adverse outcomes and to direct referral for perioperative coronary angiography and revascularization. Large-scale clinical trials are clearly needed to determine which management strategies reduce risk for perioperative adverse outcomes.

REFERENCES

1. Mangano DT: Perioperative morbidity and review. Anesthesiology 1990; 72:153–184.
2. National Center for Health Statistics: Health, United States, 1988. In: Advance data from vital and health statistics. Washington DC, Govern-

ment Printing Office, 1989; pp. 111–122(DHHS pub. no. PHS89–1232).

3. Abraham SA, Coles NA, Coley CM, et al: Coronary risk of noncardiac surgery. Prog Cardiovasc Dis 1991; 34:205–234.
4. Tarhan S, Moffitt EA, Taylor WF, Giuliani ER: Myocardial infarction after general anesthesia. JAMA 1978; 220:1451–1454.
5. Goldman L, Caldera DL, Nussbaum SR, et al: Multifactorial index of cardiac risk in noncardiac surgical procedures. N Engl J Med 1977; 297:845.
6. Zeldin RA: Assessing cardiac risk in cardiac patients who undergo noncardiac surgical procedures. Can J Surg 1984; 27:402.
7. Jeffrey CC, Kunsman J, Cullen DJ, et al: A prospective evaluation of cardiac risk index. Anesthesiology 1983; 58:462.
8. Detsky AS, Abrams HB, McLaughlin JR, et al: Predicting cardiac complications in patients undergoing non-cardiac surgery. J Gen Intern Med 1986; 1:211–219.
9. Detsky AS, Abrams HB, Forbath N, et al: Cardiac assessment for patients undergoing noncardiac surgery: a multifactorial clinical risk index. Arch Intern Med 1986; 146:2131.
10. Wong T, Detsky AS: Perioperative cardiac risk assessment for patients having peripheral vascular surgery. Ann Intern Med 1992; 116: 743–753.
11. Eagle KA, Singer DE, Brewster DC, et al: Dipyridamole thallium scanning in patients undergoing vascular surgery: optimizing preoperative evaluation of cardiac risk. JAMA 1987; 257:2185.
12. Eagle KA, Coley CM, Newell JB, et al: Combining clinical and thallium data optimizes preoperative assessment of cardiac risk before major vascular surgery. Ann Intern Med 1989; 110:859.
13. Cutler BS, Wheeler HB, Paraskos JA, et al: Applicability and interpretation of electrocardiographic stress testing in patients with peripheral vascular disease. Am J Surg 1981; 141:501–506.
14. McPhail N, Calvin JE, Shariatmadar A, et al: The use of preoperative exercise testing to predict cardiac complications after arterial reconstruction. J Vasc Surg 1988; 7:60–68.
15. Carliner NH, Fisher ML, Plotnick GD, et al: Routine preoperative exercise testing in patients undergoing major noncardiac surgery. Am J Cardiol 1985; 56:51–58.
16. Gerson MC, Hurst JM, Hertzberg VS, et al: Cardiac prognosis in noncardiac geriatric surgery. Ann Intern Med 1985; 193:832–837.
17. Kopecky Sl, Biggons RJ, Hollier LH: Preoperative supine exercise radionuclide angiogram predicts perioperative cardiovascular events in vascular surgery (abstract). J Am Coll Cardiol 1986; 7:226A.
18. Leppo J, Plaja J, Gionet M, et al: Noninvasive evaluation of cardiac risk before elective vascular surgery. J Am Coll Cardiol 1987; 9:269.
19. Lette J, Waters D, Cerino M, et al: Preoperative coronary artery disease risk stratification based on dipyridamole imaging and a simple three-step three-segment model for patients undergoing noncardiac vascular surgery or major general surgery. Am J Cardiol 1992; 69:1553.
20. Mangano DT, London MJ, Tubau JF, et al: The Study of Perioperative Ischemia Research Group: Dipyridamole thallium-201 scintigraphy as a preoperative screening test. A re-examination of its predictive potential. Circulation 1991; 84:493–502.
21. Younis LT, Aguirre F, Byers S, et al: Perioperative and long-term prognostic value of intravenous dipyridamole thallium scintigraphy in pa-

tients with peripheral vascular disease. Am Heart J 1990; 119: 1287–1292.

22. Fleisher LA, Nelson AH, Rosenbaum SH: Failure of negative dipyridamole thallium scans to predict perioperative myocardial ischaemia and infection. Can J Anaesth 1992; 39:179–183.
23. Kazmers A, Kispert JF, Rotiman L, et al: Thallium redistribution does not predict perioperative cardiac complications following vascular surgery. J Ky Med Assoc 1991; 89:279–284.
24. Hendel RC, Whitfield SS: Prediction of late cardiac events by dipyridamole thallium imaging in patients undergoing elective vascular surgery. Am J Cardiol 1992; 70:1243–1249.
25. McFalls EO, Doliszny KM, Grund F, et al: Angina and persistent exercise thallium defects: independent risk factors in elective vascular surgery. J Am Coll Cardiol 1993; 21:1347–1352.
26. Brown KA, Rowen M: Extent of jeopardized viable myocardium determined by myocardial perfusion imaging best predicts perioperative cardiac events in patients undergoing noncardiac surgery. J Am Coll Cardiol 1993; 21:325–330.
27. Pasternak PF, Imparato AM, Riles TS, et al: The value of the radionuclide angiogram in the prediction of perioperative myocardial infarction in patients undergoing lower extremity revascularization procedures. Circulation 1985; 72:II-13.
28. Goldman L, Caldera Dl, Southwick FS, et al: Cardiac risk factors and complications in non-cardiac surgery. Medicine 1978; 57:357–370.
29. Pasternak PF, Grossi EA, Baumann FG, et al: The value of silent myocardial ischemia monitoring in the prediction of perioperative myocardial infarction in patients undergoing peripheral vascular surgery. J Vasc Surg 1989; 10:617–625.
30. Kazmers A, Cerqueira MD, Zierler E: The role of preoperative radionuclide left ventricular ejection fraction in direct abdominal aortic aneurysm repair. J Vasc Surg 1988; 8:128–136.
31. Kazmers A, Cerqueira MD, Zierler RE: Perioperative and late outcome in patients with left ventricular ejection fraction of 35% or less who require major vascular surgery. J Vasc Surg 1988; 8:307–315.
32. Franco CD, Goldsmith J, Veith FJ, et al: Resting gated pool ejection fraction: a poor predictor of perioperative myocardial infarction in patients undergoing vascular surgery for infrainguinal bypass grafting. J Vasc Surg 1989; 19:656–661.
33. McCann RL, Wolfe WG: Resection of abdominal aortic aneurysm in patients with low ejection fractions. J Vasc Surg 1989; 10:240–244.
34. Lane RT, Sawada SG, Ryan T, et al: Dobutamine stress echocardiography as a predictor of perioperative cardiac events. Am J Cardiol 1991; 68:976–977.
35. Elliott BM, Robinson JG, Zellner JL, Hendrix GH. Dobutamine-201-thallium imaging: assessing cardiac risks associated with vascular surgery. Circulation 1991; 83:III-54-III-60.
36. Picano E, Lattanzi F, Orlandini A, et al: Stress echocardiography and the human factor: the importance of being expert. J Am Coll Cardiol 1991; 17:666–669.
37. Previtali M, Lanzarini L, Ferrario M, et al: Dobutamine versus dipyridamole echocardiography in coronary artery disease. Circulation 1991; 83:III-27-III-31.
38. Sawada SG, Segar DS, Ryan T, et al: Echocardiographic detection of coronary artery disease during dobutamine infusion. Circulation 1991; 83:1605–1614.

39. Martin TW, Seaworth JF, Johns JP, et al: Comparison of adenosine, dipyridamole, and dobutamine in stress echocardiography. Ann Intern Med 1992; 116:190–196.
40. Poldermans D, Fioretti PM, Forster T, et al: Dobutamaine stress echocardiography for assessment of perioperative cardiac risk in patients undergoing major vascular surgery. Circulation 1993; 87:1506–1512.
41. Davila-Roman VG, Waggoner AD, Sicard GA, et al: Dobutamine stress echocardiography predicts surgical outcome in patients with an aortic aneurysm and peripheral vascular disease. J Am Coll Cardiol 1993; 21:957–963.
42. Pepine CJ: Ambulant myocardial ischemia and its prognostic implications (editorial). Circulation 1990; 81:1136–1138.
43. Raby KE, Goldman L, Creager MA, et al: Correlation between preoperative ischemia and major cardiac events after peripheral vascular surgery. N Engl J Med 1989; 321:1296–1300.
44. Ouyang P, Gerstenblith G, Furman WR, et al: Frequency and significance of early postoperative silent myocardial ischemia in patients having peripheral vascular surgery. Am J Cardiol 1989; 64:1113–1116.
45. Mangano DT, Browner WS, Hollenberg M, et al: Association of perioperative myocardial ischemia with cardiac morbidity and mortality in men undergoing noncardiac surgery. N Engl J Med 1990; 323: 1781–1788.
46. Fleisher LA, Rosenbaum SH, Nelson AH, Barash PG: The predictive value of preoperative silent ischemia for postoperative ischemic cardiac events in vascular and nonvascular surgery patients. Am Heart J 1991; 122:980–986.
47. Pasternack PF, Grossi EA, Bauman FG, et al: Silent myocardial ischemia monitoring predicts late as well as perioperative cardiac events in patients undergoing vascular surgery. J Vasc Surg 1992; 16:171.
48. Landesberg G, Erel J: Perioperative myocardial ischemia in carotid endarterectomy under cervical plexus block and prophylactic nitroglycerin infusion. J Cardiothorac Vasc Anesth 1993; 7:259–265.
49. Kirwin JD, Ascer E, Gennaro M, et al: Silent myocardial ischemia is not predictive of myocardial infarction in peripheral vascular surgery patients. Ann Vasc Surg 1993; 7:27–32.
50. Landesberg G, Luria MH, Cotev S, et al: Importance of long-duration postoperative ST-segment depression in cardaic morbidity after vascular surgery. Lancet 1993; 341:715–719.
51. Seegobin RD, Wilmshurst TH, Johnston J, et al: Early postoperative myocardial morbidity in patients with coronary artery disease undergoing major noncardiac surgery: correlation with perioperative ischaemia. Can J Anaesth 1991; 38:1012–1022.
52. Koolen JJ, Visser CA, Reichert SL, et al: Improved monitoring of myocardial ischemia during major vascular surgery using transesophageal echocardiography. Eur Heart J 1992; 13:1028–1033.
53. Eisenberg MJ, London MJ, Leung JM, et al: Monitoring for myocardial ischemia during noncardiac surgery: a technology assessment of transesophageal echocardiography and 12-lead. JAMA 1992; 268: 210–216.
54. McPhail NV, Ruddy TD, Barber GG, et al: Cardiac risk stratification using dipyridamole myocardial perfusion imaging and ambulatory ECG monitoring prior to vascular surgery. Eur J Vasc Surg 1993; 7: 151–155.
55. Hertzer NR, Young JR, Beven EG, et al: Late results of coronary bypass in patients with infrarenal aortic aneurysms: the Cleveland Study. Ann Surg 1987; 205:360–367.

56. Stone JG, Foex P, Sear JW, et al: Myocardial ischemia in untreated hypertensive patients: effect of a single small oral dose of a beta-adrenergic blocking agent. Anesthesiology 1988; 68:495–500.
57. Pasternack PF, Grossi EA, Baumann FG, et al: Beta blockade to decrease silent myocardial ischemia during peripheral vascular surgery. Am J Surg 1989; 158:113–116.
58. Pasternack PF, Imparato AM, Baumann FG, et al: The hemodynamics of beta-blockade in patients undergoing abdominal aortic aneurysm repair. Circulation 1987; 76:III-1.
59. Godet G, Coriat P, Baron JF, et al: Prevention of intraoperative myocardial ischemia during noncardiac surgery with intravenous diltiazem: a randomized trial versus placebo. Anesthesiology 1987; 66:241–245.
60. Coriat P, Daloz M, Bousseau D, et al: Prevention of intraoperative myocardial ischemia during noncardiac surgery with intravenous nitroglycerin. Anesthesiology 1984; 61:193–196.
61. Antiplatelet Trialists' Collaboration: Collaborative overview of randomized trials of antiplatelet treatment: Parts I, II, and III. Br Med J 1994; 308:81.
62. Mangano DT, et al: Perioperative ischemia and outcome in patients undergoing noncardiac surgery. JAMA 1992; 268:233- 239.

CHAPTER 9

Acute Airway Problems

T. James Gallagher

Case Report

A 6′2″, 315-lb male patient was admitted for a decompression lumbar laminectomy. In the operating room, intubation was attempted following a sleep dose of thiopental. After determination that the patient could be ventilated by mask, paralysis was introduced with 100 mg of succinylcholine. Direct laryngoscopy was first attempted with a No. 3 Miller blade and then a No. 4 MacIntosh. The larynx could not be visualized.

The patient could be ventilated by bag and mask and therefore was allowed to awaken. Following topical analgesia and intravenous sedation of the patient, a fiberoptic bronchoscope was passed through an 8.5-endotracheal tube. Both the tube and the bronchoscope were advanced into the previously prepared right nares. During bronchoscopy, the larynx was visualized and the scope passed beyond the vocal cords. The nasal tracheal tube was then advanced over the bronchoscope and positioned within the trachea. Immediately following placement of the tube above the carina, the patient was again anesthetized with another large dose of thiopental. The cuff was inflated.

The operative procedure lasted 4½ hours and resulted in extensive blood loss. Because of the large blood loss and dependent edema as a result of the supine position, it was elected that the patient be kept intubated overnight. He was attached to a mechanical ventilator, and low-level mechanical ventilation was instituted. The cuff was inflated to a pressure of 15 mm Hg, and the inflation pressure was checked every 2 hours. During the night, the cuff required multiple attempts at inflation in order to provide an effective seal. Following each attempt to instill air, the pilot balloon showed no evidence of any increase in cuff volume or pressure. Inspection of the posterior pharynx with a laryngoscope while the patient was under thiopental sedation demonstrated that the tube and cuff had not migrated into the posterior pharynx. The ventilator manometer indicated that the level of continuous positive airway pressure (CPAP) was able to be maintained. Exhaled tidal volumes had decreased by approximately 100 ml. Because of the previous difficult intubation, it was decided not to change the tube that night.

The following day, a chest radiograph revealed infiltrative changes bilaterally in both lung bases. PaO_2 levels were judged not acceptable for extubation. Following light sedation of the patient, again with thiopental, a tube changer was passed through the endotracheal tube. A bronchoscope was on standby in case there were any difficulties. The tube was easily removed, and the new tube slid over the tube changer through the nares and into the trachea. Following confirmation of appropriate position, the cuff was inflated and the tube secured.

Twenty-four hours later, the patient's oxygenation and ventilation had improved. His chest radiograph cleared 48 hours later. Deflation of the endotracheal tube cuff revealed an air leak. Inspection of the posterior pharynx indicated no evidence of any edema. The patient was then extubated. Immediately following extubation, nebulizer therapy with 0.5 ml of racemic epinephrine was instituted in an attempt to reduce any potential edema present. The patient tolerated extubation well and was discharged from the intensive care unit (ICU) the next day.

REASONS TO DELAY EXTUBATION

Following surgery and at the conclusion of anesthesia, events may suggest that extubation be delayed until some later time, after the patient arrives in the ICU (Table 9–1). Intraoperative hypoxemia or hypercarbia, either prolonged or transient in nature and unexplained, should alert the clinician to potential airway and respiratory problems in the postoperative period. Relative hypoxemia can

Table 9–1.
Reasons to Consider a Delay of Extubation

Significant atelectasis
Large volume fluid resuscitation
Prolonged intra-abdominal operation
Inability to follow commands: obtundation
Absent gag reflex
Dependent upper airway edema
Difficult intubation
Residual neuromuscular blockade
Possible aspiration
Grossly abnormal postoperative pulmonary function studies

often be camouflaged because of the high oxygen concentrations commonly used during anesthesia. This is particularly so if monitoring only consists of pulse oximetry. A PaO_2 of 130 mm Hg with an FIO_2 of 0.7 or 0.8 will still result in a saturation of 99%, but it obviously represents significant pulmonary dysfunction. Such a patient may require positive end-expiratory pressure (PEEP) to restore lung volume to increase functional residual capacity (FRC) and thereby improve oxygenation.[1,2] Another potential cause of hypoxemia is significant atelectasis. Atelectasis can often be best treated by fiberoptic bronchoscopy for removal of plugs and secretions (Fig. 9–1). In the postoperative period, this can be done most expeditiously in an already intubated patient. The point remains that unexplained hypoxemia should result in delayed extubation and continuation of mechanical ventilatory support until it is clear that the patient's condition has stabilized and the situation has resolved. Often, this will require blood gas analysis as well as portable radiographic evaluation of the chest.

- *Fiberoptic bronchoscopy should be aggressively utilized to eliminate atelectasis. It is usually far more efficient and rapid than the chest physiotherapy.*

Modern anesthesia practice presumes that patients will not breathe spontaneously during general anesthesia, and therefore they are almost always paralyzed and ventilated in the control mode. Increases in minute ventilation will maintain $PaCO_2$ within a normal range. Therefore, the development of hypercarbia almost always suggests a mechanical problem or a significant physiologic change in the patient. For example, an increase in the metabolic rate because of hyperthermia secondary to sepsis or malignant hyperpyrexia will elevate $PaCO_2$ if minute ventilation does not increase.[3,4] Pulmonary embolic phenomena will increase dead space and therefore $PaCO_2$.[5] Any unexplained elevation in $PaCO_2$ calls for

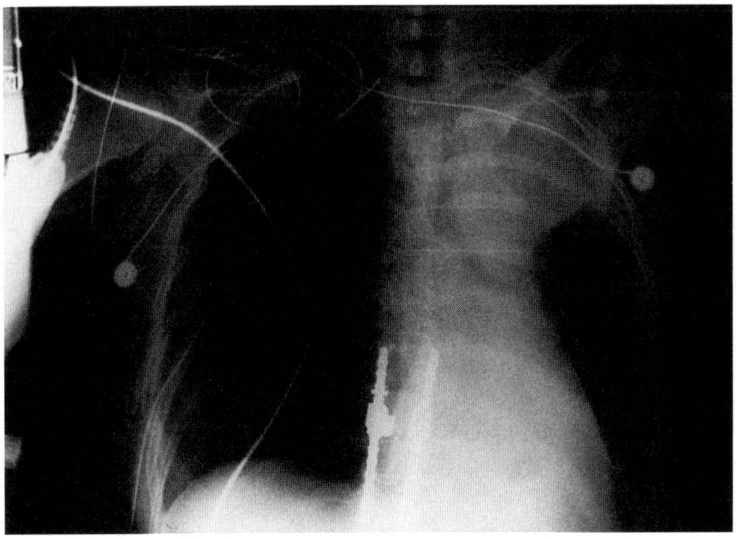

Figure 9–1.
Left upper lobe atelectasis. This had not previously responded to chest physiotherapy and position changes. Fiberoptic bronchoscopy will usually reexpand such a segment.

a delay in extubation and continued mechanical ventilation support until the problem can be identified and rectified.

Patients who have required or received large fluid administrations of either crystalloids or colloids, alone or coupled with massive blood transfusion, are also excellent candidates for delayed extubation. Such patients can shift significant amounts of fluid into the pulmonary interstitial space, with ultimate interference of oxygenation.[6] Moreover, laryngeal and postpharyngeal edema may form, with the potential for airway occlusion. Although such patients may otherwise meet the unit's criteria for extubation, it may be wise to delay extubation until the airway can actually be evaluated. The presence of a leak following endotracheal tube cuff deflation usually means minimal laryngeal edema. Direct observation of the posterior pharynx via laryngoscopy will determine the degree of edema as well as the ease of reintubation if required. The examination can be facilitated by incremental doses of etomidate or thiopental sodium.[7,8] With a tube through the larynx, the vocal cords cannot be easily evaluated.

- *Large volume fluid resuscitation does not necessarily predict development of pulmonary dysfunction.*

Prolonged intra-abdominal operative procedures invariably lead to bowel wall edema. Additionally, intraluminal fluid may accumulate. Both can result in massive bowel distention and may make abdominal closure difficult. This will often result in an increase in intra-abdominal pressure with a massively distended, tight abdomen. The increased abdominal pressure will force the diaphragm cephalad and contribute to a decreased FRC. This, in turn, mandates higher airway pressures to accomplish ventilation. These patients will not be able to breathe well on their own and will rapidly develop hypocarbia.[9] The decreased FRC will also result in relative, if not absolute, hypoxemia.[9]

- *On occasion, following abdominal closure, the abdomen may have to be reopened and packs or mesh employed so as to reduce intra-abdominal and, ultimately, airway pressures during mechanical ventilation.*

Following neurosurgical procedures, patients are usually awakened rapidly to assess neurologic status in the immediate postoperative period. This provides early feedback on the success of the surgery as well as any early complications such as edema or bleeding. For those patients who fail to awaken rapidly, extubation should almost always be delayed. An altered mental status immediately following such surgery will predictively result in hypoventilation. Furthermore, these patients will often have an immediate CT scan. In these circumstances, the airway is more easily maintained with an endotracheal tube that is already in place, particularly during transport to the CT scanner.

Certain surgical procedures also contribute to potential airway edema. These include operations in the prone or head-down position. Dependent edema will usually develop and can be further exacerbated if large fluid volumes have also been infused. This type of edema will clear rapidly within several hours, particularly if the patient's head can be kept upright in the postoperative period. However, caution should prevent any hasty decision making. The usual criteria described to ensure a patent upper airway should be followed.

Obviously, any patient in whom intubation was initially difficult should have extubation delayed. Extubation must proceed only when the patient is clearly awake and is able to support spontaneous ventilation. Moreover, any problems that may require reintubation should either not be present or not be likely to develop. At times in the immediate postoperative period, I extubate patients who have marginal gas exchange based on an expectation of further improvement. This should not be the modus operandi for patients who have already demonstrated a difficult airway.

If neuromuscular blockade cannot be adequately or easily reversed, the patient will require mechanical ventilatory support for the immediate postoperative period. Often, this may follow premature discontinuation of surgery shortly after administration of neuromuscular blockers. Hypothermia, acidosis, and aminoglycoside therapy can all contribute to an inability to reverse rapidly neuromuscular blockade.[10–12] These conditions should be reasonably corrected in advance of further attempts at reversal. The clinician should also be aware that, following infusion of reversal agents, during the circumstances described, neuromuscular blockade may appear to be adequately reversed. However, the effects of neuromuscular blockade will rapidly return.

- *Almost all instances of residual neuromuscular blockade can be traced to altered elimination of the neuromuscular blocking agents.*

Invasive procedures during surgery, such as inadvertent puncture of the carotid artery during internal jugular vein line placement, can lead to neck hematoma with potential serious compromise of the airway (Fig. 9–2). This may require direct inspection of the posterior pharynx under short-term anesthesia, such as thiopental, to ensure that there is no posterior pharyngeal edema or external compression of the airway.

An abscess in the posterior pharynx or peritonsillar area can severely compromise the airway. Following drainage, the surgeons can provide guidance as to the severity of the situation and how long edema and airway compromise may persist. However, the intensivist should ensure directly that all problems have been resolved prior to extubation. Again, direct inspection under laryngoscopy is the most efficacious way to ensure that edema is not present. This can also be accompanied by deflation of the endotracheal tube cuff, to ensure that a leak is present and that the likelihood of laryngeal edema is minimal. On occasion, an optimistic surgeon may attempt to assure the intensivist that all swelling is "anterior" and that there is no problem with the airway. One should clearly take this admonition with a grain of salt and, again, directly ascertain the situation.

Aspiration of gastric contents, either during induction or at some other time during anesthesia, will often result in significant hypoxemia.[13] Extubation should be delayed until it is clear that the situation is resolved. A severe problem will require even higher levels of mechanical ventilator support. Similarly, a chest or lung injury following penetrating or blunt trauma will almost always result in some degree of lung dysfunction and hypoxemia.[14,15] Predictively, these patients will require PEEP to ensure adequate oxygenation. Extubation should be delayed until the patient can be further assessed with a physical examination, blood gas analysis, and chest x-ray study. By then, any need for further mechanical support will be obvious.

- *Following surgery, extubation should be delayed if any doubt exists as to the patient's ability to maintain adequate oxygenation.*

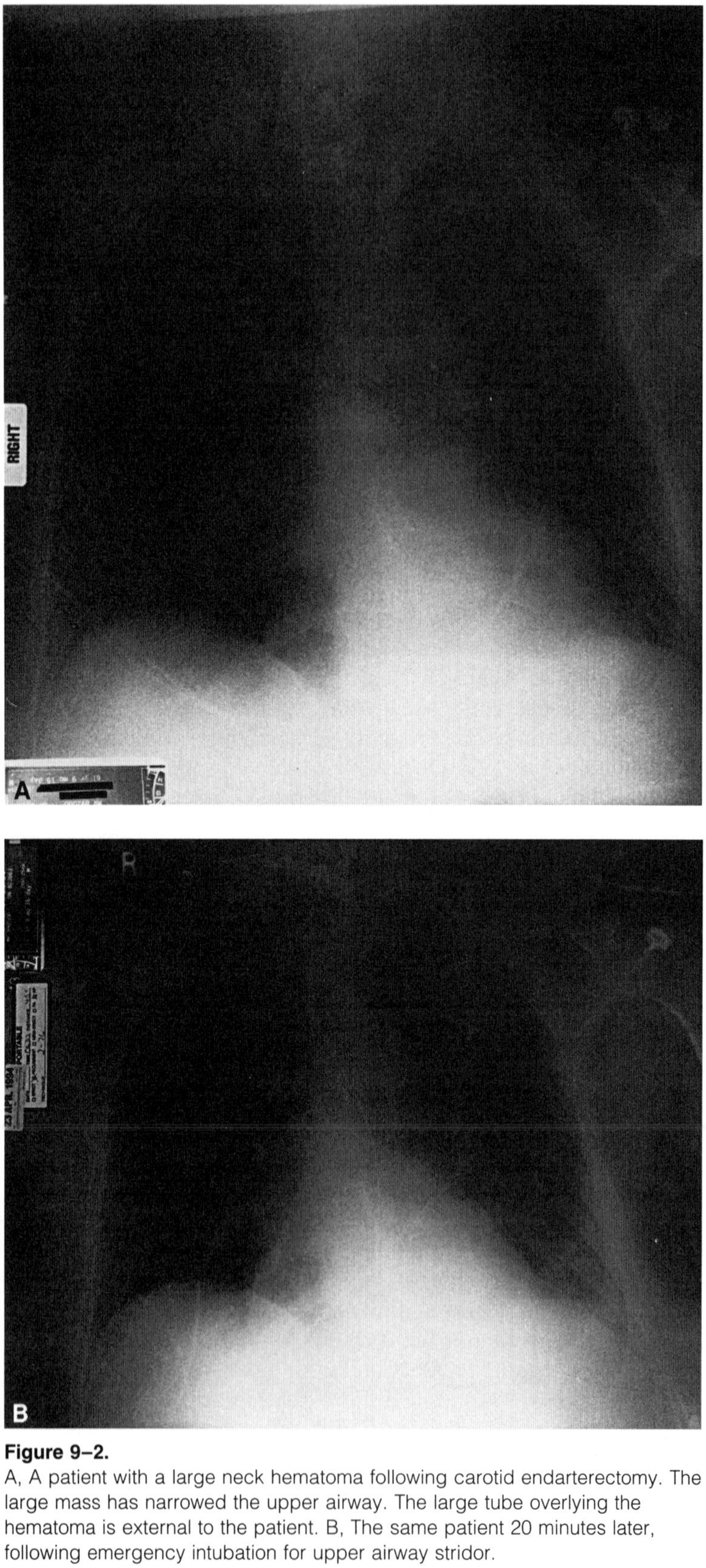

Figure 9–2.
A, A patient with a large neck hematoma following carotid endarterectomy. The large mass has narrowed the upper airway. The large tube overlying the hematoma is external to the patient. B, The same patient 20 minutes later, following emergency intubation for upper airway stridor.

Certain preoperative conditions or situations will often predict which patients will develop postoperative pulmonary complications. These problems will almost always involve either hypoxemia or hypoventilation and require mechanical ventilatory support. Prolonged upper abdominal procedures have been long known to create such situations.[16] These primarily develop because of reduction of vital capacity (VC) and FRC. Morbid obesity has been associated with central hypoventilation, sleep apnea, and CO_2 retention.[17,18] Following abdominal or thoracic surgical procedures, these patients often exhibit difficulty in resumption of effective alveolar ventilation. They may require at least short-term mechanical ventilatory support. Those with a long history of smoking often develop complications, which include atelectasis and infectious processes, and require ventilatory support. Regardless of the operative procedure, patients with severe chronic airway disease and reduction in maximum voluntary ventilation will predictably fail to maintain their usual $PaCO_2$ values.[19] This can follow a shift of the CO_2 response curve due both to anesthetics and to narcotics.[20] As such, these patients may require both adequate pain control and several days of recovery before they are able to manage their own ventilation.

Abnormal pulmonary function tests can often predict which patients will likely have postoperative difficulties. The most helpful test is an FEV_1 value less than 50% of normal.[21] Such abnormal values predict those likely to require postoperative support of alveolar ventilation. Arterial blood gas analysis, which indicates hypercarbia, also serves as a good predictor of postoperative hypoventilation. In general, pulmonary function testing can indicate which patients postoperatively will have problems with ventilation. These tests are not nearly so helpful for prediction of hypoxemia. Such situations usually develop following an event prior to or during the surgical procedure. I reserve pulmonary function screening for those with known or severe underlying lung disease. This group includes asthmatics, patients with chronic bronchitis, and long-term smokers. Other patients who require preoperative pulmonary function monitoring include the morbidly obese and those with sleep apnea, fibrotic disease, or any known chronic lung disorder.

• *It is far easier to predict which patients will have postoperative ventilation problems than which will develop altered oxygenation.*

SPECIFIC POSTOPERATIVE AIRWAY PROBLEMS

Premature extubation in many of the foregoing situations may result in an increase in $PaCO_2$ and oxygen desaturation. These may be accompanied by either a decrease in respiratory rate or a rapid, inadequate ventilatory efforts. Obvious causes include residual anesthetic effects, neuromuscular blockade, oversedation, and narcotization. Since the anesthetic's gases are not very soluble in blood, they can usually be rapidly removed by hyperventilation with 100% oxygen.

The endotracheal tube can become dislodged from the trachea. On occasion, it may be obvious that the endotracheal tube has actually been removed, usually because little of the tube is left in the

• *If the position of the endotracheal tube is in question, laryngoscopy or bronchoscopy should be performed immediately to clarify the situation.*

nose or mouth, or the patient actually speaks. At other times, the tube may still appear to be in place, but in fact is above the vocal cords. Clinical clues include a decrease in expired CO_2, if monitored, or a leak during delivery of the positive pressure mechanical breath. Additionally, minimal chest movement will be observed during the delivery of the mechanical breath.

Residual neuromuscular blockade can be quickly assessed by asking the supine patient to hold his or her head up for 5 seconds. To accomplish this requires blockade of less than 50% the neuromuscular receptors. On occasion, the neuromuscular blockade monitor can aid in assessment. However, despite an adequate twitch response or train of four, up to 70% of the neuromuscular receptors may still be blocked (Fig. 9–3).[22,23] Many clinicians believe that the head-up test is the most effective way to demonstrate adequate reversal of neuromuscular blockade. If the reversal cannot be accomplished, because of hypothermia, acidosis, or recent infusion of the relaxant, then obviously reintubation must immediately be accomplished.

Patients with residual narcotics will ventilate with a slow, spontaneous respiratory rate of 14 breaths per minute or less. They always demonstrate pinpoint pupils. Even when short-term narcotics have not been administered in several hours, their effects can still be present. Naloxone, 0.1 to 0.4 mg, will reverse the situation.[24] On occasion, a second dose may be needed within 60 minutes. Often, small doses of agents such as fentanyl or sufentanil are used for induction or maintenance of anesthesia. Since these are thought to be short-acting agents, failure to awaken several hours later may not be initially thought of as due to narcotic overdosage. However, often the effects of these drugs far outlast what is usually stated in the literature. Therefore, patients with small, constricted pupils, despite several hours having passed since last being administered narcotics, will often benefit and awaken with the use of naloxone.

• *When narcotics are combined with other drugs during anesthesia, the effects of narcotics may persist far beyond what would be normally expected.*

Benzodiazepines are often utilized as part of the preanesthetic medication or as an aid to anesthetic induction. In large doses, these agents, alone or in combination with narcotics, can depress respiration.[25] Newer drugs such as flumazenil have been developed to reverse benzodiazepine depression.[26] Flumazenil can reverse benzodiazepine-induced respiratory depression. However, the short duration of action means that dosing should usually be as a continuous infusion. The usual one-time dose is 0.5 to 2.0 mg, and 0.5 to 2.0 mg/hr when infused continuously.

Cuff failure of the endotracheal tube is usually heralded by leakage during mechanical ventilation. The problem will not be solved by inflation of more air into the cuff. The clinician must first check that the problem is not due to the pilot tube or valve failure rather than to the cuff itself. When air is inserted into the pilot tube, inability to detect any increase in pressure in the small pilot balloon attached to the valve is almost always an indicator of valve failure. Often, this problem can be easily resolved. Simply cut the pilot tube beyond the valve and pilot balloon and then attach a blunt-nosed

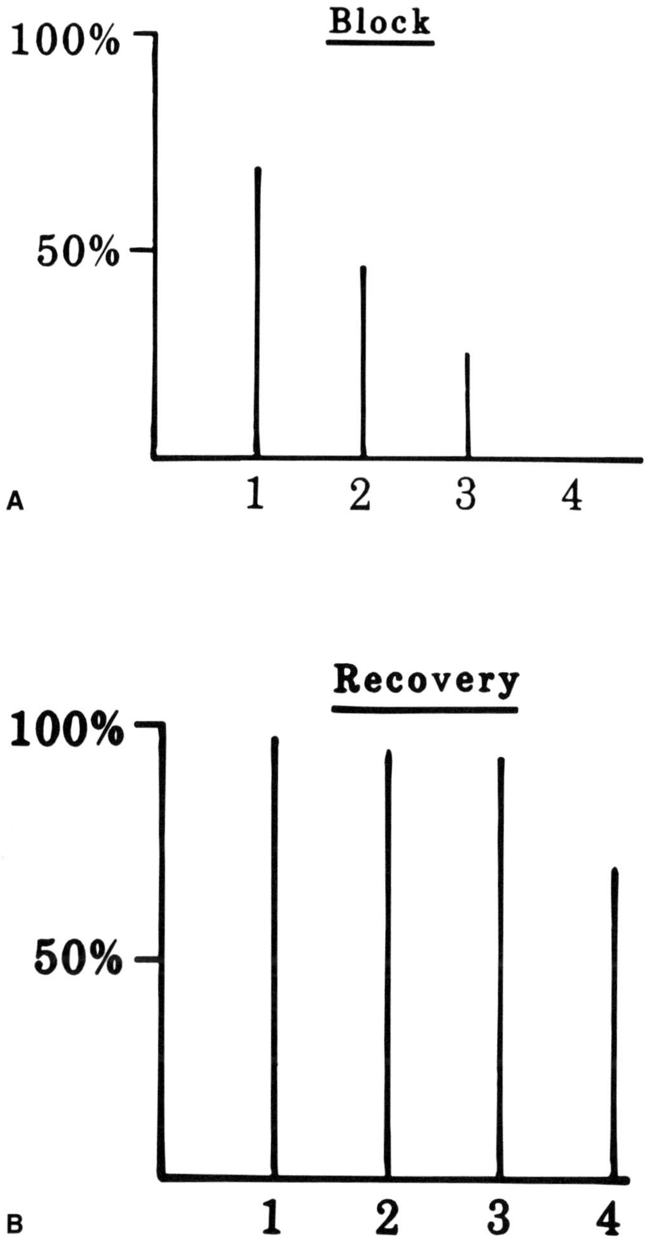

Figure 9–3.
A, The fourth response to the train of four is absent. This indicates adequate neuromuscular blockade. B, The fourth stimulus has increased to more than 50%. This indicates clinical recovery.

needle with a stopcock (Fig. 9–4). Air can then be inflated into the cuff to seal the airway.

Continued leakage may mean either a herniated or a ruptured cuff. The usual scenario of a herniated cuff is that air is injected into the cuff and temporarily appears to seal the airway. However,

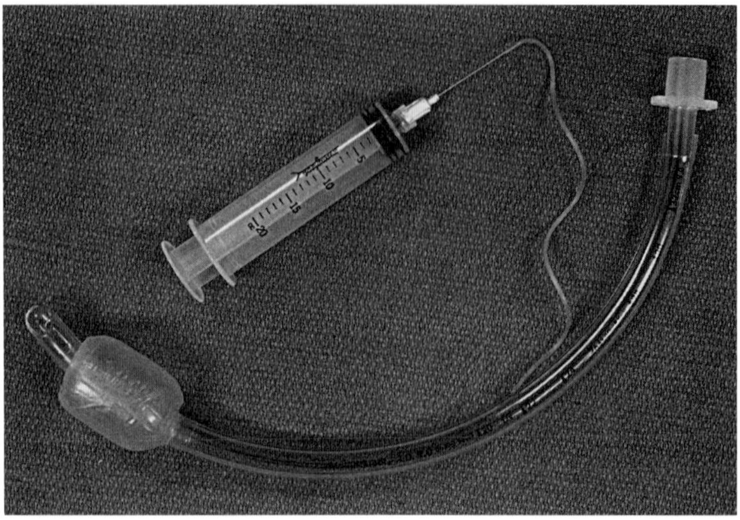

Figure 9–4.
On occasion, a pilot balloon or its tube may be cut. Moreover, the one-way valve may malfunction. Rather than changing the endotracheal tube, a blunt 18-gauge needle can be inserted into the tubing. A stopcock serves as an open-and-shut valve.

if this continues on a regular basis, it must be resolved. The problem can be addressed and diagnosed by direct laryngoscopy. If the cuff appears massively inflated or is in the posterior pharynx, deflate and reposition the cuff below the vocal cords. If the cuff is not seen and air leakage continues, the clinician can then presume that the cuff itself has been damaged and may require tube replacement. There are occasions in which it may be impossible or potentially too dangerous to consider an endotracheal tube change. Instead, pack the posterior pharynx with gauze to reduce leakage. Often, even with the leak, the patient's positive airway pressure can be maintained. An increase in the volume delivered from the mechanical ventilator will ensure that the appropriate volume is delivered to the patient. The only real risk would consist of aspiration of posterior pharyngeal contents, which is usually not of concern at this time in the patient's course.

- *Fiberoptic bronchoscopy can rapidly determine whether a tube is obstructed by a foreign body or other material.*

An obstructed or partially obstructed endotracheal tube constitutes a major emergency (Table 9–2). Usual causes include thick, tenacious secretions, blood, or clots, often coupled with a small-diameter tube usually placed in small adults or children. The prob-

Table 9–2.
Signs of Obstructed Endotracheal Tube

Signs of Obstructed Endotracheal Tube
Sudden increase in peak airway pressure
Decreased exhaled tidal volume
Increased $PaCO_2$
Lack of chest expansion
Failure of suction catheter passage

lem can be diagnosed by a rapid, sudden increase in peak inflation pressure and a decrease in exhaled tidal volume. Blood gas analysis will reveal an increase in $PaCO_2$. Chest inflation will be diminished or absent. A suction catheter will not easily pass through the endotracheal tube. If one suspects tube occlusion, rapid, fiberoptic bronchoscopy can confirm and possibly correct the situation. If the occluding contents cannot be rapidly removed during bronchoscopy, or if a bronchoscope is not available, then immediate tube replacement is indicated.

Not uncommonly, patients return from the operating room with a right main stem intubation. Clinical signs to suggest the problem include unexplained hypoxemia or hypercarbia. Breath sounds may be diminished, usually in the left lung. In the case of deep intubation, complete or almost complete collapse of the entire left lung will be evident on chest film. The situation always reverts itself by movement of the tube back above the carina and continuation of mechanical ventilation. The diagnosis should be confirmed by reexamination of blood gases as well as the chest radiograph. On occasion, if secretions have built up in the affected lung, fiberoptic bronchoscopy may be necessary to remove such secretions.

A fresh tracheostomy can present its own set of problems. The most common is dislodgement of the tracheostomy tube in the immediate postoperative period. Almost immediately, the stoma will close over and the trachea will no longer be visualized. It takes several weeks for the stoma to mature enough to remain open on its own for any length of time following inadvertent decannulation. If possible, the easiest solution may simply be to reintubate the patient by the oral or nasal route. If the surgeons have left ties on the edge of the tracheal stoma, these ties may be lifted to expose the lumen and allow placement of the tube. One should use caution and ensure that tube replacement occurs in the trachea itself and not into a false passage. The dilator present in the tracheostomy set should always be present at the bedside. Often, this can be placed into the trachea stoma to spread the tracheal lumen and permit easy tube replacement. Always remember that the trachea can be secured with an endotracheal tube as well as a tracheostomy tube.

METHODS TO ACCOMPLISH INTUBATION IN THE ICU

Although it may be apparent that intubation will be necessary in any particular patient, one should first take the steps to simply establish an airway and maintain ventilation and oxygenation. This does not require immediate reintubation. In fact, simply waiting for all the necessary equipment to be brought to the bedside for the intubation process itself may result in further desaturation and hypoxemia. A simple bag and mask, in knowledgeable hands, will provide at least short-term ventilation and oxygenation. This will stabilize the patient and permit time to gather all the necessary equipment. Self-

- *Maintenance of the airway by bag and mask should take precedence over intubation until all equipment is available.*

inflating bags can generate tremendously high airway pressures. For that reason, I advocate that they be attached to a manometer so that the operator has an idea of the pressures developed. Unlike the self-inflating bag, the Mapleson system utilizes a bag with an adjustable valve to allow maintenance of positive pressure during the expiratory phase (Fig. 9–5A). The standard self-inflating Ambu-

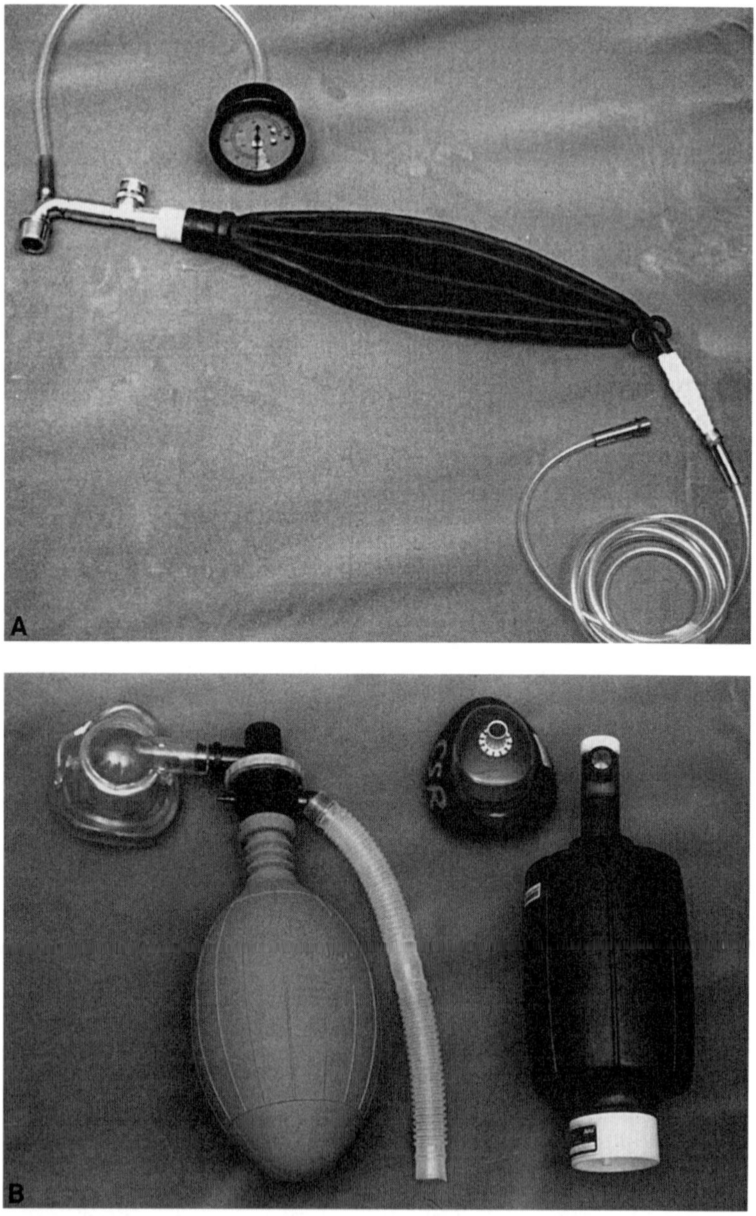

Figure 9–5.
A, Mapelson system. The valve located between the bag and the pressure manometer tubing can be opened or closed to increase the level of PEEP or CPAP. If the valve is opened too far, the room will be ventilated rather than the patient. B, Examples of bag and mask ventilation systems. The corrugated tubing can be attached to the bag to act as a reservoir and increase the FiO_2.

type bag will not allow pressure during the exhalation phase (Fig. 9–5B). However, a portable PEEP valve can be placed in line if a self-inflating bag is used. The valve on the Mapleson system requires some familiarity, and inexperienced personnel may simply ventilate the surrounding atmosphere and not the patient.[27] An oropharyngeal airway can cause more problems by pushing the tongue further into the posterior pharynx. A nasopharyngeal airway can be easily inserted and overcomes such difficulties (Fig. 9–6).

Direct vision during oral intubation provides the most rapid and safest method to secure the airway. It will also allow one immediately to confirm correct tube location. The intensivist should always ensure that the laryngoscope blade selected is large enough to accomplish the task. In adults, a MacIntosh No. 4 blade will allow intubation of the largest as well as the smallest adult patients. The axiom that it is always better to have too large than too small a blade certainly holds true here. Others may feel comfortable using the straight Miller No. 3 or No. 4 blade (Fig. 9–7). However, for those less inexperienced with intubation, the curved MacIntosh blade usually works best.

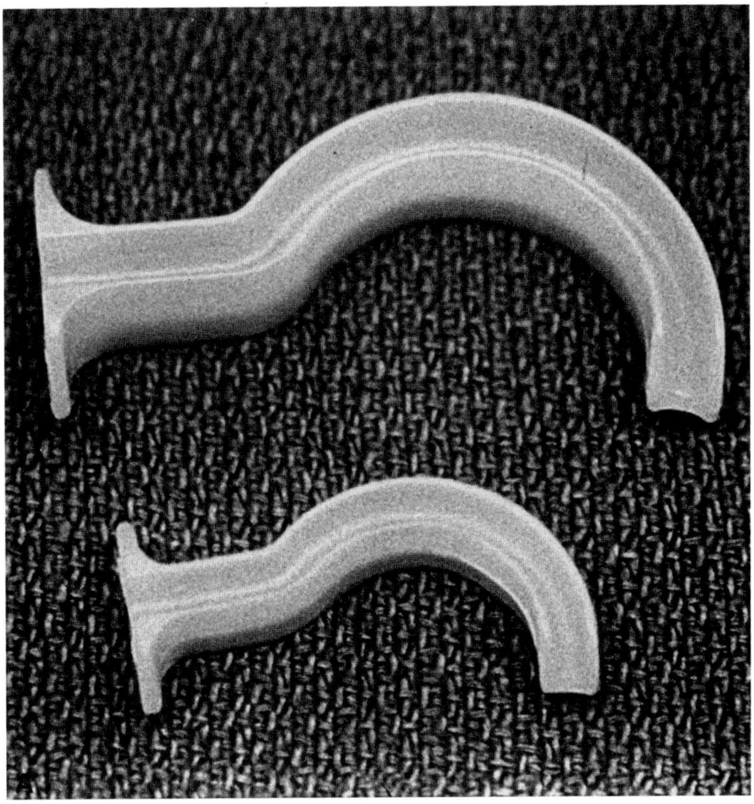

Figure 9–6.
A, An example of oropharyngeal airways. Too large an airway will simply push the tongue into the posterior pharynx. B, Bilateral and single nasopharyngeal airways. These can be easily placed. They bypass the tongue and often improve the airway. The single-lumen variety can be used to dilate the nares in preparation for nasal intubation. *(Figure continues.)*

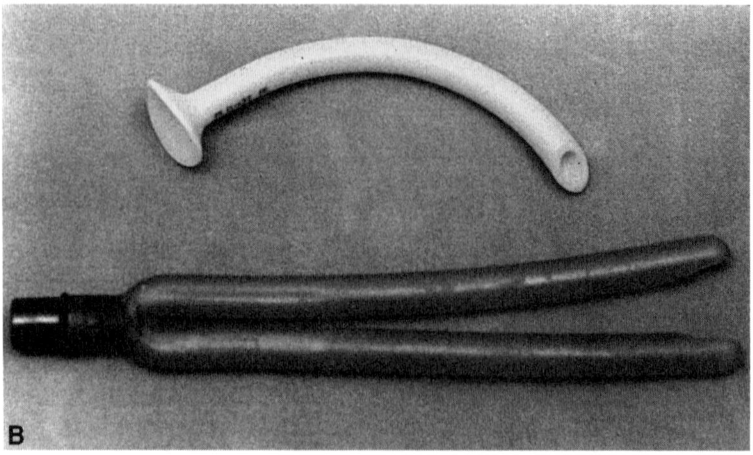

Figure 9–6.
(continued).

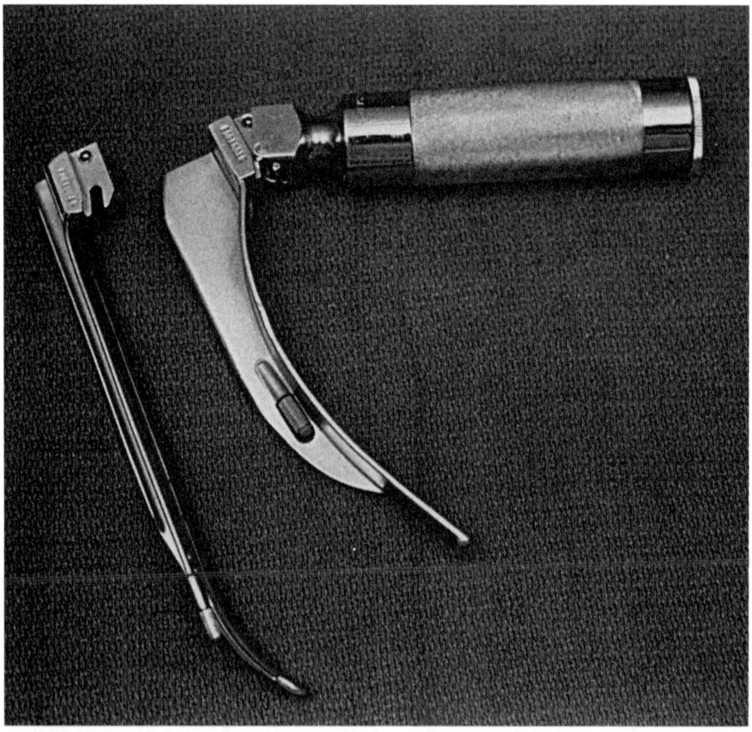

Figure 9–7.
Examples of the Miller (straight) and MacIntosh (curved) laryngoscope blades. The straight Miller blade is placed so that the tip extends into the larynx. The tongue will fall on both sides of the blade. The curved MacIntosh blade requires that the tongue be pushed to the left side of the mouth. The tip of the blade remains proximal to the valleculae.

Sedation of the patient may be required for oral intubation and laryngoscopy. This can often be accomplished with small incremental doses of short-acting agents. I believe that thiopental sodium, in 50-mg increments, or etomidate, in 20-mg increments, is ideal. Etomidate will not depress cardiovascular function to nearly the degree that thiopental will, yet both are short acting, with durations of less than 2 minutes. It is highly unlikely that neuromuscular blockade or paralysis will be required under such conditions. In an ICU, failure to intubate a paralyzed patient can lead to major complications. In less experienced hands and with less adequate equipment, the patient's airway can be easily lost. In the rare circumstances that paralysis is necessary, succinylcholine should be selected. When given in doses of 0.50 to 0.75 mg/kg, the agent has a duration of action of approximately 2 minutes and will not usually cause fasciculations. Since succinylcholine produces muscular fasciculations, some believe that it increases intracranial pressure. Even if that is so, the elevation is of very limited duration and will have no lasting effect, particularly when compared with the detrimental effects of hypoxemia. Succinylcholine may raise serum potassium levels in patients with large burns (greater than 20%) or in patients with peripheral neuromuscular disease.[28,29] In burns, this problem does not become apparent until after the first several hours. In these circumstances, a nondepolarizer such as mivacurium may be preferred. Mivacurium and other nondepolarizers do not cause any potassium release.[30] The usual dosage of 0.15 to 0.2 mg/kg will bring about paralysis in 2 to 2.5 minutes. Its effects last approximately 20 minutes.

A large-diameter endotracheal tube has less resistance and will reduce the work of breathing during spontaneous ventilation.[31] In most adult males, a size 8.0- or 9.0-mm inside-diameter (ID) tube will be adequate. Compared to a size 8.0-mm ID tube, a size 6.0-mm ID has almost twice the resistance at the same tidal volume and flow rates. In women, a 7.0- or 8.0-mm ID will work. Remember, subglottic dilatation occurs in older patients, and therefore they can accommodate larger tubes.

- *The larger the endotracheal tube diameter, the less the work of breathing.*

During direct laryngoscopy, one can mistake the esophagus for the airway. Auscultation cannot always differentiate true breath sounds from transmitted sounds following esophageal intubation. In order to confirm appropriate tube location, a CO_2 detector should be placed in line between the tube and ventilator or self-inflating bag. Disposable devices placed in line confirm the presence of CO_2 by a change in color. Since CO_2 can normally be present in the stomach, at least four or five breaths must be provided with the color change continuing to ensure that the tube is in the appropriate location (Fig. 9–8).[32] When available, a capnograph can be substituted for the disposable detector.

- *Nasal intubation cannot be safely accomplished without the necessary preparations. It should not be used in emergency situations that require immediate establishment of an airway.*

I reserve nasal intubation for those circumstances when the clinician is less skilled at laryngoscopy or when the situation is not immediately life-threatening. Blind nasal intubation requires a spontaneously breathing patient. The number one rule is to take time and proceed deliberately. The process involves several different steps.

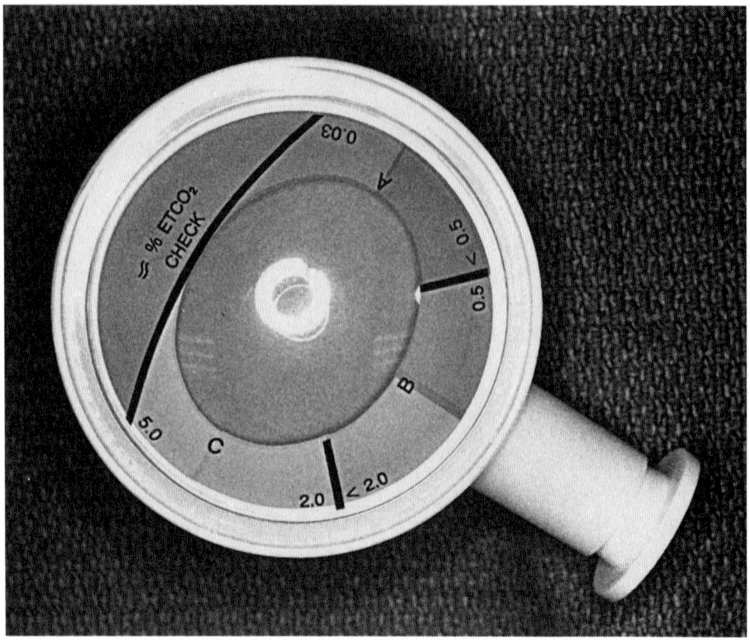

Figure 9–8.
The indicator should change color, indicating the presence of CO_2 in the exhaled gas. One should check beyond the first three breaths as the stomach can initially contain some CO_2.

First, phenylephrine (Neo-synephrine) drops are instilled to shrink the nasal mucosa. This should be followed by placement of successively larger nasopharyngeal tubes adequately lubricated with lidocaine (Xylocaine) jelly. These tubes both dilate and anesthetize the nasopharyngeal airway. One should not rush or force any of the tubes. Bleeding can follow inadvertent fracture of the nasal turbinates. The tube is then placed and advanced through the patient's nose until air exchange can be heard when the physician's ear is placed near the proximal end of the tube. On inspiration, the tube should be advanced into the airway. Advancement of the tube may be met with resistance as it intersects with the vallecula. The tube should then be pulled back, turned 90° to the right or left, and then advanced again during the next inspiratory effort. Sleep doses of sedation can be administered to the patient immediately following intubation, particularly for a patient who begins to cough and buck. Some clinicians advocate the use of local blockade including transtracheal lidocaine infusion or superior laryngeal block. While both may be helpful, they will also inhibit the patient's gag reflex and ability to protect the airway.

• *Cricothyrotomy always requires a skin incision to allow easy placement of the catheter and the cricothyrotomy tube.*

When the airway cannot be easily intubated either by the oral or nasal route, emergency cricothyrotomy may be necessary. Currently available kits rely on a modified Seldinger technique to place the tube rapidly and safely. The cricothyrotomy tube comes in several different sizes for adults and children (Fig. 9–9). Cricothyrotomy initially requires a small incision over the cricothyroid membrane.

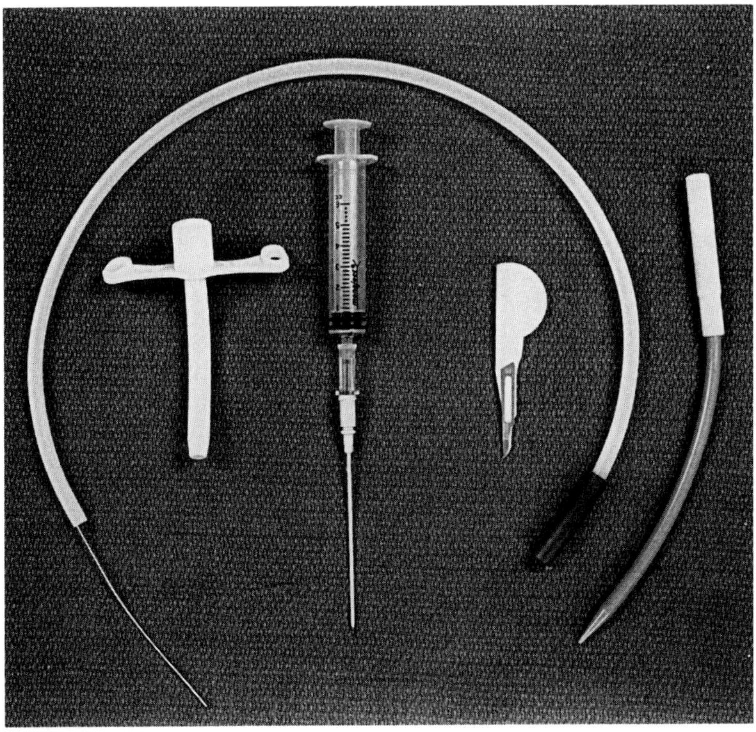

Figure 9–9.
A cricothyrotomy kit. The 20-gauge needle attached to the syringe is first placed through a small skin incision into the trachea. A wire can then be passed directly into the trachea. Attempts to remove a catheter from over the needle and into the trachea are often unsuccessful. The softness of the catheter causes it to fold up against the hard wall of the trachea and not pass into the tracheal lumen. (Courtesy of Cook, Inc., Bloomington, IN.)

A vertical incision usually causes less bleeding. Next, the needle is inserted through the skin and into the trachea. Aspiration of air confirms correct needle location. A wire is then threaded through the needle into the trachea, and the needle is removed. Some versions of these kits require that a catheter be slipped off the needle and into the airway. The enclosed guide wire will only pass through the catheter. However, the ridged tracheal wall may prevent easy passage of the catheter over the needle and into the airway. In fact, the entire airway can be lost. Once the guide wire is successfully in place, a dilator can be advanced and removed, and finally, the cricothyrotomy tube itself can be inserted into position and the wire removed. The adaptor permits easy attachment to a self-inflating bag. Ventilation should consist of rapid, small-volume breaths so as not to raise airway pressure unduly. As soon as practical, the cricothyrotomy should be converted to a tracheostomy.

In the past, a 14-gauge needle has been advocated for cricothyrotomy. However, with the availability of the cricothyrotomy kit, this technique should not be readily considered. The narrow lumen prevents adequate ventilation, and $PaCO_2$ increases with a concordant respiratory acidosis. Furthermore, although the adaptor of a

3.0-mm ID endotracheal tube will fit into the barrel, this apparatus is not usually readily available in an adult ICU.

Tracheostomy should not be considered an emergency procedure to establish an airway. It is a major operative procedure. In fact, when tracheostomy is performed under such circumstances, uncontrolled bleeding, damage to the recurrent laryngeal nerve, and other complications including injury to the thyroid gland are likely. Even under ideal circumstances, a tracheostomy cannot usually be accomplished in under 10 minutes from the time the decision is made. A cricothyrotomy can be easily done in 3 minutes.

CHANGING THE ENDOTRACHEAL TUBE

• *In some situations, it may be safer to maintain the patient with a cuff leak than to attempt to change an endotracheal tube.*

On occasion, it may be necessary to change the endotracheal tube. Circumstances can include a small tube that substantially increases the work of breathing or is partially obstructed. A damaged or leaky cuff may also necessitate reintubation. Nasal intubation with the potential for sinusitis and other problems may be an indication to convert to oral intubation.

There are several ways to safely reintubate the critically ill patient. Before any steps are undertaken, the clinician should ensure that, if all else fails, the patient can be directly and easily reintubated orally. For that reason, I always perform laryngoscopy on the patient and ensure that the larynx can be easily visualized and intubated. This maneuver may require sedation with drugs such as thiopental or etomidate. Prior to the change, patients should be preoxygenated with an $F_{I}O_2$ of 1.0 for at least 5 minutes. This provides a reservoir of time if complications develop.

One method to replace the tube utilizes the tube changer. This is simply a long, semistiff tube that acts as a stylet and is passed

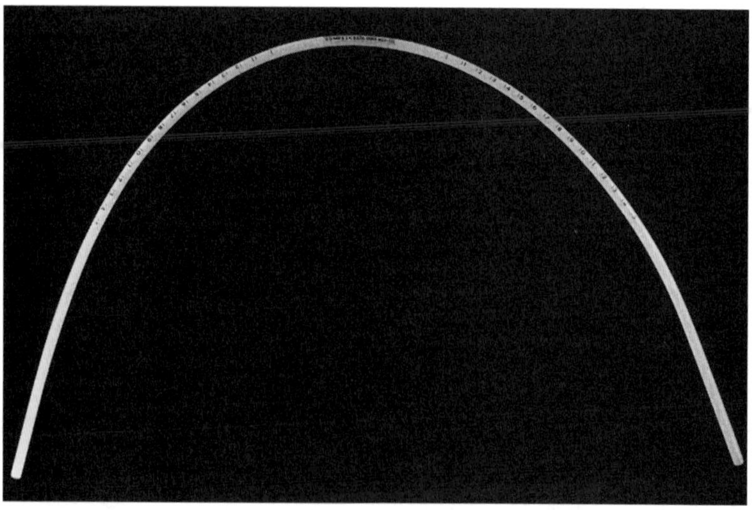

Figure 9–10.
An example of a tube changer. This is passed through the in-place tracheal tube. It should not be forced, or it may possibly perforate the tracheal wall. (Courtesy of Cook, Inc., Bloomington, IN.)

through the tube already in place (Fig. 9–10). The original tube is then removed without dislodgement of the tube changer, and a second tube previously prepared is passed over the tube changer or stylet into the airway. A tube changer without a stiff tip cannot rupture the airway.

Another method to change a tube involves direct inspection. While the laryngoscope is held in place, the tube is deflated and removed, and the second tube handed to the physician, who then rapidly intubates the patient under direct vision.

A bronchoscope can also be used to change a tube. This is somewhat more difficult than use of the tube changer. The new tube to replace the original is placed over the bronchoscope. The bronchoscope can then be passed through the already-in-place endotracheal tube. The in-place tube is then backed out of the airway while the bronchoscope remains in place in the trachea. This tube is removed from the bronchoscope by longitudinally cutting the tube as it is pulled back out of the airway. Care must be taken to not injure or dislodge the bronchoscope from the airway. With the first tube removed and the bronchoscope still in the airway, the new tube can then be advanced over the scope and secured in the appropriate position.

A tube change should always be considered a potentially dangerous undertaking. On occasion, the safer course of action may be to deal with the problems presented by the already-in-place tube and not introduce a second and perhaps life-threatening set of problems by attempting to replace the tube.

Often, patients are kept intubated for several days or longer because of upper airway edema. The clinician must rely on physical examination and judgment to decide when it is safe to extubate the patient. Therefore, prior to extubation the physician must confirm lack of cord edema, absence of postpharyngeal edema, and ability to reintubate should the need arise.

Deflation of the endotracheal cuff and detection of a leak will confirm minimal cord edema. Direct inspection of the upper airway by laryngoscopy will detect any edema and the ease or difficulty of reintubation. This can be accomplished with a dose of thiopental sodium (3 to 5 mg/kg) or etomidate (20-mg increments). Once the patient awakens, the tube can be removed.

Some individuals advocate inspection of the vocal cords with fiberoptic bronchoscopy. This can be done by placement of the scope alongside the endotracheal tube. Others advocate positioning the bronchoscope through the endotracheal tube and inspection of the upper airway during tube removal. They further advocate that, if the bronchoscope is left in place, the tube can be easily replaced if the patient develops any problems. There are several problems with that strategy. In a spontaneously breathing patient, inspection of the upper airway during extubation provides a very limited view. Furthermore, most difficulties do not occur immediately on tube removal, but some time afterward. The bronchoscope cannot be practically left in place for such a length of time.

• *Postextubation bronchoscopy usually provides little useful information on the status of the airway.*

Once the tube has been removed, the patient should be placed on supplemental humidified oxygen. Often, nebulized racemic epinephrine (0.5 ml in 5 ml saline) will reduce any upper edema contributing to stridor. The treatments may have to be repeated hourly. Care should be taken that neither hypertension nor tachycardia develops, which may then become an indication to discontinue such therapy.

On occasion, upper airway edema and stridor can be relieved with addition of helium to the gas mixture.[33] The larger upper airway uses gas flow rates that can cause turbulence when obstructions such as edema are present. Helium, in concentrations of 60 to 79%, reduces the overall gas density and the resulting turbulent flow. Helium comes in premixed cylinders with oxygen and is substituted for air. Improvement can be documented by a decrease in stridor, a reduction in $PaCO_2$ or end-tidal CO_2, and an increase in tidal volume.

In summary, rapid removal of an endotracheal tube following surgery may not be in the patient's best interest. Problems should always be anticipated during reintubation or tube change. Always proceed deliberately and have the appropriate equipment on hand.

REFERENCES

1. Gallagher TJ, Civetta JM, Kirby RR: Terminology update: optimal PEEP. Crit Care Med 1978; 6:323–326.
2. Layon J, Banner MJ, Jaeger MJ et al: Continuous positive airway pressure and expiratory positive airway pressure increase functional residual capacity equivalent. Chest 1986; 89:517–521.
3. Theuer CP, Bongard FS, Klein SR: Are blood cultures affected in the evaluation of fever in perioperative patients? Am J Surg 1991; 162: 615–619.
4. Britt BA: Malignant hyperthermia. Boston, Martinus Nijhoff, 1987.
5. Ferro TJ, Malik AB: Mechanisms of lung vascular injury and edema after pulmonary microembolism. J Crit Care 1989; 4:118–126.
6. Teplitz C: The core pathobiology and integrated medical science of adult acute respiratory insufficiency. Surg Clin North Am 1976; 56: 1091–1133.
7. Fragen RJ, Avram MJ, Henthorn TK et al: Pharmacokinetically-designed etomidate infusion regimen for hypnosis. Anesth Analg 1983; 62:654.
8. Hudson RJ, Stanski DR, Durch PG: Pharmacokinetics of methohexital and thiopental in surgical patients. Anesthesiology 1983; 59:215–219.
9. Hubmayr RD, Abel MD, Rehder K: Physiologic approach to mechanical ventilation. Crit Care Med 1990; 18:103–113.
10. Coursin BB, Kelly JS, Prielipp RC: Muscle relaxants in critical care. Curr Opin Anesthesiol 1993; 6:341–346.
11. Bevan DR, Donati S, Kopman AF: Reversal of neuromuscular blockade. Anesthesiology 1992; 77:785–805.
12. Segredo V, Caldwell JE, Matphay MA et al: Persistent paralysis in critically ill patients after longterm administration of vecuronium. N Engl J Med 1992; 327:524–528.
13. Torres A, Azne RR, Gatell JM et al: Incidence, risk and prognosis factors of nosocomial pneumonia in mechanically ventilated patients. Am Rev Respir Dis 1990; 142:523–528.

14. Graham JM, Beall AC Jr, Mattox KL et al: Systemic air embolism following penetrating trauma to the lung. Chest 1977; 72:449.
15. Sutherland GR: Anatomic and cardiopulmonary responses to trauma with associated blunt chest injury. J Trauma 1981; 21:1.
16. Biery DR, Marks JD, Schapera A et al: Factors affecting perioperative pulmonary function in acute respiratory failure. Chest 1990; 98: 1455–1462.
17. Aubier M, Murciano D, Milic-Emili J et al: Affects of the administration of oxygen on ventilation in blood gases in patients with chronic obstructive pulmonary deviation during acute respiratory failure. Am Rev Respir Dis 1980; 122:747.
18. Aubier M, Murciano D, Fournier N et al: Central respiratory drive in acute respiratory failure of patients with chronic obstructive pulmonary disease. Am Rev Respir Dis 1990; 122:191.
19. Warner MA, Offord KP, Warner ME et al: Role of preoperative cessation of smoking and other factors in postoperative pulmonary complications: a blinded prospective study of coronary artery bypass patients. Clin Proc 1989; 64:609–617.
20. Etches RC: Complications of acute pain management. Anesthesiol Clin North Am 1992; 10:417–434.
21. Frost EAM: Preanesthetic assessment of the patient with respiratory disease. Anesthesiol Clin North Am 1990; 8:657–676.
22. Rupp SM: Monitoring neuromuscular blockade "twitch monitoring". Anesthesiol Clin North Am 1993; 11:361–378.
23. Pavlin EG, Holle RH, Schoene RB: Recovery of airway protection compared with ventilation in humans after paralysis with curare. Anaesthesia 1989; 70:381–385.
24. Ready LB: Acute postoperative pain in anesthesia. In: Miller RD, ed: Anesthesia. New York, Churchill Livingstone, 1990; pp. 2140–2141.
25. Wheeler AP: Sedation, analgesia, and paralysis in the intensive care unit. 1993; Chest 104: 566–577.
26. Pepperman NL: Double-blind study of the reversal of midazolan-induced sedation in the intensive care unit with flumazenil (Ro 15–1788): effect on weaning from ventilation. Anaesth Intensive Care 1990; 18: 38–44.
27. Willis BA, Pender JW, Mapleson WW: Rebreathing in a T-piece: volunteer and theoretical studies of the Jackson-Rees modification of Ayre's T-piece during spontaneous respiration. Br J Anesth 1975; 47:1239.
28. Cooperman LH: Succinylcholine-induced hyperkalemia in neuromuscular disease. JAMA 1970; 213:1867–1871.
29. Tolmie JD, Joyce TH, Mitchell GD: Syccinylcholine danger in the burned patient. Anesthesiology 1967; 28:467–70.
30. Belmont MR, Maehr RB, Wastila WB et al: The pharmacodynamics and pharmacokinetics of benzylisoquinolinium (curare-like) neuromuscular blocking drugs. Anesthesiol Clin North Am 1993; 11: 251–281.
31. Weissman C, Askanazi J, Rosenbaum H et al: Response to tubular airway resistance in normal subjects in postoperative patients. Anesthesiology 1986; 64:353–358.
32. Murray IP, Modell JH: Early detection of endotracheal tube accidents by monitoring carbon dioxide concentration in respiratory gas. Anesthesiology 1983; 59:344–346.
33. Hill DW: Physics applied to anaesthesia, 3rd ed. London, Butterworths, 1978; pp. 157.

CHAPTER 10

Postoperative Ventilatory Support

Jukka Räsänen
John B. Downs

Case Report

The patient was a 56-year-old woman admitted to the intensive care unit (ICU) following pelvic exenteration. She had no previous medical problems. During anesthesia induction, the patient had apparently aspirated. On arrival in the ICU, she was maintained on mechanical ventilatory support. PaO_2 was 83 mm Hg on positive end-expiratory pressure (PEEP) of 10 cm H_2O, and FIO_2 was 0.5. The chest radiograph revealed minimal changes in both bases. It was decided to keep the patient intubated and ventilated until at least the next morning. Over the next 24 hours, the patient's chest radiograph continued to worsen, as did gas exchange. PEEP was increased to 18 cm H_2O, FIO_2 to 0.6. Peak inflation pressures increased from 38 to 58 cm H_2O. However, oxygenation continued to deteriorate, and the best PaO_2 was 72 mm Hg.

A pulmonary catheter had been inserted to ensure adequate oxygen delivery. Cardiac output was 6.5 L/min, with an oxygen delivery of 520 ml/min/m^2. She continued to breathe spontaneously at 32/min. Paralysis and sedation failed to provide any improvement in gas exchange.

It was elected to prolong the patient's inspiratory time and pressure limit the ventilator to minimize any risk of barotrauma. Peak airway pressure was maximized at 50 cm H_2O and PEEP was maintained at 14 cm H_2O. This resulted in a ΔP of 36 cm H_2O. Respiratory time was lengthened to 2.3 seconds. Tidal volume varied between 710 and 790 ml. Paralysis was maintained with a vecuronium infusion. Instead of improvement, oxygenation continued to deteriorate. PaO_2 was now in the mid-60s, with an oxygen saturation of approximately 90 to 91%. Mean pulmonary artery pressures varied between 45 and 58 mm Hg.

At this point, nitric oxide was added at a concentration of 20 ppm. There was an immediate improvement in oxygenation. PaO_2 increased to 80 mm Hg. Mean pulmonary artery pressure decreased to approximately 40 to 42 mm Hg. Nitric oxide was maintained over the next 8 days.

Following discontinuation of nitric oxide, the patient required a peak inflation pressure of 35 cm H_2O to deliver tidal volume of 700 ml. PO_2 was now 90 to 94 mm Hg, and FIO_2 was 0.4. During this time, the x-ray film demonstrated continued resolution of the bilateral basilar infiltrates. After 17 days of mechanical ventilatory support, the patient was successfully weaned and extubated.

Many critically ill patients will require ventilatory support in the immediate postoperative period. In most instances, this will not be due to adult respiratory distress syndrome (ARDS). Some cases may reflect a long operation coupled with the administration of large amounts of fluid and blood. Patients with a distended, tight abdomen may require ventilatory support for several days. In other patients, cardiovascular instability, arrhythmias, or hypothermia may necessitate mechanical support. The head-injured patient may require hyperventilation or may simply be intubated to protect the airway. Residual narcotics, muscle relaxants, anesthetics, or a cervical fracture may all prevent or impede ventilation. In most instances, ARDS does not immediately manifest itself. However, known risks, such as generalized sepsis, may warrant mechanical ventilatory support in the first 24 to 48 hours following surgery until it becomes clear that the patient will not develop major problems.

Although postoperative pulmonary dysfunction has many causes, in general, the lung responds in the same way. As a result, the techniques described in this chapter have wide application. Recent technologic developments have produced a confusing selection of ventilatory support modalities available to the clinician to augment alveolar ventilation, decrease the work of spontaneous breathing, and improve the oxygenation of arterial blood in patients with postoperative respiratory failure. Many of these modalities share some essential physical and physiologic characteristics and, therefore, would not be expected to alter the therapeutic end result. Since comparative studies of different techniques are lacking, the clinician must make the decision to adopt or discard a new technique with insufficient supporting information. At the same time, one must balance commercial and professional pressures to keep up with recent developments, with the financial and intellectual cost of starting a new form of treatment. The following discussion will present the principles of the most commonly used ventilatory support modalities and review their expected and documented physiologic effects, so that the reader can evaluate the usefulness of each technique in postoperative respiratory care and form an understanding of the principles of their application.

CLASSIFICATION OF AIRWAY PRESSURE THERAPY

In postoperative care, ventilators are used to accomplish two goals: (1) to produce a static increase in resting lung volume throughout the respiratory cycle; and (2) to effect dynamic, cyclic alterations in lung volume to augment alveolar ventilation mechanically. The static or dynamic change in lung volume is accomplished by altering transpulmonary pressure either by increasing airway pressure or by decreasing intrathoracic pressure. A sustained increase in transpulmonary pressure is usually effected by applying continuous positive pressure to the airway. However, the use of continuous negative extrathoracic pressure has also been described as a therapeutic modality.

• The modes of all ventilators increase overall lung volume. This is usually accomplished by delivery of positive pressure to the airway.

Mechanical ventilatory support is provided by altering transpulmonary pressure in a cyclic fashion. The techniques can be divided into four classes, depending on the method used: (1) decrease in thoracic pressure; (2) increase in airway pressure; (3) increase in intrathoracic pressure; and (4) decrease in airway pressure. These four principles have all been used, at least experimentally, in an attempt to augment alveolar ventilation (Table 10–1). For example, the cabinet ventilator increases transpulmonary pressure by reduction of extrathoracic, and thereby intrathoracic, pressure. The commonly used modes of positive pressure ventilation, such as intermittent mandatory ventilation (IMV) and pressure support ventilation (PSV), belong to group 2. Extrathoracic compression, which generates an increase in intrathoracic pressure (group 3), has been used experimentally to produce high-frequency oscillatory ventilation (HFOV). Group 4 currently includes airway pressure release ventilation (APRV) and intermittent mandatory pressure release ventilation (IMPRV), which are based on transient reductions in airway pressure from an elevated baseline.

Table 10–1.
Classification of Ventilatory Modalities

	Tidal Volume > Dead Space		**Tidal Volume < Dead Space**
Method of Lung Inflation	**Tidal Volume Modulation**	**Minute Volume Modulation**	**Minute Volume Modulation**
Decreased intrathoracic pressure	"Pneumatic chamber" 1926	"Iron lung" 1920s	NPO 1986
Increased intrathoracic pressure	"Assisted exhalation"	Resuscitation 1700s	HFTTV 1986
Increased airway pressure	AMV 1970s, PSV 1982 PAV 1992	CMV 1555 IMV 1971	HFPPV 1967, HFJV, HFFI, HFO, (CFAV)
Decreased airway pressure	IMPRV 1990	IRV 1960s APRV 1987	

NPO, negative pressure oscillation; HFTTV, high frequency transthoracic oscillation; AMV, assist-mode ventilation; PSV, pressure support ventilation; PAV, proportional assist ventilation; IMPRV, intermittent mandatory pressure release ventilation; CMV, control mode ventilation; IMV, intermittent mandatory ventilation; HFPPV, high frequency positive pressure ventilation; HFJV, high frequency jet ventilation; HFFI, high frequency flow interruption; HFO, high frequency oscillation; CFAV, continuous flow apneic ventilation; IRV, inverse ratio ventilation; APRV, airway pressure release ventilation.

Two further important factors are the magnitude of the mechanical tidal volume and the synchronization between spontaneous and mechanical respiratory cycles. When the dead space of the respiratory system is equal to or larger than the tidal volume delivered by the ventilator, mechanisms other than mass movement of gas become significant in the removal of carbon dioxide. Thus, the physiologic effects of ventilatory modalities are likely to be different, depending on whether conventional tidal volume in excess of dead space volume is delivered at a near-normal ventilatory frequency or low tidal volumes are provided at a high rate.

Spontaneous breathing and mechanical ventilation can be interfaced to modulate either minute ventilation or tidal volume. Minute ventilation can be modulated by administration of mechanical breaths in addition to spontaneous breathing. Such breaths do not attempt to support each spontaneous respiratory effort. IMV demonstrates such a technique. This technically simple interface provides a minimum minute ventilation even in the absence of spontaneous respiratory drive. However, some or all spontaneous respiratory efforts are unsupported. As such, without a readjustment, ventilatory support does not respond to an increase in ventilatory demand. Tidal volume modulation, for example, PSV, supports each spontaneous respiratory cycle. If the patient's ventilatory rate increases in response to increased ventilatory demand, the mechanical ventilatory support increases proportionately.[1] However, tidal volume modulation requires rather complex synchronization at the patient-ventilator interface, a reliable respiratory drive, and some spontaneous respiratory effort.

• *A mode such as IMV supports overall minute ventilation. However, the level of support varies based on the spontaneous breath rate.*

Three characteristics—method of transpulmonary pressure alteration, magnitude of tidal volume, and patient-ventilator interface—have been used to separate physiologically dissimilar ventilatory techniques (Table 10–1). In this discussion a ventilatory support technique is a unique method that can provide full or partial support of alveolar ventilation. Therefore, we separate only three entities among the most widely used methods that employ an increase in airway pressure to deliver conventional tidal volume: IMV, extended mandatory minute ventilation (MMV), and PSV. For example, the difference between conventional controlled mechanical ventilation (CMV) and IMV is the level of support. The techniques themselves are similar. IMV and PSV belong to the same physiologic group, but they differ in the interface between spontaneous and mechanical ventilation.

STATIC AIRWAY PRESSURE THERAPY: PEEP AND CPAP

Sustained elevation in lung volume is accomplished by the application of PEEP or continuous positive airway pressure (CPAP) to the airway. An acute parenchymal disease process or loss of negative intrathoracic pressure can reduce resting lung volume below nor-

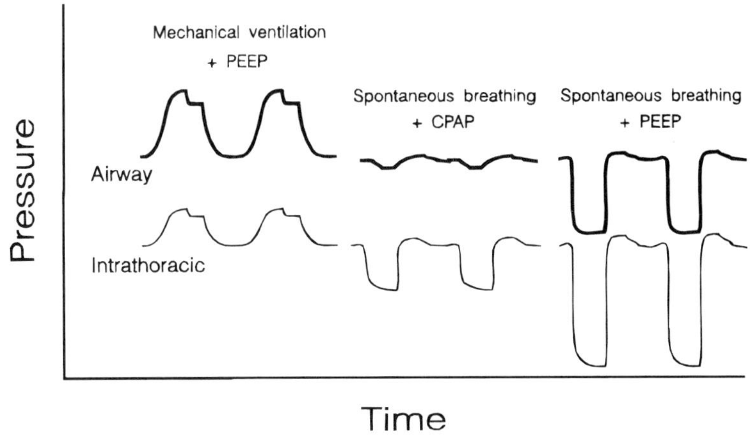

Figure 10–1.
Airway (thick line) and intrathoracic (thin line) pressure patterns during breathing with three types of positive end-expiratory pressure (PEEP). Despite a similar level of end-expiratory pressure (arrows), note that the three modalities have marked differences in airway and intrathoracic pressure. Any fall in airway pressure during spontaneous breathing with PEEP (see EPAP) is reflected in intrathoracic pressure. It will increase ventilatory work. CPAP, continuous positive airway pressure.

mal. Reinflation of the lung to a normal volume usually improves its ventilation-perfusion relationships and mechanical characteristics. Improved matching of ventilation and perfusion will correct hypoxemia. This permits a decrease in the inspired oxygen concentration (F_{IO_2}). Optimization of lung mechanics will decrease the work of breathing and often permits mechanical ventilatory support to be reduced or discontinued. It is customary to call positive expiratory airway pressure PEEP when the patient receives mechanical ventilation and CPAP when the patient breathes spontaneously. Therefore, any perceived differences between the physiologic effects of PEEP and CPAP can be attributed to the level of mechanical ventilation. From a practical standpoint, a person who takes spontaneous breaths with continuously elevated airway pressure during IMV could be considered to be breathing with CPAP. However, in this discussion, the term PEEP is used whenever mechanical breaths are or could be involved (Fig. 10–1). To avoid confusion, spontaneous breathing with positive end-expiratory but ambient inspiratory pressure is termed expiratory positive airway pressure (EPAP).

- *PEEP and CPAP both supply back pressure to the airway to restore lung volume. Commonly, PEEP is associated with mechanical ventilator breaths, while CPAP implies all spontaneous breathing.*

Ventilation, Perfusion, and PEEP

Gas exchange between the lungs and blood occurs primarily during the expiratory phase of the respiratory cycle. Consequently, when a decrease in ventilation/perfusion ratio (V_A/Q) causes arterial hypoxemia, effective improvement in arterial blood oxygenation requires correction of V_A/Q during exhalation. Mechanical ventilation is usually ineffective in improving hypoxemia in acute lung injury because it increases the V_A/Q during exhalation. In fact, a lower PaO_2 has been observed in baboons placed on CMV compared with those that received partial ventilatory support with IMV. Both groups had the same level of PEEP, which suggests that mechanical ventilation promoted a decrease in VA/Q and an increase in venous admixture.[2] The application of PEEP improves VA/Q relationships during exhalation by augmentation of ventilation in poorly aerated alveoli and reopens previously collapsed alveoli for effective gas exchange.[3] Thus, it alleviates the effects of the two major causes of hypoxemia associated with acute lung injury: mismatching of ventilation and perfusion and intrapulmonary shunting of blood. Increased alveolar volume and oxygen tension may also have a favorable effect on diffusion-related hypoxemia. Improvement in arterial blood oxygenation in response to PEEP in patients with acute lung injury has been well established in the experimental and clinical literature. Radiographic imaging studies indicate that the amount of recruitable lung tissue best correlates with improvement in oxygenation.[3,4]

- *Positive pressure breaths may recruit collapsed alveoli, but in general they do not maintain alveoli expanded between mechanical breaths. Usually, this requires the addition of PEEP/CPAP.*

Despite its beneficial effects, PEEP administered during mechanical ventilation may increase physiologic dead space and may actually decrease effective alveolar ventilation. This results from overinflation of the lungs during a positive pressure inspiration. Therefore, to minimize ventilation-perfusion mismatching in all lung regions, it is important to allow spontaneous ventilation to persist at a level comfortable to the patient. Actual mechanical ventilation is then added as necessary to prevent acidemia and excessive work of breathing.

- *PEEP/CPAP can increase dead space, particularly if levels are excessive.*

The use of PEEP and CPAP to improve oxygenation must be closely synchronized with oxygen therapy, both in a therapeutic and a diagnostic sense. An increased oxygen concentration in areas of lung with low, but finite, VA/Q can lead to absorption atelectasis, which may not be prevented even by the application of PEEP.[5] On the other hand, evaluation of pulmonary gas exchange and the appropriate airway pressure therapy in patients who receive increased concentrations of oxygen might lead to incorrect conclusions. Administration of as little as 30% oxygen may mask the hypoxemia produced by areas with low VA/Q. For example, a patient breathing 40% oxygen with a PaO_2 of 70 mm Hg might be thought to have adequate pulmonary gas exchange. A decision might then be made to wean the patient from mechanical ventilation and PEEP. However, ventilation and perfusion could be mismatched to such a degree that breathing only 30% oxygen might decrease PaO_2 to 50 mm Hg. Were the clinician unaware of this abnormality, it is likely that PEEP would be increased rather than decreased. Evaluation of pulmonary gas exchange and the rational application of PEEP are possible only when the inspired oxygen concentration remains low. The lowest possible inspired oxygen concentration that maintains acceptable arterial blood oxyhemoglobin saturation maximizes alveolar nitrogen concentration. This minimizes absorption atelectasis and right-to-left intrapulmonary shunting and theoretically may decrease the need for PEEP. To minimize potentially toxic oxygen therapy, proper PEEP must be used to make the maximum number

- *On occasion, an FiO_2 of 0.4 or 0.5 can mask some intrapulmonary shunting. However, this usually represents a minimal degree of pulmonary dysfunction.*

of alveoli accessible to oxygen. Therefore, PEEP and oxygen therapy should be considered together in the treatment of patients with arterial hypoxemia.

No therapeutic modality is more ubiquitous than oxygen in the postoperative period. Based on its perceived innocuous nature and nearly universal benefit, it is not surprising that all patients who receive ventilatory support also are subjected to an increase in inspired oxygen concentration (FIO_2). Clearly, an increased FIO_2 will elevate PaO_2. However, other maneuvers may have greater efficacy, especially when a pathophysiologic state, such as atelectasis, must be reversed. Further, an increased FIO_2 may exacerbate VA/Q mismatching by increasing blood flow to poorly ventilated lung regions or by promotion of absorption atelectasis. Obviously, sustained exposure to FIO_2 greater than 0.6 must be avoided to prevent oxygen toxicity. We suggest that a minimal increase in FIO_2 be applied until other maneuvers can establish an adequate level of oxygenation. Then, as soon as practical, the FIO_2 should be decreased.

- *A high FIO_2 can temporarily prevent hypoxemia. However, in no way should it be regarded as therapeutic.*

For nearly 3 decades, intermittent determination of PaO_2 has been the standard means of monitoring oxygen therapy. In recent years, it has been established that continuous monitoring with pulse oximetry is as accurate in most clinical situations. We recommend that SpO_2 greater than 90% be maintained for all patients except those with hypoxic ventilatory drive.

- *At least 50% of patients with an SpO_2 less than 94% can have a PaO_2 less than 60 mm Hg.*

Work of Breathing

Maximally efficient work of breathing is essential for patients with respiratory failure to breathe spontaneously. The work of breathing in patients with acute lung injury has been incompletely studied, perhaps because the techniques required to quantify work are not readily available.[6] For this discussion, only a graphic representation of the elastic work of inspiration is considered. A normal volume-pressure curve for the lung-thorax system is shown in Figure 10–2. At ambient airway pressure, the distending pressure of the lung-thorax is zero, and the lung volume is the functional residual capacity (FRC). Normal tidal breathing from FRC occurs along the volume-pressure curve. It results from a small pressure change. The elastic work of inspiration can be estimated from the shaded areas under the curve. Any alteration in the volume-pressure relationship of the lung can alter the work of breathing. This point is critical for a full understanding of the pathophysiology and therapy of respiratory failure.

- *Loss of lung volume usually results in increased work of breathing.*

In patients with acute lung injury, a shift in the volume-pressure curve decreases FRC and can increase the work of breathing. At reduced FRC, the pressure change required to achieve a normal tidal volume may be increased (Fig. 10–2). As the required pressure change increases, so does the area under the curve that represents work. The patient will then often decrease tidal volume and increase respiratory rate in an effort to minimize total work while maintaining minute ventilation unchanged. Because of these changes, clinicians often have shifted the work of breathing from the patient to

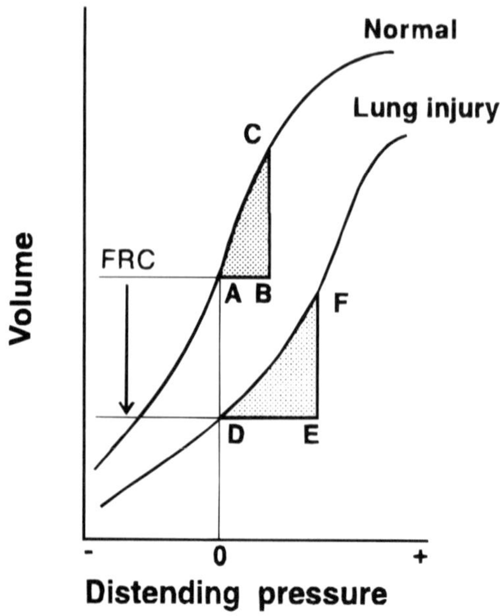

Figure 10–2.
Schematic respiratory system pressure volume curves under normal conditions and during acute lung injury. When distending pressure is zero, the expanding tendency of the chest wall and the collapsing tendency of the lungs are in equilibrium and lung volume is at functional residual capacity (FRC). When the lungs are healthy, inspiration of a tidal volume (BC) requires an increase in distending pressure (AB). Elastic work can be estimated from the area under the pressure volume curve (ABC). The injured lung operates at reduced FRC and requires a considerably larger change in distending pressure (DE > AB) for a normal tidal volume (EF). This entails more work during inspiration ($Area_{DEF} > Area_{ABC}$). See text for further details.

a machine by instituting mechanical ventilation. However, in a large number of clinical situations, the patient's work of breathing may also be decreased to an acceptable level by effecting an increase in FRC and lung compliance.

Functional residual capacity can be restored by the application of PEEP to increase the distending pressure (Fig. 10–3). Each volume-pressure curve will require a different level of PEEP to restore FRC and minimize the work of breathing. Therefore, PEEP must be individually titrated for each patient, and reassessed frequently to maintain the most effective level.[7] The use of PEEP to meet these goals, will increase FRC and which will then lie on a favorable portion of the volume-pressure curve. The required change in pressure to produce a given tidal volume will be smaller. Thus, lung compliance will be improved, work of breathing reduced and mechanical ventilatory support decreased or altogether avoided.

• *PEEP/CPAP will restore lung volumes and, as such, reduce the overall work of breathing.*

Application of PEEP also may be useful in the reduction of respiratory work related to increased upper airway resistance. An increased intraluminal airway pressure will enlarge caliber. This occurs both directly by elevation of the transmural pressure and indirectly by an increasing lung volume.[8] Continuous positive airway pressure with a nasal mask has wide usage in patients with

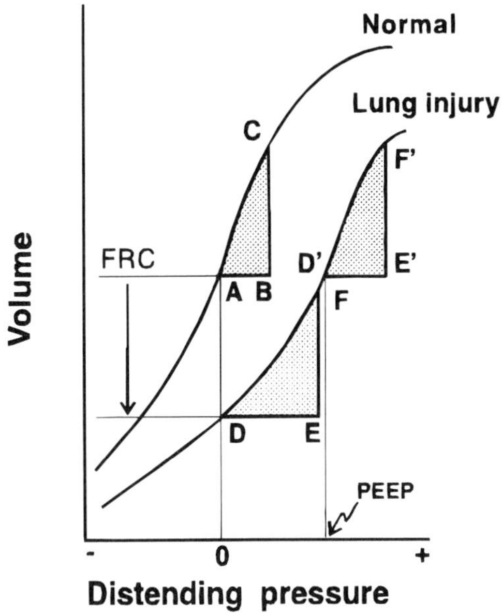

Figure 10–3.
Schematic respiratory system pressure volume curves under normal conditions and during acute lung injury. If positive end-expiratory pressure (PEEP) increases, the resting volume of the injured lung with the change in distending pressure required for a normal tidal volume decreases (D'E' < DE), and the elastic work is reduced ($Area_{D'E'F'} > Area_{DEF}$). See text for further details.

nocturnal upper airway obstruction. The application of face-mask or nasal CPAP has been successfully used in children with tracheobronchomalacia.[9,10] In these patients, the effect of CPAP simply splints open a collapsible airway with an increase in transmural pressure.

Investigations of the use of PEEP in patients with peripheral airways disease have produced conflicting results.[11] Initially, anecdotal reports of a beneficial effect of a high level of PEEP in patients with severe asthma were published, but a later controlled study showed a consistent detrimental effect.[12,13] However, individual patients with chronic airflow obstruction characterized by dynamic hyperinflation and expiratory flow limitation responded to low PEEP levels. They had improved efficiency of ventilation and decreased dyspnea, without side effects.[14,15] In such patients, PEEP may be useful as it decreases expiratory resistance by opposition to external compressive forces at the site of obstruction. This decreases the inspiratory muscle work required to overcome the resting pressure gradient between the alveoli and the airway opening.[11] The application of PEEP in excess of the positive pressure distal to the airway obstruction (intrinsic PEEP) would be expected to lead to further hyperinflation and both ventilatory and circulatory compromise. Therefore, the use of PEEP in patients with airway obstruction must be carefully contemplated and, if used, meticulously titrated. Evidence of reduced gas trapping with carefully adjusted PEEP has

- *In general, patients with asthma respond poorly to PEEP/CPAP. However, in individual cases, this modality may expand airway lumen and improve air flow.*

also been noted in patients with acute lung injury.[16] This developed despite an increase in directly measured airway flow resistance.[17]

CPAP Therapy

The beneficial effect of spontaneous breathing with elevated airway pressure in the treatment of pulmonary edema secondary to congestive heart failure was noted 6 decades ago.[18] A motor-driven blower provided an inspiratory gas source, and airway pressure was elevated with a face mask and an expiratory valve for constant positive-pressure breathing (CPPB). Shortly thereafter, the use of CPPB spread to the management of pulmonary edema secondary to traumatic lung injury[19] and pulmonary contusion.[20] Thus, there is ample historical precedent to apply elevated airway pressures to spontaneously breathing patients. Later, however, when mechanical ventilators became available, spontaneous breathing with CPPB was abandoned, and control of ventilation was emphasized for the treatment of lung injuries.[21] Over subsequent decades, mechanical ventilation became first-line therapy, so that when PEEP reappeared, it was always used in addition to positive pressure ventilation. Discontinuation of mechanical ventilatory support was, and often still is, attempted only after the need for PEEP had been alleviated. This may not be the most rational approach.

• *Acute parenchymal lung injury reduces compliance and oxygenation. Both compliance and PaO_2 will improve with PEEP/CPAP.*

An acute parenchymal lung injury decreases lung compliance and PaO_2 and increases the work of breathing. In fact, it is often the increased work of breathing that leads many clinicians to institute mechanical ventilation. By application of CPAP, resting lung volume and compliance can be increased. The increase in lung volume will improve VA/Q and arterial oxygenation. Increased compliance will decrease the work of breathing. Thus, CPAP may reduce the requirement for both mechanical ventilation and inspired oxygen supplementation. CPAP also may alleviate many problems associated with the mechanical ventilator and oxygen. We prefer to wean patients from mechanical ventilation and oxygen before removing CPAP.

• *Significant negative deflections in intrathoracic pressure during spontaneous breathing impair cardiac function in patients with underlying disease. This results from the increase in afterload on the left ventricle as intrathoracic pressure becomes more negative.*

The application of positive airway pressure to restore resting lung volume will reduce the work of breathing only if the breathing circuit is capable of maintaining a stable level of CPAP with a minimal inspiratory drop in airway pressure.[22,23] To maintain airway pressure unchanged during spontaneous breathing, gas must flow at a rate equal to or in excess of the inspiratory flow rate of the patient. With inadequate inspiratory gas flow in the circuit, airway pressure decreases during inspiration and remains elevated only during exhalation (EPAP). The inspiratory drop in airway pressure necessitates a fall in intrapleural pressure equal to the sum of the airway pressure drop and the quantity required to inflate the lung (see Fig. 10–1). The amplification of the negative inspiratory intrathoracic pressure fluctuations and an increase in the work of breathing are particularly detrimental to patients with impaired left ventricular function. The ventricle must overcome the distending effect of the negative extracardiac pressure during ejection.[24] Application of a large, negative, intrathoracic pressure has been shown to induce wall motion abnormalities in patients with coronary artery disease. When combined with enhanced blood return, this may result in acute cardiogenic pulmonary edema. The pulmonary congestion further decreases lung compliance, which in turn requires an even greater intrapleural pressure to accomplish tidal breathing. The patient may easily enter a vicious cycle of cardiopulmonary decompensation. Since our goal must be to minimize the patient's work of breathing, breathing circuits should be carefully monitored to ensure proper functioning.

When CPAP therapy is given to patients with intact, protective airway reflexes, tracheal intubation is not necessary. Equipment for the delivery of CPAP with a mask covering the patient's nose and mouth or nose only have been commercially available for 2 decades. The adverse effects of face-mask CPAP are minimal in a conscious, cooperative patient, even for several days. The most common complication is pressure-induced skin changes on the nasal bridge. Gastric distention from swallowed air has been reported in the literature, but in our practice has not constituted a significant problem. Airway pressure up to 15 cm H_2O can be successfully delivered with a mask. With higher pressure, large amounts of available air flow may be lost to leaks around the mask. A nasal mask may be somewhat more comfortable than a full-face mask.[25] However, mouth breathing during the administration of nasal CPAP may significantly lower the airway pressure. This will make the results unpredictable in some patients.[26]

Practical Aspects of PEEP/CPAP Therapy

Several published studies have attempted to find the optimum level of positive airway pressure for a given patient and clinical situation. Arterial blood oxygenation, venous admixture, oxygen delivery, lung compliance and dead space ventilation have all been proposed as end-point variables for the titration of PEEP and CPAP therapy.[27–29] However, PEEP has many effects, desirable and undesirable, on various organ systems. Therefore, it seems unlikely that a single variable that adequately reflects the physiologic effects of PEEP would ever be found or agreed on. In the assessment of PEEP therapy pulmonary gas exchange, lung mechanics and circulatory function must all be evaluated simultaneously.

• *The optimal level of CPAP can be judged in several ways. These include oxygenation, oxygen delivery, and lung compliance. Oxygen delivery probably represents the best physiologic end point.*

We utilize a combination of pulse and pulmonary artery oximetry, clinical assessment of ventilatory work, and lung mechanics to adjust PEEP. Additionally, ventilation is monitored with end-tidal carbon dioxide tension and infrequent blood gas analysis. Pulse and pulmonary artery oximetry can be used to monitor both pulmonary gas exchange and total body oxygen extraction continuously.[30] This technique has been shown to be comparable in accuracy to PEEP titration utilizing full cardiopulmonary profiles with repeated off-line blood gas analysis.[7] When small increments of PEEP are applied to a responder, arterial blood oxyhemoglobin saturation rises as ventilation-perfusion relationship improves. At the same time, improvement in arterial blood oxygen content is reflected by a decrease in the oxygen extraction ratio. A decrease in the spontaneous work of breathing effects a decrease in the spontaneous ventilatory rate and a decrease in the external signs of negative pleural pressure such as intercostal and suprasternal retractions. Secondary signs of decreased ventilatory work, alleviation of hypertension and tachycardia, are usually also evident. Excessive levels of PEEP are associated with an increase in oxygen extraction as systemic blood flow and oxygen delivery decrease. Hyperinflation of the lungs usually produces a shift in ventilatory work from inspiration to expiration. This results from a greater than normal resting lung volume. Arterial blood carbon dioxide tension may also rise. End-tidal carbon dioxide may not reflect this rise in $PaCO_2$ due to increased alveolar dead space.

Respiratory therapy must be initiated with sufficient supplemental oxygen and mechanical ventilatory support to correct hypoxemia, to provide adequate ventilation, and to eliminate excessive work of breathing. Immediately thereafter, the appropriate level of PEEP or CPAP should be determined and instituted. Subsequently, oxygen supplementation and ventilatory support are reduced to the lowest levels that maintain adequate oxygenation of arterial blood with a comfortable level of ventilatory work. After initial tailoring of respiratory support, PEEP therapy needs to be reevaluated and readjusted frequently in response to any changes in the patient's pulmonary disease.[7] Infrequent reevaluation of PEEP therapy may result in considerable overtreatment, or "bureaucratic PEEP." Conceivably, this necessitates other maneuvers to counteract the side effect of excessive airway pressure and unnecessarily prolongs the patient's stay in the ICU.[7]

• *The level of PEEP/CPAP needs to be evaluated on a frequent basis. The frequency should depend on the severity of illness and the stability of the patient.*

The use of PEEP and CPAP varies widely among practitioners of critical care medicine. In many instances, adequate arterial blood oxygenation can be achieved with oxygen supplementation, and the work of breathing can be eliminated by the use of mechanical ventilatory support. Few would argue against the use of PEEP to eliminate the need for inspired oxygen concentrations above 50%, which are known to be detrimental. Many do not consider a trade of increased PEEP for further reduction in FIO_2 or for any reduction in mechanical ventilatory support. Nelson and associates evaluated the use of PEEP and oxygen as the primary therapeutic modality to correct early hypoxemia after surgery or trauma.[31] No differences in mortality, complications, or duration of treatment were found. However, in this study, the authors did not make use of the benefits of PEEP to reduce oxygen therapy or mechanical ventilatory support; therefore, the question of the effect of early PEEP therapy on outcome remains unresolved.[32]

Adverse Effects of Sustained Positive Airway Pressure

Improper levels of PEEP and CPAP may adversely effect both the respiratory and the circulatory system. Excessive PEEP will overinflate the lungs, increase dead space ventilation, and impair blood flow in both the pulmonary and systemic circulations. Spontaneous respiratory work increases because of the low compliance of the distended respiratory system. The efficiency of respiratory muscles will also decrease because they are forced to operate at an unfavorable length-tension range.

- *Excessive PEEP/CPAP will increase dead space as well as the spontaneous work of breathing.*

An elevated mean intrathoracic pressure by the application of sustained positive airway pressure will decrease venous return and cardiac filling. This may lead to reduction in cardiac output and oxygen delivery unless fluid therapy restores preload. The magnitude of the circulatory compromise at a given level of elevated airway pressure varies with the mechanical characteristics of the respiratory system. Patients who have high lung compliance and low chest wall compliance, that is, enhanced transmission of airway pressure into the intrathoracic space, are particularly susceptible to circulatory impairment from elevated airway pressure. On the other hand, such adverse effects are unlikely to occur in patients with poorly compliant lungs, especially if the chest wall is distensible. Airway pressure transmission in these patients is attenuated.

- *Increased PEEP/CPAP will reduce venous return and ultimately cardiac output and oxygen delivery.*

The decrease in venous return seen with positive airway pressure results from a reduction in the transmural pressure of the intrathoracic veins as the pressure around them increases. Venous return can usually be restored with volume loading, but only at the expense of an elevated systemic venous pressure. An impairment in venous and lymphatic drainage, coupled with a possible decrease in arterial pressure, flow, and oxygen transport, has been reported to influence the function of several extrapulmonary tissues and organs. These include the central nervous system, the kidney, the gut, the pancreas, and the liver.[33–37] Experimental studies indicate that neural and humoral mechanisms also may mediate impairment of systemic and regional blood flow during PEEP therapy. Finally, deleterious effects of PEEP on end-organ function also depend on factors related to the patient's underlying illness. These factors include metabolic state, circulatory performance, and capillary permeability.

The effect of intrathoracic pressure on the forward flow from the right ventricle depends not only on reduction of venous return by elevated intrathoracic pressure, but also on lung volume, which is a major determinant of pulmonary vascular resistance. Elevated intrathoracic pressure affects left ventricular output because of the changes in venous return and right ventricular function. Left ventricular afterload is additionally influenced by pleural pressure. An elevation in intrathoracic pressure decreases left ventricular afterload. The net effect of the reduction in both preload and afterload brought about by PEEP or CPAP varies according to the sensitivity of the left ventricle to its loading conditions.[38] A normal left ventricle is preload sensitive and tends to respond to PEEP with a decrease in stroke volume. Hypovolemia accentuates the response. In contrast, a failing, dilated left ventricle may benefit from the afterload reduction brought about by an increase in intrathoracic pressure. Stroke volume may actually increase with PEEP. In addition to the effects of directly altered loading conditions on right and left ventricular

- *An elevated intrathoracic pressure will reduce left ventricular afterload as it reduces intrathoracic aortic pressure.*

function, mechanisms such as interventricular interaction, direct heart-lung interaction, reflex modification of cardiac function, and secondary hemodynamic effects of respiratory failure play a role.[38]

Exposure of an injured lung to positive airway pressure could easily be construed to result in further structural damage to the respiratory system. However, complications such as pneumothorax, pneumomediastinum, and interstitial pulmonary emphysema are rare in patients who breathe spontaneously with positive airway pressure. Therefore, rather than searching for a connection between pulmonary trauma and positive airway pressure therapy, the more logical culprit is mechanical ventilation, not expiratory airway pressure per se.[39,40] Application of PEEP definitely will lead to an increase in end-inspiratory airway pressure and the lung volume achieved during the mechanical breaths. However, when applied appropriately, the PEEP-associated improvement in lung mechanics should allow a reduction in mechanical ventilatory support with fewer positive pressure cycles or a smaller tidal pressure amplitude. This should reduce the risk of respiratory therapy-related lung damage.

- *PEEP does not ordinarily contribute to pulmonary barotrauma.*

A similar relationship between end-expiratory pressure and mechancial ventilation applies to the derangement in ventilation-perfusion matching that can be induced by lung overinflation with positive airway pressure. Mechanical positive pressure breaths have been shown to be inherently inefficient in the augmentation of gas exchange because of the propensity of the mechanical tidal volume to be distributed to the nondependent, least perfused regions of the lung.[41,42]

When the pulmonary parenchymal disease is severe and distinctly localized, application of positive airway pressure may not improve the ventilation-perfusion relationships of the affected area. Instead, overinflation of the unaffected regions of the lung may shift perfusion toward the nonventilated lung units. Consequently, arterial blood oxygenation may not improve following the application of PEEP but may actually deteriorate.[43] When the disease presents with large differences in the mechanical functioning of the two lungs, anecdotal reports support differential lung ventilation.[44] That is independent application of positive airway pressure to the two lungs, usually through a double-lumen tube. Controlled studies comparing this approach to conventional respiratory support are lacking.

- *For unilateral lung disease, patients require independent lung ventilation if oxygenation does not improve with PEEP/CPAP up to 15 cm H_2O.*

MECHANICAL VENTILATORY SUPPORT

Partial and Total Ventilatory Support

It is likely that patients with similar respiratory problems will be treated in a variety of ways, depending on the discipline and the background of individual practitioners. Despite these differences, the most used techniques usually allow administration of variable levels of ventilatory support. Since CMV was popular for such a long time, partial ventilatory support, when it emerged, was seen as an independent ventilatory technique. This created the colorful controversy between CMV and IMV. Objectively, conventional CMV and IMV only represent different levels of ventilatory support administered by the same basic technique. Only recently has modern respiratory care come to consider partial ventilatory support as a necessary feature of a useful ventilatory modality.

In patients with acute respiratory failure, the objectives of mechanical ventilatory support are to provide symptomatic relief of alveolar hypoventilation and to reduce respiratory work. Mechanical ventilatory support does not correct the primary cause of ventilatory failure. On the contrary, a high level of mechanical ventilatory support usually brings about some impairment in cardiopulmonary function. Control of ventilation beyond a comfortable level of spontaneous work of breathing and adequate alveolar ventilation has not been shown to have any specific advantages. Differences in hemodynamic performance between total and partial ventilatory support have not been demonstrated, even in patients with ischemic heart disease and left ventricular dysfunction.[45] Therefore, controlled ventilation is an extreme in the spectrum of ventilatory support, and its use should be justified on an individual basis.

Ventilation can be controlled only if the patient's intrinsic drive to breathe has been extinguished or if he or she has been rendered unable to breathe with neuromuscular blocking drugs. Respiratory drive can be abolished by a reduction of arterial blood carbon dioxide tension below the effective apneic threshold. To avoid induced respiratory alkalemia, sedatives are often given to raise the apneic threshold. Ventilation can then be controlled within the normal range of arterial blood carbon dioxide tension and pH. Deep sedation and prolonged neuromuscular blockade are not without side effects, however. Sedatives may adversely affect cardiovascular function, and long-term use of muscle relaxants has been reported to cause persistent abnormalities of neuromuscular function.[46] Moreover, loss of muscle tone and of spontaneous movement requires intense nursing care to prevent complications related to immobilization. Removal of spontaneous breathing activity makes accidental failure of the breathing circuit or of the ventilator life-threatening. Induced respiratory alkalosis is associated with a decrease in systemic oxygen delivery and a simultaneous increase in oxygen consumption. Cerebral hypoperfusion and bronchospasm may constitute additional hazards to critically ill patients.[47] A patient allowed to breathe spontaneously to some extent will usually regulate the arterial pH to normal.[48,49] With sufficient partial ventilatory support, the side effects of deep sedation and muscle relaxation are avoided without the need to induce respiratory alkalemia.

- *Controlled ventilation requires either induced alkalemia, paralysis, or sedation. The absence of spontaneous breathing can contribute to disuse muscle atrophy.*

Spontaneous respiratory efforts cause a more efficient distribution of inspired gas and perfusion.[42] This decreases physiologic dead space and results in a greater percentage of total ventilation as part of gas exchange. Even minimal respiratory effort, by decreasing dead space ventilation, can produce a significant increase in effective alveolar ventilation.[50] Unpublished data we collected revealed a sig-

- *Compared to controlled ventilation, spontaneous ventilation will reduce the overall amount of physiologic dead space.*

nificant increase in physiologic dead space during controlled ventilation. It further increased depending on the ventilatory rate (Fig. 10–4). In contrast, when partial support is provided, dead space increases, but to a lesser extent. When tidal volume is reduced to physiologic levels (i.e., 6 ml/kg), mechanical ventilation is unable to produce a desirable $PaCO_2$ at any rate (Fig. 10–4). This explains why substantially greater than physiologic minute ventilation has been the norm during controlled ventilation. Normally, VE of the spontaneously breathing subject is 5 to 6 L/min. However, tidal volume of 1000 ml delivered 10 to 12 times per minute is not unusual during full ventilatory support. The method of partial ventilatory support may be critical to derive beneficial effects. Experimental studies have shown that partial ventilatory support with PSV provides no advantages in pulmonary gas exchange over controlled ventilation. In contrast, purely spontaneous breaths even with minimal tidal volume were associated with increased ventilatory efficiency and improved circulatory performance.[50]

Prolonged CMV has been reported to reduce respiratory muscle strength and to result in discoordinated breathing on resumption of spontaneous ventilation.[51] Long after the initial cause of respiratory failure has disappeared, impaired strength and coordination of the respiratory system may lead to protracted ventilatory insufficiency and difficulty in weaning to spontaneous breathing. Maintenance of some spontaneous breathing activity during the course of ventilator

• *Even when patients are allowed to breathe spontaneously, methods such as PSV can contribute to disuse atrophy of respiratory muscles.*

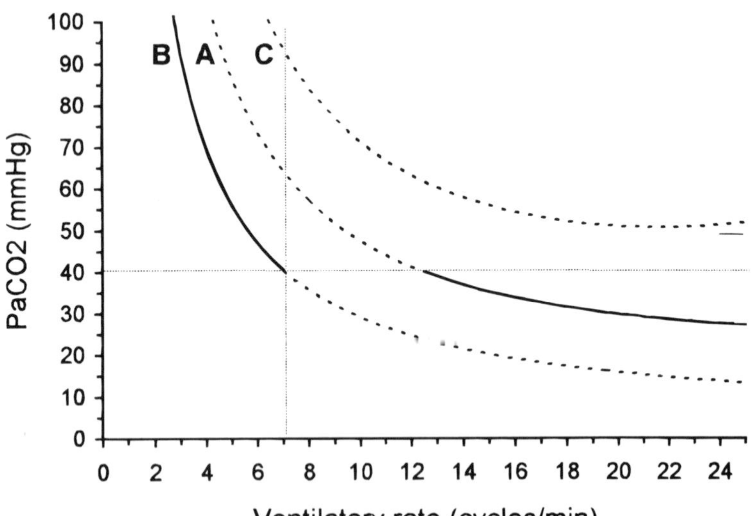

Figure 10–4.
Effect of ventilatory rate on arterial blood carbon dioxide. This is based on the association between rate and dead space during full ventilatory support (A) and spontaneous breathing (B) with a tidal volume of 700 ml. The reduced dead space ventilation allows normoventilation at a lower rate during spontaneous breathing. Extrapolation of these measurements to a lower tidal volume (600 ml) during mechanical ventilation (C) demonstrates that under these conditions normoventilation cannot be achieved with any ventilator frequency. Carbon dioxide production is assumed to be 200 ml/min.

therapy is likely to better maintain respiratory muscle strength and coordination. However, since an excessive work load also may decrease muscle strength, ventilatory support must always maintain the spontaneous work of breathing within a tolerable range.[52]

When mechanical ventilatory support increases airway and intrathoracic pressure, it reduces venous blood return to the heart.[53] In patients with normal or low circulatory filling volume, decreased ventricular filling usually causes a fall in stroke volume and systemic oxygen delivery. The circulatory depression may make it difficult to apply adequate PEEP during controlled ventilation. To reestablish adequate systemic blood flow after initiation of positive pressure ventilation, volume loading and pharmacologic support of the circulation may be required. However, hemodynamic compromise during positive pressure ventilation can be reduced by limitation of ventilatory assistance to an adequate level while maintaining some spontaneous breathing activity.[54] A decrease in intrathoracic pressure during spontaneous breaths augments venous return and increases systemic blood flow. The need for compensatory volume transfusion or inotropic support may be unnecessary, and appropriate CPAP to correct pulmonary mechanics may be applied without significant circulatory depression.

Theoretically, the decrease in intrathoracic pressure during spontaneous breathing with partial ventilatory support should be detrimental to patients with left ventricular dysfunction. Any decrease in intrathoracic pressure increases left ventricular afterload. Moreover, the dilated, failing ventricle may not respond favorably to increased filling secondary to augmented venous return. In such patients, adequate ventilatory support and CPAP must be urgently initiated and maintained at all times.[45,54] However, studies in patients with acute myocardial infarction and heart failure have shown that even patients with heart failure can tolerate the normal work of breathing, and support of circulatory function per se does not constitute an indication for control of all ventilation.[45]

- *Spontaneous breathing by itself does not impair performance in patients with left ventricular dysfunction. This only develops if severe changes in intrathoracic pressure accompany the respiratory exchange.*

The exact association between structural damage to the pulmonary parenchyma and mechanical ventilator support remains obscure. However, it is reasonable to assume that trauma secondary to hyperinflation or overpressurization of the respiratory system would be minimized during spontaneous breathing and maximized during controlled positive pressure ventilation with large tidal volumes. This claim is substantiated to some extent by clinical studies that show an association between high-peak airway pressure and pulmonary barotrauma.[40] The possible significance of a reduced number of positive pressure lung inflations is suggested by a study in which partial ventilatory support with IMV appeared to lower the incidence of barotrauma in adult patients.[39] The most convincing evidence of ventilator-related lung injury results from studies that demonstrate a reduced risk of bronchopulmonary dysplasia in neonates with respiratory failure and on extracorporeal membrane oxygenation.[55] The lungs appear best protected against ventilator-induced pulmonary injury with the application of the least amount of partial ventilatory support. Whether ventilatory modalities other

- *Pulmonary barotrauma appears most related to high peak inflation pressures and large tidal volumes. In general, this includes airway pressures in excess of 60 cm H_2O and tidal volumes in excess of 12 ml/kg.*

than conventional positive pressure ventilation reduce the risk of pulmonary trauma at a given level of support remains to be seen.

Partial ventilatory support provides the basis for weaning the patient from the ventilator. The flexibility of partial support permits gradual reduction rather than sudden discontinuation of ventilatory support and is an essential feature of a clinically useful modern ventilatory support technique. Problems were formerly caused by abrupt T-piece trials in patients who were not able to assume spontaneous ventilation. The tendency now is to apply slowly tapering mechanical ventilation with frequent blood gas analysis even to postoperative patients who are awake after recovering from general anesthesia and have normal pulmonary function.[56–58] While the latter practice is inappropriate and cost-ineffective, it presents little danger. However, to abruptly discontinue full ventilatory support in a patient recovering from cardiogenic respiratory failure would be both highly inappropriate and extremely dangerous.[45]

Ventilation with an Increase in Airway Pressure

Three major ventilatory techniques generate tidal volume with an increase in airway pressure: IMV, MMV, and PSV. The differences among them involve the method of interfacing spontaneous and mechanical ventilation. When used to provide near-total ventilatory support, these techniques produce very similar physiologic effects. It is noteworthy that PSV cannot be used to provide full ventilatory support because mechanical breaths occur only when triggered by a spontaneous effort.

- *PSV requires a spontaneously breathing patient.*

Assisted mechanical ventilation (AMV) and inverse inspiratory: expiratory ratio ventilation (IRV) are often considered to be independent modes of ventilatory support. However, neither technique allows adjustment of ventilatory support and, therefore, they cannot be used independently. Actually, they represent special applications of PSV and APRV, respectively. We present them separately for historical reasons.

Intermittent Mandatory Ventilation

During IMV, positive pressure breaths are delivered with an operator-adjusted mechanical rate while unassisted spontaneous breathing can occur simultaneously. In the absence of spontaneous breaths, the ventilator delivers the set number of breaths automatically. The mechanical breaths can be cycled, or limited in any way. Mechanical ventilatory support from 0 to 100% of total minute ventilation or ventilatory work can be delivered with IMV. Full control of ventilation can be obtained by an increase in the frequency of mandatory breaths until the $PaCO_2$ decreases below the apneic threshold and the patient stops spontaneous breathing. Weaning occurs by a gradual decrease in the frequency of mechanical breaths.

- *IMV can supply any underlying level of ventilator support required.*

The use of combined mechanical and spontaneous ventilation was first reported in infants in 1971.[59] Shortly thereafter, IMV was described as a weaning technique in 6 adult patients with lung injury who could not tolerate T-tube trials.[59] Also described were 3 patients with chronic obstructive pulmonary disease.[60] A study by Downs and associates in 1974 compared weaning with IMV to simple discontinuation of CMV in 24 patients with ventilatory failure of variable etiology.[61] The results indicated that IMV allowed more rapid weaning with better control of acid-base status and did not increase oxygen consumption. The finding that IMV shortened the duration of weaning received considerable criticism and was debated thereafter for at least a decade.[57,58]

• *IMV should not be considered a weaning technique.*

Even though introduced as a weaning technique, IMV rapidly became the standard technique for mechanical ventilation in most ICUs worldwide. This occurred despite the ongoing debate in regard to the usefulness of IMV, primarily because clinical experience quickly demonstrated IMV's superior advantages to CMV. The effects of controlled ventilation and IMV on pulmonary function, cardiovascular performance, and oxygen cost of breathing have been compared.[62–64] However, the results of these studies assess the effects of different levels of mechanical ventilatory support, that is, different levels of IMV, not the usefulness of IMV itself. The studies that compare IMV and AMV are similarly irrelevant to present-day respiratory care because the level of ventilatory support was not controlled. At the present time, IMV can be considered the standard ventilatory technique. Therefore, in this discussion, the advantages and disadvantages of newer methods of partial ventilatory support, such as PSV, MMV, and APRV, are compared with those of IMV in their respective sections.

The delivery of tidal volume is predictable because it depends on a limited number of physiologic variables that are easy to measure and monitor. Consequently, physiologic effects of different levels of IMV usually follow the expected course. The level of mechanical ventilatory support can be calculated, given the ventilator frequency and tidal volume. Changes in the patient's spontaneous ventilatory mechanics can be assessed because some spontaneous breaths occur without ventilator support. Therefore, evaluation of the patient's pulmonary function and the effects of therapy on ventilatory mechanics can be performed during any level of partial support. During ventilation with HFV and PSV, the amount of ventilatory assistance is much more difficult to document, and spontaneous ventilatory mechanics can be assessed only by turning off mechanical ventilation. The simple IMV breathing circuit does not necessarily require complex synchronization.

The major disadvantage of IMV involves a design that provides ventilatory support by augmentation of minute ventilation and not tidal volume. Not all spontaneous breaths are assisted, so one requires a well-designed breathing circuit and considerable expertise. A circuit with high resistance and low maximum flow, or an insensitive demand valve, may so increase the work of breathing that spontaneous ventilation becomes next to impossible.[65] Failure to wean a patient from a poorly designed IMV ventilator may be erroneously interpreted to result from the patient's pulmonary disease. Proper

• *A ventilator circuit that increases the flow resistance can negate the advantages of IMV.*

use of PEEP to improve pulmonary mechanics and to reduce the patient's intrinsic respiratory work must be employed during IMV. This ensures effective ventilation during the unassisted spontaneous breaths and prevents intolerable respiratory work, increased oxygen consumption, and deterioration of circulatory performance. All, reported during IMV, frequently result from use of improper breathing circuits or inappropriate end-expiratory pressure.[45,64] However, in some cases, even with optimum breathing circuit design, spontaneous ventilatory work may remain high and may require full ventilatory support.

Another shortcoming of IMV is the fixed nature of ventilatory support. Patients' ventilatory requirements change with carbon dioxide production and efficiency of gas exchange. For a given adjustment of rate and tidal volume, IMV contributes a fixed volume to minute ventilation. If the patient's ventilatory demand increases, the relative ventilatory support can decrease as the patient increases his or her own spontaneous minute ventilation. If the ventilatory demand decreases below the set IMV minute volume, hyperventilation results. Large changes in the relative ventilatory support are likely to be prevented with careful observation and frequent readjustment of the ventilator. However, the changing support ratio is a disadvantage of any minute volume-based support modality when compared with tidal volume-based techniques.

At the present time, IMV remains the ventilatory technique most widely used in critically ill patients. The wide range of ventilatory support availvable with IMV means there are few patients who cannot be managed with IMV alone. No scientific data indicate that a more favorable outcome would result from any alternative ventilatory modality. Therefore, IMV will likely remain the basic ventilatory technique well into the future.

Mandatory Minute Ventilation

• MMV has not proved satisfactory in clinical use. Patients can breathe at low tidal volumes that simply ventilate dead space. This can confuse the ventilator, and it does not supply any necessary supplemental support.

Mandatory minute ventilation operates in a fashion similar to an on-demand cardiac pacemaker. It fulfills a certain preset ventilatory goal not met by the patient's own spontaneous ventilation. In the original MMV circuit of Hewlett, two separate gas reservoirs, one for spontaneous breathing and the other for the ventilator, received fresh gas from a common source.[66] The total flow of gas to these reservoirs was adjusted to the desired minute ventilation. When spontaneous minute ventilation was lower than the fresh gas flow, the excess gas was diverted to the ventilator reservoir. Once an amount equal to the preset tidal volume had been collected, it was then delivered to the patient with a mandatory positive pressure breath. Therefore, a patient whose spontaneous ventilation matched the desired level received no mechanical ventilation. An apneic patient received the predetermined minute volume in a fashion indistinguishable from conventional CMV. If the patient breathed spontaneously less than the preset minute volume, the ventilator provided for the difference. Some ventilator manufacturers use the term extended MMV (EMMV) to denote a modification that allows spontaneous breathing beyond the set minute ventilation. However, this was possible even in Hewlett's original design. A safety valve permitted spontaneous breathing of room air regardless of the minute ventilation adjustment. Newer modifications of MMV use respiratory rate rather than minute volume as the target variable. To date, these have not been widely evaluated.[67] The mechanical breaths during MMV theoretically can be delivered using any technique. Originally, IMV was used, but MMV with PSV is now offered in some ventilators.

The technical aspects of MMV were described in 1977 by Hewlett and colleagues.[66] A case report by Higgs and Bevan later described successful postoperative weaning of a patient with myasthenia gravis using MMV.[68] Mandatory minute ventilation was designed to provide smooth transition from controlled ventilation to spontaneous breathing following anesthesia and surgery. Later, this technique was advocated as an alternative to IMV in order to provide ventilatory support for patients with acute lung injury. It provides a higher backup level of ventilation, if the patient's spontaneous respiratory activity becomes inadequate. Theoretically, MMV could provide automatic weaning from ventilatory support in patients recovering from anesthesia. However, its use in other clinical situations that require ventilatory assistance may be associated with problems related to the very mechanism of operation.

- *In theory, MMV supplies the level of minute ventilation that the patient cannot provide on his or her own.*

It may not be possible to accomplish weaning from ventilatory support with MMV without adjustment of the MMV. The relative amount of dead space ventilation may decrease when spontaneous breathing contributes more of the total minute ventilation.[69] As the amount of mechanical ventilation decreases, the total ventilatory requirement should decrease as well. In patients with respiratory failure due to acute lung injury, adequate ventilatory support is that which corrects respiratory acidosis and transfers a necessary amount of respiratory work to the ventilator. If the mandatory minute volume is set below the patient's spontaneous minute ventilation, the ventilator will not cycle until true ventilatory failure results in a reduction of spontaneous minute volume. Setting the minute volume above the patient's spontaneous minute ventilation may easily result in CMV. Therefore, in patients with lung injury, MMV may not provide a comfortable decrease in respiratory work. It is noteworthy that no scientific data support or refute the usefulness of MMV in any patient group. Therefore, discussion of this modality remains theoretic.

Inverse Ratio Ventilation

Inverse inspiratory: expiratory ratio ventilation is mechanical ventilation with an inspiratory-to-expiratory time ratio greater than 1. The prolonged inspiration will maintain a high mean alveolar pressure to maximally recruit alveolar units with long time constants and will not generate a high peak airway pressure. Inverse ratio ventilation can be either volume controlled (VC-IRV) or pressure-controlled (PC-IRV). During VC-IRV, inspiratory time can be ex-

- *IRV can be delivered by control of either the volume or the pressure.*

tended with slow inspiratory flow, an end-inspiratory pause, or decelerating inspiratory flow. During PC-IRV, constant pressure is applied to the airway for the duration of the inspiration. This results in decelerating gas flow into the lungs. Several practical differences exist between VC-IRV and PC-IRV.[70] Volume-controlled IRV permits precise control of minute ventilation and inspiratory flow. It requires careful monitoring of the airway and alveolar pressures. Pressure-controlled IRV allows exact adjustment of airway pressure, but it may result in considerable variation in tidal volume and minute ventilation. Almost any ventilator can be adjusted to deliver VC-IRV, whereas PC-IRV requires a specifically designed ventilator. Nevertheless, most of the data regarding the use of IRV in adults have been generated with PC-IRV. Pressure-controlled IRV resembles airway pressure release ventilation (APRV) when APRV is used to control ventilation. The relationship between PC-IRV and APRV is similar to that between conventional controlled positive pressure ventilation and IMV. The two may be viewed as different levels of one ventilatory technique.

- *IRV maintains the appropriate mean airway pressure necessary to ensure oxygenation. The prolonged inspiratory time usually better distributes gas to poorly ventilated alveoli.*

Inverse ratio ventilation was first used in neonates in the late 1970s, with encouraging results.[71,72] In adult patients, the interest in IRV was probably reduced by the simultaneous introduction of IMV and CPAP. Experimental and clinical studies suggested that the beneficial effects of IRV resulted from increased mean transpulmonary pressure and lung volume. This could be accomplished equally efficiently with PEEP. This probably contributed to the disuse of IRV in adults.[73–75] However, it is difficult to write off numerous reports that claim improved oxygenation, lower peak airway pressure, and reduction in dead space-tidal volume ratio during IRV.[76,77] Tharratt and associates compared IRV and volume-limited conventional ventilation in 31 patients with ARDS,[77] and they found that, during IRV, peak airway pressure was lower by 20 cm H_2O. PEEP could be reduced by 12 cm H_2O, while PaO_2 improved by 11 mm Hg, and minute ventilation was lower by 7 L/min. $PaCO_2$ remained unchanged, and mean airway pressure increased by 5 cm H_2O. These results were later confirmed by Chan and Abraham,[78] who were also able to associate the benefit with the I:E ratio and not the pressure limitation of the ventilator breaths. Unfortunately, the observed improvement in pulmonary function did not carry over to overall cardiopulmonary performance, oxygen delivery, or oxygen extraction. This suggests that depression in circulatory function by elevated mean intrathoracic pressure or lung volume associated with IRV counterbalanced the improvement in oxygenation. A decreased in the I:E ratio to minimize cardiovascular side effects will also weaken the efficacy of alveolar recruitment. Therefore, the advantages of IRV may be limited to an improvement in lung function.

- *IRV usually requires that the patient be paralyzed.*

The long inspiratory phase of IRV frequently makes this technique difficult to interface with spontaneous breathing. Sedation or even neuromuscular blockade often must be instituted to ensure patient acceptance of IRV. Consequently, IRV classically administers CMV during the peak impairment of the patient's pulmonary function. Weaning following recovery of lung function requires another technique.

Rapid pressurization of the airway, an increase in mean alveolar pressure, and air trapping during the short expiratory time may predispose the lung to injury during IRV. An incidence of pneumothorax up to 24% has been reported during PC-IRV.[77] Depending on whether a volume-variable or pressure-variable technique delivers IRV, airway pressure or tidal volume remains uncontrolled and requires close monitoring. An increased ventilator rate may cause air trapping due to the excessive reduction in expiratory time.

Available data indicate that in some patients with severe acute respiratory failure, IRV may improve ventilation and oxygenation. Favorable effects reported from the use of airway pressure release ventilation support the results obtained with PC-IRV.[79,80] A combination of spontaneous ventilation with IRV-type mechanical support could obviate the need for heavy sedation, minimize cardiovascular impairment, allow use of lower airway pressure and tidal volume without alveolar hypoventilation, and extend the use of IRV to cover any level of ventilatory assistance.

Assisted Mechanical Ventilation

During AMV, the ventilator responds to each spontaneous breathing effort with a positive pressure mechanical breath. The ventilator breath may be delivered by any form of cycling and with or without positive expiratory airway pressure. Ventilation with AMV requires a spontaneous drive to breathe. Therefore, full ventilatory support or support to an apneic patient cannot be provided with this technique. Therefore, a backup is usually provided (assist-control ventilation). The tidal volume delivered by the ventilator depends on the ventilator settings and not on the patient. Therefore, AMV does not allow transition from mechanical ventilation to spontaneous breathing. Weaning requires discontinuation of mechanical ventilation or another technique.

- *AMV usually requires a backup mode to guard against apnea.*

Assisted mechanical ventilation was developed in an attempt to improve synchronization between the ventilator and the patient. Since the patient determines the ventilatory rate, it was believed to allow nearly full ventilatory support without the need for massive sedation or hyperventilation. However, it has since been demonstrated that a patient receiving AMV usually does not terminate the spontaneous breathing effort after the ventilator is triggered, but continues it throughout the mechanical cycle. This contributes significantly to total work of breathing.[81,82] Under favorable conditions, the patient's ventilatory work contributes 33 to 50% of the energy required for passive inflation of the respiratory system. Under less favorable conditions, work may even exceed that of passive lung inflation. Therefore, AMV provides breath-to-breath partial ventilatory support that varies in an uncontrolled fashion.

- *In some patients, even during assisted ventilation, the spontaneous work of breathing remains high.*

Assisted mechanical ventilation was the first modality that allowed mechanical ventilatory support to patients with an intact spontaneous drive to breathe. However, AMV did not abolish the problem of hyperventilation during mechanical support. Adjustment of AMV to provide a large mechanical breath in response to a spontaneous effort, will cause $PaCO_2$ to remain close to the apneic threshold. Respiratory alkalosis usually will develop.[48,49,83] The acid-base status will remain normal only if the patient can independently regulate the spontaneous tidal volume, as is the case during IMV or PSV.

If flow cycling and a pressure limit are in effect during AMV, then AMV is identical to fixed-level PSV.[84] Assisted mechanical ventilation has no physiologic advantage over PSV. PSV allows the patient more control of tidal volume and the possibility to alter the level of ventilatory support when necessary. A comparison of volume-controlled AMV and PSV in patients with acute lung injury demonstrated that PSV resulted in significantly lower ventilatory rate and peak airway pressure, a higher tidal volume, and improved oxygenation.[85]

The inflexibility of AMV and the availability of other ventilatory modalities have resulted in a transition to IMV, PSV, or APRV. Since it has no practical or theoretic benefits over these newer techniques, we do not recommend the use of AMV.

Pressure Support Ventilation

Pressure support ventilation, also termed inspiratory assist or assisted spontaneous breathing, was originally developed to augment spontaneous tidal volume. It also overcomes the high circuit resistance during spontaneous breathing with MMV.[86] Inefficient, rapid, shallow spontaneous breathing that contributed little to alveolar ventilation was detected by MMV ventilators and counted as part of the mandatory minute volume. This resulted in inadequate ventilatory support in some cases and prompted a modification that provided an additional gas flow up to an adjustable pressure limit during spontaneous breathing. In 1984, Hansen and colleagues disassociated PSV from MMV and employed it as a weaning technique.[87] This initiated its use as a new ventilatory support modality.[87]

During PSV, the patient's spontaneous inspiratory effort triggers the ventilator to open a variable gas flow that increases rapidly until airway pressure reaches a preselected level above baseline. A feedback mechanism maintains the flow so that inspiratory airway pressure remains constant. When the patient's inspiratory effort wanes, flow decreases and terminates when the patient's inspiratory flow is sufficiently reduced. Airway pressure then returns to baseline. Thus, during each spontaneous respiratory effort, the patient receives assisted ventilation with a mechanism that is pressure limited and flow cycled. The inspiratory work of breathing performed by the ventilator during PSV depends on the pressure level selected and on the patient's respiratory mechanics. With a sufficiently high pressure support level, the ventilator performs most of the respira-

• *During PSV, the actual volume received by the patient depends on his or her spontaeous effort as well as on the level of pressure support selected.*

tory work. This mode is similar to AMV.[84,87] The major theoretic advantage of PSV is adjustable breath-to-breath ventilatory assistance. Each respiratory cycle has a similar configuration and is equally assisted by the ventilator. This may facilitate adaptation of the patient to the ventilator and may allow smoother weaning from ventilatory support. Since the patient controls respiratory rate and the duration of inspiration, the development of respiratory alkalosis should be less likely during PSV than during AMV.

Hansen and associates administered PSV with pressures ranging from 5 to 30 cm H_2O above CPAP to 10 patients recovering from ARDS.[87] When the pressure support level exceeded 10 cm H_2O, tidal volume increased and inspiratory time decreased. This suggested that the patients received a high degree of mechanical ventilatory support. In order to reduce the spontaneous respiratory rate, a pressure support level of at least 20 cm H_2O was required in 5 of 10 patients. Despite the absence of any data, all patients were reported to have failed an attempt to wean using IMV and CPAP. Weaning was accomplished in 12 hours to 4 days utilizing PSV. Prakash and Meij compared IMV and PSV in 26 patients who were recovering from coronary artery bypass surgery.[88] The authors claimed that use of PSV was associated with shorter intubation time. However, this result was not tested with adequate statistical analysis. The different weaning protocols used for PSV and IMV, not the techniques themselves, explained most of the differences. MacIntyre compared synchronized IMV and PSV in 15 patients who required mechanical ventilatory support.[89] Pressure support ventilation was administered with the pressure limit (range from 13 to 41 cm H_2O) adjusted to minimize respiratory rate. During PSV, the patient's respiratory rate was lower than the total respiratory rate during SIMV, despite similar minute ventilation. Peak airway pressure was lower and mean airway pressure higher during PSV. All but one patient expressed a subjective preference for PSV. Lung model studies suggest that PSV may alter the pressure-volume characteristics of the lung and decrease respiratory muscle work. Compared with IMV, this occurs with a smaller change in pressure and a larger change in volume.[89]

- *PSV may aid as a weaning tool if it overcomes the imposed work in the ventilator circuit, which normally increases the patient's work of breathing.*

The level of pressure support is normally adjusted to achieve a desired tidal volume, ventilatory rate, and patient comfort. During PSV weaning, the patient will maintain an adequate tidal volume and acceptable ventilatory rate by an increase in his or her relative spontaneous ventilatory effort as the pressure support level is gradually decreased. While it is clear that spontaneous respiratory work can be reduced using PSV, the actual level of ventilatory assistance provided by a given level of pressure support cannot be easily determined. However, in selected cases, the adequacy of mechanical support can usually be confirmed by clinical evaluation of the work of breathing, supplemented by esophageal pressure monitoring. Since PSV provides breath-to-breath ventilatory support, it responds to an increase in ventilatory demand with more support, as long as the patient increases ventilatory rate or duration of inspiration.

• *PSV is a form of positive pressure ventilation.*

It is essential to understand that PSV delivers variable positive pressure mechanical ventilatory support. It is not a form of spontaneous breathing. Although the patient triggers all PSV breaths, high levels of pressure support provide nearly full ventilatory assistance. Even low levels of pressure support may contribute significantly to the patient's tidal volume and minute ventilation.

• *PSV negates the effects of spontaneous breathing and associated negative changes in intrathoracic pressure.*

Some breathing circuits with high flow resistance during spontaneous breaths may require PSV. When IMV is the primary ventilatory mode, PSV levels should be adjusted to overcome circuit resistance only. Higher levels of PSV will likely defeat the purpose of partial ventilatory support. For patients who do not require mechanical ventilation, a well-designed low-resistance CPAP system may be a more efficacious and simpler alternative than application of low-level PSV to balance a poor ventilator circuit.

Cardiovascular and pulmonary complications, like other forms of mechanical ventilation of PSV, result from increased airway pressure. The patient-triggered nature of PSV means that it does not provide ventilatory support unless the patient makes an effort to breathe. Furthermore, the ventilatory effort must be sustained. Short, nonsustained inspiratory efforts may result in premature termination of the pressure support and, possibly, inadequate ventilatory assistance.[90] As with all pressure-limited ventilatory modalities, the ventilatory support of PSV depends on the functional state of the respiratory system. When lung compliance or airway resistance changes, adjustment of the pressure support level may be necessary. A self-adjusting form of PSV that maintains ventilatory rate below a set limit has been described, but its feasibility has not been evaluated on a large scale.[67]

Available data demonstrate that PSV can provide ventilatory support to patients with respiratory failure and existing ventilatory drive, and weaning from ventilatory support may be accomplished using decremental PSV. There are no comparative investigations that establish PSV as the method of choice for ventilatory assistance or for weaning from ventilatory support. However, PSV, along with IMV, has become one of the two major ventilatory modalities currently in use. Its major advantages over other techniques include breath-to-breath ventilatory support and a close interface with spontaneous breathing.

Ventilation by Decrease in Airway Pressure

Airway Pressure Release Ventilation

• *APRV does not employ positive pressure delivery of gases to the airway. APRV appears to work best with modest degrees of pulmonary impairment.*

Airway pressure release ventilation, introduced in 1986,[91] was the first ventilatory technique that augmented alveolar ventilation by decrease in airway pressure and lung volume. During APRV, a CPAP circuit maintains the baseline airway pressure above ambient. Lung volume changes following rapid intermittent release of CPAP (Fig. 10–5). This is accomplished by a release valve situated in the circuit's expiratory limb. The release valve must have minimal flow resistance to allow adequate emptying of the lungs during pressure

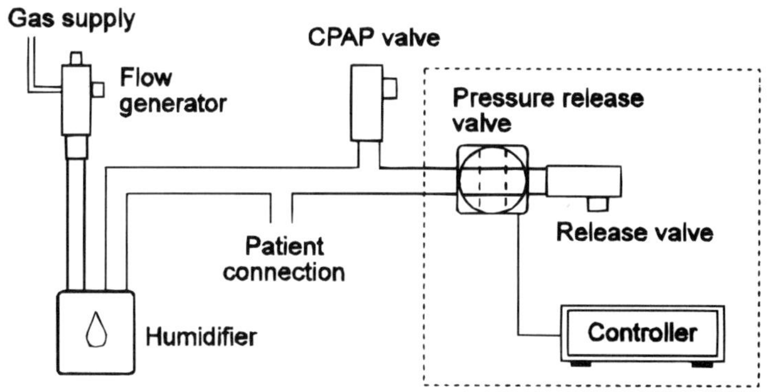

Figure 10–5.
Diagram of the original airway pressure release ventilation (APRV) circuit. Modifications include adding a timer-controlled airway pressure release valve and a second threshold resistor valve to the circuit (dotted box). A high flow of humidified gas maintains a nearly constant level of continuous positive airway pressure (CPAP) during spontaneous inspiration and during exhalation. To assist breathing, CPAP is interrupted briefly by a pressure release valve, which opens to allow a transient decrease in lung volume to a level detemined by the release pressure valve. Closure of the pressure release valve reestablishes functional residual capacity (FRC).

release. The release valve controller adjusts the duration and frequency of pressure release. This method was designed to augment alveolar ventilation during spontaneous breathing with CPAP.[92] Alveolar ventilation during APRV is determined by the APRV rate and tidal volume. The tidal volume depends on lung compliance, airway resistance, release time, and the difference between CPAP and the airway pressure during the release phase. The patient can breathe spontaneously at any time during the APRV cycle. If the release frequency and tidal volume lower the patient's arterial blood carbon dioxide below apneic threshold, controlled ventilation similar to PC-IRV will result. Weaning from APRV requires reduction of the release frequency.

Initial experimental and clinical investigations have demonstrated that alveolar ventilation and arterial oxygenation can be effectively maintained during APRV.[91,93] Experimental investigations that compared APRV and conventional positive pressure ventilation found no significant differences in oxygenation or ventilation. These were studies in animals with normal lung function. The two modalities utilized similar airway pressure, tidal volume, and ventilator rate. In an oleic acid dog model, APRV produced significantly lower arterial blood carbon dioxide tension and higher arterial blood oxygen tension than positive pressure ventilation. These results suggested that the airway pressure pattern of APRV may favor a more uniform distribution of ventilation than positive pressure ventilation in injured lungs. In another study, dogs with oleic acid-induced lung injury were allowed to breath spontaneously on APRV or positive pressure ventilation. Both methods corrected ventilatory failure and arterial desaturation equally effectively.[94] Systemic oxygen delivery was far superior during APRV.

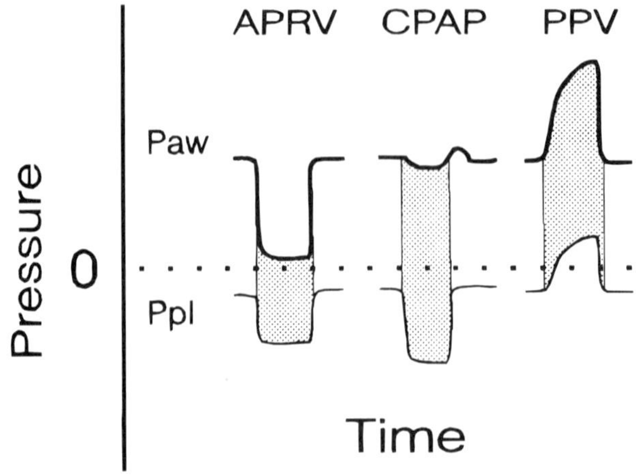

Figure 10–6.
Changes in airway (Paw) and intrathoracic pressure (Ppl) during spontaneous breathing with continuous positive airway pressure (CPAP), during airway pressure release ventilation (APRV), and positive pressure ventilation (PPV). Note the similarity in the intrathoracic pressure pattern between spontaneous breathing and APRV, the decrease in transpulmonary pressure (dotted area) during APRV, and the high peak airway pressure during PPV.

Peak airway pressure during APRV equals the CPAP level (Fig. 10–6). Augmentation of alveolar ventilation with low peak airway pressure and without overdistention of the lung parenchyma appears to be a consistent major advantage of APRV. Clinical and laboratory studies demonstrate that conversion from positive pressure ventilation to APRV will cause a 30 to 75% reduction in peak airway pressure.[79,80,91]

As expected, studies that employed similar levels of mean airway pressure between APRV and positive pressure ventilation did not show any differences in circulatory function. This holds regardless of the presence or absence of acute lung injury or the volume status of the experimental animal or the patient.[79,80,91,93] When added to existing CPAP therapy, the hemodynamic advantages of APRV become obvious. An experimental investigation in dogs with induced lung injury revealed that APRV ventilation caused no depression of stroke volume, cardiac output, and tissue oxygen delivery compared with spontaneous breathing with CPAP. Positive pressure ventilation caused significant reductions in stroke volume and oxygen delivery.[94]

The use of APRV in the clinical setting has been evaluated in four studies. Garner and colleagues compared APRV and positive pressure ventilation with similar mean airway pressures. Patients had mild acute lung injury following cardiopulmonary bypass. The two modalities were equally effective in providing ventilation and oxygenation.[93] Peak airway pressure, however, was significantly reduced during APRV. There were no differences in circulatory function. All patients were weaned successfully from ventilatory support using APRV without complications.

- *APRV can often significantly reduce the peak airway pressure that develops during more standard modes of mechanical ventilatory support.*

A prospective short-term study of 50 adult patients with moderate-to-severe acute respiratory failure demonstrated that 47 were adequately ventilated with APRV.[79] Changeover from conventional ventilation to APRV effected a reduction in peak airway pressure by 55 ± 17%. Again, no significant effects on oxygenation or circulatory function were documented.

Cane and associates reported data from 18 adult patients with severe acute respiratory failure, sequentially ventilated with continuous positive pressure ventilation and APRV.[80] APRV provided effective ventilatory support to 17 of the 18 patients with peak airway pressure significantly lower than that during positive pressure ventilation. One patient developed unexplained cardiopulmonary decompensation after initiation of APRV. Six patients who initially responded well to APRV were later returned to positive pressure ventilation because of lobar atelectasis (2), hypoxemia (2) and inadequate ventilation (2). The authors attributed the development of atelectasis to the volume-variable nature of APRV.

Valentine and colleagues compared APRV, IMV, and PSV in eight patients recovering from open-heart operations. APRV provided adequate ventilation with the lowest peak airway pressure and dead space ventilation.[95] No differences in oxygenation of arterial blood and no complications were seen during APRV.

Available data indicate that a marked reduction in peak airway pressure seems to be the major advantage of APRV. Depending on the method of application, mean airway and mean intrathoracic pressure may be reduced as well. APRV could potentially lower the incidence of airway pressure or lung volume-related pulmonary trauma as well as cardiovascular impairment. The optimum pressure levels and the duration of pressure release during ventilation with APRV have not yet been determined. Therefore, further development of this technique deserves attention.

Intermittent Mandatory Pressure Release Ventilation

Intermittent mandatory pressure release ventilation (IMPRV) combines PSV and APRV.[96] The IMPRV cycle begins with a pressure support breath, which is followed by airway pressure release below the initial level of CPAP (Fig. 10–7). Although patient-triggered, IMPRV does not necessarily support each spontaneous respiratory effort. The desired amount of mechanical ventilatory support requires adjustment of both the pressure variables of the mechanical breath and the ratio of spontaneous and IMPRV breaths. Breath-to-breath ventilatory support, synchronization of mechanical breaths to spontaneous breathing, and the ability to alter airway pressure independent of CPAP may constitute advantages of IMPRV over APRV.[97] IMPRV requires a microprocessor-controlled ventilator programmed to deliver this mode of ventilation. The feasibility of IMPRV has been demonstrated in patients with acute respiratory failure.[98] Results of comparisons between IMPRV and other modalities of mechanical ventilatory support are not yet available.

Even though a large number of ventilatory modalities are already available, new techniques continue to be introduced. It is likely that

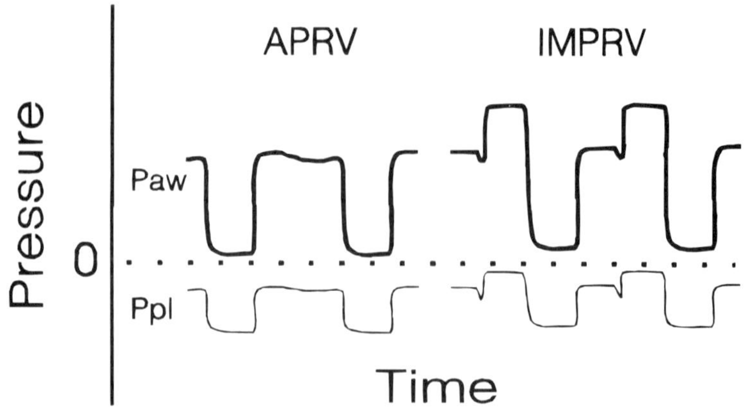

Figure 10–7.
Changes in airway (Paw) and intrathoracic pressure (Ppl) during mechanical ventilation with airway pressure release ventilation (APRV) and intermittent mandatory pressure release ventilation (IMPRV). The IMPRV cycle is triggered by the patient's initiation of a small decrease in airway pressure. After a pressure support phase, the airway pressure is released below the initial continuous positive airway pressure (CPAP) level. It then returns following completion of the APRV phase.

sophisticated controlling techniques designed to better adapt ventilator function to the patient may offer an improvement in ventilator therapy. However, the clinical value of any new ventilatory technique will require demonstration of therapeutic efficacy, safety, ease of operation, and cost-effectiveness. Since such data are not currently available, extensive research will be necessary to establish the basis for the clinical use of most already existing ventilatory modalities and for any new techniques yet to come.

Nitric Oxide

• *Nitric oxide is a specific pulmonary vasodilator. It improves ventilation-perfusion relationships and oxygenation.*

• *Nitric oxide is a support modality and as such reduces the required level of airway pressures and* F_{IO_2}.

No current discussion of postoperative mechanical ventilation would be complete without an inclusion of nitric oxide. An important element of respiratory dysfunction often includes pulmonary hypertension. The addition of nitric oxide to the inspired gas mixture can dramatically reduce pulmonary artery pressures and yet have a minimal effect on systemic pressures.[99,100] In most instances, inspired gas concentrations of 2 to 20 ppm have effectively reduced pulmonary artery pressure and increased oxygenation. No doubt ventilation-perfusion matching improves and pulmonary blood flow redistributes.

The major benefit of nitric oxide appears to be its ability to reduce the required level of ventilatory support. As PaO_2 improves, both ventilatory pressures and F_{IO_2} can be reduced. The gas itself does not have any therapeutic effect but merely improves gas exchange.

As improvement takes place, nitric oxide can be slowly weaned. One must judge the patient's response to weaning and titrate levels accordingly.

In conclusion, any number of techniques are available to support oxygenation and ventilation in the postoperative critically ill patient. Part of this represents engineering advancements, while the large number of choices indicates that none is ideal for every circumstance. Rather, the clinician must be familiar with all the concepts so when the usual modalities prove ineffective, the correct alternative can be quickly substituted.

REFERENCES

1. Räsänen J, Leon MA, Cane RD: Adaptation of pressure support ventilation to increasing ventilatory demand during experimental airway obstruction and acute lung injury. Crit Care Med 1993; 21:562–566.
2. Zarins CK, Bayne CG, Rice CL: Does spontaneous ventilation with IMV protect from PEEP induced cardiac output depression? J Surg Res 1977; 22:299–304.
3. Gattinoni L, Pesenti A, Bombino MEA: Relationships between lung computed tomographic density, gas exchange, and PEEP in acute respiratory failure. Anesthesiology 1988; 69:824–832.
4. Gattinoni L, D'Andrea L, Pelosi P: Regional effects and mechanism of positive end-expiratory pressure in early adult respiratory distress syndrome. JAMA 1993; 269:2122–2127.
5. Douglas ME, Downs JB, Dannemiller FJ: Change in pulmonary venous admixture with varying inspired oxygen. Anesth Analg 1976; 55:688–695.
6. Gherini S, Peters RM, Virgilio RW: Mechanical work on the lungs and work of breathing with positive end-expiratory pressure and continuous positive airway pressure. Chest 1979; 76:251–256.
7. Räsänen J, Downs JB: Optimum versus clinically established continuous positive airway pressure in respiratory therapy. J Clin Monit 1988; 4:235–239.
8. Cormier Y, Couture J, Desmeules M: Changes in upper airway resistance with lung inflation and positive airway pressure. J Appl Physiol 1990; 68:1075.
9. Sotomayor JL, Godinez RI, Borden S et al: Large-airway collapse due to acquired tracheobronchomalacia in infancy. Am J Dis Child 1986; 140:367–371.
10. Ferguson GT, Benoist J: Nasal continuous positive airway pressure in the treatment of tracheobronchomalacia. Am Rev Respir Dis 1993; 147:457–461.
11. Marini JJ: Should PEEP be used in airflow obstruction? Am Rev Respir Dis 1989; 140:1–3.
12. Qvist J, Anderson JB, Pemberton M: High-level PEEP in severe asthma. N Engl J Med 1982; 307:1347–1348.
13. Tuxen DV: Detrimental effects of positive end-expiratory pressure during controlled mechanical ventilation of patients with severe airflow obstruction. Am Rev Respir Dis 1989; 140:5–9.
14. Smith TC, Marini JJ: Impact of PEEP on lung mechanics and work of breathing in severe airflow obstruction. J Appl Physiol 1988; 65: 1488–1499.
15. Petrof BJ, Legare M, Goldberg P: Continuous positive airway pressure reduces the work of breathing and dyspnea during weaning from

mechanical ventilation in severe chronic obstructive pulmonary disease. Am Rev Respir Dis 1990; 141:281–289.

16. Dall'ava-Santucci J, Armaganidis A, Brunet F: Mechanical effects of PEEP in patients with adult respiratory distress syndrome. J Appl Physiol 1990; 68:843–848.
17. Pesenti A, Pelosi P, Rossi N: The effects of positive end-expiratory pressure on respiratory resistance in patients with the adult respiratory distress syndrome and in normal anesthetized subjects. Am Rev Respir Dis 1991; 144:101–107.
18. Barach A, Martin J, Eckman M: Positive pressure respiration and its applications to the treatment of acute pulmonary edema. Ann Intern Med 1938; 12:754–759.
19. Burford TH, Burbank B: Traumatic wet lung: observations on certain physiologic fundamentals of thoracic trauma. J Thorac Surg 1945; 14:415–422.
20. Jensen NK: Recovery of pulmonary function after crushing injuries of the chest. Dis Chest 1952; 22:319–325.
21. Ashbaugh DG, Petty TL, Bigelow DG: Continuous positive-pressure breathing (CPPB) in adult respiratory distress syndrome. J Thorac Cardiovasc Surg 1969; 57:31–41.
22. Douglas ME, Downs JB: Cardiopulmonary effects of PEEP and CPAP. Anesth Analg 1978; 57:347–350.
23. Sturgeon CL Jr, Douglas ME, Downs JB: Cardiopulmonary effects during spontaneous ventilation. Anesth Analg 1977; 56:633–641.
24. Scharf SM, Bianco JA, Tow DE: The effects of large negative intrathoracic pressure on left ventricular function in patients with coronary artery disease. Circulation 1981; 63:871–875.
25. Putensen C, Hörmann C, Baum M: Comparison of mask and nasal continuous positive airway pressure after extubation and mechanical ventilation. Crit Care Med 1993; 21:357–362.
26. Thomas AN, Ryan JP, Doran B: A nasal CPAP system: description and comparison with facemask CPAP. Anaesthesia 1992; 47: 311–315.
27. Downs JB, Klein EFJ, Modell JH: The effect of incremental PEEP on PaO_2 in patients with respiratory failure. Anesth Analg 1973; 52: 210–215.
28. Kirby RR, Downs JB, Civetta JM: High level positive end expiratory pressure (PEEP) in acute respiratory insufficiency. Chest 1975; 67: 156–165.
29. Suter PM, Fairley HB, Isenberg MD: Optimum end-expiratory airway pressure in patients with acute airway pressure in patients with acute pulmonary failure. N Engl J Med 1975; 292:284–289.
30. Räsänen J, Downs JB, Hodges MR: Continuous monitoring of gas exchange and oxygen use with dual oximetry. J Clin Anesth 1988; 1:3–8.
31. Nelson LD, Civetta JM, Hudson-Civetta J: Titrating positive end-expiratory pressure therapy in patients with early, moderate arterial hypoxemia. Crit Care Med 1987; 15:14–19.
32. Downs JB, Räsänen J: Confirming the null hypothesis. Crit Care Med 1987; 15:82–83.
33. Cooper KR, Boswell PA, Choi SC: Safe use of PEEP in patients with severe head injury. J Neurosurg 1985; 63:552–555.
34. Marquez JM, Douglas ME, Downs JB: Renal function and cardiovascular responses during positive airway pressure. Anesthesiology 1979; 50:393–398.

35. Matuschak GM, Pinsky MR, Rogers RM: Effects of positive end-expiratory pressure on hepatic blood flow and performance. J Appl Physiol 1987; 62:1377–1383.
36. Kahle M, Lippert J, Willemer S: Effects of positive end-expiratory pressure (PEEP) ventilation on the exocrine pancreas in minipigs. Res Exp Med 1991; 191:309–325.
37. Arvidsson D, Almquist P, Haglund U: Effects of positive end-expiratory pressure on splanchnic circulation and function in experimental peritonitis. Arch Surg 1991; 126:631–636.
38. Weber KT, Janicki JS, Hunter WC: The contractile behavior of the heart and its functional coupling to the circulation. Progr Cardiovasc Dis 1982; 24:375–400.
39. Mathru M, Rao TL, Venus B: Ventilator-induced barotrauma in controlled mechanical ventilation versus intermittent mandatory ventilation. Crit Care Med 1983; 11:359–361.
40. Petersen GW, Baier H: Incidence of pulmonary barotrauma in medical ICU. Crit Care Med 1983; 11:67–69.
41. Froese AB, Bryan AC: Effects of anesthesia and paralysis on diaphragmatic mechanics in man. Anesthesiology 1974; 41:242–255.
42. Wolff G, Brunner JX, Grädel E: Gas exchange during mechanical ventilation and spontaneous breathing. Chest 1986; 89:11–17.
43. Hawker FH, Torzillo PJ, Southee AE: PEEP and "reverse mismatch": a case where less PEEP is best. Chest 1991; 99:1034–1036.
44. Adoumie R, Shennib H, Brown R et al: Differential lung ventilation: applications beyond the operating room. J Thorac Cardiovasc Surg 1993; 105:229–233.
45. Räsänen J, Nikki P, Heikkilä J: Acute myocardial infarction complicated by respiratory failure: the effects of mechanical ventilation. Chest 1984; 85:21–28.
46. Hansen-Flaschen J, Cowen J: Neuromuscular blockade in the intensive care unit: more than we bargained for. Am Rev Respir Dis 1993; 147:234–236.
47. Kilburn KH: Shock, seizures, and coma with alkalosis during mechanical ventilation. Ann Intern Med 1966; 65:977–984.
48. Hudson LD, Hurlow RS, Craig KC: Does intermittent mandatory ventilation correct respiratory alkalosis in patients receiving assisted mechanical ventilation? Am Rev Respir Dis 1985; 132:1071–1074.
49. Culpepper JA, Rinaldo JE, Rogers RM: Effect of mechanical ventilator mode on tendency towards respiratory alkalosis. Am Rev Respir Dis 1985; 132:1075–1077.
50. Putensen C, Lopez F, Räsänen J: Effect of interfacing between spontaneous breathing and mechanical cycles on VA/Q distributions in canine lung injury (abstract). Am Rev Respir Dis 1994; 77:A291.
51. Pontoppidan H, Geffin B, Lowenstein E: Acute respiratory failure in the adult. N Engl J Med 1972; 287:743–752.
52. Roussos C: Respiratory muscle fatigue and ventilatory failure. Chest 1990; 97:89S-96S.
53. Cournand A, Motley HL, Werkö L et al: Physiologic studies of the effects of intermittent positive pressure ventilation on cardiac output in man. Am J Physiol 1948; 152:162–174.
54. Räsänen J, Heikkilä J, Downs JB et al: Continuous positive airway pressure by face mask in the treatment of cardiogenic pulmonary edema. Am J Cardiol 1985; 55:296–300.
55. Bartlett RH, Toomasian JM, Roloff D et al: Extracorporeal mem-

brane oxygenation (ECMO) in neonatal respiratory failure: 100 cases. Ann Surg 1986; 204:236–244.

56. Downs JB, Douglas ME: Intermittent mandatory ventilation: why the controversy? Crit Care Med 1981; 9:622–623.
57. Petty TL: IMV vs. IMC. Chest 1975; 67:630–631.
58. Weisman IM, Rinaldo JE, Rogers MH: Intermittent mandatory ventilation. Am Rev Respir Dis 1983; 127:641–647.
59. Kirby RR, Robison EF, Schultz C: A new pediatric volume ventilator. Anesth Analg 1971; 50:533–537.
60. Downs JB, Block AJ, Vennum KB: Intermittent mandatory ventilation in the treatment of patients with chronic obstructive pulmonary disease. Anesth Analg 1974; 53:437–443.
61. Downs JB, Perkins HM, Modell JH: Intermittent mandatory ventilation. Arch Surg 1974; 109:519–523.
62. Räsänen J: Conventional and high frequency controlled mechanical ventilation in patients with left ventricular dysfunction and pulmonary edema. Chest 1987; 91:225–229.
63. Downs JB, Mitchell LA: Pulmonary effects of ventilatory pattern following cardiopulmonary bypass. Crit Care Med 1976; 4:295–300.
64. Prakash O, Meij S: Oxygen consumption and blood gas exchange during controlled and intermittent mandatory ventilation after cardiac surgery. Crit Care Med 1985; 13:556–559.
65. Mecklenburgh JS, Latto IP, Al-Obaidi TAA et al: Excessive work of breathing during intermittent mandatory ventilation. Br J Anaesth 1986; 58:1048–1054.
66. Hewlett AM, Platt AS, Terry G: Mandatory minute volume: a new concept in weaning from mechanical ventilation. Anaesthesia 1977; 32:163–168.
67. Boyer F, Jay S, Gaussorgues P et al: A new approach to mandatory ventilation: pressure support mandatory minute frequency. Intensive Care Med 1988; 14:262.
68. Higgs BD, Bevan JC: Use of mandatory minute volume ventilation in the perioperative management of a patient with myasthenia. Br J Anaesth 1979; 51:1181–1184.
69. Douglas ME, Downs JB: Cardiopulmonary effects of intermittent mandatory ventilation. Int Anesthesiol Clin 1980; 18:97–121.
70. Marcy TW, Marini JJ: Inverse ratio ventilation in ARDS: rationale and implementation. Chest 1991; 100:494–504.
71. Boros SJ, Matalon SV, Ewald R et al: The effect of independent variations in inspiratory: expiratory ratio and end-expiratory pressure during mechanical ventilation in hyaline membrane disease: the significance of mean airway pressure. J Pediatr 1977; 91:794–798.
72. Boros SJ: Variations in inspiratory: expiratory ratio and airway pressure waveform during mechanical ventilation: the significance of mean airway pressure. J Pediatr 1979; 94:114–117.
73. Berman LS, Downs JB, VanEeden A: Inspiration:expiration ratio: Is mean airway pressure the difference? Crit Care Med 1981; 9: 775–777.
74. Gattinoni L, Marcolin R, Caspani ML et al: Constant mean airway pressure with different patterns of positive pressure breathing during the adult respiratory distress syndrome. Clin Respir Physiol 1983; 27:273–279.
75. Cole AG, Weller SF, Sykes MK: Inverse ratio ventilation compared with PEEP in adult respiratory failure. Intensive Care Med 1984; 10: 227–232.

76. Gurevitch MJ, VanDyke J, Young ES: Improved oxygenation and lower peak airway pressure in severe adult respiratory distress syndrome: treatment with inverse ratio ventilation. Chest 1986; 89: 211–213.
77. Tharratt RS, Allen RP, Albertson TE: Pressure controlled inverse ratio ventilation in severe adult respiratory distress syndrome. Chest 1988; 94:755–762.
78. Chan K, Abraham E: Effects of inverse ratio ventilation on cardiorespiratory parameters in severe respiratory failure. Chest 1992; 102: 1556–1561.
79. Räsänen J, Cane RD, Downs JB et al: Airway pressure release ventilation during acute lung injury: a prospective multicenter trial. Crit Care Med 1991; 19:1234–1241.
80. Cane RD, Peruzzi WT, Shapiro BA: Airway pressure release ventilation in severe acute respiratory failure. Chest 1991; 100:460–463.
81. Marini JJ, Capps JS, Culver BH: The inspiratory work of breathing during assisted mechanical ventilation. Chest 1985; 87:612–618.
82. Marini JJ, Rodriguez RM, Lamb V: Bedside estimation of the inspiratory work of breathing during mechanical ventilation. Chest 1986; 89:56–63.
83. Downs JB, Douglas ME, Ruiz BC: Comparison of assisted and controlled mechanical ventilation in anesthetized swine. Crit Care Med 1979; 7:5–8.
84. Banner MJ, Kirby RR: Similarities between pressure support ventilation and intermittent positive-pressure ventilation. Crit Care Med 1985; 13:997–998.
85. Tokioka H, Saito S, Kosaka F: Comparison of pressure support ventilation and assist control ventilation in patients with acute respiratory failure. Intensive Care Med 1989; 15:364–367.
86. Norlander O: New concepts of ventilation. Acta Anaesth Belg 1982; 33:221–234.
87. Hansen J, Wendt M, Lawin P: Ein neues weaning-Verfahren (inspiratory flow assistance—IFA). Anaesthesist 1984; 33:428–432.
88. Prakash O, Meij S: Cardiopulmonary response to inspiratory pressure support during spontaneous ventilation vs. conventional ventilation. Chest 1985; 88:403–408.
89. MacIntyre NR: Respiratory function during pressure support ventilation. Chest 1986; 89:677–683.
90. Zeravik J, Borg U, Pfeiffer UJ: Efficacy of pressure support ventilation dependent on extravascular lung water. Chest 1990; 97:1412–1419.
91. Stock MC, Downs JB, Frolicher DA: Airway pressure release ventilation. Crit Care Med 1987; 15:462–466.
92. Downs JB, Stock MC: Airway pressure release ventilation: a new concept in ventilatory support. Crit Care Med 1987; 15:459–461.
93. Garner W, Downs JB, Stock MC: Airway pressure release ventilation (APRV): a human trial. Chest 1988; 94:779–781.
94. Räsänen J, Downs JB, Stock MC: Cardiovascular effects of conventional positive pressure ventilation and airway pressure release ventilation. Chest 1988; 93:911–915.
95. Valentine DD, Hammond MD, Downs JB et al: Distribution of ventilation and perfusion with different modes of mechanical ventilation. Am Rev Respir Dis 1991; 143:1262–1266.
96. Rouby JJ: Pressure release ventilation. In: Vincent JL, ed: Update in intensive care and emergency medicine, vol 10. New York, Springer-Verlag, 1990, pp. 185–195.

97. Räsänen J: IMPRV: synchronized APRV or more? Intensive Care Med 1992; 18:65–66.
98. Rouby JJ, Ben Ameur M, Jawish D: Continuous positive airway pressure vs. intermittent mandatory pressure release ventilation (IMPRV) in patients with acute respiratory failure. Intensive Care Med 1992; 18:69–75.
99. Fratacci MD, Frostell CG, Chen TY et al: Inhaled nitric oxide: a selective pulmonary vasodilator of heparin-protamine vasoconstriction in sheep. Anesthesiology 1991; 75:990–999.
100. Rossaint R, Falke K, Lopez F et al: Inhaled nitric oxide for the adult respiratory distress syndrome. N Engl J Med 1993; 328:399–405.

CHAPTER 11

The Postoperative Patient and Sepsis

Robert F. Wilson

Case Report

A 52-year-old black woman was admitted to the intensive care unit (ICU) following a drainage procedure for a perforated colon. Her previous history included a renal transplant that had been functioning well for the last 4 years. Current therapy included cyclosporine.

On arrival in the surgical ICU, the patient had a blood pressure of 80/50 mm Hg and a heart rate of 122/min. To maintain cardiac stability, the patient required aggressive fluid resuscitation with lactated Ringer's solution and blood. Dopamine was also used to increase cardiac output to maintain a supernormal (optimal) oxygen delivery. The initial antibiotic was imipenem. The patient also required mechanical ventilatory support.

Intravenous central hyperalimentation was begun the next day. Over the ensuing 4 days, the patient's course continued to improve. By day 4 she was afebrile. A small feeding tube was placed through the nose and advanced over the next 24 hours into the proximal duodenum. She was started on half-strength feedings at 10 ml/hr. These were progressively increased until, by the fourth day, she was tolerating full-strength feedings at 60 ml/hr. On the eighth postoperative day, the patient again became febrile. New cultures of blood, urine, and sputum were obtained. All central lines were changed. A CT scan of the abdomen revealed an abscess in the right lower quadrant. A percutaneous drain guided by CT was placed, and cultures revealed the organism Morganella morganii, which was resistant to the current drug imipenem. For that very reason the patient was then placed on tobramycin therapy.

Over the next 3 days, the patient's fever fell, and she showed no further signs of sepsis. She was extubated 2 days later and was discharged from the ICU on the 17th postoperative day.

The treatment of sepsis in critically ill surgical patients involves two distinct subsets. First are critically ill patients who require operation, usually intra-abdominal or intrathoracic, to drain or remove a known septic source. The second group includes those patients who develop signs of sepsis while in the ICU.

GENERAL PRINCIPLES

• *Handwashing may be the most effective way to prevent cross-contamination among patients.*

To prevent the spread of infection among ICU patients, certain standard procedures are followed. These include the so-called universal precautions. Perhaps the principal violation involves handwashing between patient contacts. For whatever reason, almost all hospitals and hospital infectious disease personnel report difficulty in maintenance of high compliance rates for this relatively simple task. Unwashed hands serve as a primary mode of bacterial transmission among patients. A second major goal should be to ensure sterile performance of all invasive procedures. This means that physicians should don masks and sterile gowns and gloves for such procedures. All other personnel should at least wear a face mask and use sterile gloves. Certain invasive procedures such as tracheostomy should usually be performed in the operating room where sterility can be maintained more thoroughly and all the required instruments are readily available. Obviously, multiuse vials of various drugs should not be used. Furthermore, all intravenous injections should be given through a sterile site, and, at a minimum, a wipe with an alcohol pledget should precede injection through any intravenous port. Simple acts such as placement of an endotracheal tube can introduce a large inoculum of bacteria into the airway.

Patients returned to the ICU following a surgical procedure to drain or remove a septic source represent a reasonably straightforward management problem. In fact, the majority of this book is devoted to such critically ill patients. Specifics such as the management of pulmonary problems and maintenance of oxygen delivery are addressed in other chapters. However, the new onset of sepsis or its recurrence can present its own problems and requires an organized approach for both diagnosis and definitive therapy.

The close monitoring available in the ICU provides the best opportunity to detect early sepsis as exhibited by various signs and symptoms. Fever is probably the most common finding that initiates a search for infection. Ordinarily, we diagnose a true fever as a temperature higher than 38.5°C (101.3°F). However, not all patients are able to produce or sustain a febrile response. This can be particularly evident in debilitated, older patients or those who are on immunosuppressive therapy, such as steroids. If chills or rigor are present, the fever often indicates a major abscess and/or a large bacteria load in the blood.

Other early hallmarks of sepsis include altered mental status. The patient may become confused and disoriented to person, place, time, or any combination of these. The patient may still follow simple commands, but with questioning, the confusion is generally readily apparent. This situation may be due to cytokines interfering with normal neurotransmitter function.

Hypotension and tachycardia are also frequent early cardiovascular signs of sepsis. Various cytokines including tumor necrosis factor (TNF) and interleukin 1 and 6 (IL-1, IL-6) help to mediate these changes.[1,2] TNF, IL-1 and IL-6 have the greatest effects on hemodynamic performance. Blood pressures as low as 70 mm Hg systolic and heart rates in excess of 120/min are not uncommon. Although interference with TNF, IL-1, and IL-6 can improve cardiovascular function,[3] other more mundane measures may be of enormous benefit. A simple reduction of the patient's temperature by external cooling (alcohol, fans, cooling blanket) or antipyretics can at least partially reverse the vasodilatation and improve blood pressure.

• *Cytokines IL-1 and tumor necrosis factor may be responsible for many of the hemodynamic changes seen in sepsis.*

DIAGNOSIS OF A SEPTIC SOURCE

To be of maximum benefit, the physical examination of the possibly infected patient must be carefully performed. A change in abdominal findings such as loss of bowel sounds or development of peritoneal signs (tenderness, guarding, and/or rigidity) may point to an intra-abdominal source. Production of copious or purulent sputum may be the initial evidence of a pneumonic process. In addition, one should inspect all central and peripheral intravenous access sites. Induration or redness around a central line indicates a need to remove that line. If an intravenous line is still necessary, a replacement should be inserted at a new site. A culture of the catheter tip can help one to diagnose line contamination or sepsis. Any thrombosed peripheral vein site should be carefully examined. If pus can be expressed, the involved portion of vein should be resected. On occasion, we have found sepsis in unexpected sites such as a retained tampon, epididymitis, or perirectal abscess. Urinary tract infections are usually diagnosed by culture. Occasionally, pyelonephritis causes ileus. Meningitis may result in not only mental confusion, but also a stiff neck. A wound infection may not be apparent until it begins to drain.

• *The diagnosis of sepsis should begin with a thorough history and physical examination.*

When one suspects sepsis, certain laboratory tests may be helpful. Systemic infections ordinarily cause white blood cell counts to rise in excess of 12,000/mm^3. However, in some severe cases or for patients in the midst of chemotherapy or radiation therapy, the bone marrow may respond very poorly. In such situations, the white blood cell count may not exceed 4000/mm^3, and on occasion, it may be less than 1000/mm^3. However, the white blood cell count usually exhibits a left shift, and immature band cells form more than 10% of the count.

Other diagnostic studies include cultures of urine, sputum, and blood. Body fluids such as cerebrospinal fluid (CSF), pleural fluid, and peritoneal fluid should be cultured when clinically indicated. Blood cultures should be obtained percutaneously following sterilization of the proposed puncture site. When feasible, the blood cultures should be drawn from at least two different sites. Cultures should be drawn for both anaerobic and aerobic bacteria.[4] Blood cultures should not ordinarily be drawn through arterial or venous lines that have been in place. Positive results under such circumstances may only indicate colonization of the line.

- *If at all possible, blood cultures should never be drawn through a central or arterial line.*

Infiltrates on a chest radiograph are often nonspecific but may be helpful in terms of diagnosis. Pneumonia is typically evident as lobar or diffuse infiltrate. In my experience, in most surgical patients, pneumonia usually presents as an interstitial process. This is in contradistinction to the lobar involvement commonly seen in community-acquired pneumonias. A diffuse process consistent with adult respiratory distress syndrome (ARDS) may also develop and can make the radiographic diagnosis of pneumonia extremely difficult. In ARDS, the pulmonary dysfunction is usually the first evidence of the diffuse organ changes often identified with generalized sepsis.[5] However, patients with ARDS can easily develop secondary bacterial infections.

- *Pulmonary changes during sepsis may represent a wide variety of processes besides pneumonia or ARDS.*

Sophisticated studies are often required to diagnose intra-abdominal sepsis. Free air, secondary to bowel perforation, may be noted on an upright chest film or lateral decubitus film of the abdomen. A kidney-ureter-bladder study (KUB) may demonstrate abnormal air fluid levels or displacement of bowel loops. An elevated right hemidiaphragm may indicate a subphrenic abscess. On occasion, contrast studies of the bowel may demonstrate extrinsic pressure from an intra-abdominal abscess.

In surgical patients, central nervous system infections rarely cause a picture of generalized sepsis. Meningitis usually follows earlier invasive procedures such as intracranial pressure (ICP) monitoring. With generalized sepsis, the patient's level of consciousness is often depressed, but without any localizing signs. Generally the diagnosis requires a lumbar spinal tap and culture. Therapy often involves administration of systemic antibiotics that demonstrate good cerebrospinal fluid (CSF) penetration such as gentamicin, tobramycin, and ceftazidime. Local instillation into the CSF may also occasionally be needed.

An ultrasound examination can often enable the clinician to identify abnormal collections of fluid within the abdomen or chest. This noninvasive study has the advantage of being able to be performed at the bedside. However, gas within bowel can interfere with ultrasound examination. Abdominal ultrasound can permit accurate diagnosis of conditions such as acute cholecystitis, acalculous cholecystitis, or appendiceal or tubo-ovarian abscess.[6]

- *Excess bowel gas interferes with an ultrasound study of the abdomen.*

Computed tomographic (CT) scans, particularly with intravenous and oral contrast material can help greatly in the diagnosis of intra-abdominal infection. However, 5 to 7 days must usually elapse after the initial trauma or surgery before a CT scan is of particular benefit.[7] This should always be kept in mind during the search for a recurrent source of sepsis. At our hospital, the incidence of false negative CT scans has remained between 10 and 15%.

• *A CT scan is unlikely to demonstrate an abscess less than 6 days after the initial insult.*

Radionuclide scanning with gallium or indium is used occasionally in a final attempt to locate a septic source not detectable by other means.[8] Both gallium and indium studies require 24 to 72 hours to complete. These radionuclide agents should localize in areas of sepsis because they bind to leukocytes or tissue proteins.

• *Gallium and indium are usually nonspecific in their ability to define a septic site.*

If ascitic fluid is present, it can be aspirated or diagnostic peritoneal lavage may be performed. Care must obviously be taken to be sure that the aspirated fluid is from the peritoneal cavity and not bowel lumen. The presence of large numbers of polymorphonuclearcytes (PMNs) and bacteria on smears of the abdominal fluid is diagnostic of an intra-abdominal infection.

In patients who have had abdominal surgery or trauma and who become increasingly septic and have not demonstrated another source of sepsis in spite of all the previously mentioned tests, a "blind laparotomy" can be considered a diagnostic procedure. Fry's group found a 44% intraperitoneal infection rate in patients who had such a nondirected laparotomy.[9] Patients with the usual signs of sepsis and multiple organ deterioration but without any other specific evidence of intra-abdominal abscess may also benefit from such a procedure.

Sutherland and associates analyzed their results with an aggressive approach in 80 patients who had finally undergone nondirected laparotomy for sepsis and/or organ failure. The nondirected laparotomies detected fewer cases (21/36 = 58%) of abdominal sepsis than did directed laparotomies (52/64 = 81%).[10] However, the high positive rate for the blind laparotomies indicates that they should be considered in selected patients. Once multiple system organ failure develops, it is unlikely that the patient will survive, even if the intra-abdominal abscess is eventually drained.[11]

TARGET ORGANS IN SEPSIS

The lungs often become a secondary target organ for sepsis. The increased capillary permeability and resultant accumulation of pulmonary interstitial fluid makes lung compliance progressively worse. Tachypnea is usually the first sign. The increased lung water and elevated interstitial fluid pressures cause a deterioration of oxygenation.[12] These findings are different from those seen with pneumonia. However, both problems may interfere with gas exchange.

• *ARDS is simply another manifestation of a generalized inflammatory response.*

Pulmonary infection can be very difficult to diagnose in critically ill patients, even though over 20% of intubated patients develop nosocomial pneumonia (Table 11–1). In general, patients should demonstrate a large number of PMNs and a preponderance of a single bacterial organism recovered from the lower respiratory tract,

Table 11–1.
Aids in the Diagnosis of Pneumonia

Temperature < 35.5°C (95.9°F) or < 38.5°C (101.3°F)
WBC < 4000/mm^3 or > 12,000/mm^3
Bandemia > 10%
New infiltrate on chest radiograph
Polymorphonuclearcytes on sputum gram stain
Single organism isolated on sputum culture
Bronchoalveolar lavage
Brush biopsy
Transthoracic aspiration

• *Pulmonary infections may either be an interstitial process or tracheobronchitis.*

accompanied by a new infiltrate on a chest radiograph.[13] Other confirmatory signs include fever and leukocytosis, especially with an increase in immature band forms.

In many cases, the only pulmonary cultures used are those obtained by suctioning through an endotracheal tube. Some investigators argue that this may represent colonization rather than a true infection. However, recovery of a single organism in large numbers and the presence of many PMNs, coupled with the other evidence previously mentioned, should be considered indicative of pneumonia. Some believe that it is preferable to obtain the cultures from bronchial washings via a catheter wedged into a bronchus associated with a pulmonary infiltrate. Brushing the involved bronchi to obtain material to culture represents another important way to diagnose pulmonary infections. This procedure also requires a fiberoptic bronchoscope and a specially protected brush to avoid contamination in the upper airway. Transthoracic aspiration has been done on occasion, but it may be impractical to use in most critically ill patients requiring high ventilatory pressures.[14]

Renal dysfunction due to systemic sepsis may exhibit itself in several ways. Initially, urine volume may decrease because of a reduced effective renal blood flow despite a normal or increased cardiac output. Patients with preexisting renal disease may have vessels that have lost the ability to autoregulate. As such, renal blood flow becomes pressure dependent. Parenchymal damage, either due to sepsis or to nephrotoxic agents, results in an elevation of blood urea nitrogen (BUN) and a reduced creatinine clearance. Serum creatinine levels may only rise late in the course.

Patients who have had secondary peritonitis due to a bowel leak or injury and who fail to control the infection adequately may develop "tertiary peritonitis" caused by microorganisms that are resistant to the usual standard antibiotic regimens.[15] This superinfection often involves candida or antibiotic-resistant bacteria such as acinetobacter, pseudomonas, serratia, and enterobacter. Patients who have had intra-abdominal sepsis and have received a 10- to 14-day course of broad-spectrum antibiotics and who still appear septic without obvious other sites of infection fit this pattern. In addition to surgical drainage and the use of more potent antibiotics, the clinician should consider empiric treatment with an antifungal regimen. Additionally, early oral nystatin therapy may help prevent candida infections from developing in the gastrointestinal tract.

Pancreatitis, although primarily an inflammatory process, can sometimes mimic an intra-abdominal infection. Such patients may exhibit all the usual signs of sepsis.[16] Cytokine release, secondary to the pancreatic inflammation, probably mediates these findings. Furthermore, acute pancreatitis can lead to an infectious process as a result of pseudocyst development or frank necrosis. Since clinically, delineation of sepsis from pancreatitis can be a difficult problem, blood cultures at the time of each fever spike should be obtained. Free fluid in or around the pancreas should also be aspirated for smear and culture studies.

Bilirubin increases that occur within 3 to 5 days of trauma usually develop because of transfusions, hemolysis, hematomas, or liver ischemia. In most cases, this results in relatively high levels of indirect bilirubin and only modest elevations of alkaline phosphatase. If aspartate aminotransferase (AST) and/or alanine aminotransferase (ALT) levels are markedly elevated, some element of hepatic damage has probably also occurred. Such findings usually require close monitoring of liver function studies.

Jaundice that develops 8 to 12 days after surgery or trauma usually indicates a septic complication, particularly peritonitis with Bacteroides fragilis.[17] This hyperbilirubinemia may persist for some time, even after control of the apparent sepsis. The mechanism of "septic jaundice" is not known. However, in addition to hepatocellular dysfunction, electron microscopy can demonstrate evidence of bile stasis in the smallest canaliculi.

- *Hyperbilirubinemia may be due to sepsis-induced hepatic dysfunction sepsis. Sepsis-induced liver dysfunction does not usually occur until at least 8 days after surgery or trauma.*

A patient who has been unable to use his or her intestinal tract for nutrition and has relied on total parenteral nutrition (TPN) for more than 2 to 3 weeks has a good chance of developing some hepatic steatosis.[18] Factors that seem to be associated with this fatty infiltration of the liver include the use of carbohydrate as the sole source of calories in TPN, infusion of excess calories, and deficiencies of essential fatty acids or carnitine. High rates of glucose infusion stimulate hyperinsulinemia, which in turn stimulates lipogenesis and inhibits lipid mobilization from fat stores. A respiratory quotient (RQ) greater than 1.0 indicates that carbohydrate nutrients are being converted to fat, and some of this is likely to accumulate in the liver. Essential fatty acid deficiency can be caused by inadequate intake or by high insulin levels that suppress endogenous fatty acid mobilization.[18] Carnitine deficiency leads to impaired transport and subsequent mitochondrial oxidation of lipids.

Liver biopsy does not usually demonstrate intrahepatic cholestasis until after at least 3 to 4 weeks of TPN.[18] Jaundice preceded by an elevated alkaline phosphatase level is often the only evidence that this is occurring. Histologically, the lesion presents as periportal canalicular bile plugging, bile staining of surrounding hepatocytes, and some degree of triaditis with a predominately lymphocytic infiltration. This triaditis may persist for several months following discontinuation of TPN.

Gallbladder sludge commonly is seen after 3 to 4 weeks of TPN and is present in almost all patients after 6 weeks of TPN. Continued use of TPN increases the risk of acalculous cholecystitis or gallstone formation.

• *The majority of spontaneous bleeding in patients receiving massive transfusions results from diminished platelets rather than from reduction of other factors.*

Several other factors can cause abnormal bleeding in patients with postoperative sepsis. Diagnostic efforts begin with a review of all current medications, particularly aspirin-containing agents. In addition, one should look for evidence of hepatic failure, renal failure, and disseminated intravascular coagulation (DIC).[19]

The physical examination should attempt to determine whether the process is localized or diffuse and whether bleeding involves mucosal surfaces. Increased bleeding from mucosal surfaces, needle sticks, and any open wounds, especially in areas that were previously dry, suggests the presence of DIC. Increased postoperative bleeding from the abdomen or operative site alone suggests a technical error, especially if the operation was completed while the patient was hypotensive.

Blood samples drawn through an indwelling vascular cannula almost invariable have some heparin present. This may cause spurious thrombin (TT), prothrombin (PT), and partial thromboplastin (PTT) times as well as increased levels of fibrin degradation products (FDP). Ideally, blood for clotting studies should be drawn directly from an uncannulated vein. If blood must be taken from a vascular catheter, a minimum of 20 ml of blood should be withdrawn through the cannula before obtaining a specimen for analysis.[20] Most suspected bleeding disorders can be confirmed using readily available tests including: (1) peripheral blood smear and platelet counts; (2) bleeding time; (3) PT, PTT, and TT; (4) fibrinogen levels; (5) fibrin degradation products; and (6) D-dimers.

• *Septic patients with DIC will usually require control of the sepsis plus continued replacement of factors including platelets.*

The combination of prolonged PT and PTT, hypofibrinogenemia, and thrombocytopenia in patients with sepsis or prolonged shock establishes the diagnosis of DIC in most cases. Very severe hepatic insufficiency can produce an almost identical laboratory profile. However, FDP greater than 40 μg/ml and/or elevated D-dimer levels can help confirm DIC.[21] Full-blown DIC has an extremely poor prognosis in spite of correction of the primary process and restoration of the deficient platelets and clotting factors.

In patients with severe liver disease, factor VII activity levels usually decrease first and result in a prolonged PT. As the severity of liver disease increases, the PTT can also be affected. Fibrinogen levels are usually maintained above 100 mg/dl until terminal hepatic failure. The D-dimer assay should be negative if no abnormal intravascular clotting is present.[19] If the PT remains elevated more than 5.0 seconds above control in spite of vitamin K repletion, it may take more than 8 to 12 units of fresh frozen plasma (FFP) to bring the PT within 3.0 seconds of control.

The patient who bleeds because of massive transfusions tends also eventually to have diffuse bleeding from all surgical wounds and puncture sites. The most frequent severe laboratory abnormality in patients receiving massive blood transfusions is thrombocytopenia. However, patients with a clinical coagulopathy usually also have prolonged PT, PTT, and TT.[22] Fibrinogen levels with massive transfusions tend to be only moderately decreased, and FDP does not usually exceed 40 mg/ml unless the patient has concurrent DIC. Hypothermia ($< 35°C$) makes all these abnormalities much worse.[23] Nevertheless, the most common cause of postoperative bleeding after massive transfusions is still inadequate surgical control of bleeding vessels.

A brain abscess could conceivably develop following an operative procedure. More often it follows a septic embolic event from a distant site. Patients usually exhibit localizing signs, based on the abscess location. In addition to the antibiotic therapy described for meningitis, removal or drainage is usually required.

The principal cardiac lesions seen with sepsis, especially in patients with underlying valve disease, are valvular vegetations of either bacterial or fungal origin. Such lesions can then seed other areas, especially the brain and spleen. Development of these lesions can sometimes be detected by appearance of a new cardiac murmur. Echocardiography, especially by the transesophageal route, can usually confirm the diagnosis. If untreated, these lesions can obviously destroy the valve and cause acute severe cardiac failure and death.

On occasion, a gallstone can become impacted in an hepatic duct. This can rapidly lead to ascending cholangitis. The typical triad seen with this problem is jaundice, right upper quadrant pain, and chills and fever (Charcot's triad). If the patient also has hypotension and mental changes, the combination is referred to as Reynold's pentad. The appearance of dilated bile ducts on ultrasound or endoscopic retrograde cholangiopancreatography in addition to the triad or pentad is virtually diagnostic.[24] Placement of a drainage catheter to decompress the biliary system can initially stabilize the situation.

Urine should be cultured on a regular basis in patients apt to become septic. Patients with bladder infections are often asymptomatic. However, when colony counts reach 100,000/ml, we consider this a sign of infection. Antibiotic therapy should be instituted and, if possible, the catheter should be removed. When fungi such as candida are recovered, either continuous irrigation of the bladder with amphotericin B or administration of a systemic agent such as fluconazole can be initiated.

- *Treatment of urinary tract infections includes removal of an indwelling catheter as soon as possible or practical.*

Multiple organ failure still causes the greatest number of deaths from sepsis in surgical patients.[25] Once organ failure develops, these patients can be expected to demonstrate continuing deterioration, even if various infections are finally eradicated. The critical care physician must attempt to diagnose and control infections before organ failure develops.

PERIOPERATIVE MANAGEMENT OF THE SEPTIC PATIENT

The perioperative management of septic patients involves early hemodynamic resuscitation and correction or any pulmonary, renal, electrolyte, or coagulation abnormalities. One study of high-risk patients demonstrated that preoperative optimization of cardiac output by increasing intravascular volume, guided by either pulmonary artery wedge pressure (PAWP) or end-diastolic volume (EDV), reduced the incidence of significant postoperative complications from 79 to 14%.[26] I routinely obtain arterial and mixed venous gases at the time of the cardiac output determinations in these patients and then calculate oxygen delivery (DO_2) and oxygen consumption (VO_2). Data now suggest that a DO_2 level of 600 ml/min/m^2 or more is associated with a significantly greater likelihood of survival.[27,28]

• *The outcome in patients who may become septic or who are septic improves by achieving a DO_2 of > 600 ml/min/m^2 and a $VO_2 > 170$ ml/min/m^2.*

• *In sepsis, early maintenance of a supernormal oxygen consumption and oxygen delivery is extremely important.*

The DO_2 should be progressively increased by increasing cardiac output, hemoglobin levels, and/or arterial oxygen saturation (SaO_2). If DO_2 is less than 600 ml/min/m^2 in spite of an optimal preload, I seriously consider the addition of inotropic support. This presumes that the hemoglobin levels have already been increased to 11 to 12 g/dl. VO_2 should also be raised to a minimum of 170 ml/min/m^2. Urine output should be at least 1.0 ml/kg/hr, and core temperature also is best normalized. I institute appropriate empiric antibiotic therapy preoperatively, and an additional dose may be required during the operation if there has been much blood loss or if the patient has required large quantities of fluid. Additional doses may also be required in the immediate perioperative period to ensure that adequate tissue concentrations are achieved and maintained during and after surgery.[29]

At the time of this writing, at least three different types of monoclonal antibodies have been developed in an attempt to combat sepsis. These antibodies have been specifically targeted against endotoxin, interleukin-1α (IL-1α) receptor, and tumor necrosis factor (TNF). Although these agents have contributed to improved outcome in small subgroups, to date, large, multi-institutional studies have failed to yield convincing results.[30–32] Therefore, antibiotics and antifungal agents continue to be the mainstay of pharmacologic therapy against sepsis.

ANTIMICROBIAL THERAPY

A wide variety of antibiotics is available for treating infected patients. Determining which antibiotics to use should be based both on sensitivity of the infecting organisms and their ability to develop resistance to the chosen antibiotic (Table 11–2). If equally effective agents are available, cost should be taken into consideration. When the organism has not yet been identified, almost all physicians initially begin with broad coverage. However, once culture and sensitivity results become available, the selection should be narrowed as rapidly as possible and any unnecessary drugs removed. This helps to delay or prevent resistance in any other organisms that may be present. Broad coverage for us for empiric therapy of intra-abdominal infections includes an aminoglycoside to cover gram-negative bacilli, such as E. coli, and clindamycin or metronidazole to cover

• *Although a logical goal, narrowing the spectrum of antibiotic therapy is often difficult in septic, surgical patients.*

Table 11–2.
Most Common Gram Negative Organisms Recovered in Sepsis

Klebsiella pneumoniae
Escherichia coli
Enterobacter cloacae
Proteus mirabilis
Pseudomonas aeruginosa
Acinetobacter

anaerobic organisms, such as Bacteroides fragilis. Because most ICUs have high rates of staphylococcal resistance to methicillin or oxacillin, vancomycin is included if there is any suggestion that these organisms may also be involved. After 72 hours, if no organisms have been recovered, a judgement must be made in regard to continued coverage. If the clinical picture more likely represents a systemic inflammatory response, antibiotics may not be required. On the other hand, prompt antibiotic administration may make it difficult to obtain positive cultures in the operating room. Usually, the patient's fever, white blood cell count and differential, and overall clinical course help one to decide on the need for continued antibiotic therapy.

It is essential to monitor antibiotic dosages, particularly when using potentially toxic agents, such as vancomycin or aminoglycosides. Patients with severe sepsis often have a greatly expanded volume of distribution.[33] As such, they may require dosages 50 to 100% higher than normally recommended to achieve therapeutic levels. One recent study in an ICU demonstrated that aminoglycosides, in dosages recommended by standard clinical guidelines, produced significantly lower peaks than did dosages determined by pharmacokinetic methods. Many more patients were able to achieve therapeutic levels with revised pharmokinetically determined dosage protocols. The data indicate that the higher dosages resulted in higher initial blood levels with increased killing power.[34] In clinical practice, accurate tracking of peak drug concentrations is extremely difficult. These levels depend on the drug's being administered over a specific interval and the levels' being drawn at precise times following the completion of the infusion. This is rarely practical. Trough levels prior to the next dose provide information on potential toxicity of the agent. High drug trough levels usually indicate a need to lengthen the interval between doses.

- *Aminoglycosides appear to work better when administered in higher doses with longer interdose intervals. This results from higher blood levels and therefore, better killing power.*

If the patient is still on antibiotics but continues to demonstrate signs of sepsis, this may mean inadequate drainage of an abscess, a new infection, or ineffective antibiotic coverage. If no other causes for the signs of sepsis can be found, the clinician should consider discontinuation of all the antibiotics. Blood cultures can be drawn over the next several days in the hopes of obtaining positive cultures. Appropriate antibiotic therapy can then be reinstituted.

Many hospitals track drug resistance and sensitivities to the microorganisms recovered from patients. Selection of a specific antibiotic should be based not only on the laboratory sensitivity findings, but also on the resistance patterns of the bacteria in that hospital.

Patients who are critically ill and immunocompromised and continue to be septic after 10 to 14 days of treatment should be considered for empiric treatment with antifungal agents.[35] Candida infections have become the third or fourth most common cause of nosocomial pneumonia. Aggressive antifungal therapy should begin immediately if demonstrated histologic evidence of an invasive fungal infection is present or if blood cultures are positive. I also initiate antifungal therapy in critically ill patients when fungi are recovered from two or more sites.

Selective gut decontamination (SGD) has been popular in some centers in Europe (Table 11–3). Such therapy has two basic goals.[36,37] These are stomach decontamination to minimize pulmonary contamination secondary to microaspiration and decontamination of the rest of the gut to reduce or prevent bacterial translocation. However, such therapy has not improved survival rates. In one study, when stomach decontamination was obtained, the incidence of pneumonia did decrease.[38] Nevertheless, this type of empiric therapy is perhaps best suited to specific high-risk populations.

• *Selective gut decontamination may reduce the incidence of pneumonia. However, it does not appear to have any effect either on outcome or length of ICU stay.*

Selective decontamination of the remainder of the gut may be a treatment in search of a disease. Although bacterial translocation does occur in many animal species, it has not been documented convincingly in humans beyond the lymphatic system.[39]

The decreased incidence of pneumonia following SGD without reductions in the mortality rate and length of ICU stay may be explained by the definition of pneumonia.[40] Most authorities recognize the wide variety of infiltrative changes that may be seen on the chest radiograph that can also cause fever and white blood cell elevation. However, sputum cultures obtained through an endotracheal tube are not considered as diagnostic as a protected brush specimen or bronchoalveolar lavage.

Newer nonantibiotic agents, such as granulocyte colony-stimulating factor (GC-CSF), were introduced to aid patients with bone marrow depression due to chemotherapy.[41] These agents have also been used in some neutropenic patients with cancer who become infected. Such an agent seems to be most effective when the total

• *Granulocyte colony-stimulating factor may be efficacious in septic patients with severely depressed white blood cell counts.*

Table 11–3.
Examples of Agents Used for Selective Gut Decontamination

Suspension or Paste (usually qid)	Posterior Pharynx and Stomach
Amphotericin B	500 mg
Polymyxin E	200 mg
Tobramycin	80 mg
Norfloxacin	50 mg
Colistin sulfate	100 mg
Neomycin	1 g
Parenteral	
Cefotaxime	70 mg/kg/day

white blood cell count remains less than $1000/mm^3$. However, there has been no demonstrated improvement in outcome with the use of these agents.

In addition to cultures done prior to or at the time of a temperature spike, some rationale exists to perform cultures on a regular or daily basis. In critically ill infected patients, the flora may continually change. In addition, various antibiotic resistance patterns can develop. Although the yield may be low, repeated Gram stains of all possible infected material and culture and sensitivity are the best and quickest way to determine a change in antibiotic resistance patterns. Moreover, some patients are so immunosuppressed that they may not exhibit either a fever spike or a change in white blood cell count. Other candidates for surveillance cultures include patients who have had a known septic source and have demonstrated little or no progress toward recovery. Often, these patients have an occult infection and may require multiple cultures before the other source or organisms are identified.

• *Daily surveillance cultures can help provide early notification of change in either the bacteria present or antibiotic resistance.*

Positive cultures from central lines often reflect line colonization. Only when these cultures have the same bacteria and resistance profiles as simultaneous cultures from a direct percutaneous blood culture can line infection be documented. Nevertheless, colonization of a line or a catheter tip is an indication to change the line. If the catheter represents the only source of bacteria, antibiotics are not usually required.

The frequency of central line changes in septic patients has been a source of endless debate. In the septic patient, line colonization has been reported as early as 72 hours following line placement.[42] Most authorities believe that the skin entry site serves as the primary source of bacterial colonization.[43] Some data also suggest that, when properly cared for, central lines, including pulmonary artery catheters, may be left in place up to 7 days.[44] Most ICUs change such lines at intervals of 3 to 7 days.

• *Central lines can probably be safely changed as infrequently as every 6 or 7 days if they are inserted in a sterile manner and used with great care.*

Central lines can be changed over a guide wire. Since, as mentioned, most line contamination occurs at the entry site, such methodology may be problematic. Obviously, an indurated site should not be wired unless extenuating circumstances exist. These include unavailability of other sites such as in a burn patient or one with severe coagulopathy.

The more manipulation of a central line or pulmonary artery catheter, the greater the risk of contamination. Such manipulations include multiple injections or blood withdrawals. However, multiple-lumen catheters do not necessarily become colonized more frequently than single-lumen catheters.[45]

Septic patients become malnourished much more rapidly than those who simply fast.[46] Protein loss also occurs at rates 1.5 to 3.0 times faster.[47] The effects of this rapid protein loss on host defenses and wound healing may be devastating. In addition, muscle mass and organ function in critically ill trauma victims can be rapidly reduced. In a normal, fasting adult, infusion of 100 to 150 g of glucose per day can reduce urine urea nitrogen losses to less than 5 g per day. Unfortunately, in septic patients the protein losses are much greater, and glucose does not suppress proteolysis in these patients to nearly the degree that it does in normal individuals. As a consequence, we attempt to provide 2.0 to 2.5 g of amino acids/kg/day to our septic patients.

A meta-analysis compared early total enteral nutrition (TEN) with TPN.[48] The incidence of postoperative infectious complications was lower with TEN (16% = 19/118) than with TPN (35% = 39/112). The TEN group also had a lower incidence of pneumonia (15 versus 6), intravenous catheter sepsis (7 versus 0), bacteremia (5 versus 2), and urinary tract infection (3 versus 1).

• *Enteral feeding appears to reduce overall septic complications. This effect does not appear to be due simply to a decrease in catheter sepsis.*

Sepsis was originally thought to increase resting energy expenditure (REE) by at least 30 to 60% even in the absence of fever.[47] However, more recent data from indirect calorimetry suggest that the REE may only increase by 15 to 30% in such patients.

• *To be maximally effective, enteral nutrition should be started within 12 to 14 hours of surgery or trauma.*

We believe that enteral feeding should be initiated as early as possible in all critically ill or injured patients. Moore and associates have shown the advantages of early jejunostomy feeding, frequently within 24 to 48 hours of major abdominal trauma.[49] Anticipation of a prolonged delay in oral feeding results in a feeding jejunostomy with or without a decompressive gastrostomy performed during the initial surgical procedure or within 4 to 5 days. Such tubes can reduce the discomfort and irritation of an indwelling oral or nasal tubes. They also reduce pulmonary secretions and the incidence of sinusitis.

If the patient has not or should not have a laparotomy, a percutaneous endoscopic gastrostomy (PEG) tube can be helpful. However, one must be concerned about possible reflux of gastric contents into the lungs, particularly if the gastric residual volumes cannot be checked. To help prevent such reflux, a catheter can be inserted via the PEG and advanced into the jejunum. This procedure can significantly reduce the amount of gastric regurgitation, as long as the tube does not retract back into the stomach.

• *Enteral feeding-associated diarrhea in septic patients should be considered due to antibiotic-induced colitis until proved otherwise.*

About 25 to 40% of enterally fed critically ill patients develop some diarrhea.[50] If the patient has been on broad-spectrum antibiotics, Clostridium difficile enterocolitis should be suspected. Stool specimens can then be sent to the laboratory for a toxin screen. Other causes of diarrhea can include mucosal breakdown due to malnutrition. When diarrhea does develop, I stop or reduce all feedings for 24 hours and then try a new or more dilute formulation. The use of opioids to reduce or eliminate diarrhea usually only masks symptoms and can cause an ileus.

A multitude of enteral feeding formulations is currently available (Table 11–4). Many are compounded to deal with specific organ dysfunction such as the liver, lungs, or kidney. However, few if any objective data exist to support their claims of superiority to the more standard formulations.

The amount of bulk or fiber present in the enteral formula can improve overall gut function. Fiber stimulates gut hormone release, and intestinal mucosal blood flow and overall function can significantly improve.

For enteral nutrition in septic critically ill patients, I attempt to

Table 11–4.
Examples of Enteral Feeding Formulations

Product	Protein Source	Fat Source	Carbohydrate Source	cal/ml	Osmolality (mOsm/kg H_2O)	Protein (%)	Fat (%)	Carbohydrate (%)
Osmolite	Soy protein Sodium and calcium caseinate	Safflower oil MCT oil	Cornstarch	1.06	300	14	31	54
Tolerex	Free amino acids	Safflower oil	Glucose	1.0	550	8	1	91
Perative	Sodium caseinate L-arginine	Canola oil MCT oil Corn oil	Cornstarch	1.3	385	20	25	54
Pulmocare	Sodium and calcium caseinate	Canola oil MCT oil Corn oil Oleic safflower oil	Sucrose Cornstarch	1.5	475	16	55	28
Traumacal	Sodium and calcium caseinate	Soy oil MCT oil	Corn syrup Sugar	1.5	490	22	40	38
Criticare HN	Hydrolyzed casein amino acids	Safflower oil	Cornstarch	1.06	650	14	4.5	81.5

provide increased amounts of arginine and nucleic acids. When added as a nutritional supplement, the amino acid arginine has been shown experimentally to improve protein synthesis, wound healing, and immune function.[51] Although arginine is normally a nonessential amino acid in mature mammals, under conditions of immaturity or severe stress, it becomes necessary for adequate nitrogen balance. Arginine also improves host immunity. Its use results in a less severe depression and an earlier return to normal of peripheral T-lymphocyte mitogen stimulation response and a greater expression of the T-helper cell phenotype.

• *Supplemental nucleic acids may improve macrophage function in immunosuppressed patients.*

When host immunity is depressed, supplemental nucleic acids, particularly the purine and pyrimidine bases of ribonucleic acid (RNA) and deoxyribonucleic acid (DNA), experimentally appear to improve indices of delayed hypersensitivity and macrophage function and also to reduce mortality rates.[52] This dependence on exogenous nucleotides for proper immune function appears to be most characteristic of cells such as lymphocytes and intestinal cells, which are metabolically hyperactive and exhibit rapid turnover.

Experimental studies have shown that diets supplemented with omega-3 fatty acids improve a variety of nutritional indices and immune responses.[53] Following burn injury, diets containing fish oil appear to preserve weight and transferrin levels better and to result in lower metabolic rates and better cell-mediated immune responses than diets that contain omega-6 fatty acids. Dietary supplementation with omega-3 fats also attenuates the inflammatory mediator responses that increase thromboxane A_2 and prostacyclin in experimental sepsis.[53]

Non-septic adults may burn up to 5 to 6 g of intravenous glucose/kg/day.[54] However, if larger amounts of glucose are given to septic

• Septic patients tend to use endogenous protein as an energy source.

patients, a substantial proportion of the glucose administered will be converted to fat and these patients will continue to consume endogenous protein.[55] I have noted the phenomenon of a respiratory quotient (RQ) higher than 1.0 with a negative nitrogen balance in some of our most septic patients who are receiving TPN. This phenomenon may result from cellular enzymatic blocks of pyruvate dehydrogenase[56] or carnitine acyl-CoA transferase.[57] It has been hypothesized that medium-chain triglycerides and/or branched-chain amino acids (isoleucine, leucine, and valine) can circumvent these metabolic blockades and serve as a preferred fuel in sepsis.[58]

Theoretically, weight changes should help one monitor the patient's nutrition. However, accurate daily weights can be difficult to obtain in patients with multiple tubes, even when the clinician uses bed scales. Furthermore, weight gain or loss usually follows changes in water balance and not lean body mass.

Plasma albumin levels may fall rapidly in injured or septic patients. However, this change is largely due to a shift of albumin into the interstitial fluid space.[59] Furthermore, during the anabolic phase of nutritional therapy, albumin blood levels tend to rise slowly because of the prolonged half-life. Absolute lymphocyte counts (ALC) may also reflect visceral protein changes and host-defense capabilities. An ALC lower than 800/mm^3 is generally evidence of anergy, but ALC levels can widely vary on a day-to-day basis.

We determine nitrogen balance at least twice weekly in our critically ill patients. We calculate nitrogen intake by totaling all the grams of protein or amino acid intake and dividing by 6.25. Thus, 3 L of a 4.25% amino acid solution provide 127.5 g of amino acids or 20.4 g of nitrogen. The grams of urine urea nitrogen (UUN) in a 24-hour urine sample plus 4 (2 g for other nitrogen loss in urine and 2 g of nitrogen loss from skin and feces) usually provide a reasonable estimate of the total nitrogen output. The difference between nitrogen output and intake provides the nitrogen balance, which we would like to be slightly positive (2 to 3 g/day). For each 10 mg/dl that the BUN rises in a 70-kg man, 4.2 g must also be added to the nitrogen loss. Although nitrogen balances can be extremely variable from day to day, they seem to be our best guide to the adequacy of the patient's nutrition.

The availability of a metabolic cart to measure oxygen consumption (VO_2) and carbon dioxide production (VCO_2) permits calculation of the patient's REE. The metabolic rate (kcal/day) is equal to (3.94)(VO_2 L/day) plus (1.11)(VCO_2 L/day).[60] One can convert the VO_2 in milliliters per minute to liters per day by multiplying by 1.44 (Table 11–5).

• A metabolic cart study requires a steady state for at least 1 hour before and during measurement. Repeat determinations can provide more accurate data on the patient's actual metabolic state.

The RQ, which is the ratio of carbon dioxide production to oxygen consumption, can easily be obtained by indirect calorimetry from the metabolic cart. Each substrate has its own RQ (carbohydrates = 1.0; fat = 0.7; protein = 0.82). Theoretically, the RQ for lipogenesis from excess carbohydrate equals 8.0, but clinically it seldom exceeds 1.25.[61] Conversion of fat to ketones consumes oxygen, and ketones are burned like fat with an RQ of 0.7. However, with ketonuria, the RQ is less than 0.7. If at all possible, pa-

Table 11–5.
Calculation of Metabolic Rate

Measured:	VO_2—250 ml/min VCO_2—200 ml/min
Calculated:	$RQ = \frac{200}{250} = 0.8$ Metabolic rate = $3.94 \times (VO_2 \text{ ml/min}) \times 1.44 = VO_2$ in L/min $1.11 \times (CO_2 \text{ ml/min}) \times 1.44 = VCO_2$ in L/min Therefore: $3.94 \times 1.44 \times (VO_2 \text{ ml/min}) + 1.11 \times 1.44 \times (VCO_2 \text{ ml/min})$ = number kcal/day Total kcal/day = $3.94 \times 1.44 \times (250) + 1.11 \times 1.44 \times (200)$

tients should have an RQ of 0.90 or less, and the REE should be supplied with nonprotein calories.

As a general rule, metabolic carts are considered accurate if the patient's activity and ventilation are quiet and uniform. The cart's accuracy deteriorates if the patient is hyperactive and when the FIO_2 exceeds 0.60. Sufficient accuracy for clinical management has been obtained with a variety of commercially available instruments.

OPERATIVE INTERVENTIONS

When patients require an operation because of sepsis, the operative intervention should be directed at identification and eradication of the cause of that sepsis. The most severe cases of sepsis that require surgery are usually due to peritonitis secondary to a gastrointestinal tract leaks, particularly of the colon or distal small bowel.

During surgery, care must be taken to prevent additional spillage or spread of either gastrointestinal contents or any suppurative material. When complete eradication of necrotic or infected tissue cannot be done safely or easily, or when continued drainage of pancreatic secretions or bile into the peritoneal cavity is likely, closed drainage should be provided. Bowel anastomosis in patients with peritoneal contamination carries a high risk. In fact, it may be far more judicious to exteriorize the involved bowel. In areas other than the abdomen or chest, removal of dead or devitalized tissue along with any pus should suffice. Complete removal of all infected or necrotic material is essential.

- *Following large bowel perforation, any attempts to perform a primary anastomosis lead to a high rate of anastomotic leakage and breakdown.*

Careful, complete irrigation of all infected material from the peritoneal cavity may require multiple liters of fluid, preferably with pulsating pressure. Some surgeons believe that the addition of antibiotics to the irrigant can be of great value because of the high local antibiotic concentration that can be achieved. One gram of cephalothin per liter of irrigant works effectively against virtually all gram-positive, gram-negative, and anaerobic bacteria. Following irrigation, the fluids should be removed as completely as possible, to enhance maximal efficiency of peritoneal macrophages.

The skin and subcutaneous tissue are not closed in the presence of moderate or severe contamination. The risk of necrotizing fasciitis makes it dangerous even to close fascia in the presence of severe infection. Closure of the abdomen in a patient with severe, generalized suppurative peritonitis has resulted in mortality rates exceeding 70%.[62] Consequently, in such cases, we believe that the abdomen should be packed open with sterile dressings held in place by an abdominal binder. The open abdomen can be explored daily for 3 to 5 days until the peritoneal cavity is clear, and the fascia is then closed.[63] This protocol has resulted in a greatly reduced mortality rate in our patients.

• *Leaving the abdomen open in patients with diffuse suppurative peritonitis allows easy access for continued daily irrigation and debridement and greatly reduces mortality rates.*

In summary, septic patients or those at risk of sepsis require rapid and focused intervention. Sources must be exhaustively searched for and aggressively treated, drained, or removed. Antibiotic coverage must be broad, but focused to minimize the development of resistance. Unfortunately, other nonantibiotic pharmacologic therapies have not yet lived up to early expectations.

REFERENCES

1. Moldawer LL: Biology of pro-inflammatory cytokines and their antagonists. Crit Care Med 1994; 22:S3–7.
2. Song Y, Moldawer LL, Shires GT et al: The biology of cytokines and their implication in surgical injury. Surg Gynecol Obstet 1990; 170: 363–378.
3. Fisher CJ Jr, Opal FN, Dhainaut JFA et al: Influence of an antitumor necrosis factor monoclonal antibody on cytokine levels in patients with sepsis. Crit Care Med 1993; 21:318–327.
4. Chandrasekar PH, Brown WJ: Clinical issues of blood cultures. Arch Intern Med 1994; 154:841–849.
5. Bernard GR, Artigas A, Brigham KL et al: Report of the American-European consensus conference of acute respiratory distress syndrome: definitions, mechanisms, relevant outcomes, and in clinical trial coordination. J Crit Care 1994; 9:72–81.
6. Mirvis SE, Vainright JR, Nelson AW et al: The diagnosis of acute acalculus cholecystitis: a comparison of sonography, scintigrapy and CT. AJR Am J Roentgenol 1986; 147:1171.
7. Norwood SH: An approach to the febrile ICU patient. In: Civetta JM, Taylor RW, Kirby RR, eds: Critical care. Philadelphia, JB Lippincott, 1988, pp. 745–756.
8. Moir C, Robin R: The role of ultrasonography, gallium scanning and computed tomography in the diagnosis of intraabdominal abscess. Am J Surg 1982; 143:582.
9. Fry DE, Pearlstein L, Fulton RL et al: Multiple system organ failure. Arch Surg 1980; 115:136–140.
10. Sutherland FR, Temple WJ, Snodgrass T et al: Predicting the outcome of exploratory laparotomy in ICU patients with sepsis or organ failure. J Trauma 1989; 29:152–157.
11. Norton LW: Does drainage of intraabdominal pus reverse multiple organ failure? Am J Surg 1985; 149:347–350.
12. Bone RC, Balk R, Slotman G et al: Adult respiratory distress syndrome: sequence and importance of development of multiple organ failure. Chest 1992; 101:320–326.
13. Kolles MH: Ventilator-associated pneumonia: a multivariant analysis. JAMA 1993; 165:1965–1970.

14. Palmer DL, Davidson M, Lusk R: Needle aspiration of the lung in complex pneumonias. Chest 1980; 78:16.
15. Ahrenholz DH, Simmons RL: Peritonitis and other intra-abdominal infections. In: Howard RJ, Simmons RL, eds: Surgical infectious diseases, 2nd ed. Norwalk, CT, Appleton & Lange, 1988; pp. 605–646.
16. Sarles H: Definitions and classification of pancreatitis. Pancreas 1991; 6:470–474.
17. Champion HR, Jones RT, Trump BF et al: Post-traumatic hepatic dysfunction as a major etiology in post-traumatic jaundice. J Trauma 1976; 16:650–657.
18. Barton RG, Cerra FB: Metabolic and nutritional support. In: Moore EE, Mattox KL, Feliciano DV, eds: Trauma, 2nd ed. Norwalk, CT, Appleton & Lange, 1991; pp. 965–994.
19. Farmer JC, Parker RI: Coagulation disorders. In: Civetta JM, Taylor RW, Kirby RR, eds: Critical care. Philadelphia, JB Lippincott, 1988; pp. 1469–1480.
20. Poon MC: Coagulation testing of Hickman catheter blood in patients with acute leukemia. Arch Intern Med 1986; 146:2165–2169.
21. Bang NU: Diagnosis and management of thrombosis. In: Shoemaker WC, Ayres S, Grenvik A et al, eds: Textbook on critical care. Philadelphia, WB Saunders, 1989; pp. 886–895.
22. Wilson RF, Dulchavsky SA, Soullier G et al: Problems with 20 or more blood transfusions in 24 hours. Am Surg 1987; 53:410–417.
23. Valeri CR, Feingold H, Cassidy G et al: Hypothermia-induced platelet dysfunction. Ann Surg 1987; 205:175–181.
24. Roslyn JJ, Zinner MJ: Biliary ducts. In: Levine BA, Copeland EM, Howard RJ et al, eds: Practice of surgery. New York, Churchill Livingstone, 1993.
25. Deitch EA: Overview of multiple organ failure in critical care state of the art. In: Lough DS, Traystman RJ, eds: Anaheim, CA, Society of Critical Care Medicine, 1993; pp. 131–168.
26. Shoemaker WC Appel PL, Kram HB et al: Prospective trial of supranormal values of survivors as therapeutic goals in high risk surgical patients. Chest 1988; 94:1177–1186.
27. Hayes MA, Yau EHS, Pinmins AC: Response of critically ill patients to treatment aimed at achieving supranormal oxygen delivery and consumption: Relationship to outcome. Chest 1993; 103:886–895.
28. Yu M, Levy MM, Smith P et al: Effective maximizing oxygen delivery on morbidity and mortality rates in critically ill patients: a prospective, randomized, controlled study. Crit Care Med 1993; 21:830–838.
29. Ericcson CD, Fisher RP, Rowlands BJ et al: Prophylactic antibiotics in trauma: the hazards of underdosing. J Trauma 1989; 29:1356–1361.
30. Ziegler EG, Fisher CJ, Sprung CL et al: Treatment of gram negative bacteremia and septic shock with HA-1A human monoclonal antibody endotoxin: HA-1A Sepsis Study Group. N Engl J of Med 1991; 324: 429–436.
31. Greenman RL, Schein RM, Martin MA et al: A controlled clinical stress trial of E5 murine monoclonal IgM antibody to endotoxin in treatment of gram negative sepsis: XOMA Sepsis Study Group. JAMA 1991; 266:1097–1102.
32. Fisher CJ Jr, Dhainaut JFA, Opal FM et al: Recrecombinant human interleukin-1 receptor antagonist in the treatment of patients with sepsis syndrome: results from a randomized, double-blind, placebo-controlled trial. JAMA 1994; 271:1836–1843.
33. Reed RL III, Wu AH, Miller-Crotchett P et al: Pharmacokinetic moni-

toring of nephrotoxic antibiotics in surgical intensive care patients. J Trauma 1989; 29:1462–1470.
34. Dilbert BN: Once-daily aminoglycoside therapy. Antimicrob Agents Chemother 1991; 35:399.
35. Solomkin JS: Pathogensis and management of candida infection syndromes in nonneutropenic patients. New Horizons 1993; 1:202–213.
36. Vandenbroucke-Grauls CMJE, Vandenbroucke JP: Effective selected decontamination of the digestive tract on respiratory tract infections and mortality in the intensive care unit. Lancet 1991; 338:859–862.
37. Martinez-Pellus AE, Merino P, Bru M et al: Can selected digestive decontamination avoid the endotoxemia in cytokine activation promoted by cardiopulmonary bypass? Crit Care Med 1993; 21: 1684–1691.
38. Petteroo GWM, Wagenvoort JHT, Mulder PGH et al: Decreased mortality rate in length of hospital stay in surgical intensive care unit patients with successful selected decontamination of the gut. Crit Care Med 1994; 21:1692–1698.
39. Moore FA, Moore EE, Poggetti R et al: Gut bacterial translocation via the portal vein: a clinical perspective with major torso trauma. J Trauma 1991; 31:629–638.
40. Heyland DK, Cook DJ, Jaeschke R et al: Selected decontamination of the digestive tract: An overview. Chest 1994; 105:1221–1229.
41. Abraham E, Stevens P: Effective granular site colony stimulating factor in modifying mortality from pseudomonas aeruginosa pneumonia after hemorrhage. Crit Care Med 1992; 20:1127–1133.
42. Applefeld JJ, Caruthers TE, Reno DJ et al: Assessment of the sterility of long-term cardiac catheterization using a thermodilutions Swan-Ganz catheter. Chest 1978; 74:377.
43. Dickinson GM, Bisno AL: Infections associated with indwelling devices: concepts of pathogenesis, infections associated with intravascular devices. Antimicrob Agents Chemother 1989; 33:597.
44. Eyer S, Brummitt C, Crossley K et al: Catheter-related sepsis: prospective, randomized study of three methods of long-term catheter maintenance. Crit Care Med 1990; 18:1073–1079.
45. Powell C, Fabri PJ, Kudsk KA: Risk of infection accompanying the use of single lumen versus double lumen subclavian catheters: a prospective, randomized study. JPEN J Parenter Enteral Nutr 1988; 12: 127–129.
46. Schlictig R: Nutritional assessment, requirements and monitoring. In: Civetta JM, Taylor RW, Kirby RR, eds: Critical care. Philadelphia, JB Lippincott, 1988; pp. 503–511.
47. Long CL, Schaffel N, Geiger JW et al: Metabolic response to injury and illness: estimation of energy and protein needs for calorimetry and nitrogen balance. JPEN J Parenter Enteral Nutr 1979; 3:452–456.
48. Moore FA, Feliciano DV, Andrassy RJ: Early enteral feeding, compared with parenteral, reduces postoperative septic complications. Ann Surg 1992; 216:172–183.
49. Moore EE, Jones TN: Benefits of immediate jejunostomy feeding after major abdominal trauma: a randomized prospective study. J Trauma 1986; 26:874–881.
50. Brinson RR, Pitts VL, Taylor AE: Intestinal absorption of peptide enteral formulas in hypoproteinemic (volume-expanded) rats: a paired analysis. Crit Care Med 1989; 17:657–660.
51. Kirk SJ, Barbul A: Role of arginine in trauma, sepsis and immunity. JPEN J Parenter Enteral Nutr 1990; 14:226S.

52. Rudolph FB, Kulkarni AD, Fanslow WC et al: Role of RNA as a dietary source of pyramidines and purines in immune function. Nutrition 1990; 61:45.
53. Maukkassa FF, Koruda MJ, Ramadan FM et al: Effect of dietary fish oil on plasma thromboxane B_2 and 6-keto-prostaglandin $F_1\alpha$ levels in septic rats. Arch Surg 1991; 126:179–182.
54. Elwin DH, Kinney JM, Malayappa J et al: Influence of increasing carbohydrate intake on glucose kinetics in injured patients. Ann Surg 1979; 190:117–127.
55. Giovannini I, Boldrini G, Castagneto M et al: Respiratory quotient and patterns of substrate utilization in human sepsis and trauma. JPEN J Parenter Enteral Nutr 1983; 7:226–230.
56. Vary TC, Siegel JH, Nakatani T et al: Regulation of glucose metabolism by altered pyruvate dehydrogenase activity. I. Potential site of insulin resistance in sepsis. JPEN J Parenter Enteral Nutr 1986; 10:351–355.
57. Vary TC, Siegel JH, Nakatani T et al: A biochemical basis for depressed ketogenesis in sepsis. J Trauma 1986; 26:419–425.
58. Siegel JH, Cerra FB, Coleman B et al: The effect of normalization of plasma amino acids on hepatic encephalopathy in man. Surgery 1976; 80:77–91.
59. Dawson CW, Lucas CE, Ledgerwood AM: Altered interstitial fluid space dynamics and postresuscitation hypertension. Arch Surg 1981; 116:657–662.
60. Agarwal NR, Savino JA, Feldman M et al: The automated metabolic profile. Crit Care Med 1983; 11:546–550.
61. Barrett TA, Robin AP, Armstrong MK et al: Nutrition and respiratory failure. In: Bone RC, George RB, Hudson LD, eds: Acute respiratory failure. New York, Churchill Livingston, 1987; pp. 265–303.
62. Dunn DL, Barke RA, Ahrenholz DH et al: The adjuvant effect of peritoneal fluid in experimental peritonitis. Ann Surg 1984; 199:37–43.
63. Duff JH, Moffat J: Abdominal sepsis managed by leaving the abdomen open. Surgery 1981; 90:774–778.

CHAPTER 12

Oxygen Delivery and Utilization

T. James Gallagher

Case Report

The patient was a 58-year-old woman admitted to the intensive care unit (ICU) in apparent septic shock. On arrival, blood pressure was 80/58 mm Hg, pulse was 126/min, and respiratory rate was 38/min. Six days previously, the patient had had an esophagogastrectomy with colonic interposition. This was done as a palliative procedure for carcinoma of the esophagus. At the time of ICU admission, the source of sepsis was unclear, but concerns included an intra-abdominal leak or mediastinitis. The patient's initial oxygen saturation by pulse oximetry was 84%. The patient was rapidly intubated orally under direct vision. This procedure was chosen to avoid any possible disruption of the suture line in the neck.

Resuscitation was initiated following placement of large-bore intravenous access. Fluids included normal saline and plasma protein fraction. An arterial line was placed in the right radial artery, while simultaneously the left subclavian vein was cannulated and a pulmonary artery catheter was placed. Initial laboratory work revealed a hematocrit of 27% and a hemoglobin of 8.9 g/dl. Further initial data included a cardiac output of 3.6 L/min with an index of 2.7 L/min/m^2. Wedge pressure was 9 mm Hg. Systemic vascular resistance was calculated at 1480 dyn·sec·cm^{-5}. Dopamine was begun and titrated to 8 μg/kg/min. Two units of packed red blood cells were administered to elevate hemoglobin. Fluids were continued in the form of crystalloids to expand intravascular volume in hopes of improving the patient's cardiac output.

After 2 hours of resuscitation, wedge pressure was 16 mm Hg and cardiac output was 6.7 L/min. Urine output improved from 20 to 45 ml/hr. At the time of line placement, blood cultures had been drawn and sputum and urine samples had been obtained. Broad-spectrum antibiotics were initiated against gram-positive and gram-negative organisms and anaerobes. Drugs included imipenem, vancomycin, and metronidazole. The patient's initial chest radiograph revealed bilateral infiltrates that were greater on the right. Because of the colonic intraposition, it was somewhat difficult to adequately assess the mediastinum.

On a ventilator rate of 8/min (F_IO_2 0.8), 5 cm H_2O of CPAP, the PaO_2 was 170 mm Hg, and $PaCO_2$ was 36 mm Hg. Adjustments were made, and the F_IO_2 was decreased to 0.5 while the continuous positive airway pressure (CPAP) was increased to 12 cm H_2O. The ventilator rate was reduced to 6 breaths/min. Repeat blood gases revealed a PaO_2 of 92 mm Hg and a $PaCO_2$ of 39 mm Hg; pH was 7.32. Lactic acid remained less than 2.0 mEq/L. Further stabilization efforts included reduction of temperature with antipyretics and a cooling blanket. Following the blood infusions, the patient's cardiac output remained in the same range, and oxygen delivery was now calculated at 940 ml/min. This was indexed to 630 ml/min/m^2.

After the patient appeared initially stabilized, contrast material was instilled and the patient taken to the computed tomographic (CT) scanner. The CT scan revealed an intra-abdominal abscess, which was reached by a percutaneous, CT-guided drain.

With fluid administration, the patient's blood pressure had improved to 100/74 mm Hg. The nursing staff was instructed that, as long as the patient's systolic pressure remained greater than 90 mm Hg with a cardiac output of 6 to 7 L/min, it was not necessary to increase pressors in an attempt to raise pressures any higher. The patient appeared to maintain good perfusion, as indicated by her ability to follow simple and complex commands. After 4 days, the patient was afebrile and hemodynamically stable. The pulmonary artery catheter was then discontinued. Six days following admission to the ICU, the patient's respiratory status had resolved so extubation could proceed without difficulty. The patient was discharged from the ICU on the eighth day following admission.

In earlier times, it was enough for clinicians to concern themselves, in the immediate postoperative period, with blood pressure. If systemic blood pressures were within a normal range and the patient had a reasonable urinary output, the assumption was that perfusion and, one hoped, oxygen delivery were adequate. The next stage found the introduction of the pulmonary artery catheter.[1] Clinicians could now follow cardiac output in addition to or in lieu of blood pressure. It soon became apparent that there was often little correlation between blood pressure and perfusion, as indicated by thermodilution cardiac output measurements.[2] Over the ensuing years, the emphasis shifted to cardiac output as the main determinant of the adequacy of cardiac function and oxygen delivery in a postoperative period. We have now begun to recognize that cardiac output itself may not be the final answer. Increasing evidence suggests that oxygen consumption ($\dot{V}O_2$) and its relationship to oxygen delivery (DO_2) should demand more attention from the physician.[3]

All patients in the immediate postoperative and post-traumatic period have predictably increased metabolic demands.[4] These elevated metabolic rates reflect the increased catecholamine release following major insults. However, the exact cause or stimulus of the increased demands remains unclear. Sufficient data and knowledge have accumulated to support the concept as valid. The elevated metabolic rate usually persists for at least 24 hours following such events. Specific patient populations, including those with greater than 30% surface area burns and generalized sepsis, may persist with increased oxygen requirements for prolonged periods of time.[5]

• *Postoperative metabolic demands may remain elevated for several days. The specific illness usually determines their duration.*

As our understanding has increased, it has become apparent that the ideal postoperative cardiac output cannot be represented by any one particular number. Rather, cardiac output represents one other measurable parameter that makes up the constellation of factors that serve to provide adequate oxygen to meet all tissue metabolic demands. In general, all other things being even and if the system is working properly, one might expect that, as metabolic demands increase, cardiac output and therefore oxygen delivery also increase. Furthermore, data have begun to emerge that would suggest that, in septic patients, outcome appears to be associated with the ability to reach threshold levels of both oxygen delivery and demand.

METHODS TO MEASURE OXYGEN DELIVERY AND CONSUMPTION

In critically ill patients, oxygen delivery will continue to change throughout the course of the patient's illness (Fig. 12–1). For instance, we know that the effects of anesthesia tend to reduce not only oxygen requirements, but also oxygen delivery.[6] Most inhalation and many intravenous anesthetic agents have depressant effects on the myocardium and can also cause systemic hypotension.[7] During the recovery phase, metabolic demands will return to and increase above the original baseline levels. As a result, to maintain homeostasis, oxygen delivery will also of necessity increase. As we shall see later, several methods are available to effect these changes.

In order to understand the basic relationships, the clinician needs to be aware of and calculate oxygen delivery on a relatively frequent basis. The actual number of measurements will relate to the patient's stability and response. In the past assumptions, have been made that factors such as hemoglobin and cardiac output remain relatively constant. This cannot be assumed for the critically ill, postoperative patient. Fluid shifts, bleeding, the varying effects of residual anesthetics, the impact of analgesics, and fluid requirements all impact

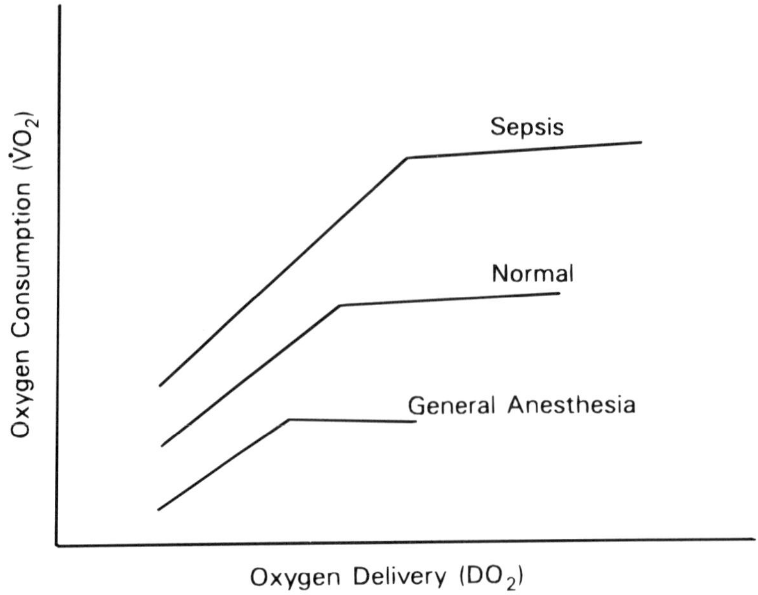

Figure 12–1.
Idealized representation of oxygen delivery and consumption. In general, sepsis results in a linkage between oxygen delivery and consumption at higher levels than would be seen under normal circumstances.

on and alter cardiac output and hemoglobin values. Oxygen delivery can be calculated from the following formula:

$$DO_2 = CO \cdot Ca$$

where Ca = arterial oxygen content.

Because of the relatively small contribution of dissolved oxygen, PaO_2 calculations are not always taken into account when attempting rapid and repeated measurements of oxygen delivery.

• *Blood pressure provides little reliable information about oxygen delivery.*

We have available a number of parameters to aid the clinician in monitoring the adequacy of oxygen delivery. Systemic blood pressure has often been substituted for cardiac output. One presumes that blood pressure changes are directly related to cardiac output, and hence, oxygen delivery. In fact, blood pressure has almost no relationship with flow or stroke volume. For instance, patients may have a decrease in intravascular volume by as much as 20% before any observed changes in systemic blood pressure occur.[8] The body simply responds by intense vasoconstriction. Likewise, it is not uncommon to see patients who are somewhat hypertensive postoperatively, with blood pressures in excess of 160 mm Hg, yet, when actually measured, have quite low cardiac outputs. Therefore, to attempt to judge oxygen delivery and tissue perfusion based on blood pressure represents a large leap of faith on the part of the clinician.

• *Direct evidence of adequate perfusion such as urinary output may be altered by many coexisting factors.*

Indirect evidence of normal organ function and perfusion relies on a number of clinical signs. Reasonable urinary output has been thought to indicate adequate renal perfusion resulting from overall adequate blood and flow oxygen delivery. However, the quality and type of urine should be considered as important as the volume when judging the adequacy of perfusion. Obviously, if patients have received diuretic therapy, the resultant volume of urine bears little if any relationship to organ perfusion. Patients who have glucosuria because of hyperglycemia also cloud the evidence in regard to their organ function and perfusion. High urinary outputs will also be present in patients with diabetes insipidus, and occasionally patients develop high-output renal failure.

In some patients, mental status may reflect the adequacy of oxygen delivery. The awake, alert, oriented patient obviously has reasonable cerebral perfusion. However, even such situations do not necessarily indicate the overall adequacy of organ perfusion to meet most of the body's metabolic demands. The fact that the patient is awake and oriented, however, represents a move in the right direction.

Of less help in determining oxygen delivery and utilization, but still of some benefit, is the myocardium with or without evidence of ischemia. Multiple factors can lead to ischemia, particularly in patients with underlying coronary artery disease. However, ischemia can also indicate inadequacy of perfusion, at least to the myocardium. Since the heart under normal conditions utilizes all oxygen delivered,[9] it can be presumed that if ischemia develops, other organs may also be at risk in that oxygen delivery may be inadequate to meet metabolic demands. A number of specific factors can contribute to inadequate oxygen delivery and myocardial ischemia. Tachycardia will significantly increase myocardial metabolic demands (Fig. 12–2).[10] This is particularly true when heart rate exceeds 100/min. Patients with underlying coronary artery disease and therefore a fixed flow are at increased risk for development of ischemia. Hypertension will cause the heart to pump against an increased impendance. The resultant increase in wall tension may cause myocardial oxygen consumption to outpace oxygen delivery. An elevated end-diastolic pressure, particularly when coupled with diastolic hypotension, will reduce myocardial perfusion pressure possibly to inadequate levels and set the stage for ischemia.

• *The electrocardiogram does not always provide reliable information about the onset or degree of ischemia.*

None of the other organs appears to respond rapidly enough to provide much clinical information on a frequent basis about oxygen delivery and perfusion. For example, changes in the liver are relatively slow. Bilirubin elevation and enzyme changes may take 24 hours or more to develop. Moreover, they can represent events other than hypoperfusion and reduced oxygen delivery.

We can on occasion find some useful information by examination of peripheral perfusion. This includes the color of the extremities. For instance, blue or mottled lower extremities in a hypertensive postoperative patient usually indicate inadequate organ perfusion. Some clinicians have advocated evaluation of skin or big toe temperature as another perfusion indicator.[11] At best, these are qualitative markers and serve only as an early warning system. In addition, these factors can be modified by many events and therefore may be of only minimal value.

• *Physical examination cannot always indicate cardiac output, but it often can detect inadequate oxygen delivery.*

When measured, cardiac index may range in resting normal patients between 1.9 and 3.0 L/min/m^2. It then becomes the clinician's

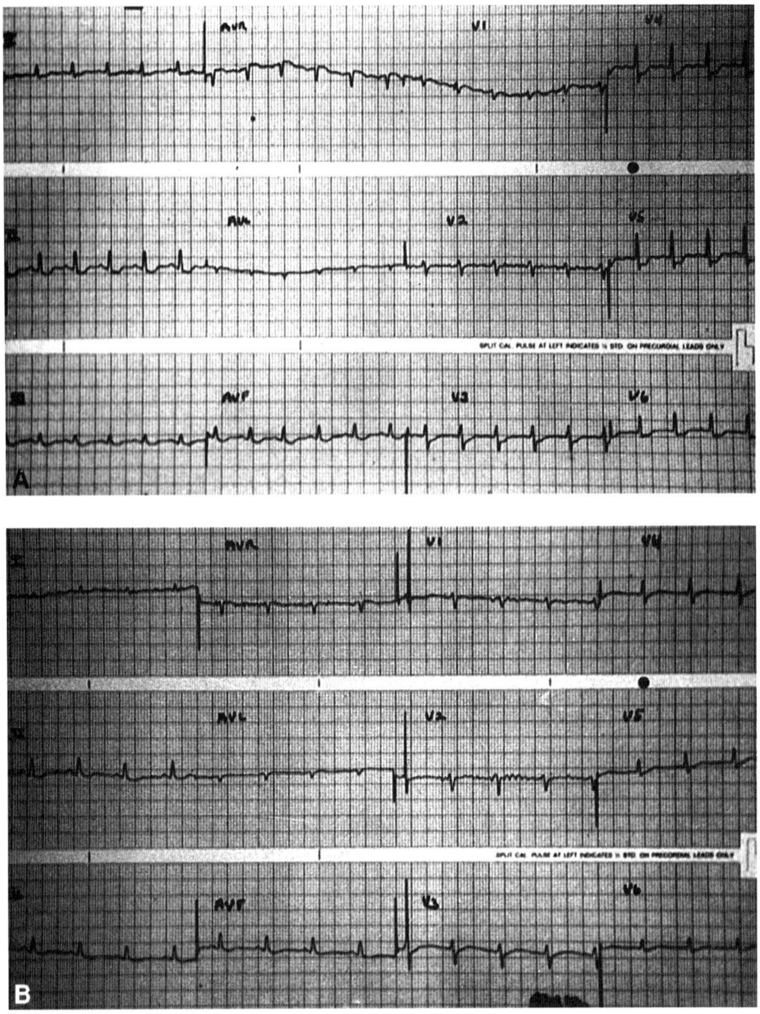

Figure 12–2.
A, Tachycardia-related ischemia. Note the ST-T-wave changes. B, Following beta blockade, the heart rate has slowed and the ischemia has improved.

duty to determine when that specific output meets metabolic demands. Therefore, knowledge of only cardiac index or cardiac output cannot of itself provide all of the necessary information. In general, a recognizably low cardiac index usually provides reliable information that things are not well. However, patients who are hypothermic, paralyzed, or sedated may all be able to tolerate a lower than normal cardiac index and oxygen delivery because of the concomitant decrease in oxygen consumption.

Mixed venous oxygen saturation (SvO_2) has been touted as a clinical method to determine the adequacy of oxygen delivery to meet metabolic demands.[12] The underlying principle states that venous oxygen content will reflect changes in oxygen delivery and uptake (Table 12–1). An increase in cardiac index, without a change in oxygen consumption, indirectly means an increase in oxygen de-

Table 12–1.
Factors That Independently Affect SvO_2

Fever
Patient movement or agitation
Cardiac Output
Hemoglobin
Metabolic rate
Paralysis
Shivering
Hypothermia

livery resulting in an elevated mixed venous oxygen content or venous oxygen saturation (SvO_2). On the other side, if delivery does not increase in the face of increased demands, then oxygen extraction must increase to make up the difference. An increase in oxygen extraction will result in lowered venous oxygen content or SvO_2. Therefore, a reduction in SvO_2 could reflect a decrease in oxygen delivery and by inference a decrease in cardiac index. We now know that fully 20% of changes in SvO_2 can occur independent of any change in oxygen delivery.[13] That is, oxygen consumption can increase or decrease without any compensatory response on the part of the body to maintain oxygen delivery. We also know that in a number of instances, roughly between 15 and 20%, an increase in oxygen delivery may still be paradoxically associated with a decrease in SvO_2.[13] This likely develops when oxygen consumption increases over and above the ability of oxygen delivery to increase to meet the demands. Therefore, a change in SvO_2 may at times reflect a change in oxygen delivery, but not necessarily a change in the direction presumed, and is not necessarily related to cardiac index. At most, one can say that a change in SvO_2 indicates that there has been some alteration of the balance between oxygen delivery and consumption and bears further investigation.

- *Changes in SvO_2 can represent alteration of either the demand side or the supply side of the equation.*

Currently, two different methods are used by clinicians to calculate oxygen consumption. The indirect Fick method requires placement of a pulmonary artery catheter.[14] The calculation of oxygen content in arterial and mixed venous blood is carried out using the following formulas:

$$Ca = (Hgb \times 1.34)(art\ O_2\ sat) + 0.0031)(PaO_2)$$

$$Cv = (Hgb \times 1.34)(ven\ O_2\ sat) + 0.0031(PvO_2)$$

$$\text{then } VO_2 = C.O. \times (Ca - Cv)$$

The Fick calculation of oxygen consumption relies on a single point in time to make the determination. Various other measurement techniques have demonstrated, however, that oxygen consumption does not necessarily stay constant. In fact, it may vary by as much as 20% over the course of the day in any critically ill patient.[15] Many multiple factors affect instantaneous oxygen consumption.[16] These include such simple maneuvers as moving the

- *The Fick equation can estimate oxygen consumption. However, oxygen consumption changes considerably throughout the day and the course of the patient's illness.*

patient in the bed or bathing. Suctioning the patient can impact on oxygen consumption. Furthermore, it takes as much as 1 hour after the precipitating event before the patient returns to baseline. Errors during blood gas analysis or collection of the sample can affect results.

- *While a metabolic cart can provide useful information about oxygen consumption, it is only a window on a constantly changing parameter.*

Metabolic carts have become available and are in wide clinical use (Fig. 12–3). These carts permit on-line direct calculation of oxygen consumption. All of the devices rely on precise metering of the amount of oxygen taken up on a breath-to-breath basis, as well as the amount exhaled with each breath. The difference over time obviously represents the oxygen uptake or consumption. These devices also have a number of potential errors. Most cannot accurately calculate oxygen consumption if the FiO_2 is above 0.6. Leaks in the system will also interfere with measurements.[17] They are less accurate in the nonintubated patient. At times it may be difficult to obtain a steady-state analysis. Therefore, at best one can come up with a mean value of oxygen consumption over the time of the measurements. Metabolic carts should only be used when it is clear that the patient has not been recently stimulated and is in some type of steady state that resembles the usual clinical condition of the patient.

ADEQUACY OF OXYGEN DELIVERY

- *Most clinicians prefer to minimize demands rather than to let extraneous factors continue to drive oxygen consumption upward.*

Once information on oxygen delivery becomes available, it is then incumbent on the physician to determine whether, in fact, the current delivery is sufficient to meet the patient's present and future metabolic needs. A number of different conditions can and will affect the oxygen requirements. A hypermetabolic state following surgery, trauma, or ongoing sepsis illustrates one example. Fever will increase oxygen requirements by about 14% per 1°C elevation.[18] Hypothermia, on the other hand, can reduce oxygen requirements by about 7% per 1°C drop.[19] Shivering, which can accompany hypothermia, can paradoxically increase oxygen requirements by 200 to 300%.[20] We also now recognize that overfeeding patients can drive metabolic rate to higher than needed levels.

- *Minimal levels of oxygen delivery and not consumption appear to have some relation to outcome in critically ill patients.*

Investigators have recently suggested that survival in critically ill patients appears linked to some critical threshold level of oxygen delivery.[21–24] Currently, the data seem to be consistent in patients labeled as septic. Those include those who have displayed the usual hemodynamic criteria such as hypotension, elevated cardiac output, fever, and proven septic source. The data indicate that high oxygen deliveries are associated with enhanced survival. For that reason, many clinicians now strive to maintain oxygen delivery above 600 ml/min/m^2. From a larger perspective, it seems unlikely that for a clinical condition such as sepsis, in which the patient remains ill for a prolonged period of time, that a specific level of oxygen delivery will prove critical to survival. It may simply be that the oxygen delivery threshold serves as an indicator of the adequacy of underlying total body function and its ability to maintain and support such levels of delivery.

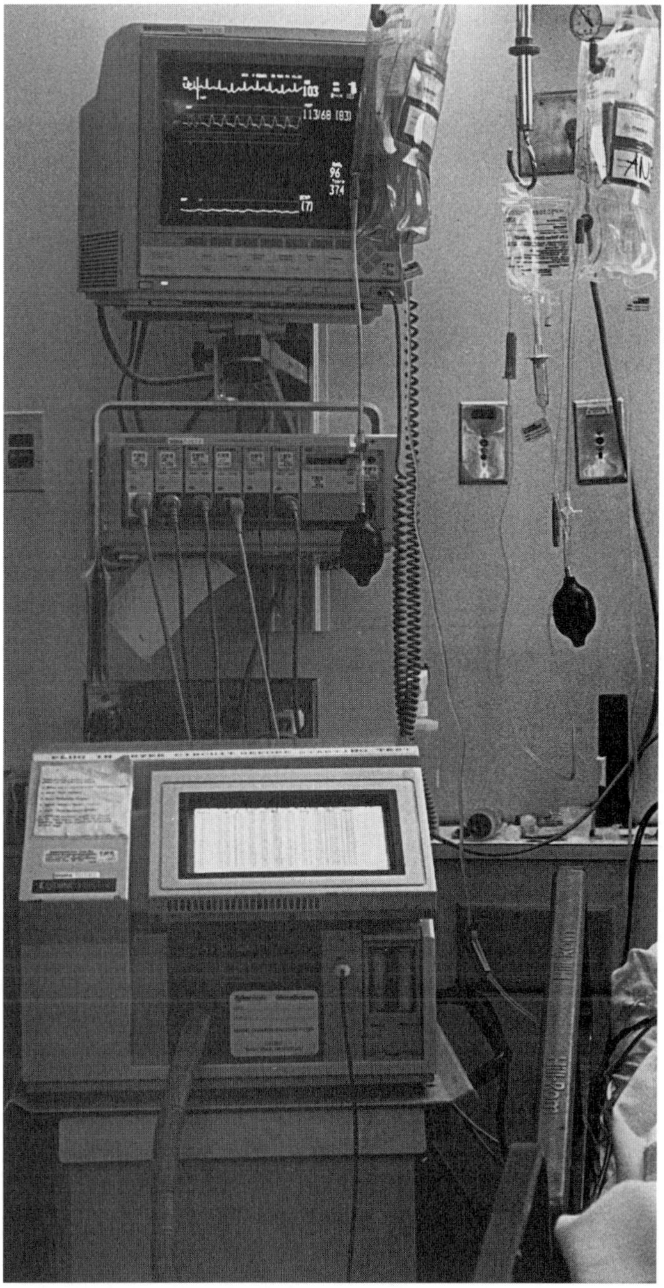

Figure 12–3.
A bedside metabolic cart. The device directly measures oxygen consumption and CO_2 production. A formula calculates actual caloric requirements. (Courtesy of Cybermedic, Inc., Louisville, CO.)

The oxygen delivery data are much less solid in regard to nonseptic patients and their outcome. Therefore, it does not seem reasonable that, in all patients judged to be critically ill (by itself a highly subjective decision), that oxygen delivery should be maintained at these high threshold levels. In fact, one can presume that in other sick patients with known cardiac disease, attempts to do so may result in more cardiac damage and lessen the chances for survival. As in all areas of medicine, enthusiasm for increased oxygen delivery needs to be tempered and selected for the appropriate patient. In some cases specific organ damage, such as advanced cirrhosis, may be a better predictor of outcome.

In nonseptic patients, I rely on the arterial-venous oxygen content difference (Ca-vDO_2) to provide information on oxygen delivery. One can presume that if oxygen delivery meets current demands, extraction and therefore the Ca-vDO_2 will remain within an acceptable range, ordinarily 3.5 to 5.5 ml/dl. If oxygen extraction must increase to meet elevated metabolic demands because of insufficient oxygen delivery, then the Ca-vDO_2 will widen. A widened Ca-vDO_2 signals that steps must be undertaken to correct the situation and to increase the availability of oxygen for peripheral uptake. If DO_2 is not maximized, the patient's position on a plot of DO_2 versus VO_2 will often be on the ascending limb. Oxygen consumption remains linked to oxygen delivery. Based on other organs' function and their ability to respond, attempts to improve delivery if necessary should be done with caution so as not to place any system, particularly the heart, in jeopardy. A decreased pH and elevated lactate are late findings and indicate that the patient has significantly deteriorated and requires prompt attention.

- *At the very least, critically ill patients should have the Ca-vDO_2 kept within the normal range.*

New data have suggested that in some septic states the inability of lactate to be handled by pyruvate has resulted in increased lactate levels, despite normal pH and oxygen delivery.[25] Therefore, lactate must not be judged alone but only in view of the pH. Moreover, lactate levels and their reduction may be dependent on both liver function and perfusion.

Always remember that Ca-vDO_2 is a global determinant of DO_2 and VO_2. Widening of the Ca-vDO_2 can serve as an indicator that other organs may be at increased risk. For example, the myocardium normally operates at maximal oxygen extraction. This results in an Ca-vDO_2 of 9 to 11 ml/dl. If total body Ca-vDO_2 has widened, then the heart may be at an even greater risk because it already maximally extracts all of the available oxygen.

METHODS TO INCREASE OXYGEN DELIVERY

One way to balance the metabolic demands is obviously to increase oxygen delivery. The clinician should attempt this in a manner that minimizes myocardial stress. Often the patients who most need attention are those with the greatest degree of underlying cardiac disease and who will not tolerate, or are unable to effect an increased cardiac output.

From a physiologic standpoint, one of the cheapest and most effective methods to improve oxygen delivery involves an increase of hemoglobin. Current practice advocates minimal numbers of blood transfusions. However, in the critically ill patient, the opposite approach should be taken. An increased oxygen-carrying capacity secondary to an elevated hemoglobin can have dramatic influence on

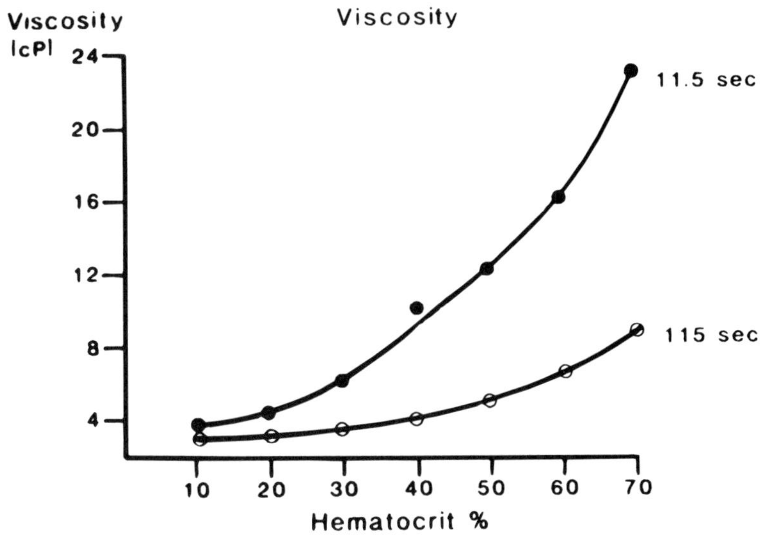

Figure 12–4.
In the arterial circulation, viscosity remains relatively constant through the usual hematocrit range. This presumes normothermia.

the cardiovascular system's ability to meet metabolic demands without placing undue stress on the heart. In such patients, we normally maintain hemoglobin levels between 11 and 12 g/dl. Hemoglobin values in this range have no effect on viscosity and microcirculatory flow. In normothermic patients, viscosity does not become important until hemoglobin exceeds 15 to 16 g/dl (Fig. 12–4). While the risk of AIDS remains at about 1 per 200,000 units of blood and hepatitis non-A, non-B at 6 to 8%,[26] the risks seems warranted given the likelihood of either a protracted course or a fatal outcome. Furthermore, in terms of the physiologic impact, it is cheaper to increase hemoglobin than to expect the heart to increase cardiac output. One additional gram of hemoglobin roughly represents a 1-L increase in cardiac output.[27] Hemoglobin also expands the intravascular volume, particularly in patients with leaky capillaries, because it is more likely than other fluids to stay within the intravascular space.

• *In critically ill patients, the risk from blood transfusions given to increase oxygen delivery is frequently less than the risk associated with other methods used to increase cardiac output.*

The physician also has some latitude with the oxyhemoglobin dissociation curve. Based on the Bohr effect, a rightward shift of the curve, present during hyperthermia and acidosis, contributes to offloading of oxygen in peripheral tissues.[28] This effect can prove beneficial. Furthermore, most enzyme systems, if given a choice, function more effectively in an acid than an alkaline medium. Therefore, correction of alkalosis can have an important impact on the availability of oxygen for the peripheral tissues. Clinically, we have few other methods to influence the shift of the curve. The fresher the blood the less the depletion of 2,3-diphosphoglycerate (2,3-DPG).[29] Reduced 2,3-DPG levels cause a leftward shift in the curve, and peripheral oxygen extraction becomes more difficult.

• *Critically ill patients' metabolic needs are better met in an acidotic than an alkalotic state.*

Obviously, the clinician's ability to influence the shape of the oxyhemoglobin dissociation curve remains limited. Therefore, the

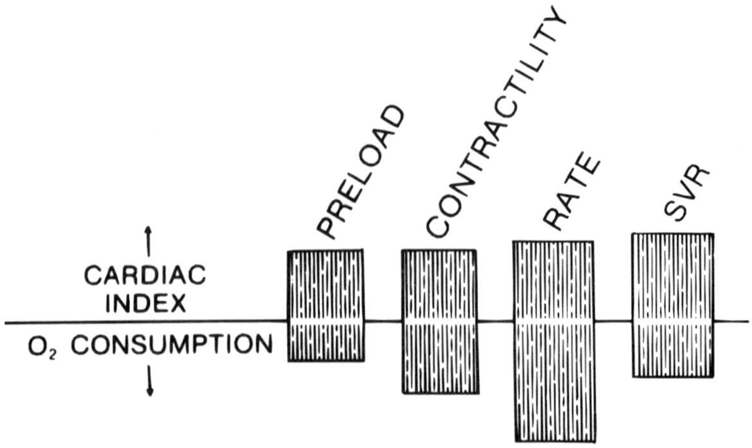

Figure 12–5.
A schematic representation of the relative increase in myocardial oxygen consumption following various therapeutic interventions.

majority of efforts involve manipulation of cardiac output. Rate-related increases in cardiac output should be avoided in older patients at all costs. Such patients most often have underlying coronary artery disease and, therefore, limited myocardial oxygen delivery potential. They have demonstrated time and again that an elevated heart rate above 100 beats/min will frequently lead to myocardial ischemia. Therefore, we should direct our efforts at other methods to increase cardiac output.

The easiest and most effective method to boost cardiac output involves maintenance of intravascular volume or preload (Fig. 12–5). On a comparative basis, an increase in cardiac output following preload enhancement requires less oxygen than does increased heart rate or contractility. Many arguments have been advanced for various fluid regimens. In general, balanced electrolyte solutions, such as Ringer's lactate or normal saline, or colloid-containing solutions can all be effectively utilized. Compared to crystalloids, colloids will usually result in less overall volume infusion, but significantly increase the cost.

Clinically, we do not directly measure afterload. At best, it is inferred from the changes in systemic vascular resistance. An elevated systemic vascular resistance results in ventricular dilatation with a concomitant increase in wall tension or afterload. The increased afterload significantly increases myocardial oxygen requirements. Systemic vascular resistance is calculated from the equation:

$$SVR = (MAP - CVP)/CO \cdot 80$$

Where SVR is systemic vascular resistance, MAP is the mean arterial pressure, CVP is the central venous pressure, and CO is the cardiac output. This can be indexed by substituting cardiac index for cardiac output. The normal values for SVR index (SVRI) = 500 to 800 $dyn \cdot sec \cdot cm^{-5}/m^2$.

Because systemic vascular resistance and systemic vascular resistance index are calculated values, anything that results in a low cardiac output will tend to cause these calculations to be elevated. Therefore, not all elevations of these parameters reflect an increase in afterload. Instead it may be a mathematical finding due to the reduced cardiac output. A high systemic vascular resistance associated with systolic blood pressures above 110 mm Hg usually means that the high systemic vascular resistance is a true value and follows intense primary vasoconstriction. On the other hand, high systemic vascular resistance accompanied by low blood pressure (< 110 mm Hg systolic) often points toward a primary problem with cardiac contractility. These patients do not have intense primary vasoconstriction, but only a calculated value due to the low cardiac output.

- *Information on systemic vascular resistance should be used cautiously because it is a derived value, rather than a directly measured value.*

Clinically, we do not directly measure cardiac contractility. There are no methods currently available to permit placement of a strain gauge on the myocardium. Instead, we generally presume altered contractility when cardiac output is depressed in the face of normal preload and afterload. Several different drugs are available to improve cardiac contractility. Those most often used and most reliable include epinephrine, dopamine, and dobutamine (Table 12–2).

Dopamine remains the most popular agent. This no doubt reflects its dose-response range. In most patients, beta or inotropic effects will occur between 4 and 12 μg/kg/min.[30] However, one must remember that this represents a bell-shaped response curve. Some patients, particularly the elderly, may have an improvement in contractility even at rates between 2 and 5 μg/kg/min. Other patients, particularly if young, may demonstrate ionotropic enhancement even at levels up to 30 μg/kg/min.[31] In my own practice, since dopamine relies upon release of norepinephrine, if patients do not respond appropriately at levels up to 12 μg/kg/min, I generally shift to another agent. Failure to respond often indicates depletion of norepinephrine, as can occur in a severely stressed patient.

Dobutamine has been promoted as an agent with both ionotropic and vasodilating properties.[32] The promotional literature also suggests that it will not increase heart rate. However, most clinicians would agree that dobutamine will often increase heart rate even as it improves cardiac output. The degree of vasodilatation will vary but may be more pronounced, particularly in patients already septic. Dobutamine works best in ranges between 5 and 15 μg/kg/min.

Table 12–2.
Vasoactive Agents

Drug	**Effective Dose Range (μg/kg/min)**	**Inotrope**	**Chronotrope**
Dopamine	3–15	yes	yes
Dobutamine	5–15	yes	yes
Epinephrine	0.01–0.5	yes	yes
Phenylephrine (Neo-synephrine)	0.1–8.0	no	no

• Epinephrine remains the most reliable inotropic agent.

Epinephrine remains the mainstay of inotropic therapy, particularly in the severely ill. Nonresponders to dopamine and dobutamine will ordinarily still increase cardiac output and blood pressure following epinephrine infusion. Although I normally start out at low ranges, between 0.01 and 0.02 μg/kg/min, it is not unusual to utilize doses as high as 0.5 μg/kg/min. I have gone even higher on occasion.

When the initial agent chosen has not been adequate and another deemed necessary, several methods are available to add that second agent. It is not advisable simply to stop the first and begin titration of the second. This will almost always result in a blood pressure and cardiac output reduction with possible detrimental results. Rather the second agent should be added and titrated until ultimately the desired response has been achieved. At that point, the first agent can be weaned back and removed. In the case of dopamine, I will almost always continue infusion in a low-dose, dopaminergic range of 2 to 4 μg/kg/min in an attempt to maintain renal perfusion.

• Strictly alpha-agonist agents have little role in the critically ill patient who requires an increase in oxygen delivery and cardiac output.

I see little if any role for any other agents, such as phenylephrine and norepinephrine. These agents primarily have alpha properties and as such are usually not effective agents to improve cardiac contractility. In the case of septic patients with vasodilatation and hypotension, they may on occasion be useful to maintain systolic blood pressures above 80 mm Hg. However, in no way should they be thought of as agents to improve contractility.

• Incremental doses of propranolol can effectively reduce heart rate without depressing cardiac contractility.

Fast heart rates, as previously stated, can produce ischemia and ultimately reduce cardiac output. Rates above 140/min will reduce ventricular filling times and also decrease cardiac output. Similarly, as heart rates increase over 100/min, myocardial oxygen requirements significantly increase. Often, it may be desirable to reduce heart rate. Beta blockade with continuous agents such as esmolol in doses of 50 mg, and propranolol given intermittently in 1-mg doses up to a total of 6 mg at any one time, will usually reduce heart rate without an alteration of cardiac contractility. This can and should be tested by calculation of stroke volume before and after administration of such agents. Stroke volume is almost always preserved or increased. Beta blockade may be contraindicated in some patients, such as those with reactive airway disease. Continuous infusion of the calcium channel blocker, diltiazem, in doses of 10 to 25 mg/hr will effectively slow heart rate without a reduction of cardiac contractility or development of bronchoconstriction.

METHODS TO REDUCE METABOLIC DEMANDS

• Although it is often advisable to reduce a fever, hyperthermia may in fact enhance the immune response.

Of late, attention has been directed at ways to reduce the metabolic demands rather than simply raise oxygen delivery to meet them. Fever causes an increase in oxygen consumption as much as 14% per 1°C elevation. In patients whose condition is marginal, this can be important. Such situations call for liberal use of antipyretics. Additionally, surface cooling can also be utilized. This may involve alcohol baths, surface ice on the patient, and the use of fans. However, care must be utilized to ensure that during the temperature reduction phase that shivering does not begin. Shivering will have the opposite of the desired effect and will probably worsen the situation. In fact, VO_2 may increase by 200 to 300%. Fever should be aggressively treated when temperatures are above 39°C (102.2°F).

As indicated, shivering should be avoided and stopped. Often, shivering will be gross and readily apparent. On other occasions, a hand placed on a large muscle mass of the patient feels the presence of fine tremors. Warming will ultimately reduce shivering, but often takes too long. In such situations muscle paralysis should be instituted. Once the patient is warmed, the muscle relaxant can be discontinued. Obviously, such patients require intubation and mechanical ventilation.

If patients are allowed to become hypothermic during surgery and anesthesia this may have serious repercussions in the postoperative state. The hypothermia usually results in intense vasoconstriction as blood is shifted from the periphery in an attempt to prevent further heat loss. In a patient with compromised cardiac function this vasoconstriciton may impede cardiac output. The result will be a cool patient with mottled extremities indicative of poor peripheral perfusion.

Rewarming causes vasodilation. If fluids are not rapidly infused, hypotension will ensue. The response will be further exaggreated if antihypertensives are used to either reduce the elevated systemic vascular resistance or systemic blood pressure secondary to the vasoconstriction.

Acidosis may often be noted. This can represent inadequate perfusion secondary to a reduced intravascular volume as vasodilation begins. At times, reperfusion during warming may cause washout and acidosis from tissue beds that were shut down during the intense vasoconstriction.

Agitation should also be actively treated. A patient who moves and thrashes about in the bed clearly elevates his or her metabolic demands. Several different agents are available to treat postoperative agitation. One must obviously examine the patient to ensure that the agitation is not due to inadequate pain relief, hypoxemia, pneumothorax, head injury, or some other correctable problems. Sedatives can be used either on an intermittent or a regular basis. I find midazolam quite satisfactory when given in incremental doses of 1 mg or a continuous infusion up to 4 mg/hr.[33] Propofol, a nonbenzodiazepine, is also administered by continuous infusion. The agent has a rapid onset and rapid dissipation of action when discontinued. It has become quite popular in the treatment of critically ill patients. Propofol does have some minor vasodilator properties evident at initiation of the infusion. Therefore, it should be used with caution in hypovolemic patients.

Some postoperative patients are clearly so sick that they remain in a marginal state. Despite all attempts, oxygen delivery may be barely adequate or inadequate to meet all metabolic demands. Under those circumstances, even if there are no other specific reasons it may be reasonable to paralyze and sedate the patient, at least initially. This will contribute to a further reduction in the metabolic oxygen requirement. The muscles of respiration, including the diaphragm, may consume as much as 20% of overall oxygen demands during this period.[34] Therefore, short-term paralysis may be of benefit until the situation has stabilized.

In conclusion, if a steady state is to be achieved, oxygen delivery must meet metabolic demands. Demands increase during sepsis. The ability to maintain a high delivery appears to result in an improved survival rate. When feasible, oxygen consumption should be reduced using the appropriate aids.

REFERENCES

1. Ganz W, Donoso R, Marcus HS et al: A new techique for measurement of cardiac output by thermodiluation in man. Am J Cardiol 1971; 27: 392–396.
2. Connors AF Jr, Dawson NV, McCaffree DR et al: Assessing hemodynamic status in critically ill patients: do physicians use clinical information optimally? J Crit Care 1987; 2:174–180.
3. Phang PT, Russell JA: When does VO_2 depend on DO_2? Respir Care 1993; 38:618–627.
4. Vermeij CG, Feenstra BWA, Bruining HA: Oxygen delivery and oxygen uptake in postoperative and septic patients. Chest 1990; 98:415–420.
5. Wilmore DW, Aulick L: Metabolic changes in burn patients. Surg Clin North Am 1978; 58:1173.
6. Shibutani K, Komatsu T, Kubal K et al: Critical level of oxygen delivery in anesthetized man. Crit Care Med 1983; 11:640–643.
7. Pavlin EG, Su JY: Cardiopulmonary pharmacology in anesthesia. In: Miller RD, ed: Anesthesia. New York, Churchill Livingstone, 1990; pp. 105–134.
8. Holcroft JW, Blaisdell FW: Shock: Causes and management of circulatory collapse. In: Sabiston DC Jr, ed: Textbook of surgery. Philadelphia, WB Saunders, 1991; pp. 4–56.
9. Weber KT, Janicki JS: The metabolic demand in oxygen supply of the heart: physiologic and clinical considerations. Am J Physiol 1979; 44: 726.
10. Slogoff S, Keats AS: Further observations on perioperative myocardial ischemia. Anesthesiology 1986; 65:539–542.
11. Joly HR, Weil MH: Temperature of the great toe as an indication of the severity of shock. Circulation 1969; 39:131.
12. Viale JP, Annat G, Lehot JJ et al: Relationship between oxygen uptake and mixed venous oxygen saturation in the immediate postoperative period. Anesthesiology 1994; 80:278–283.
13. Gallagher TJ: Unpublished data.
14. Weg JG: Oxygen transport in adult respiratory distress syndrome and other acute circulatory problems: relationship of oxygen delivery and oxygen consumption. Crit Care Med 1991; 19:650–657.
15. Buskirk ER, Hodgson J, Blair D: Assessment of daily energy balance: some observations on the methodology for indirect determinations of energy intake and expenditure. In: Kinney JN, ed: Assessment of energy metabolism and health and disease. Report of the First Ross Conference on Medical Research. Columbus, OH, Ross Laboratories, 1980; pp. 113–117.

16. Brandi LF, Grana M, Mazzanti T et al: Energy expenditure and gas exchange measurements in postoperative patients: thermol dilution versus indirect calorimetry. Crit Care Med 1992; 20:1273–1283.
17. Ronco JJ, Phang PT: Validation of an indirect calorimeter to measure oxygen consumption in ranges seen in critically ill patients. J Crit Care 1991; 6:36–41.
18. Landsberg L, Saville NE, Young JB: Sympathoadrenal system and regulation of thermogenesis. Am J Physiol 1984; 247:E181.
19. Roe CF, Goldberg MJ, Blair CS et al: The influence of body temperature on early postoperative oxygen consumption. Surgery 1966; 60: 85–92.
20. Ralley FE, Wynands JE, Ramsa JG et al: The effects of shivering on oxygen consumption and carbon dioxide production in patients rewarming from hypothermic cardiopulmonary bypass. Can J Anesth 1988; 35:332–337.
21. Ronco JJ, Fenwick JC, Tweeddale MG et al: Identification of the critical oxygen delivery for anaeorbic metabolism in critical ill septic and nonseptic patients. JAMA 1993; 270:1724–1730.
22. Hayes MA, Yau EHS, Timmins AC et al: Response of critically ill patients to treating and achieving supranormal oxygen delivery and consumption: relationship to outcome. Chest 1993; 103:886–895.
23. Yu M, Levy MM, Smith P et al: Effect of maximizing oxygen delivery on morbidity and mortality rates in critically ill patients: a prospective, randomized, controlled study. Crit Care Med 1993; 21:830–838.
24. Boyd O, Grounds RM, Bennett ED: A randomized clinical trial of the effect of deliberate perioperative increase of oxygen delivery on mortality and high risk surgical patients. JAMA 1993; 270: 2699–2707.
25. Curtis SE, Cain SM: Regional and systemic oxygen delivery/uptake relations and lactate flux in hyperdynamic, indotoxin-treated dogs. Am Rev Respir Dis 1992; 145:348–364.
26. Alter HJ, Purcell RH, Shih JW et al: Detection of antibody to hepatitis C virus in prospectively followed transfusion recipients with acute and chronic non-A non-B hepatitis. N Engl J Med 1989; 321:1494–1500.
27. Steffes CP, Bender JS, Levison MA: Blood transfusion oxygen consumption in surgical sepsis. Crit Care Med 1991; 19:512–517.
28. Greenburg AG, Elia C, Levine B: Hemoglobin solution and the oxyhemoglobin dissociation curve. J Trauma 1975; 15:943–950.
29. MacDonald R: Red cell 2,3,-diphosphoglycerate in oxygen infinity. Anesthesia 1977; 32:544–553.
30. Maestracci P, Grimaud D, Livrelli N et al: Increase in nephrotic blood flow and cardiac output during dopamine infusion in man. Crit Care Med 1981; 9:14–16.
31. Berk JL, Hagen JF, Tong RK et al: The use of dopamine to correct the reduced cardiac output resulting from positive and expiratory pressure: a two edge sword. Crit Care Med 1977; 5:269–271.
32. Shoemaker W, Appel P, Kram H et al: Comparison of hemodynamic and oxygen transport effects of dopamine and dobutamine in critically ill surgical patients. Chest 1989; 96:120.
33. Ronan KP, Gallagher TJ, George B, Hamby B: Comparison of propofol and midazolam for sedation in ICU patients. J Crit Care 1995; 23: 286–293.
34. Roussos C: Function and fatigue of respiratory muscles. Chest 1985; 88: 1245–1325.

CHAPTER 13

Post-Traumatic Head Injury

Robert J. Schultz
Kent S. Pearson

Case Report

A 17-year-old male was involved in a motor vehicle accident in which his compact car was struck head on by a semitrailer truck. He suffered extensive injuries, including head trauma, multiple facial and skull fractures, fractures of the radius and ulna of one arm, pelvic fractures, femur fractures on both legs, blunt abdominal trauma, and four fractured ribs with underlying lung contusions. At the scene, he was apneic and profoundly hypotensive. Initial resuscitation, including blind nasotracheal intubation, fluid resuscitation, and fracture immobilization was carried out at the local hospital before transfer for further evaluation and treatment.

On admission to our hospital, the patient had a blood pressure of 135/75 mm Hg, a pulse of 140/min, and oxygen saturation of 96% on 100% oxygen with controlled ventilation. He exhibited flexor posturing of the upper extremities and withdrawal of the lower extremities in reponse to noxious stimuli. His right pupil was 3.5 mm and reactive, while the left pupil was 6 mm and unreactive. A computed tomograph (CT) of the head revealed cerebral edema throughout and a small right frontal subdural hematoma (Fig. 13–1A). The Glasgow coma score was 7 at the time of admission, and intracranial pressure (ICP) measured with a fiberoptic intraparenchymal catheter ranged between 18 and 20 mm Hg.

The patient was admitted to the surgical intensive care unit (ICU) for monitoring and treatment. Because of the serious head injury, initial therapy was directed toward treatment of elevated ICP. It was decided that further management of the patient's fractures would wait until the acute cerebral edema resolved. Meaures to control ICP included fluid restriction, hyperventilation to a $PaCO_2$ of 26 mm Hg, and mannitol as needed to ensure an

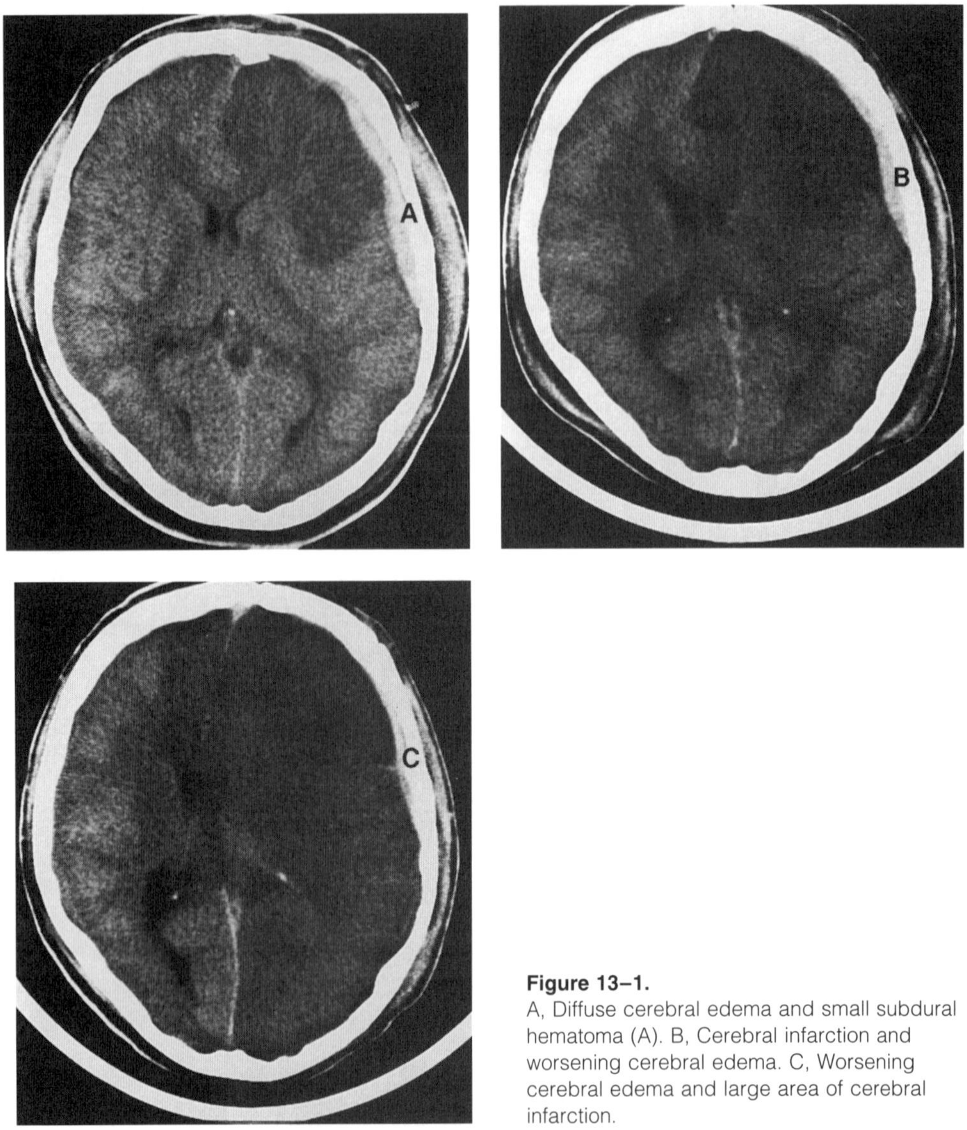

Figure 13–1.
A, Diffuse cerebral edema and small subdural hematoma (A). B, Cerebral infarction and worsening cerebral edema. C, Worsening cerebral edema and large area of cerebral infarction.

ICP of less that 20 mm Hg. With this therapy, the patient's condition stabilized for 6 hours. The patient developed a sudden episode of hypotension, with systolic blood pressure of 40 mm Hg and cerebral perfusion pressure of 15 mm Hg. He was treated with colloid and blood administration and an epinephrine infusion to achieve a blood pressure of 90 mm Hg. Repeat physical examination revealed no obvious source of hemorrhage, and transthoracic echocardiography did not demonstrate any evidence of pericardial tamponade. After stabilization, a repeat CT showed an early cerebral infarct and continued cerebral edema (Fig. 13–1B).

Within the next 2 days, the patient had high outputs of very dilute urine. Electrolyte determination showed diabetes insipidus, and aqueous pitressin was titrated to control his polyuria. In addition, the patient's ICP rose to 30 to 35 mm Hg in spite of maximal therapy. The decision to start barbiturates for ICP control was made. A pentobarbital infusion decreased the ICP to 15 to 17 mm Hg. The patient remained in this condition for 2 more days. Repeat head CT on the fourth hospital day showed worsening and progression of the cerebral infarcts (Fig. 13–1C). In spite of this maximal therapy with dehydration to a serum osmolality of 325 mOsm, hyperventilation to a $PaCO_2$ of 25 mm Hg, and 30 seconds of burst suppression on the electroencephalogram (EEG), clinical deterioration continued. In light of this deterioration, decision was made to stop aggressive therapy, and the patient met brain death criteria on the fifth day of hospitalization.

Contemporary society is fast paced and occasionally violent. Trauma is an unfortunate consequence of these facts. One of the most costly and potentially devastating injuries that a person may suffer is head trauma. Regardlesss of one's practice, all practitioners must be familar with at least the principles of initial patient evaluation and stabilization. Because of the high degree of invasive monitoring and labor involved in the care of critically ill trauma patients, it is likely that a significant percentage of trauma patients cared for in an average ICU will have some degree of head injury. This chapter will provide the reader with a review of the pathophysiology of head injury and then apply these physiologic principles to describe the interventions that may be required in the care of these severely ill patients.

Obviously, the magnitude of the head-injured patient population in an ICU depends on the unit's location and physician staffing patterns, but it is likely that virtually all critical care practictioners will be faced with head-injured patients at least occasionally in their practices. It is estimated that approximately 300 patients suffer head injury for each 100,000 population.[1] This would result in approximately 500,000 head injuries occurring annually in the United States. Andrews estimated that up to 20% of these injuries are severe.[2] Up to 2000 patients annually suffer from such severe injury that they are left in a persistent vegetative state.[3] Brain injury is also a common finding in patients who have died of traumatic injuries. Shackford and associates found that neurologic injuries caused death in 48% of their patients suffering from multiple trauma.[4] Injuries included cerebral contusion, skull fracture, subarachnoid hemorrhage, subdural hematoma, epidural hematoma, laceration, and secondary injury due to hypoxia or hypoperfusion.[4] Thus, the importance of dealing with such a large population of critically ill patients is clear. Aggressive intensive care of head-injured patients has been demonstrated to decrease both morbidity and mortality.[5] As discussed later in this chapter, it is often the goal of critical care physicians to provide support for the head-injured patient while performing maneuvers to limit any secondary injury that may take place in the postinjury period.

• *Following head injury, 2000 patients in the United States annually remain in persistent vegetative state; 48% of multitrauma deaths result from neurologic injury.*

MECHANISMS OF INJURY

The human brain is relatively well protected by floating in cerebrospinal fluid (CSF) and while enclosed in the rigid bony shell of the skull. The human's upright position with the head on the end of the mobile spinal column does, however, expose the brain to significant rotational, flexion extension, and shearing forces in the event of trauma.[6] Additionally, impact of the brain on the overlying bone can result in neuronal damage, tissue laceration, and tearing of blood vessels.[6] This type of damage is referred to as primary injury. The magnitude of this primary injury is an important determinant of the likelihood of ultimate survival.

Multiple forces can act on the brain to produce unconsciousness. These forces can be divided into static and dynamic forces, where static forces are those forces applied slowly (over > 200 msec), while dynamic forces are applied over a shorter time interval (over < 200 msec).[7] Static loading leading to injury is rare; dynamic loading is the most common cause of damage. This dynamic loading can be caused both by direct blows to the head or by sudden movement of the head in response to impact.[7] These forces can lead to a wide spectrum of injury that ranges from a brief episode of unconsciousness with no long-term residual effects to injuries so severe that the patient either dies or remains in a persistent vegetative state.

• *Rotational or diffuse axonal injury causes the most severe type of closed head injury.*

Rotational injury may cause diffuse injury throughout the brain. Animal models and human pathologic studies demonstrate the importance of this diffuse injury. The extent of postinjury dysfunction is correlated well with the degree of axonal damage.[8–10] This axonal injury is characterized by axonal beading and retraction balls.[11,12] This type of axonal impact is very important to determine the extent of permanent disability. Adams and associates demonstrated significant axonal injury in a large series of patients who died of head injury.[12]

CEREBRAL EDEMA

• *Vasogenic or interstitial edema more frequently develops after closed head injury than does cytotoxic or cellular edema.*

Primary damage to the brain cells at the time of injury is not the only cause of neurologic injury. Following injury, the damaged cells often develop edema that leads to cellular hypoperfusion and further worsening of cellular function. Cerebral edema represents an increase of water content within the brain. This edema can occur in one of two areas, either within the cell or within the extracellular space.[13] Cytotoxic edema refers to fluid that accumulates within the cells of the brain. This type of edema is often found after local cellular damage causes the cell to no longer be able to pump water from the cell. It may be present after many insults, including trauma or localized ischema.[14] In contrast, vasogenic edema results from from an ultrafiltrate of plasma into the cerebral parenchyma at a greater than normal rate.[13] This type of change follows injury at the level of the capillary. The types of edema are schematically illustrated in Figure 13–2.

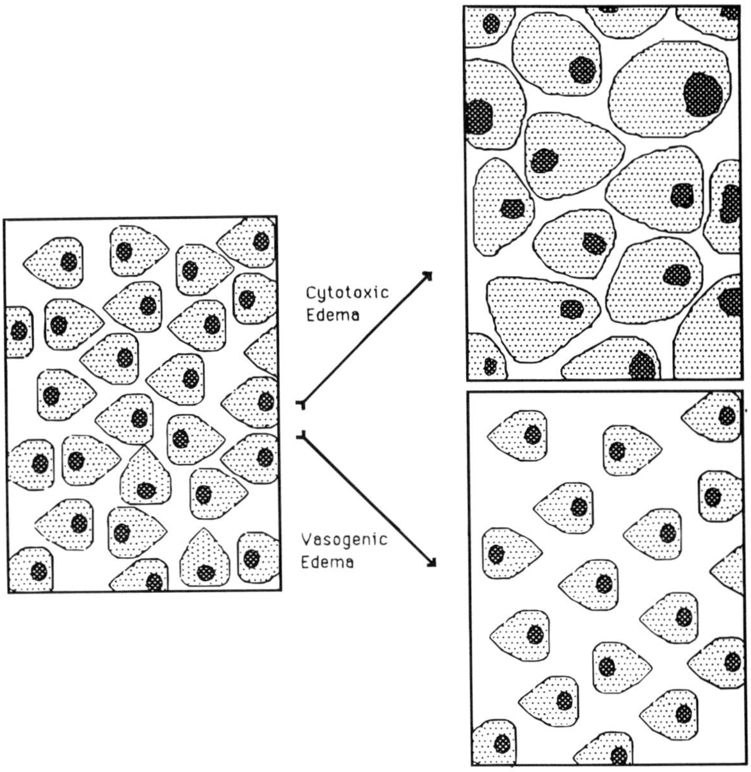

Figure 13–2.
Comparison of types of cerebral edema that develops after cerebral trauma. (From Rosner MJ: Pathophysiology and management of increased intracranial pressure. In: Andrews BT, ed: Neurosurgical intensive care. New York, McGraw-Hill, 1993.)

In terms of potential therapeutic options, cytotoxic edema can be thought of as being secondary to metabolic damage that would be difficult to treat, while vasogenic edema can be thought of as being secondry to more mechanical problems. These problems may be easier to address after injury. Of course these two processes often exist together, and the differentiation between them is artificial. The net result of the two processes is ultimately cell death if the edema continues untreated.

CEREBRAL BLOOD FLOW AND METABOLISM

A steady supply of energy is required for brain survival. The brain relies mainly on the aerobic oxidation of glucose to provide cellular energy.[15] If, for some reason, cerebral blood flow decreases, the brain will switch to anaerobic metabolism. This type of metabolism is much less efficient at providing energy than aerobic metabolism. It also results in the formation of lactic acid, which can cause cellular injury.[16] Much of the therapy applied to the head-injured patient involves limitation of factors that increase cell damage, coupled with simultaneous maintenance of cerebral blood flow.

• *Cerebral autoregulation may not remain intact following closed head injury.*

The brain has evolved a complex mechanism to *autoregulate* its blood flow. It achieves a constant blood flow regardless of the blood perfusion pressure that feeds the brain.[17] Generally, cerebral blood flow is regulated within the normal range of 50 ml/100 g/min as long as perfusion pressure is within the range of 50 to 150 mm Hg.[18] Autoregulation is probably due to intrinsic tone in the cerebral vessels themselves, with some modulation by the sympathetic nervous system.[18,19] This protective mechanism may be altered by head trauma, which leaves the brain vulnerable to additional injury due to inadequate blood flow in the post-trauma period.

The cerebral metabolic rate of oxygen utilization ($CMRO_2$) depends on cerebral blood flow. If the arterial-venous oxygen content difference ($Ca\text{-}vDO_2$) and cerebral blood flow are known, the $CMRO_2$ may be calculated by the following relationship:

$$CMRO_2 = CBF \times Ca\text{-}vDO_2 \tag{1}$$

where CBF = cerebral blood flow. Normal $CMRO_2$ is 3.2 ml/100 g/min.[20] Approximately half of this energy is required for synaptic function; 25% is required for maintaince of normal cellular sodium and potassium homeostasis, and the remaining energy is used for unknown processes.[21,22]

Several adaptive mechanisms exist for the maintenance of near-normal $CMRO_2$ in the face of injury. First, the normal $Ca\text{-}vDO_2$ gradient may be increased.[21] Second, cerebral blood flow may change while $Ca\text{-}vDO_2$ remains constant. This change in blood flow can come about in response to changed metabolic demands through metabolic autoregulation.[23] This regulation of cerebral blood flow takes place through alteration of the diameter of cerebral blood vessels, most probably the cerebral arterioles.[24] The release of vasodilator metabolites, perhaps adenosine or adenosine triphosphate, may cause metabolic regulation of blood flow.[21]

Changes in arterial CO_2 also cause significant change in cerebral blood flow. The cerebral arterioles dilate in response to increased CO_2 and constrict in response to decreased CO_2. Because of this response, $PaCO_2$ influences vascular resistance, cerebral blood flow, and cerebral blood volume.[25] Unlike other autoregulatory changes, the change of cerebral blood flow in response to CO_2 change is passive, rather than an active adaptation to stimuli. The clinical application of hyperventilation therapy is addressed later in this chapter.

• *CO_2 reactivity usually remains intact following head injury.*

The mechanisms necessary for regulation of cerebral blood flow may be altered after head injury. It is generally true that CO_2 reactivity remains intact after head injury.[26,27] Lost CO_2 reactivity indicates a poor prognosis.[28] This suggests that early after injury, manipulation of the patient's CO_2 could favorably influence cerebral blood flow and thus ICP.

In contrast to CO_2 responsiveness, autoregulation may be altered acutely after head injury. Response to changes in intracerebral pressure is often altered after injury. Several studies have shown that approximately half of patients with severe head injury may have abnormal cerebral autoregulation, as measured by response to infusions of vasopressors.[29,30] The presence or lack of autoregulation does not, however, appear to be a predictor of final outcome.[29,30] The cause of defective autoregulation is not apparent. One study did not demonstrate a relationship between the site of a lesion, as demonstrated by evoked potentials, and the presence of abnormal autoregulation.[31] Additionally, the duration of autoregulation loss after head injury is uncertain.

The ability of a patient to maintain autoregulation does have important implications for therapy following brain injury. For example, treatment of systemic hypertension could have different results, depending on the state of autoregulation present. If a patient with defective autoregulation is treated for hypertension, a direct decrease in ICP will result from decreased cerebral blood volume and decreased transmural pressure gradients. This assumes that baseline cerebral blood flow is adequate. However, without adequate baseline flow, cerebral ischemia may result. In contrast, with intact autoregulation, treatment of arterial hypertension lowers cerebral perfusion pressure and causes cerebral vasodilation. Coupled with increased cerebral blood volume, this can lead to increased brain stiffness.[30] Optimal treatment of systemic hemodynamics, therefore, would benefit from a knowledge of the state of autoregulation. If facilities for the measurement of cerebral blood flow, such as ^{133}xenon techniques, are available, it is possible clinically to assess the brain's response to induced alterations in cerebral blood flow. This will help determine the patient's state of autoregulation prior to initiation of therapy.[31,32] If such measurements are not available, the clinician must keep in mind the possibility that autoregulation may be defective and evaluate responses to therapy accordingly.

CEREBRAL COMPLIANCE

It is obvious that the brain may suffer multiple insults after injury and that the brain's ability to compensate for traumatic changes will partially determine the extent of a patient's injury. The brain is enclosed within the rigid skull, bathed in CSF, and fed with a rich blood supply. Because of this rigid container, the brain demonstrates limited ability to swell before permanent harm occurs. The concept that the craniocerebral axis represents a rigid container of fixed volume is termed the Monro-Kellie doctrine.[13] Because both brain tissue and CSF are noncompressible, any increase in volume of the intracranial space, such as with acute hematoma or edema, results in the rapid increase in pressure within the skull, as schematically illustrated in Figure 13–3. The focus of therapy in the critically ill head-injured patient is minimization of such pressure increases.

- *Because of the closed cavity, any brain swelling will result in a reduction of either blood or CSF volume within the intracranial vault.*

SECONDARY INJURY

Little can be done to salvage brain cells directly damaged at the time of an accident. The clinician can, however, attempt to minimize

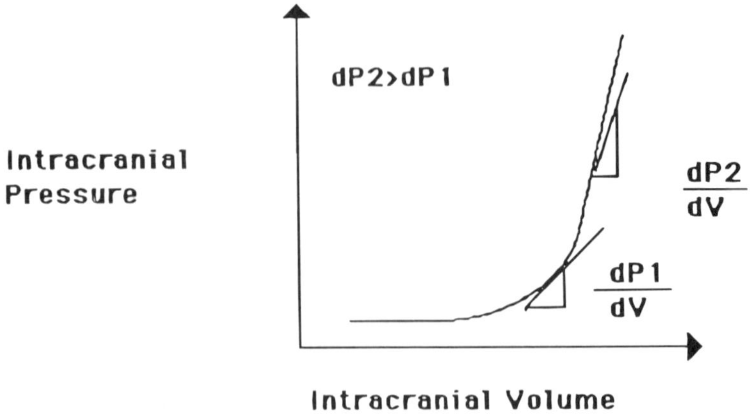

Figure 13–3.
Relationship of alterations of intracerebral volume in response to pressure changes.

• *Following closed head injury, the majority of efforts are directed at treatment of the secondary injuries that result from hypoxemia and ischemia.*

secondary damage that occurs as a result of intracranial or systemic insults. These insults include an expanding hematoma or cerebral edema. Hypoxic-ischemic cerebral injuries result from systemic causes, such as hypoxia, hypercarbia, hypotension, and acidosis.[2] The importance of secondary injury was recognized by Dandy over 50 years ago. He wrote: "The effects of injuries to the head are both immediate and late. During the stage of cerebral injury the first concern is for preservation of life; the second, for preservation of function. In acute stages, life is lost almost entirely because of intracranial pressure; and intracranial pressure is due to hemorrhage and edema."[33] Patients suffering from secondary injury have been shown to have worse outcomes than patients with a similar degree of brain injury, but free of secondary injury. This is true both when patients are admitted with hypoxia and hypotension[34] or develop hypotension after stabilization.[35] This worsening of injury has been linked to metabolic derangements that result in anaerobic glycolysis and the accumulation of lactate.[36] This observation is supported by the fact that cerebral blood flow measured early after injury demonstrated ischemia in severely brain injured patients, and mortality and the degree of residual damage were greatest in the group of patients with the lowest cerebral blood flow.[37] Clearly, the goals of intensive care should include the minimalization of any possible secondary insults after head injury.

• *Various neurotransmitters that are released following head injury may alter the blood-brain barrier permeability.*

Multiple mediators have been proposed in the propagation of secondary injury. Following head injury, there appears to be a release of a variety of neurotransmitters that cause changes in permeability of the blood-brain barrier, and altered receptor activation leads to altered intracellular signal transduction. This all culminates in pathologic damage to the brain cells.[38] This process is schematically represented in Figure 13–4. A variety of mediators have been proposed as responsible for the alteration of normal cellular physiology. These include, but may not be limited to, excitatory amino acids,[39] acetylcholine,[40] lactic acid,[41,42] endogenous opioids,[43,44]

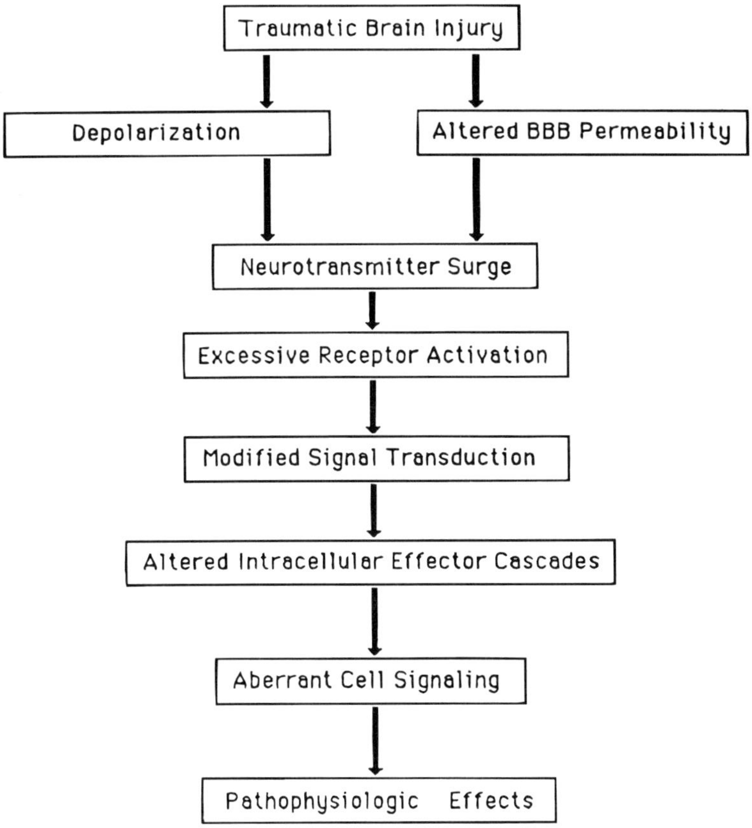

Figure 13–4.
Schematic illustration of brain mediator response following trauma. (From Lyeth BG, Hayes RL: Cholinergic and opioid mediation of traumatic injury. J Neurotrauma 1992.)

calcium,[45] bradykinin,[46,47] and free radicals.[48,49] The exact cascade of mediators remains under intensive investigation. When such a cascade is determined, clinicians may have access to specific agents to block injury propagation. Unfortunately, at present no specific therapy is available clinically.

INITIAL EVALUATION OF THE HEAD-INJURED PATIENT

Since the majority of head injuries are the result of some form of multisystem trauma, the initial evaluation requires diligent application of the principles of trauma resuscitation. The physician needs to avoid focusing on the needs of one system at the expense of overlooking life-threatening injuries or other injuries that will cause significant morbidity. It often requires a great deal of effort, as well as excellent communication skills, in order to appropriately prioritize the patient's problems and needs when each specialty consultant believes that his or her focus is the most important.

It is important to recognize that not even the best therapy aimed at saving a severely injured brain will be effective in an unstable patient. For this reason, the focus in the first minutes needs to be on the basics of resuscitation. Evaluation of the ABCs is most important.

Evaluation of the airway should include consideration of not only adequate ventilation and oxygenation, but also of the patient's level of consciousness. When in doubt, it is always better to secure the airway by endotracheal intubation than to risk aspiration of gastric contents or secondary injury to the central nervous system secondary to hypoxia or hypercarbia.

• *Most head-injured patients will require intubation to prevent risk of aspiration.*

There are multiple indications for endotracheal intubation. These include loss of ventilatory drive, loss of the ability to maintain a patent airway, and loss of protective airway reflexes. Therapeutic indications for intubation are not limited to hyperventilation for acute management of ICP or to tracheal access for pulmonary hygiene. Any unresponsive patient probably should be intubated in order to ensure optimum levels of oxygenation and ventilation. It will also assure a patent, protected airway.

Head-injured patients can have multiple problems that make endotracheal intubation difficult. Most patients with head injury will have had insufficient evaluation to rule out injury to the cervical spine. Furthermore, maxillofacial trauma can result in swelling or distortions of the oral, pharyngeal, and laryngeal structures. This makes visualization of the airway by direct laryngoscopy difficult and positive pressure ventilation by mask airway also difficult or impossible. Blood or secretions in the airway also impair visualization. The possibility of a basilar skull fracture raises questions about the appropriateness of nasal techniques. All of these issues make the choice of technique for intubation problematic, with few, if any, clearly defined rules to follow. Similarly, there are few absolute contraindications to the various techniques. The decision requires clinical judgment based on the situation presented.

Two principles are important. First, airway management in these patients should be the responsibility of the available person with the most experience in this field. The management of these airways might require complex techniques for intubation,[50] and should be performed by an anesthesiologist, intensivist, or emergency room physician with previous training in the management of difficult airways. Second, it is important to remember that the singular objective is to obtain a secure airway. A strong association exists among hypoxemia, head injury, and poor outcome. For this reason, any approach that secures the airway quickly and safely is acceptable. A search for the ideal method based on cerebrovascular effects often promotes delay, further hypoxia, and secondary brain damage.

• *There is no best method to secure the airway. However, speed is of the essence in order to prevent the devastating effects of hypoxemia on secondary brain injury.*

The selection of awake intubation or a standard or modified rapid sequence induction is dictated by the individual clinical situation. While it may be theoretically better to perform an awake intubation in patients with cervical spine injury, an uncooperative patient who thrashes about may indeed do more damage than a careful direct laryngoscopy in an anesthetized patient. Similarly, while an anesthetized patient may better tolerate intubation in regard to intracranial hypertension, loss of the airway following anesthetic induction will clearly do more damage than brief hypertension in response to an awake technique. Careful assessment of the situation and a flexible response are key points.

Through the years, succinylcholine, because of its effects on ICP, has been labeled as contraindicated in head-injured patients. This is a moot point and should not be a factor in the decision-making process. The effects on ICP are quite transient. Furthermore, they are likely insignificant when considered in the context of the clinical use of succinylcholine. In the setting of a rapid sequence induction, succinylcholine is combined with a rapid-acting intravenous anesthetic agent, and all such agents, except ketamine, lower ICP. This will thus attenuate the effects of the succinylcholine. In addition, the effects of ongoing hypoxia or hypercarbia are much more detrimental. Therefore, the ability provided by succinylcholine to facilitate the clinician's rapid control of the airway may make its use desirable. Some would argue that by use of the priming principles, nondepolarizing muscle relaxants can be used for a rapid sequence induction. However, the prolonged effect from this dosing method, combined with the potential for unanticipated difficulty during intubation, contraindicates the use of such agents.

- *Succinylcholine has transient and minimal effects on ICP elevation. If the intubation is difficult, nondepolarizing muscle relaxants may unnecessarily prolong the block and cause airway management to be more difficult.*

At times, severe maxillofacial injuries may make endotracheal intubation by any means difficult or impossible. Percutaneous cricothyrotomy with commercially available kits can rapidly provide airway access. They can then be converted to a formal tracheostomy.

After establishment of a secure airway, the circulation stabliza-tion assumes the highest priority. A large percentage of severe head injuries develop hypotension at some point early in the course of care. These hypotensive episodes have been linked to eventual poor outcome by several investigations.[51] They may lead to secondary injury, which compounds the primary insult to the central nervous system. There are very few if any intracranial injuries that directly cause hypotension, therefore systemic causes should be aggressively sought. Again, attention to the basics of trauma resuscitation is most important in order to detect a potentially correctable life-threatening injury.

- *Closed head injury rarely causes hypotension.*

Frequently, these patients have significant blood loss associated with injuries that do not appear to be severe. Scalp lacerations, long bone fractures, and pelvic fractures will cause a significant blood loss. Use of diuretics such as mannitol and furosemide in order to provide cerebral dehydration can further contribute to hypovolemia and hemoconcentration. The onset of hypotension can sometimes be very sudden, as these patients tend to be young and can compensate for large volume loss before supine hypotension develops. The hypotension can coincide with the administration of medications or anesthetics used for endotracheal intubation or the onset of positive pressure ventilation.

The focus of the initial resuscitation should be to return the patient to a euvolemic state. There has been considerable dogma passed down through the years in regard to appropriate fluid management. Much has led to misunderstandings regarding the goals of therapy. The following will summarize the current approach to the fluid management of these patients.

Fluid Management

In order to understand the fluid management of the head-injured patient, it is important to understand the factors that control cerebral blood flow, intracranial volume, and ICP and that are affected by fluid management. ICP control is attempted by minimizing intracranial volume and edema formation while striving to maintain adequate levels of cerebral perfusion. The most important variable to control is the serum osmolality. Changes in the total sodium load or colloid oncotic pressure have little effect.[52,53]

- *Intracranial fluid movement is principally controlled by osmolality.*

Osmolality, a physical property of solutions, is a function of the number of particles present in solution. It is a reference to the osmotic pressure that a solution produces toward the movement of solvent across a semipermeable membrane. In vivo, the solvent is water while the membrane can be vascular endothelium or cell membrane. The osmotically active substances include the normal electrolytes, glucose, urea, and serum proteins, as well as exogenous molecules such as mannitol, glycerol, or ethanol.

Osmolality has the largest effect on cerebral fluid shifts. The reason lies in the pore size difference present in the cerebral vasculature. In the cerebral capillaries, the apparent pore size of 8 angstroms differs markedly from the 65-angstrom apparent pore size of the systemic capillaries.[54] What this means is that while electrolytes such as sodium can easily equilibrate across the capillary endothelium elsewhere in the body, they are effectively excluded by the vascular endothelium in the brain. Instead, they can act to produce osmotic gradients by changes in their concentration across the endothelial membrane.

While colloid oncotic pressure is a significant factor in the production of peripheral edema, it does not appear to affect the production of cerebral edema.[53,55,56] The reason has to do with the relative permeabilities as noted previously. In the systemic capillaries, the small molecules present in high concentrations equilibrate across the membrane, and therefore, only the large molecules responsible for the colloid oncotic pressure can exert effects on fluid translocation. Large reductions in colloid oncotic pressure therefore favor fluid movement into the interstitium. In the normal brain, the small molecules such as serum electrolytes are present in much higher concentrations than the colloid molecules. Since osmolality is a function of the number of particles, and not their size, the effect of the colloid particles becomes negligible. It has been estimated that the normal total colloid oncotic pressure of about 20 mm Hg is equivalent to about 1 mOsm/kg. Furthermore, the extracellular space is very noncompliant in normal brain leading to resistance to expansion in excess of peripheral tissues. Therefore, even a 50% reduction in colloid oncotic pressure has negligible effect on free water accumulation in normal brain.

- *The oncotic pressure has little effect on brain fluid movement.*

These effects have been well described in normal and damaged brain tissue. In damaged tissue, the blood-brain barrier becomes permeable to even the colloid molecules, as demonstrated in animal models by the extravasation of albumin-bound Evans blue dye. In these areas of the brain, neither osmotic nor oncotic gradients can be established. Thus, the tissue water content can be neither increased nor decreased by manipulation of the osmolality or colloid oncotic pressure.

These findings lead to the conclusion that isotonic crystalloid infusions used in the resuscitation of trauma victims will not lead to exacerbations of cerebral edema *as long as appropriate serum osmolality is maintained.* However, those fluids commonly thought of as isotonic are, in reality, slightly hypotonic. For example, a liter of Ringer's lactate lists the calculated osmolality of 273 mOsm/L. This is a theoretical value based on the amount of solute in the solution. Because of molecular interactions within the solution, the actual measured value is 246 mOsm/L. Therefore, Ringer's lactate is not really isotonic, but indeed slightly hypotonic. Therefore, in situations when large amounts of Ringer's lactate are administered for resuscitation, serum osmolality will fall. The reduced osmolality will lead to increased accumulation of free water in the brain and increased ICP.

- *Ringer's lactate is not an isotonic fluid.*

Normal saline is closer to isotonicity than Ringer's lactate, but is hyperchloremic and raises concerns over aggravation of acidosis. A potential solution is hetastarch, which is slightly hypertonic and an excellent volume expander. However, because of concern over the development of coagulation defects, hetastarch should be limited to 20 ml/kg per 24-hour period. It is the measured osmolality however, and not the colloid nature, that gives hetastarch its advantage over crystalloid solutions.

It is important to point out that the data listed are heavily weighted with animal studies that used cryogenic lesions over time periods less than 24 hours. These experiments assume that the model is applicable to humans with head injury. However, as the blood-brain barrier repairs itself, colloid oncotic pressure may have a significant effect. Thus, while crystalloid solutions appear safe, it is probably best to avoid excessive dilution of colloid proteins.

- *Isotonic solutions may be best if the blood-brain barrier remains intact. However, following head injury, if the integrity of the blood-brain barrier is unknown, colloid solutions with high sodium content may be preferable.*

Neurologic Examination

After the appropriate steps have been taken to support the airway and circulation, a more thorough evaluation of the patient's other injuries can be undertaken. At this point, a neurologic examination can be performed. It is neither practical nor possible to perform an entire neurologic examination in all of its subtle detail in the patient with a recent head injury and multiple other serious injuries. In the comatose patient, the examination revolves around assessment of the level of consciousness, evaluation of external signs that might be clues to more serious injury, evaluation of motor responses to external stimuli, and evaluation of brain stem responses. Focal neurologic injuries are sought by comparison of responses between sides and by impairment of brain stem reflexes.

If patients are awake at the time of examination, the presence or absence of post-traumatic amnesia should be sought. Generally, amnesia will persist longer than confusion, and even short periods of amnesia are signs of diffuse brain injury. In patients who are comatose, attempts should be made to determine whether the patient was awake and speaking at some time after the accident. If they were awake at some time after, then diffuse impact injury can be excluded and some secondary cause for the current condition must be sought. Eighty percent of these patients have a mass lesion that potentially will require surgery.[57] It must be emphasized that the level of consciousness will vary with the degree of hemodynamic stability. Even neurologically intact patients will develop impairment of consciousness associated with poor perfusion. Therefore, any assessment of the neurologic condition should be repeated once the patient has been adequately resuscitated.

- *Patients awake immediately after head injury do not have a diffuse impact injury, but usually some secondary cause for their later mental status changes.*

The Glasgow coma scale,[58] developed in 1974, has become a standard tool in the assessment and description of the level of consciousness in patients with neurologic injury. It assigns a numeric score to the best response of the patient in each of three areas, including motor activity, eye opening, and vocalization. The scale has been useful because of its simplicity and unambiguous nature, allowing multiple health care providers of different backgrounds to evaluate patients and obtain consistent results.[59,60] The numeric score for each response is listed in Table 13–1. It should be noted that the patient's response often fluctuates at the time of the examination. Therefore, the best response is recorded. The three individual scores are added, to give a total score that ranges from 3 to 15; however, all three scores are significant and should be reported, as opposed to simply the total.

While the total from the Glasgow coma scale is a useful snapshot of the patient's level of consciousness, the description should not end there. Often, the best and worst responses are significant, especially in the evaluation of motor response. Focal neurologic injury can cause differences between the right and left side, as well as between the upper and lower extremities. One should record the stimulus used to elicit the response, such as direct nail bed pressure, sternal rub, or pressure on the supraorbital notch, and the extent of the response. The more accurately the information can be recorded, the easier it will be to follow the patient for changes in neurologic status over a period of hours to days, particularly with multiple examiners.

During assessment of the level of consciousness, external signs of more severe injury should be sought. Bruises and lacerations should be noted. Signs of basilar skull fracture should be sought. These include CSF rhinorrhea, CSF otorrhea, hemotympanum, bilateral periorbital hematoma, or mastoid hematoma (Battle's sign). Each of these can be a clue to the presence of a significant skull fracture, which causes a 20- to 30-fold increase in the risk of intracranial hematoma.[61] Care should be taken to evaluate these injuries

- *A skull fracture increases the likelihood of intracranial hematoma 20- to 30-fold. Almost all patients with any impairment of consciousness require a CT scan.*

Table 13–1.
Glasgow Coma Scale

Motor response	
Obeying commands	6
Localizing response	5
Withdraws from noxious stimulus	4
Flexor response	3
Extensor posturing	2
No response	1
Verbal Response	
Oriented	5
Confused conversation	4
Inappropriate speech	3
Incomprehensible speech	2
No verbal response	1
Eye Opening	
Spontaneous	4
In response to speech	3
In response to pain	2
None	1

and not allow impairment of consciousness to be attributed to other less serious conditions such as concomitant intoxication. One study from 1976 reported that 10% of patients with a significant traumatic intracranial hematoma were initially considered to have suffered a stroke, and a similar percentage were considered intoxicated.[62] All patients with impairment of consciousness should undergo CT scanning.

Evaluation of brain stem function is undertaken next and is heavily dependent on the eye examination (Table 13–2). The eyes

Table 13–2.
Brain Stem Examination

Eye Finding	Area of Involvement or Drug
Miosis	Pontine Opioids Metabolic
Horner's syndrome	C-spine Carotid sheath
Mydriasis	↓ Cerebral perfusion Atropine Scopolamine
Absent light response	Oculomotor nerve injury
Tonic horizontal deviation	Eyefields Pons
Skew Deviation (ventricle)	Brain stem
Oculocephalic (doll's eyes)	Pons Vestibular nuclei Oculomotor nerve Abducens nerve
Caloric testing	Pons Vestibular nucleus

are observed for size and reactivity of the pupils as well as any differences. Other parameters include position, movement, and vestibulo-ocular reflexes. Peripheral nerve, muscle, and bone injuries can influence eye findings in head injury, as can various drugs administered during resuscitation. All findings must be considered in terms of the entire clinical picture, without focusing on isolated issues, such as dilated pupils, which might stand out as inconsistent with the remainder of the examination.

The pupils are first carefully examined for size and equality. Bilateral small pupils can be caused by pontine lesions, drugs including opioids, and certain metabolic encephalopathies. Small pupils may represent an early sign of central cephalic herniation. A unilateral, small pupil may be caused by a traumatic Horner's syndrome due to interruption of sympathetic innervation anywhere along the outflow from the brain, spinal cord, or sympathetic pathways in the neck. Ipsilateral ptosis serves as a clue to the presence of a Horner's syndrome and should prompt a search for causes, especially injury to the cervical spine or carotid sheath, both of which require immediate evaluation. The ciliospinal reflex, which consists of ipsilateral pupillary dilation caused by painful stimuli delivered to the body, can be used to determine the location of the lesion causing traumatic Horner's syndrome. The ciliospinal reflex is present in preganglionic lesions and absent in postganglionic lesions.

Mydriasis, as with miosis, can be either bilateral or unilateral. Bilateral mydriasis without reaction to light implies inadequate cerebral perfusion. Atropine and scopolamine, either administered for resuscitation or as adjuncts to anesthetics, can cause significant bilateral mydriasis, with a blunted response to light. This can lead to incorrect conclusions about cerebral perfusion. The use of a strong light, a dark room, and a magnifying lens such as that found on an ophthalmoscope may help to make the distinction between a nonreactive and a sluggish pupil. Unilateral mydriasis can be caused by direct trauma to the globe, damage to the ipsilateral oculomotor nerve, or by ipsilateral uncal or temporal lobe herniation.

Of note is the phenomenon of hippus. Hippus is an oscillation in the size of the pupil when stimulated with light. The presence of hippus is a normal variant and indicates preservation of the sympathetic and parasympathetic pathways.

Light response, as with pupillary size, can be affected both by injuries to the brain and brain stem, or by cranial nerve damage. Damage to the optic nerve leads to a pupil that constricts with illumination of the contralateral pupil, but does not react to direct illumination. This condition is confirmed with the swinging flashlight test. The light is first directed at the affected pupil, then moved directly to the contralateral pupil which causes constriction of the affected pupil. When the flashlight is moved directly back to the affected pupil, there is loss of consensual response and the appearance of dilation. Damage to the oculomotor nerve will lead to an absent light response on both direct and consensual stimulation.

Further information about brain stem function can be obtained from ocular movement examination. First, the resting position of the eyes should be noted. Tonic deviation of the eyes in either horizontal gaze implies a lesion that affects either the ipsilateral frontal eye fields or the contralateral pons. Skew deviation, in which the patient demonstrates divergence of vertical gaze, implies damage to the brain stem. However, localization of the lesion is not possible. Divergence in the horizontal plane is a nonspecific finding either due to coma or induction of anesthesia.

If comatose patients have no ocular deviation on the initial examination, the ocular motions can be investigated by evaluation of the oculovestibular response. Either the oculocephalic maneuver or caloric testing can be used. These diagnostic interventions test the function of horizontal gaze. Loss of horizontal gaze in a comatose patient indicates significant injury and requires urgent evaluation. In the oculocephalic maneuver, the cervical spine is first evaluated to establish that it has not sustained an injury. Once this is established, the patient's head is positioned 30° above the horizontal plane and rotated from side to side. With the intact response, the patient's eyes will maintain a forward gaze, adjusting for the rotation of the head as if fixed on an object. This indicates that the pathway controlling the response is intact from the semicircular canal, through the pons, vestibular nuclei, oculomotor nuclei and nerves, and abducens nuclei and nerves.

In patients with impaired response to the oculocephalic maneuver, caloric testing can be performed to confirm the finding. Some patients with impairment of the oculocephalic response will have intact caloric testing. In order to perform this test, first the external auditory canal must be cleared of obstructing debris, and the tympanic membrane evaluated for evidence of perforation.

Calorics should not be performed if there is evidence of dural perforation. Otherwise, in the event of a basilar skull fracture, contaminants can be forced into the brain. With intact membranes and cervical spine, the patient's head is again elevated 30°, and cold water is flushed into the external canal. A temperature gradient is established in the endolymph. This causes nystagmus in the awake patient, with slow deviation toward the tested side, and in the fast phase returning toward the midline. In the comatose patient, depression of the reticular activating system that controls saccadic eye motion results in loss of the fast phase and therefore tonic deviation of the eyes to the affected side. The response usually occurs within 1 minute of irrigation, and loss of the response can be due to injury to the labyrinthine system, neural pathways within the brain stem, or cranial nerves involved. Performance of bilateral warm and cold calorics can rule out unilateral injury to the semicircular canals.

- *Caloric testing should not be performed in the presence of tympanic membrane perforation. This can lead to infection, particularly if the patient has a basilar skull fracture.*

Evaluation of motor response requires some standardization in approach in order to obtain reproducible results. First, the patient is prompted with verbal instructions. Care must be taken to evaluate motor function in the cranial nerves as well as in the body. Injuries to the cervical spine can give the appearance of a nonresponsive patient when, in fact, the patient may have no cranial nerve injury but only loss of facial muscle control. For patients unable to respond to verbal stimuli, application of deep nail bed pressure with a pen,

- *Cervical spine injury can impair the motor portion of the neurologic examination.*

reflex hammer, or some other object will provide a reproducible stimulus. For patients unresponsive to these stimuli, application of pressure in the supraorbital notch can evaluate motor response in a patient paralyzed by a cervical spine injury.

Motor responses can be characterized as intact, purposeful, semipurposeful, or abnormal posturing. Intact responses appropriately follow simple commands. Purposeful responses consist of brisk and full withdrawal of the affected limb away from the stimulus or movement of the contralateral limb across the midline in response to pain. When stimuli are applied to the head, the limb should be flexed which will bring the hand above the level of the shoulder. Semipurposeful responses are of the same nature but are incomplete. These include slow, incomplete withdrawal, or failure to reach across the midline or above shoulder level. Abnormal posturing can be either decorticate or decerebrate. Decorticate posturing consists of adduction of the shoulders, flexion of the elbows and wrists, adduction and extension of the legs. Decerebrate posturing includes adduction of the shoulders, internal rotation of the arms, extension at the elbow, adduction of the legs with extension at the knee, and plantar flexion at the ankle.

MONITORING THE CENTRAL NERVOUS SYSTEM

For many years, the only practical measure used to monitor the central nervous system was the neurologic examination. Over the last 30 years, ICP monitoring has gone from an experimental technique to a standard of care. Monitoring of venous oxygen saturation from the jugular bulb is currently under development and shows promise as a potential improvement in monitoring technique.

Intracranial Pressure Monitoring

Monitoring of ICP has been accepted as standard practice in the management of patients with severe head injury. It is used in combination with CT scanning and frequent neurologic examination to guide the management of these patients.

While measurement of ICP was described in 1951,[63] the most widely known early description was by Lundberg in 1960.[64] Lundberg described the use of ventricular catheters to monitor ICP in 143 patients. This investigator systematically described the variations of the pressure waves over time, as well as documenting the risks and relative safety of the procedures involved. By 1964, Lundberg and colleagues had monitored 368 patients using ventricular catheters, as well as 30 patients with traumatic brain injury.[65]

Although ICP monitoring is now routine in most modern day ICUs, its use has not been without past criticism. Proponents of monitoring argue that elevations of ICP are associated with poor outcome, and only with actual knowledge of the ICP can one aggressively treat elevations and hope to improve outcome. Clinical signs such as bradycardia, hypertension, dilation of the pupils, and abnormal motor posturing may be absent when the ICP is elevated and can be present with normal ICP. Therefore, such signs are unreliable indicators of intracranial hypertension.[66] Furthermore, since many of the therapeutic options provide diminishing effectiveness, one needs accurate assessment of the ICP such that interventions can be timed in order to maximize their benefits.

Critics have argued that the correlation between elevated ICP and poor outcome simply represents an association, and not a cause and effect phenomenon. They argue that marked elevations merely indicate more severe underlying injuries. Thus, the severity of those injuries, and not the elevation of the ICP, leads to the poor outcome. Furthermore, they argue that monitoring of the ICP has never been definitively shown to improve outcome, but does carry definite risks to the patient.

The indications for placement of an ICP monitor will vary among neurosurgeons, but several general principles exist. First, ICP monitoring is not necessary in patients who can follow simple commands. These patients can be adequately followed by frequent neurologic examinations. In those who cannot follow simple commands, ICP monitoring is limited to patients likely to have elevations in ICP, and not in those in whom elevated ICP is unlikely. In those unable to follow commands, the next step proceeds to evaluation of the CT scan. Patients with abnormal CT scans who are unable to follow commands should have an ICP monitor placed. One study found that with normal CT scans, 98% had normal ICP through the first 24 hours, and 15% later developed increased ICP.[67] We recommend ICP monitoring when any of the following risk factors are present: age over 40, history of hypoxemia, or history of hypotension.[68] In patients with normal CT scans without the foregoing risk factors, ICP monitoring may be unnecessary. In those patients, however, repeat CT scanning should be performed at 24 hours after injury, or earlier if there is a decline in clinical status. The need for monitoring should then be reevaluated.

• *ICP monitoring should be reserved for patients with an abnormal CT scan or who are unable to follow commands.*

The normal ICP is less than 10 mm Hg. The measured value is not alone in importance, but must be evaluated in terms of the patient's intracranial compliance. Although not frequently used clinically, attempts to describe the intracranial compliance have included the volume pressure response[69] and the pressure volume index.[70] The volume pressure response is the rise in ICP which results from the injection of 1 ml of fluid over 1 second. Normal value varies between 0 and 2 mm Hg. The pressure volume index is the theoretic volume of fluid that would be required to produce a 10-fold increase in ICP. It is calculated as the volume of fluid injected divided by the log of the ratio of the initial to final ICP. The normal value for the pressure volume index is 22 to 30 ml. With poor intracranial compliance, the value of the pressure volume index is less than half the normal value. While not clinically used, these values are helpful concepts to understand intracranial compliance.

Lundberg defined three types of ICP waves: A, B, and C waves (Table 13–3). C waves are similar in appearance to the arterial pressure wave form and reflect minor variations in ICP based on

Table 13–3.
Brain Wave Forms

A: Plateau; ICP elevation
B: Respiratory cycle reflection
C: Arterial pressure wave

• *ICP A wave forms represent large decremental changes in pressure. They are usually related to changes in cerebral perfusion.*

arterial pressure pulsatility. B waves are slower oscillations occurring several times per minute and reflect changes in ICP due to the respiratory cycle. When marked, B waves can be a sign of decreased intracranial compliance. A waves, otherwise referred to as plateau waves, are abnormal, large elevations in the ICP over baseline. They persist from a few minutes to a half-hour, then abruptly end. They represent severe decrements of intracranial compliance and may reflect a response to decreased perfusion pressure. The cerebral vessels dilate in order to maintain blood flow. This leads to further increases in ICP and the development of a self-perpetuating cycle. At least one author has suggested that elevation of the systemic blood pressure in order to raise the cerebral perfusion pressure will break the cycle of plateau waves once started.[71]

Intracranial pressure measurements should be taken within the compartment of interest. The tentorium and the falx divide the intracranial contents into multiple compartments. Expanding mass lesions interrupt the free communication of CSF. This contributes to the development of pressure gradients among the individual compartments. These gradients can be significant and can lead to underestimation of the ICP if it is measured in the contralateral supratentorial compartment.[72] Similarly, lesions in the posterior fossa or in the temporal fossa can cause a significantly elevated intracompartmental pressure, yet not be detected by monitors in the supratentorial compartments.[73] Herein lies a weakness of current measurement techniques, and one should not be lulled into a false sense of security by a monitor that displays a relatively normal value.

There have been many devices developed to monitor ICP. They have been placed in many different locations, including intraventricular, subarachnoid, epidural, and intraparenchymal locations. Each has advantages and disadvantages.

The two most common forms of ICP monitors are the ventricular catheters and transducer-tipped fiberoptic systems. Because of performance limitations, the classic subarachnoid bolt has been largely replaced by the newer fiberoptic systems. Epidural systems, while popular in the past, are also rarely used due to performance limitations when compared to other systems.

Intraventricular Catheters

For years, the standard against which other methods of measurement have been compared has been the intraventricular catheter. In this method, following placement of a bur hole through the skull, a catheter is introduced into the lateral ventricle of the nondominant or nonaffected side, traversing the parenchyma of the brain. This method measures CSF pressure by connection of the lateral ventricle of the CSF via a continuous column of fluid to a pressure transducer located at a specified level, such as the external auditory meatus.

There are several advantages to intraventricular catheters. In addition to the measurement of ICP, this method also allows withdrawal of CSF in efforts to decrease ICP, or in the therapy of hydrocephalus before placement of a shunt. Furthermore, the ventricular catheter can be used to measure compliance of the intracranial compartment by injecting small volumes and measuring the ICP response.

There are also several disadvantages to ventricular catheters. These include infection, hemorrhage, and failure due to occlusion. They can also be difficult to place when the elevated ICP has produced ventricular narrowing or displacement. Accurate data collection requires that the transducer level be adjusted when the patient is moved. Nurses must be able to maintain the system and interprete the wave form.

The infection risk attributable to ventriculostomies has been estimated to be between 0 to 27%.[64,65,74–76] This is higher than any of the other methods used to monitor ICP. It can take the form of ventriculitis or meningitis. Factors that can lead to development of infection include intraventricular hemorrhage, neurosurgical operation, ICP higher than 20 mm Hg, ventricular catheterization for more than 5 days, and irrigation of the system.[76] Some clinicians recommend that the catheters be removed after 5 days and reinserted in a different site in order to minimize the infection risk. However, it is unclear whether this adequately accounts for the risks associated with the placement of a new catheter. Furthermore, it is unclear whether prophylaxis with parenteral antibiotics is beneficial. Many clinicians, however, initiate prophylaxis against the pathogens that commonly cause ventriculostomy-related infections. These clinicians argue that the potential severity of the infection justifies the risk.

- *Intraventricular catheters allow removal of CSF to help reduce ICP. They may increase the risk of infection or hemorrhage.*

The second major problem of intraventricular catheters is hemorrhage. This primarily relates to placement and can occur in epidural, subdural, intraventricular, and intraparenchymal locations. While normally a low risk, the incidence can be unacceptably high when a coagulopathy is present. For example, in the case of hepatic encephalopathy, the incidence can reach 20%,[77] frequently with devastating results. Every effort should be made to correct any coagulation defect before placement of an ICP monitor.

Failure of intraventricular catheters due to clot occlusion or ventricular narrowing due to tissue impingement on the catheter tip is a common occurrence. This can result in failure to identify rising ICP. This can usually be identified by an abnormal ICP wave form. Occlusion will also be indicated by the abrupt cessation of CSF drainage from the catheter.[78] In addition to occlusion, incorrect values are obtained if measurements are taken when the ventriculostomy system is opened to the drainage collection system[79] (Fig. 13–5). As a result, intraventricular catheters require more skill on

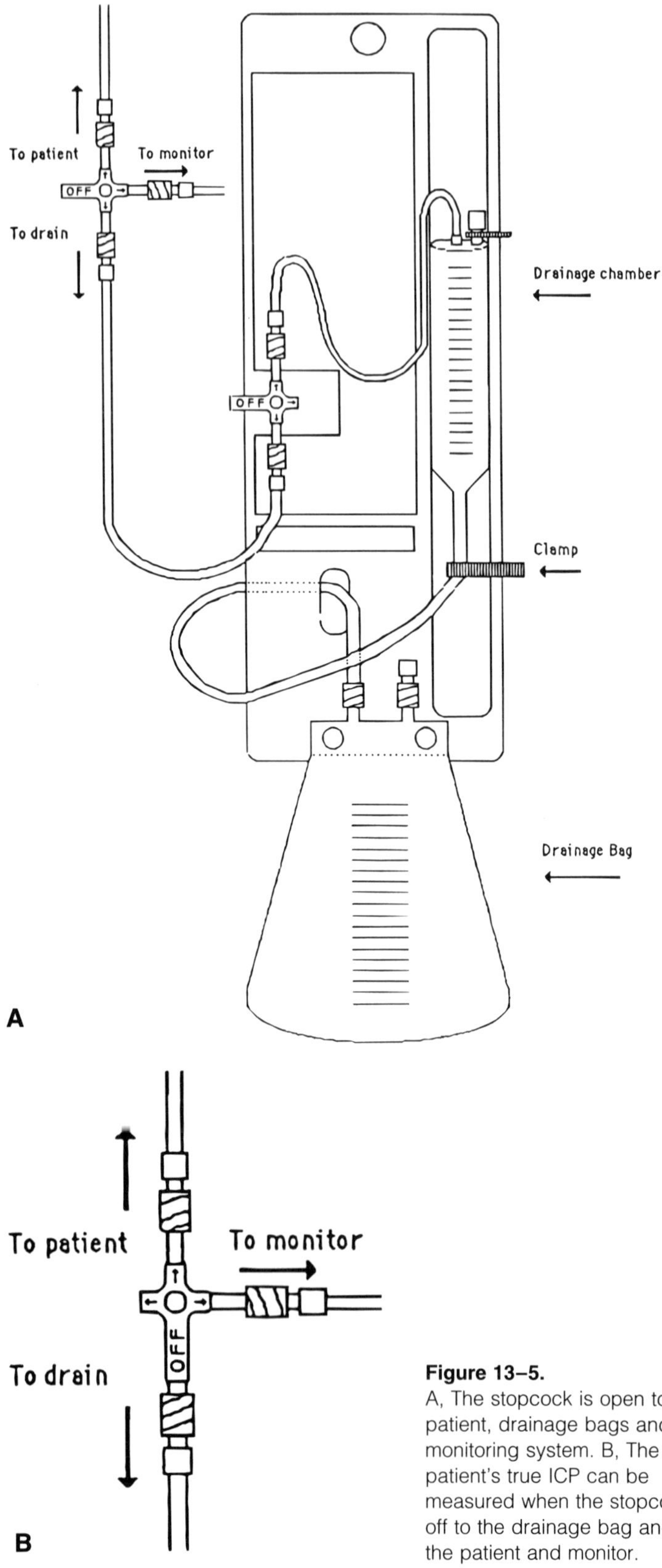

Figure 13–5.
A, The stopcock is open to the patient, drainage bags and monitoring system. B, The patient's true ICP can be measured when the stopcock is off to the drainage bag and onto the patient and monitor.

the part of the nursing staff than with other devices currently in use.

Transducer-Tipped Fiberoptic Catheters

Recent years have seen the proliferation of fiberoptic ICP monitoring systems (Camino Laboratories, San Diego, CA). These systems rely on transducer-tipped fiberoptic strands. ICP is determined by use of reflected light and a semirigid, mirrored membrane at the catheter tip. Pressure against the membrane causes alteration in the amount of reflected light returned by the fiberoptic strands. They can be placed in the ventricle or subdural space, but most often are located about 1 cm into the parenchyma of the brain. They are compact systems that, because of the location of the transducer in the tip, can accurately follow the ICP. The transducer does not require a new zero each time the head position changes. Since they are closed systems, the infection risk is lower than with ventriculostomy or Richmond bolt. As a result of the intraparenchymal location, these devices are easy to place in patients with narrowed ventricles. They are subject to the same risk of bleeding as ventriculostomies.

There are several disadvantages to intraparenchymal fiberoptic catheters. Since the transducer is at the tip, the system cannot be recalibrated once it is placed. This fact, coupled with the tendency for the system to drift, leads to significant errors in the measurement of ICP after several days. Some physicians recommend replacement of the system after 5 days. Drift averages about 0.6 mm Hg per day or about 2.1 mm Hg over 5 days. The maximum drift at 5 days in three sample catheters was 6 mm Hg.[80] Furthermore, unlike ventricular catheters, intraparenchymal fiberoptic catheters cannot be used to drain CSF. Last, the fiberoptic strands can break if mishandled which then require replacement of the entire system.

- *Once placed, transducer-tipped intraparenchymal catheters do not permit recalibration.*

Several studies have compared the values obtained from the fiberoptic system with those from ventricular catheters. Conflicting results have been obtained. Crutchfield and associates found good correlation with intraventricular catheters in dogs with experimental mass lesions.[80] Ostrup and colleagues found slight differences,[81] but Schickner and Young found significant elevations of the value obtained from the fiberoptic system relative to ventricular catheters.[82] These differences were sometimes as much as 40 mm Hg. These investigators found 66% of the measurements to be greater than those obtained from ventriculostomy and 21% to be lower.[82] Drift did not appear to be a factor in their trial. The authors speculated that the differences may in part reflect true differences in measured pressures between the two compartments in which the pressures were measured. Despite these few negative results, the system has gained acceptance as a reliable and accurate monitoring system.

- *Since they measure different compartments, there may not necessarily be close correlation between intraventricular and intraparenchymal catheters.*

Subarachnoid Bolt

Of historical note is the subarachnoid screw, often referred to as a Richmond bolt. This is a hollow tube which is placed through an opening produced by a twist drill or bur hole. It is a fluid-coupled system that links the fluid in the subarachnoid space to an external transducer. The transducer is leveled similarly to that of a ventricular catheter. The simple bolt shares the advantage of simplicity in placement with the intraparenchymal fiberoptic system. In some cases, it can be used to drain small amounts of CSF for decompression, but it is not as effective as a ventricular catheter.

There are several disadvantages to subarachnoid screws which have led to their decreased utilization as monitoring devices. First, they are easily obstructed by blood, debris, or by brain tissue itself. Ordinarily, the subarachnoid space is 2 to 3 mm deep. With edema formation, the space can be severely compressed, causing brain tissue to impinge on the bolt. This causes loss of coupling, wave form damping, and inaccurate ICP values. These effects can be most significant in patients with marked elevation in ICP and often cause significant underestimation of the ICP.

Jugular Bulb Venous Saturation Monitoring

A new experimental monitor that has shown some promise is venous oxygen saturation in the jugular bulb ($SjvO_2$). The technique involves percutaneous placement of a 4-Fr fiberoptic oxygen saturation catheter into the jugular vein ipsilateral to the most severely injured area of the brain. The catheter is then advanced to the level of the jugular bulb. Placement is confirmed radiographically.

With this system, the saturation of the venous effluent from the intracranial compartment can be continuously monitored. Analogous to the mixed venous saturation, the jugular bulb saturation provides a functional measure of cerebral oxygen supply relative to demand. The normal value for $SjvO_2$ is 65%,[83] and should be equal bilaterally.[84] Desaturation of the jugular venous blood implies that the level of cerebral perfusion is less than optimal for the given patient. This assumes that other system variables remain constant. These episodes of desaturation are not clinically detectable, nor are they prevented by maintenance of empiric cerebral perfusion pressure levels. For these reasons it is believed that monitoring the $SjvO_2$ will benefit patients by optimization of cerebral blood flow.

There are other causes of jugular venous desaturation beside cerebral blood flow effects. In one study, almost half of the episodes of jugular venous desaturation were artifactual. This necessitates that blood from the jugular catheter be drawn for analysis to confirm the value before initiating changes in therapy.[83] Other causes of desaturation include systemic hypoxemia and anemia, and these must be sought. Once these causes are ruled out, the level of cerebral blood flow can be addressed.

• *The $SjvO_2$ does not always provide continually reliable information on the status of brain metabolic function.*

There are limitations to the use of the catheter. Sheinberg and associates found that $SjvO_2$ did not change with increasing intracranial hypertension until signs of tentorial herniation were apparent.[83] Thus, $SjvO_2$ does not replace ICP monitoring, but instead serves as an adjunct. As mentioned, there were a large number of artifactual decreases in the value obtained from the fiberoptic catheter. No determination was made as to whether the catheter identified all episodes of desaturation. Furthermore, when cerebral blood flow falls to extremely low levels, the jugular bulb can be contaminated by extracerebral blood which leads to higher than expected values. This could be inappropriately interpreted as an indication of adequate cerebral blood flow.

There frequently is concern expressed about placement of lines in the jugular veins of patients with poor intracranial compliance. Potentially, the catheter might obstruct venous outflow, with a resultant rise in ICP. One study found no effect on ICP due to placement or maintenance of these catheters in the jugular bulb.[85]

Other Monitoring Modalities

In the past, therapy for severe head injury has been largely empiric, based on neurologic examination, CT findings, and ICP measurement. In recent years, the search has begun for other monitoring techniques that would provide information for therapy to control abnormal physiologic parameters.

Transcranial Doppler ultrasonography (TCD) can measure flow velocity in cerebral vessels, usually the middle cerebral artery. It is currently widely used for the evaluation of vasospasm following subarachnoid hemorrhage. Recently, studies have been undertaken to evaluate its potential as a monitor in traumatic brain injury. While the work is still in its infancy, some recent work with TCD combined with jugular venous oxygen monitoring and ICP measurement suggest that adequacy of cerebral perfusion pressure can be noninvasively monitored using middle cerebral artery flow velocity.[86,87]

- *TCD can provide reliable information on middle cerebral artery flow and cerebral perfusion pressure.*

Other past work evaluated somatosensory evoked potentials (SSEP), EEG, and cerebral blood flow measurements. SSEPs, initially believed to be promising, have not passed the test of time as a useful monitor.[88] Recent interest has focused on new methods of signal analysis and may result in a clinically useful monitor, but only time will tell. EEG is useful in the detection of seizure activity, but it is not sensitive enough to detect much of the clinically relevant regional ischemia present in head-injured patients. Last, cerebral blood flow measurement remains a useful research tool, but is not practical for widespread bedside use.

CONTROL OF THE INTRACRANIAL PRESSURE

Central to the control of ICP is control of the volume of the three compartments defined in the Monro-Kellie doctrine. These compartments include the CSF, intravascular volume, and brain tissue. Traditionally, control of these compartments has been achieved through maintenance of venous drainage, hyperventilation, cerebral dehydration, temperature control, seizure control, CSF drainage, and in severe cases, neuromuscular blockade and sedation. Barbiturates and surgical decompression via craniectomy or resection of contusion have been reserved for refractory cases with unacceptable ICP despite more conservative measures.

Venous Drainage

Appropriate attention to head position cannot be emphasized enough. It is the least invasive, has low risk, and is the most easily accomplished of the therapeutic measures available for treatment of intracranial hypertension. The head should be elevated between 15 and 30°[89] and maintained in the neutral position. Elevation of the head allows for free drainage of blood through the venous system. It prevents increases in the intracranial blood volume due to venous congestion. Similarly, maintenance of the head in the neutral position prevents stretch on the jugular veins, which leads to narrowing of these veins and impairment of venous drainage of the head. Since most of the intracranial blood volume is contained on the venous side of the capillaries, small increases in back pressure can lead to substantial changes in the vascular volume and the ICP.

In addition, care must be taken to avoid external compression of the patient's neck by items such as tape, electrocardiogram leads, or poorly fitting cervical collars. In a similar fashion, external pressure on the neck can lead to increased ICP through impaired venous drainage and venous congestion.

• When patients are kept in a head-up position, the arterial line transducer should be zeroed at the level of carotid bifurcation. This provides more accurate assessment of cerebral perfusion pressure.

Cerebral perfusion pressure will be affected by elevation of the head of the patient, reaching a maximum between 15 and 30° of elevation.[89] For a given level of arterial pressure, as the head is elevated, the pressure transmitted to the intracranial vessels will fall due to the effect of gravity on the column of blood. The effect of head elevation on venous drainage, however, should reach a maximum when the vertical distance from the right atrium to the intracranial venous sinuses is greater than the central venous pressure in centimeters of water. At that point, static pressure in the jugular veins falls to a minimum, and further elevation of the patient's head does not increase venous outflow further. However, intracranial arterial pressure continues to fall with further elevation. There may also be a contribution to a lower ICP by hydrostatic displacement of CSF from the cranial cavity to the spinal subarachnoid space resulting from head elevation. Again, this effect probably diminishes as the patient's head is elevated further. This means that maximization of cerebral perfusion pressure usually occurs between 15 and 30° of elevation. In patients with ICP monitors in place, this point can usually be easily determined.

Hyperventilation

Hyperventilation is a very effective therapeutic maneuver for the acute reduction of ICP through its ability to produce cerebral vasoconstriction. Indeed, the short-term use of hyperventilation can be lifesaving following detection of impending herniation. It is quick to take effect, and it is effective in all but the most traumatized of the population. The long-term use of hyperventilation is controversial, however, because of concern over the potential adverse effects of protracted cerebral vasoconstriction.

The mechanism of action of hyperventilation relates to the ability of carbon dioxide to diffuse out of the CSF because of a concentration gradient induced by the hyperventilation. This creates an alkalosis in the CSF, which, in turn, is a potent stimulus for vasoconstriction. The vasoconstriction reduces cerebral blood volume and thus causes a lowering of the ICP. Cerebral blood volume changes by about 0.05 ml/100 g tissue for each mm Hg change in the $PaCO_2$.[90] The lowered pressure will reduce the tendency for intercompartmental shifting of the intracranial contents due to pressure gradients, reducing the possibility of catastrophic herniation.

• The resultant CSF alkalosis from hyperventilation serves as the primary stimulus for cerebral vasoconstriction.

While hyperventilation can reduce the tendency toward herniation, its effects on regional blood flow are less certain. The hope is that, when ICP is lowered, marginal perfusion in regions with locally high tissue pressures will improve. However, globally hyperventilation reduces blood flow, and some regions will most certainly have reduced perfusion. This is supported by at least one study where cerebral blood flow, as measured by radioactive xenon, was reduced to below 20 ml/100 g tissue/min in multiple regions following hyperventilation.[91] Studies that measured jugular venous oxygen saturation have demonstrated venous desaturation when arterial carbon dioxide tension is lowered into currently recommended ranges.[83] It currently is unclear if this is harmful. Clearly there is not enough information at this time to draw conclusions in regard to regional blood flows and on whether some areas are adversely affected to a significant degree during hyperventilation.

• Hyperventilation may significantly reduce cerebral blood flow to the point of ischemia development.

Further problems occur due to compensation of the central nervous system for the alkalosis induced by hyperventilation. Over a period of 24 to 72 hours, the CSF pH returns toward normal.[92–94] This, in turn, causes a loss of vasoconstriction. Moreover, the cerebral blood vessels will demonstrate vasodilation beyond their baseline state when arterial carbon dioxide tension is returned toward normal and can produce an increase in ICP. Thus, the patient who has been chronically hyperventilated must be cautiously weaned when the decision is made to normalize arterial carbon dioxide tension. Neurologic decompensation can develop secondary to a rapid increase in cerebral blood volume and ICP.

Some investigators have attempted to utilize the buffer tromethamine (THAM), in order to avoid the loss of CSF alkalosis over time in the hyperventilated patient. Tromethamine is administered intravenously as a 0.3-mEq/ml solution, with a loading dose in milliliters equal to the patient's body weight times the base deficit necessary to raise the arterial pH to 7.6. This is followed by a maintenance infusion of 1 ml/kg/hr. Their results seem to indicate that tromethamine is effective in attenuating compensation by the CSF, thus allowing the maintenance of cerebral responsiveness to hypocapnia.[93]

• Tromethamine may effectively maintain CSF alkalosis and the resultant vasoconstriction.

Tromethamine and hyperventilation have been evaluated in a fluid percussion model of experimental brain injury in cats.[95] The authors concluded that tromethamine can effectively reduce tissue acidosis and ameliorate the adverse effects of hyperventilation. In a similar model, mortality at 7 days was significantly lower in tromethamine-treated cats than in those untreated.[96]

Because of concern of the effects of prolonged hyperventilation, a prospective comparison of hyperventilation with and without tromethamine versus normocapnic management was undertaken. Patients in the group that received hyperventilation without tromethamine were noted to have poorer outcome at 6 months than the other two groups, however at 1 year no differences were reported. The authors concluded that hyperventilation slowed recovery from severe head injury.[93] This was a small study, however, and generalization to clinical practice should await further confirmation.

What recommendations can then be made regarding the use of hyperventilation? Since it can effectively reduce ICP, until further information is available, one would continue to recommend its use as an adjunct to other measures in the control of ICP. In the acute setting, it can be lifesaving. However, it appears prudent to limit its use to those patients in whom the benefits in lowering ICP would outweigh the possible risks, and also to limit its use to the minimum duration possible.

Cerebral Dehydration

- *Cerebral dehydration should involve brain water removal without the development of systemic hypovolemia.*

- *Osmotic gradients, not diuresis per se, produce changes in blood brain water.*

Another mainstay in the therapy of intracranial hypertension is cerebral dehydration. This form of therapy attempts to remove free water from the intracranial compartments in order to reduce ICP. It is a commonly misunderstood phenomenon, especially by those who do not specialize in the treatment of neurosurgical problems. The point of confusion rests in the distinction between removal of volume from the intracranial compartment utilizing osmotic gradients and depletion of the intravascular volume. The goal is to perform the first without the second, that is, remove water from the brain while maintaining euvolemia.

The principle behind cerebral dehydration is that water will move across boundaries such as the cell membrane in response to osmotic gradients. As stated previously, osmolality is a function of the total number of particles dissolved in a given mass of solvent. In vivo, the solvent is water, and the particles include both the usual electrolytes, glucose, and proteins in the compartment of interest, as well as any exogenous molecules added to the system such as mannitol, ethanol, or glycerol. In addition, description of the in vivo system often times separates that part of the osmolality resulting from the presence of colloidal proteins and labels it as the colloid oncotic pressure. An increase in the concentration of an osmotically active substance in one compartment (blood), will raise the osmolality of that compartment, and water will diffuse across the cell membranes into the vascular space. This will decrease the extravascular volume and therefore the ICP. While this form of therapy is directed at the brain, it also results in loss of free water from other tissues as well and causes vigorous diuresis with loss of intravascular volume due to the osmotic diuretic action of the agents involved. However, it must be remembered, that it is the production of osmotic gradients, and not the diuretic action per se, that produces the reduction of ICP.

It is also important to note that the osmotic agents used in the therapy of intracranial hypertension rely on removal of water from areas of relatively normal brain, and have little effect on areas where injury has broken down the blood-brain barrier. This is because the relatively tight junctions in areas where the blood-brain barrier is intact exclude the active agent from the extravascular compartments, thus creating the osmotic gradients. When this barrier is broken down, the agent is free to leave the vascular compartment; thus, no gradient can be formed and water will not move out of the cell.

Historically, the agents used have included urea, mannitol, and glycerol. Mannitol has nearly totally replaced the other agents for this mode of therapy. Mannitol is supplied as a 25% solution and is administered intravenously. Initial dosing is 0.5 to 1.0 g/kg, followed by repeat doses of 0.25 g/kg as needed, guided by ICP and measurement of serum osmolality. Effective lowering of ICP occurs within 10 to 20 minutes,[97] and peak effect on ICP occurs between 20 minutes and 1 hour after administration. It has been demonstrated that no additional benefit is obtained by administration of more mannitol than needed to control the ICP. In fact, use of larger doses of mannitol have been found to lead to the need for continued large doses,[98] and may cause problems with rebound increases in ICP following discontinuation of mannitol. It is therefore recommended that the minimum dose needed to obtain control be administered, rather than adherence to fixed dosing schedules.

- *Mannitol is preferred over furosemide for brain water reduction therapy.*

A secondary effect may account for some of the ICP reduction obtained after mannitol administration. Due to changes in blood viscosity, vasoconstriction occurs in those cerebral beds where autoregulation is intact.[99] This effect has been implicated as the cause of early reductions in ICP, which occur shortly after administration, before the osmotic effects could be manifested. Supporting this is the finding that ICP reduction is less in patients with impaired autoregulation, as measured by radioactive xenon inhalation.[100] Further support comes from the finding that ICP reductions are also greater in patients with cerebral perfusion pressure higher than 70 mm Hg, a situation in which the cerebral vasculature is already partially vasoconstricted.[101]

It is widely known that rapid administration of mannitol can produce hypotension; however, it is usually safe when administered at the rate produced by free flow through a large-bore intravenous line. It should never be given by rapid intravenous push. The initial increase in the intravascular volume following mannitol infusion and prior to the onset of diuresis does not seem to be clinically significant except at the fastest rates of administration. Clinically significant expansion of the intravascular volume can develop in the patient with decreased glomerular filtration rate in whom a brisk diuresis does not ensue.

There is concern that osmotic agents can cause a rebound effect which refers to an increase in ICP over pretreatment levels following withdrawal of the osmotic agent. The clinical relevance of this phenomenon has been subject to debate. Possible causes include some degree of diffusion of the osmotic agent into the interstitium and intracellular compartment,[102] as well as an increase in osmolality of the intracellular compartment. This causes reabsorption of free water as the serum osmolality falls upon withdrawal of the osmotic agent. It is difficult to prove the significance of this phenomenon since such studies occur when brain edema has worsened and ICP would be expected to be increased. One would therefore expect that ICP would be higher after the effects of the osmotic agent have disappeared than they were before treatment. Further support of the concept are studies that indicate that the amount of mannitol necessary to control ICP depends on the amount of mannitol given in preceding doses.[98,103]

• *There is no strong clinical evidence that rebound brain hypertension develops following mannitol therapy.*

Hyperosmolarity resulting from overuse of osmotic agents can be detrimental, possibly resulting in renal failure,[104–106] hemolysis, rhabdomyolysis, neurologic deterioration, and even death. Renal failure during mannitol administration presents with oliguria or anuria, as well as hyponatremia, intravascular volume overload, or congestive heart failure. The cause of renal failure is not understood, and may result from loss of osmotic gradients within the kidney or loss of filtration pressure from afferent arteriolar vasoconstriction.[106] Mannitol-induced renal failure appears to be reversible through removal of the agent, usually by dialysis. For this reason, we recommend that serum osmolality be maintained below 320 mOsm/L. There is some concern that a serum osmolality above 320 mOsm/L will cause breakdown of the blood-brain barrier in normal brain areas and increased edema formation. However, no such evidence exists in the current literature.

• *Serum osmolalities above 320 mOsm/L can lead to renal failure.*

Loop Diuretics

Historically, loop diuretics have been used in multiple ways in the therapy of head injury. They have been used as primary agents for ICP reduction, combined with albumin in "oncodiuretic therapy," and used to potentiate the effect of osmotic diuretics.

As primary agents, their appropriate role remains unclear. Loop diuretics have reduced ICP in patients who undergo elective surgery.[107] Loop diuretics have been used with some success in the treatment of head injury in patients with elevated ICP. The presumed mechanism of action involves alterations in membrane sodium transfer which ultimately reduces cellular volume. They also interfere with CSF production.[108] While loop diuretics provide reduction of ICP over longer periods of time, that is, hours. They do not appear to cause reductions quickly enough to warrant their use in the setting of acute ICP elevation. When compared to mannitol, furosemide requires a longer time to peak effect, produces a lesser effect on ICP, and a shorter duration of action.[109,110] Because of their presumed alternate mechanisms of ICP reduction, loop diuretics may be beneficial in patients who have elevated ICP and in

• *Furosemide is inferior to mannitol as a rapid method to reduce ICP.*

whom maximal elevations in serum osmolality have already been achieved with osmotic agents.

Loop diuretics have also been used in combination with intravenous administration of colloid solutions, that is, albumin, 2 g/kg, and referred to as "oncodiuretic" therapy, with some reported success.[111] Interestingly, these authors found that dehydration of normal brain tissue did not occur, which contradicts work done with osmotic diuretics. Furthermore, it is unclear if the addition of the albumin significantly improved the results, or if the results simply reflect the effects of high-dose loop diuretics.

The use of loop diuretics for head-injured patients is best supported as adjunctive to therapy with osmotic diuretics.[112–115] Loop diuretics are effectively prolong the elevation in serum osmolality, and can extend the interval between doses of the osmotic agent. When administered prior to the osmotic diuretic, they minimize any tendency of the osmotic agent to expand the intravascular volume. They are useful in patients with impaired cardiac function when osmotic agents might precipitate transient symptoms of congestive heart failure.

- *A loop diuretic can effectively prolong elevated serum osmolality.*

Fluid Restriction

Tradition dictates that, when possible, all patients with significant head injury should be fluid restricted. This recommendation can be made only for patients who are hemodynamically stable without abnormal fluid losses. It is not unusual to find a hypotensive patient due to bleeding or excessive volume loss from diuretics or diabetes insipidus. Such a patient may not be appropriately resuscitated due to an inexperienced physician's desire to maintain fluid restriction.

It is unclear whether fluid restriction helps in the management of head injury. Most neurosurgeons believe that strict fluid restriction minimizes development of cerebral edema. While the mechanism of this effect has not been conclusively elucidated, there are several physiologic effects which may contribute. A reduced central venous pressure will reduce back pressure to the vessels in the area of injury. This will result in a lower static pressure which ordinarily contributes to fluid translocation into the extracellular space. Second, the renal compensation for volume loss will gradually increase osmolality. This prevents normalization of osmolalities which were raised by previous osmotic diuretic treatment. These effects may contribute to any beneficial effects following fluid restriction.

There are, however, studies that indicate no effect on edema formation from either salt load or fluid volume.[116] In one study animals were administered maintenance, 66% maintenance, and 133% maintenance, with no change in cerebral water content after experimental injury. The high-maintenance fluid group did show a 13% gain in total body weight, presumably secondary to fluid retention. Again, this leads to the conclusion that while volume overload is to be avoided, attention to serum osmolality is probably most important, and fluid restriction per se is probably less so.

- *Rather than dehydration, maintenance of serum osmolality may better protect brain function.*

Temperature Control

Cerebral metabolic rate increases by 5 to 7% for every degree centigrade increase in brain temperature. In patients with intact coupling of blood flow to cerebral metabolic rate, any increase in temperature will result in increases in blood flow and possibly increases in ICP. As a result, when control of the ICP is an issue, fever must be treated aggressively in patients. This is best directed at the source. However, adjuvant measures including cool forced-air convection, lowered room temperature, and antipyretic medications are required.

• *Mild hypothermia may improve outcome in brain-injured patients.*

Some have attempted to take this idea one step further and have induced deliberate hypothermia in head injury patients. Primarily, they hoped to improve ICP and possibly promote some degree of cerebral protection. Three small randomized studies recently published demonstrate reductions in ICP with mild hypothermia to core temperatures of 32 to 33°C.[117–119] Cerebral blood flow and cerebral metabolic rate were reduced in the hypothermic group relative to the normothermic group, and outcome at 3 months improved. In general, there were no more increases in complications in the hypothermia group. However, one study did find an increased incidence of sepsis in the hypothermic group; it did not reach statistical significance.

The benefits and complications of mild systemic hypothermia are still not well elucidated. Multicenter trials will hopefully soon provide clearer information on this form of therapy.[120] Until further studies are performed, the use of mild hypothermia must be considered experimental. The poorly defined risk of immunosuppression must be weighed against the potential benefits of ICP reduction. The current results do emphasize the importance of aggressive control of hyperthermia and the potential detriment to patient status that follow development of fever.

CSF Drainage

Drainage of CSF is a safe and effective method for the acute reduction of ICP in patients with functioning intraventricular catheters. It can be difficult in patients with small or slit ventricles due to impingement of the brain parenchyma on the catheter tip. During the acute phase of injury, the reductions of ICP are of limited duration; more prolonged reductions occur with its use several days after injury. Indeed, within the first 72 hours, CSF subtraction has little influence on the clinical course, while after 72 hours, CSF withdrawal can often times completely control ICP.[121]

Muscle Relaxants and Sedation

• *Sedation and neuromuscular blockade can reduce the overall cerebral metabolic rate.*

Many neurotrauma services routinely administer muscle relaxants and sedatives to head-injured patients in order to facilitate their care, as well as help control ICP. Neuromuscular blockade is useful in the initial management as it ensures a motionless patient for diagnostic studies such as CT. Furthermore, it allows for fully controlled ventilation and thus facilitates therapeutic hyperventilation. Sedation helps reduce increases in cerebral metabolic rate associated with arousal. This minimizes metabolically linked cerebral blood volume changes.

We avoid muscle relaxants as much as possible, since their use precludes assessment by serial evaluation of motor response. Since no consensus exists on this subject, their use must be guided by the clinical situation and the judgment of an experienced physician.

Anticonvulsants

The use of anticonvulsants in head injury remains controversial, especially the decision to discontinue use. Their use takes one of three forms: (1) acute seizure therapy; (2) prophylaxis of early seizure activity; and (3) prophylaxis of late seizure activity.

The incidence of post-traumatic epilepsy varies with the severity of the head injury. It ranges from 5% in patients hospitalized for head injury to as high as 35% in patients with hematoma or those comatose for 3 weeks or more. Seizures are defined as early or late, depending on their timing of their occurrence. Early seizures occur in the first 7 days following injury, and late seizures develop on or after the eighth day. Several studies have looked at risk factors for the development of seizure activity after head trauma. The most substantial risk for early seizures appears to be intracranial hematoma or brain contusion. The risk appears to be greater for subdural than for epidural hematomas. Other risk factors include prolonged post-traumatic amnesia, depressed skull fracture, and focal neurologic deficits. The risk factors associated with the development of late seizures include early seizures, intracranial hematoma, depressed skull fracture, and prolonged post-traumatic amnesia. The relative importance of these factors varies considerably among published series.

- *Early seizures are more likely to occur in patients with a hematoma or contusion. A depressed skull fracture or subdural hematoma further increases the risk.*

The use of anticonvulsants in the acute management of seizure activity is basic to critical care skills and has generally agreed upon principles. Seizure activity is detrimental as it creates a marked increase in cerebral metabolic activity and cerebral blood flow. It can therefore raise ICP. Furthermore, it creates hemodynamic instability that can further aggravate cerebral ischemia and acidosis. First-line drugs for the acute management of seizures include rapid-acting benzodiazepines and barbiturates. Diazepam, 10 mg by intravenous bolus, remains an inexpensive and effective traditional first-line agent. However, other benzodiazepines including midazolam and lorazepam are also effective. Rapid-acting barbiturates such as thiopental sodium effectively suppress seizure activity. The disadvantage of the rapid-acting barbiturates, however, is the termination of effect due to redistribution. This can lead to recurrence of the seizure as blood levels fall below therapeutic levels.

- *Seizures should be prevented or controlled since they increase overall brain metabolic rate and ICP.*

The use of anticonvulsants in the prophylaxis of early seizures has been controversial. The reason lies in the large percentage of patients who never experience seizures and who would unnecessarily be exposed to medication complications if all head-injured patients received anticonvulsant prophylaxis. Arguments in favor of prophylaxis point out that not all seizure activity is readily apparent, especially in patients who require muscle relaxants in the management of their ICP. For these reasons, some argue that only those patients at high risk of seizures should receive prophylaxis. Others administer such prophylaxis to all patients with severe head injuries.

The effectiveness of anticonvulsants for prophylaxis against early seizures has been subject to debate; some studies demonstrated no effect. These studies failed to reach adequate statistical power and did not always maintain customary therapeutic blood levels. Retrospective studies have suggested benefit. One prospective study of appropriate statistical power found that prophylactic phenytoin reduced the incidence of early seizures from 14.2 to 3.6%.[122] It therefore seems, at this time, that early-seizure prophylaxis in high-risk patients does provide benefits.

• *Seizure prophylaxis in higher risk patients does appear to be beneficial.*

The recommended dosage of phenytoin in the head-injured patient is 20 mg/kg administered slowly as an intravenous load, at a rate of no more than 30 mg/min. Alternatively, many clinicians administer 1 g intravenously as a standard adult loading dose. This is followed by a maintenance dose that can be varied from patient to patient and should be adjusted to maintain serum levels between 15 and 20 μg/ml.

Late-seizure prophylaxis provides even more controversy. The basis for prophylaxis in the past related to early seizures as a risk factor for late seizures. For this reason, it was hoped that prevention of early seizures would reduce the incidence of late seizures. While studies have shown that early seizures are reduced with use of prophylactic phenytoin, late seizures are not.[122] Since many late posttraumatic seizures are partial seizures, perhaps phenytoin may not be the best drug. Furthermore, it is not clear as to the optimal time to discontinue anticonvulsants administered purely for prophylaxis.

Barbiturates

The use of barbiturates in the treatment of head injury remains controversial. Barbiturates have been of interest in the field of neuroanesthesia because of their ability to lower cerebral metabolic rate, cerebral blood flow, and cerebral blood volume. They also provide potential cerebral protective effects during ischemia that are independent of their effect on cerebral metabolic rate. Potential mechanisms include reduction of cerebral blood volume, and therefore ICP, and cerebral vasoconstriction, which, in turn, reduces the rate of edema formation. Barbiturates also act as free radical scavengers to prevent cellular damage from oxygen-derived free radicals.

At the heart of the controversy surrounding barbiturates is the question of benefits. This is a difficult question to answer. Ethical issues have prevented a large prospective trial of barbiturates versus conventional therapy with crossover following failure of conventional therapy. In the United States, a multicenter, randomized prospective trial compared conventional therapy with pentobarbital plus conventional therapy. About twice as many patients had con-

• *Barbiturate therapy can reduce ICP, but it is unclear whether it changes outcome.*

trolled ICP in the pentobarbital-treated group than in the conventionally treated group. Furthermore, of nonresponders in the conventional-therapy group, 27% responded when pentobarbital was administered. This study concluded that barbiturates are beneficial in the control of ICP, but it did not comment on neurologic outcome or survival.[123] Furthermore, it suggests that there is a small subpopulation in which barbiturates are beneficial in control of ICP. Unfortunately, because of its cross-over design, long-term outcome could not be assessed in regard to the benefits of barbiturate.

In a prospective study of the effect of barbiturates and hyperventilation, Cold found that the barbiturate effects on cerebral blood flow could be correlated with global $CRMO_2$.[124] Barbiturate effects on cerebral blood flow were abolished at low levels of $CRMO_2$, ranging between 1.0 and 1.1 ml O_2 per 100 g/min. This is in agreement with the known effect of barbiturates on cerebral metabolic rate and cerebral blood flow and suggests that their best use is in patients with preserved cerebral metabolic rate and preserved coupling of cerebral blood flow to cerebral metabolic rate.

• Barbiturates may work best in patients in whom the cerebral metabolic rate is still related to cerebral blood flow.

There are also retrospective studies that suggest a benefit to barbiturate therapy in head injury. In most studies, failure to respond to conventional therapy plus barbiturates has been associated with a very poor prognosis, with nearly 100% mortality. A variable percentage of responders do progress to an eventual good outcome, as defined by Jennett and Bond.[125] This leaves one with the question whether barbiturates are truly beneficial or whether response to barbiturates is simply a marker for patients with less severe injury.

Several studies have failed to show benefit with barbiturate treatment. Ward and associates, in a study of prophylactic barbiturates, failed to demonstrate any benefit.[126] In this study, patients in whom conventional treatment had failed did not receive barbiturates; however, the small study size precluded identification of a small subpopulation who might benefit. Furthermore, Schwartz and colleagues studied barbiturates versus mannitol as adjunctive therapy to hyperventilation and muscle relaxants. These investigators found that mannitol controlled ICP better than pentobarbital.[127] This study included all patients with head injury, and because of its size it did not distinguish whether a small subset of patients would benefit from barbiturate therapy.

While the current literature is inconclusive, there may be a small group of patients in whom high-dose barbiturates are beneficial. Clearly, there are subgroups of patients in whom conventional therapy has failed, but in whom ICP control can be achieved with the addition of barbiturates. It is not known, however, whether this improves long-term outcome.

Barbiturate administration has significant side effects. Hypotension has been reported in over 50% of cases.[126] It occurs due to peripheral vasodilation, and in high doses secondary to myocardial depression and suppression of vasomotor reflexes. These effects can lower blood pressure more than ICP which results in a lowered cerebral perfusion pressure. Administration of volume expanders and vasopressors are commonly required in patients treated with

• Barbiturates can significantly depress cardiac function. Often invasive hemodynamic monitoring is required to stabilize the patient.

high-dose barbiturates. Because of the sometimes complex cardiovascular effects of barbiturates, osmotic diuretics, and vasoactive drugs, a pulmonary artery catheter should be placed whenever there is any doubt about the patient's cardiovascular status. We recommend monitoring with a pulmonary artery catheter in almost all patients in need of high-dose barbiturate therapy in order to optimize cardiac output and cerebral perfusion pressure.

Other side effects occur as well. Local tissue destruction can occur due to the highly alkaline pH, if infiltrated. Therefore, administration through a secure central line is recommended. Possibly, infectious complications increase in patients treated with high-dose barbiturates, because of effects on lymphocyte function.[128] Drugs administered concurrently with barbiturates can have increased clearances. These include theophylline, or metoprolol. Last, patients in barbiturate coma have impaired thermoregulation that can lead to hypothermia if they are not adequately monitored and supported.

Pentobarbital is the most common agent employed. Various dosing regimens have been used, with the usual loading dose of 3 to 10 mg/kg. Maintenance doses range from 1 to 3 mg/kg/hr. The EEG is usually monitored for evidence of burst suppression, and serum levels should be drawn daily. Acute tolerance to the EEG effects has been reported, and the authors suggest that the barbiturate dose titrated to EEG findings can lead to serum levels associated with cardiac toxicity.[129]

• *The end point of barbiturate therapy is burst suppression on the EEG.*

CONCURRENT AND EVOLVING PROBLEMS

In many respects, the head-injured patient presents the clinician with unique management problems. Some therapeutic measures that can be routinely applied to other critically ill patients must be modified in head injured patients. This section will focus on evolving systemic problems that are common in this patient population.

Diabetes Insipidus

The combination of dilute urine and hypertonic plasma is characteristic of diabetes of insipidus (DI). There are multiple causes of this disorder, but only DI secondary to head injury will be considered in this discussion. Most patients suffering from post-traumatic DI have suffered from significant head injury.[130] The diagnosis of DI is suspected when a patient develops polyuria. Prior to making the diagnosis of DI, it is necessary to exclude other causes of polyuria, such as excessive diuretic or fluid administration. Solute diuresis due to glucosuria, mannitol, or radiographic contrast administration must also be ruled out. In the case of solute diuresis, the urine is usually isotonic or slightly hypertonic to plasma. Neurogenic DI is associated with urine osmolality that is hypotonic to plasma.[131] If the polyuria is present for any length of time, the patient will also exhibit hypernatremia.

Table 13–4.
Replacement Therapy for Diabetes Insipidus

Agent	Dose	Route	Duration (hours)
Desmopressin	1–2 μg	SC	12–24
DDAVP	5–20 μg	Intranasal	12–24
Aqueous vasopressin	5–10 U	SC, IM	4–6
Vasopressin tannate (in oil)	2.5–50 U	IM	24–72

SC, Subcutaneous; IM, intramuscular.
(From Hall JB, Robertson G: Diabetes insipidus. In: Hall JB, Schmidt GA, Wood LH, eds: Principles of critical care. New York, McGraw-Hill, 1992.)

Treatment of neurogenic DI is based on replacement of the missing antidiuretic hormone and ongoing fluid losses. Several agents are available for hormone replacement and are summarized in Table 13–4. Aqueous vasopressin may be used for conformation of the diagnosis of DI and for initial therapy. Because of its longer therapeutic half-life and ease of administration, desmopressin (DDAVP) is usually preferred for long-term management of DI. It is necessary to carefully assess and replace intravascular fluid losses caused by DI. The replacement of fluid losses with the necessary hypotonic fluids may result in increased cerebral edema, as discussed previously. Therapy must be individualized to provide adequate resuscitation without further damage to the injured brain.

Pulmonary Injury

Patients with head injuries often suffer from a wide variety of associated pulmonary injuries. The diagnosis and treatment of pulmonary injuries are discussed elsewhere in this book and are not repeated in this chapter. Two complications, neurogenic pulmonary edema and pneumonia, are reviewed in this section.

A rare complication of severe head injury is neurogenic pulmonary edema. Early autopsy studies reported marked lung congestion and some pulmonary edema in many patients who died shortly after massive head injury.[132,133] This edema was rarely seen in patients who suffered from less severe head injury.[134] It has been proposed that severe head injury causes a massive transient increase in sympathetic nervous system activity that leads to generalized vasoconstriction and elevated systemic vascular resistance. Pulmonary vascular engorgement, pulmonary vasoconstriction, and elevated pulmonary vascular pressures all follow.[135,136] These transient high pressures are thought to lead to pulmonary endothelial injury and ultimately to pulmonary edema, even in the presence of normal pulmonary filling pressures.[137] Treatment is mainly supportive, with special attention to the treatment of the underlying cerebral pathology being paramount. It has been suggested that the sympathetic response may be modified by the use of alpha and beta blocking agents.[138,139] Therapy with such agents will have to be balanced

- *Neurogenic pulmonary edema is an extremely rare and questionable event.*

against the possible deleterious hemodynamic effects that these agents might induce.

Pulmonary infection is commonly present in patients with head injury. Helling and associates found that pneumonia was the most common source of infection in this patient group.[140] Another retrospective study demonstrated that 41% of patients with severe head injury developed pneumonia. This pneumonia tended to occur early in the patient's hospital stay (64% within 3 days of admission), and that the pneumonia tends to lengthen ICU and hospital stay while not affecting mortality.[141] The investigators suggested that this early development of pneumonia could be due to aspiration of gastric or orophyaryngeal contents at the time of injury.[141] Other studies have been unable to demonstrate any role for the use of prophylactic antibiotics in this patient population.[142] Therapy should be based on prevention of pneumonia whenever possible through strict attention to bronchial hygiene and culture-directed therapy when an infecting organism has been identified.

• *Head-injured patients as a group have the highest incidence of nosocomial pneumonia.*

Nutritional Issues

It is widely recognized that adequate nutrition is necessary to optimize a patient's chances of recovery following major trauma. Patients with head injuries are no exception to this dictum. In fact, severe head injury has been associated with a marked hypermetabolic state.[143,144] Energy expenditures of up to 200% of predicted have been reported.[145–147] The actual magnitude of this hypermetabolism appears to be directly related to the severity of injury. It is at least partially due to the release of endogenous mediators, such as catecholamines, cytokines, and cortisol.[148] Available data suggest that these patients will benefit from early alimentation.

Multiple questions must be addressed before initiaton of nutritional therapy. These include the choice of feeding methods, avoidance of hyperglycemia, and limitations of its deleterious side effects. Hyperglycemia has been associated with worsening of outcome in multiple experimental studies when cerebral ischemia was induced in hyperglycemic animals.[149,150] Clinical reports have also linked hyperglycemia to poor outcome.[151,152] As Robertson and associates point out, this hyperglycemia could just represent a marker of severity of injury, or it could be an important mechanism of secondary injury.[148] Until the exact relationship between hyperglycemia and head injury is determined, it would appear prudent to provide a nutritional formula that would minimize the appearance of hyperglycemia.

• *Nutritional support should be monitored closely to prevent the development of hyperglycemia and its detrimental effects on brain function.*

The appropriate feeding route for these critically ill patients must be established. Early reports that compared early parenteral therapy with delayed enteral nutrition found an improved outcome and decreased mortality in those who received parenteral nutrition.[153,154] If, however, enteral therapy was started early after injury, there was no difference in outcome, even though patients with enteral nutrition received fewer calories and less protein and were more likely to have negative nitrogen balances.[155] Thus, it appears that the route of nutritional delivery is less important than the fact that nutrition is delivered as early as feasible after injury. Most experts today recommend use of the gut if at all possible.

OUTCOME

Studies of outcome from severe head injury serve two purposes. First, knowledge of expected outcome allows physicians to evaluate the various therapeutic options in order to improve management. Second, this information provides physicians with prognostic information for families of patients with severe head injuries.

As health care costs become a larger part of the equation, interest in outcome from severe head injury has turned toward efforts to predict outcome. Prediction of nonsurvivors might allow for a reduction of resuorce expenditures on patients who would not benefit. Unfortunately, the sensitivity and specificity of the current prediction models are inadequate for such purposes.

Classification of outcome typically follows the Glasgow outcome scale, as defined by Jennett and Bond in 1975.[125] This scale distinguishes five categories for outcome. Good recovery implies resumption of normal life. Moderate disability means that the patient can function independently despite some degree of disability. The categories of good recovery and moderate disability are many times combined together as favorable outcomes. The category of severe disability describes a conscious patient but dependent on daily support because of mental or physical impairment. The category of persistent vegetative state includes those patients who remain unresponsive and never improve. Death is the final category.

Multiple studies have explored outcomes. Many of these studies have evaluated specific patient factors such as outcome, age, type of injury, radiologic findings, neurologic presentation, ICP, or physiologic abnormalities. The reader is referred to an excellent review by Torner.[156] Key points will be summarized here.

Data from the Traumatic Coma Data Bank (TCDB) from 1984 through 1987 indicate that the mortality rate, based on postresuscitation Glasgow coma score, varied from 76% in patients with a total score of 3 to 18% in patients with a score of 6, 7, or 8.[157] Total Glasgow coma score in some studies is no better than motor score alone,[158] perhaps because of conditions such as endotracheal intubation that confound the total but not the motor score.

Age has clearly been shown to adversely affect outcome, with higher morbidity and mortality with advanced age.[159] Other studies have related other physical findings to outcome. The most accurate predictors of outcome within a given patient are age, best motor response, and bilateral pupillary responses.[158] The two most important factors that modify the outcome based on these factors were the amount of time the patient had ICP measurements over 20 mm Hg and the amount of time the patient had a systemic blood pressure less than 80 mm Hg.[160]

- *Important factors for outcome determination include the patient's age and Glasgow coma score, as well as the duration of elevated ICP and hypotension.*

Radiographic criteria have been correlated with outcome. The worst prognosis occurred in patients with brain stem injury (66% mortality), nonevacuated mass lesions (53% mortality), and evacuated mass lesions (40% mortality). The TCDB data also allow the division of diffuse injury into four grades based on radiographic findings and relate outcome to these grades. While grade IV diffuse injury had a 56% mortality, grade I injury yielded a 90% survival.[161]

Morbidity from severe head injury tends to parallel mortality. The chances of a good recovery, as determined by the Glasgow outcome score, vary from 27% for patients with grade I diffuse injury to about 3% for diffuse injury III, diffuse injury IV, and nonevacuated mass lesions.[161] If a favorable outcome is defined to be a categorization of good or moderately disabled, then the percentage of favorable outcomes varies from 51% for diffuse injury I to 6.2% for diffuse injury IV.

Unfortunately, to date, studies have failed to validate a prognostic system that conclusively distinguishes patients who will have a favorable outcome from those with an eventual unfavorable outcome. In the worst prognostic categories, about 5% of people will have a favorable outcome, despite predictions to the contrary. What confuses matters for intensive care physicians, is that a significant number of these patients will remain unresponsive for weeks to months after injury, and will leave the ICU comatose, or at best poorly responsive.[162] This gives many in critical care environments a skewed and pessimistic view of outcome from these injuries. These findings make prediction of outcome for purposes of resource allocation problematic at best.

Care of the patient with severe head injury can be difficult because of the complexity of their associated injuries, as well as the emotional aspects of the tragedy of a potentially devastating injury in a previously healthy, vital individual. The severity of the injury, combined with the fact that the average intensive care physician often discharges the patient from the ICU before the patient has made a functional recovery, and rarely has long-term follow-up, can make care of these patients unsatisfying. Reassurance, though, may be had by the knowledge that many patients do make a favorable, functional recovery, perhaps largely because of the efforts of the critical care team in the early postinjury period.

While a significant part of the long-term prognosis is determined by the initial injury sustained before entering the emergency medical system, secondary injury can be very significant for outcome prognosis. Attention to the details presented here can make a significant difference to the patient.

The basic therapy for elevated ICP that has stood the test of time revolves around attention to details, including ICP measurement, cerebral perfusion pressure, arterial oxygen and carbon dioxide tension, blood pressure, serum osmolality, head position, and temperature. Adjunctive therapies include anticonvulsants, barbiturates, hypothermia, and tromethamine are more controversial and must be applied with knowledge of the clinical situation. While recommendations can be made based on review of the current literature, its limitations must be recognized. This is reflected by a 1989 study of the practices of academic neurosurgeons that showed a significant lack of uniformity in how they handled basic care.[163]

Medicine is entering an exciting time in research of mechanisms of brain injury and cerebral protection. Knowledge of excitatory neurotransmitters and of chemical substances that modify their effects in the production of brain injury is beginning to show potential for therapeutic interventions. In addition, with new monitoring techniques, therapy targeted at specific physiologic abnormalities is becoming possible. Over the next decade, therapeutic practice has the potential to change significantly.

REFERENCES

1. Zwimpfer TJ, Moulton RJ: Neurologic trauma concerns. Crit Care Clin 1993; 9:727–739.
2. Andrews BT: The intensive care management of patients with head injury. In: Andrews BT, ed: Neurosurgical intensive care. New York, McGraw-Hill, 1993; pp. 227–242.
3. Committee on Trauma Research: Injury: magnitude and characteristics of the problem. In: Injury in America. Washington, DC, National Academy Press, 1985; pp. 18–24.
4. Shackford SR, Mackersie RC, Davis JW et al: Epidemiology and pathology of traumatic deaths occurring in a level I trauma center in a regionalized system: the importance of secondary brain injury. J Trauma 1989; 29:1392–1397.
5. Duffy KR, Becker DP: State of the art: management of severe closed-head injury. J Intensive Care Med 1988; 3:291–302.
6. Richards P: Management of head injuries. Curr Anaesth Crit Care 1990; 1:99–104.
7. Ommaya AK, Gennarelli TA: Cerebral concussion and traumatic unconsciousness. Brain 1974; 97:633–654.
8. Gennarelli TA, Thibault LE, Adams LH: Diffuse axonal injury and traumatic coma in the primate. Ann Neurol 1982; 12:564–574.
9. Lighthall JW: Controlled cortical impact: a new experimental brain injury model. J Neurotrauma 1988; 5:1–17.
10. Adams JH, Doyle D, Ford I et al: Diffuse axonal injury in head injury: definition diagnosis and grading. Histopathology 1989; 15:49–59.
11. Lighthall JW, Goshgarian HG, Pinderski CR: Characterization of axonal injury produced by controlled cortical impact. J Neurotrauma 1990; 7:65–76.
12. Adams JH, Mitchell DE, Graham DI, Doyle D: Diffuse brain damage of immediate impact type. Brain 1977; 100:489–502.
13. Roser MJ: Pathophysiology and management of increased intracranial pressure. In: Andrews BT, ed: Neurosurgical intensive care. New York, McGraw-Hill, 1993; pp. 57–112.
14. Hovda DA, Becker DP, Katayama Y: Secondary injury and acidosis. J Neurotrauma 1992; 9:S47-S60.
15. Muizelaar JP: Cerebral blood flow cerebral volume and cerebral metabolism after severe head injury. In: Becker DP, Gudema SK, eds:

Textbook of head injury. Philadelphia, WB Saunders, 1988; pp. 221–240.
16. Pulsinelli WA, Petito CK: The neurotoxicity of hydrogen ions. Stroke 1983; 14:13.
17. Paulson OB, Strandgaard S, Edvinsson L: "Cerebral autoregulation." Cerebrovasc Brain Metab Rev 1990; 2:161–192.
18. Todd MM, Warner DS: Neuroanesthesia: a critical review. In: Rogers M et al, ed: Principles and practices of anesthesiology. St. Louis, Mosby-Year Book, 1993.
19. Edvinsson L, Owman C, Siesjo B: Physiological role of cerebrovascular nerves in the autoregulation of cerebral blood flow. Brain Res 1976; 117:519–523.
20. Kennedy C, Sokoloff L: An adaptation of the nitrous oxide method to the study of cerebral circulation in children: normal values for cerebral blood flow and cerebral blood volume in childhood. J Clin Invest 1957; 36:1130–1140.
21. Muizelaar JP: Cerebral blood flow, cerebral blood volume and cerebral metabolism after severe head injury. Philadelphia, WB Saunders, 1989; 221–240.
22. Astrup J: Energy requiring cell function in the ischemic brain. J Neurosurg 1982; 56:482–497.
23. Raichle ME, Grubb RL, Gado MH et al: Correlation between regional cerebral blood flow and oxidative metabolism. Arch Neurol 1976; 33:523–526.
24. Kontos HA, Wei EP, Navari EM et al: Response of cerebral arteries and arterioles to acute hypotension and hypertension. Am J Physiol 1978; 234:H371-H383.
25. Bouma GJ, Muizelaar P: Cerebral blood flow, cerebral blood volume, and cerebrovascular reactivity after severe head injury. J Neurotrauma 1992; 9:S333-S348.
26. Cold GE: Measurement of CO_2 reactivity and barbiturate reactivity in patients with severe head injury. Acta Neurochir 1989; 98:153–163.
27. Messeter K, Nordstrom CH, Sundburg HM et al: Cerebral hemodynamics in patients with acute severe head trauma. J Neurosurg 1986; 64:231–237.
28. Nordstrom CH, Messeter K, Sundburg G et al: Cerebral blood flow vasoreactivity and oxygen consumption during barbiturate therapy in severe traumatic brain lesion. J Neurosurg 1988; 68:424–431.
29. Muizelaar JP, Lutz HA, Becker DP et al: Effect of mannitol on ICP and CBF and correlation with pressure autoregulation in severely head injured patients. J Neurosurg 1984; 61:700–706.
30. Bouma GJ, Muizelaar JP: The relationship between cardiac output and cerebral blood flow in patients with intact and impaired autoregulation. J Neurosurg 1990; 73:368–374.
31. Muizelaar JP, Ward JD, Marmarou A et al: Cerebral blood flow and metabolism in severely head-injured children. Part II: Autoregulation. J Neurosurg 1989; 59:822–828.
32. Lassen NA, Inguar GH: Regional cerebral blood flow measurement in man. Arch Neurol 1963; 9:615.
33. Dandy WE: Diagnosis and treatment of injuries of the head. JAMA 1933; 101:772–775.
34. Miller JD, Becker DP: Secondary insults to the injured brain. J Royal Coll Surg Edinb 1982; 27:292–298.
35. Marmarou A, Anderson RL et al: Impact of ICP instability and out-

come in patients with severe head trauma. J Neurosurg 1991; 75: S59-S66.
36. Graham DI, Adams JH, Doyle D: Ischemic brain damage in fatal non-missile head injuries. J Neurol Sci 1978; 39:213–234.
37. Bouma GJ, Muizelaar JP, Choi SC, et al: Cerebral circulation and metabolism after severe traumatic brain injury: the elusive role of ischemia. J Neurosurg 1991; 75:685–693.
38. Hayes RL, Jenkins LW, Lyth BD, et al: Neurotransmitter-mediated mechanism of traumatic brain injury: acethylcholine and excitatory amino acids. J Neurotrauma 1992; 9:S173-S187.
39. Nilsson P, Hillered L, Ponten V, Ungerstedt V: Changes in extracellular levels of energy-related metabolites and amino acids following concussive brain injury in rats. J Cereb Blood Flow Metab 1990; 10: 631–637.
40. Sajia A, Hayes RL, Lyeth BG, et al: The effect of concussive cerebral injury on central cholinergic neurons. Brain Res 1988; 452:303–311.
41. De Salles AAF, Muizelaar JP, Young HF: Hyperglycemia, cerebrospinal fluid lactic acidosis and cerebral blood flow in severely head-injured patients. Neurosurgery 1987; 21:45–50.
42. Marmarou A: Intracellular acidosis in human and experimental brain injury. J Neurotrauma 1992; 9:S551-S562.
43. Zimmerman RS, Hayes RL, Morris DL, et al: Exogenous and endogenous opioids after severe head injury. Neurosurgery 1990; 26: 764–770.
44. Yao JJ, Cheng Z, CE CC, et al: Endorphin like immuoreactivity increases in cerebrospinal fluid of acute head injured patients. Neuropeptides 1988; 12:177–179.
45. Young W: Role of calcium in central nervous system injuries. J Neruotrauma 1992; 9:S9-S25.
46. Unterberg A, Dautermann C, Baethmann A, Muller-Esterl W: The kallikrein-kinin system as mediators in vasogenic brain edema. J Neurosurg 1986; 64:269–276.
47. Davis KD, Dostrovski JO: Cerebrovascular application of bradykinin excites central sensory neuron. Brain Res 1988; 446:401–406.
48. Flamm ES, Demopoulos HB, Seligman ML, et al: Free radicals in cerebral ischemia. Stroke 1978; 9:445–447.
49. Demopoulos HB, Flamm ES, Pietronigro DD, Seligman ML: The free radical pathology and the microcirculation in the major cerebral nervous system disorders. Acta Physiol Scand (suppl) 1980; 492:91–109.
50. Benumof JL: Management of the difficult adult airway: with special emphasis on awake tracheal intubation. Anesthesiology 1991; 75: 1087–1110.
51. Marmarou A, Anderson R, Ward J et al: Impact of ICP instability and hypotension on outcome in patients with severe head trauma. J Neurosurg 1991; 75:S59-S66.
52. Schmoker J, Shackford S, Wald S, Pietropaoli J: An analysis of the relationship between fluid and sodium administration and intracranial pressure after head injury. J Trauma 1992; 33:476–481.
53. Kaieda R, Todd MM, Cook LN, Warner DS: Acute effects of changing plasma osmolality and colloid oncotic pressure on the formation of brain edema after cryogenic injury. Neurosurgery 1989; 24: 671–678.
54. Fenstermacher J, Johnson J: Filtration and reflection coefficients of the rabbit blood-brain barrier. Am J Physiol 1966; 211:341–346.
55. Zornow M, Scheller M, Todd M, Moore S: Acute cerebral effects of

isotonic crystalloid and colloid solutions following cryogenic brain injury in the rabbit. Anesthesiology 1988; 69:180–184.

56. Kaieda R, Todd M, Warner D: Prolonged reductions in colloid oncotic pressure do not increase brain edema following cryogenic injury in rabbits. Anesthesiology 1989; 71:554–560.
57. Lobato R, Rivas J, Gomez P et al: Head-injured patients who talk and deteriorate into coma: analysis of 211 cases studied with computerized tomography. J Neurosurg 1991; 75:256–261.
58. Teasdale G, Jennett B: Assessment of coma and impaired consciousness: a practical scale. Lancet 1974; 2:81–84.
59. Teasdale G, Knill-Jones R, Van der Sande J: Observer variability in assessing impaired consciousness and coma. J Neurol Neurosurg Psychiatr 1978; 41:603–610.
60. Braakman R, Avezaat C, Maas A et al: Inter-observer agreement in the assessment of the motor response on the Glasgow coma scale. Clin Neurol Neurosurg 1977; 80:100–106.
61. Mendelow A, Teasdale G, Jennett B et al: Risks of intracranial hematoma in head injured adults. Br Med J 1983; 287:1173–1176.
62. Gailbraith S: Misdiagnosis and delayed diagnosis in traumatic intracranial hematoma. Br Med J 1976; 1:1438–1439.
63. Guillaume J, Janny P: Manometrie intracranienne continue: intérêt de la méthode et premiers résultats. Rev Neurol 1951; 84:131–142.
64. Lundberg N: Continuous recording and control of ventricular fluid pressure in neurosurgical practice. Acta Psychiatr Neurol Scand 1960; 36:1–193.
65. Lundberg N, Troupp H, Lorin H: Continuous recording of the ventricular fluid pressure in patients with severe acute traumatic brain injury: a preliminary report. J Neurosurg 1965; 22:581–590.
66. Bruce D, Berman W, Schut L: Cerebrospinal fluid pressure monitoring in children: physiology, pathology and clinical usefulness. Adv Pediatr 1977; 24:233–290.
67. Kishore PR, Lipper MH, Becker DP, et al: Significance of CT in head injury: correlation with intracranial pressure. AJR Am J Roentgenol 1981; 137:829–833.
68. Narayan RK, Kishore PR, Becker DP et al: Intracranial pressure: to monitor or not to monitor? A review of our experience with severe head injury. J Neurosurg 1982; 56:650–659.
69. Miller J, Pickard J: Intracranial volume pressure studies in patients with head injury. Injury 1974; 5:265–269.
70. Marmarou A: Progress in the analysis of ICP dynamics and application to head injury. In Becker D, Povlishock J, eds: CNS trauma status report. Bethesda, MD, National Institute of Neurological and Communicative Disorders and Stroke, 1985; pp. 79–88.
71. Rosner MJ, Becker DP: Origin and evolution of plateau waves: Experimental observations and a theoretical model. J Neurosurg 1984; 60:312–324.
72. Weaver D, Winn H, Jane J: Differential intracranial pressure in patients with unilateral mass lesions. J Neurosurg 1982; 56:693–699.
73. Rosenwasser RH, Kleiner LI, Krzeminski JP, Buchheit WA: Intracranial pressure monitoring in the posterior fossa: a preliminary report. J Neurosurg 1989; 71:503–505.
74. Wyler, Kelly W: Use of antibiotics with external ventriculostomies. J Neurosurg 1972; 37:185–187.
75. Smith R, Alksne J: Infections complicating the use of external ventriculostomy. J Neurosurg 1976; 44:567–570.

76. Mayhall C., Archer NH, Lamb VA et al: Ventriculostomy-related infections: a prospective epidemiologic study. N Engl J Med 1984; 310:553–559.
77. Blei AT, Olafsson S, Webster S, Levy R: Complications of intracranial pressure monitoring in fulminant hepatic failure. Lancet 1993; 341: 157–158.
78. Boulard G, Ravussin P, Guerin J: A new way to monitor external ventricular drainage. Neurosurgery 1992; 30:636–638.
79. Wilkinson H, Yarzebski J, Wilkinson E, Anderson F: Erroneous measurement of intracranial pressure caused by simultaneous ventricular drainage: a hydrodynamic model study. Neurosurgery 1989; 24: 348–354.
80. Crutchfield JS, Narayan RK, Robertson CS, Michael LH: Evaluation of a fiberoptic intracranial pressure monitor. J Neurosurg 1990; 72: 482–487.
81. Ostrup RC, Luerssen TG, Marshall LF, Zornow MH: Continuous monitoring of intracranial pressure with a miniaturized fiberoptic device. J Neurosurg 1987; 67:206–209.
82. Schickner DJ, Young RF: Intracranial pressure monitoring: fiberoptic monitor compared with the ventricular catheter. Surg Neurol 1992; 37:251–254.
83. Sheinberg M, Kanter MJ, Robertson CS et al: Continuous monitoring of jugular venous oxygen saturation in head-injured patients. J Neurosurg 1992; 76:212–217.
84. Gibbs E, Lennox W, Gibbs F: Bilateral internal jugular blood: comparison of A-V differences, oxygen-dextrose ratios and respiratory quotients. Am J Physiol 1945; 102:184–190.
85. Goetting MG, Preston G: Jugular bulb catheterization does not increase intracranial pressure. Intensive Care Med 1991; 17:195–198.
86. Chan KH, Dearden NM, Miller JD: The significance of posttraumatic increase in cerebral blood flow velocity: a transcranial Doppler ultrasound study. Neurosurgery 1992; 30:697–700.
87. Chan KH, Miller JD, Dearden NM, et al: The effect of changes in cerebral perfusion pressure upon middle cerebral artery blood flow velocity and jugular bulb venous oxygen saturation after severe brain injury. J Neurosurg 1992; 77:55–61.
88. Marschall L: Evoked potentials: a decade later. Crit Care Med 1991; 19:1337.
89. Feldman Z. Kanter M, Robertson C et al: Effect of head elevation on intracranial pressure, cerebral perfusion pressure, and cerebral blood flow in head injured patients. J Neurosurg 1992; 76:207–211.
90. Greenberg JH, Alavi A, Reivich M et al: Local cerebral blood volume response to carbon dioxide in man. Circulation Res 1978; 43: 324–331.
91. Cold GE: Does acute hyperventilation provoke cerebral oligaemia in comatose patients after acute head injury? Acta Neurochir 1989; 96: 100–106.
92. Muizelaar JP, van der Poel HG, Li ZC et al: Pial arteriolar vessel diameter and CO_2 reactivity during prolonged hyperventilation in the rabbit. J Neurosurg 1988; 69:923–927.
93. Muizelaar J, Marmarou A, Ward J et al: Adverse effects of prolonged hyperventilation in patients with severe head injury: a randomized clinical trial. J Neurosurg 1991; 75:731–739.
94. Severinghaus J: Role of cerebrospinal fluid pH in normalization of

cerebral blood flow in chronic hypocapnia. Acta Neurol Scand (suppl) 1965; 14:116–120.

95. Yoshida K, Marmarou A: Effects of tromethamine and hyperventilation on brain injury in the cat. J Neurosurg 1991; 74:87–96.
96. Rosner MJ, Becker DP: Experimental brain injury: successful therapy with the weak base, tromethamine: with an overview of CNS acidosis. J Neurosurg 1984; 60:961–971.
97. Mendelow AD, Teasdale GM, Russell T et al: Effect of mannitol on cerebral blood flow and cerebral perfusion pressure in human head injury. J Neurosurg 1985; 63:43–48.
98. McGraw CP, Howard G: Effect of mannitol on increased intracranial pressure. Neurosurgery 1983; 13:269–271.
99. Muizelaar JP, Wei EP, Kontos HA, Becker DP: Mannitol causes compensatory cerebral vasoconstriction and vasodilation in response to blood viscosity changes. J Neurosurg 1983; 59:822–828.
100. Muizelaar JP, Lutz HA, Becker DP: Effect of mannitol on ICP and CBF and correlation with pressure autoregulation in severely head-injured patients. J Neurosurg 1984; 61:700–706.
101. Rosner MJ, Coley I: Cerebral perfusion pressure: a hemodynamic mechanism of mannitol and the postmannitol hemogram. Neurosurgery 1987; 21:147–156.
102. Kaufmann AM, Cardoso ER: Aggravation of vasogenic cerebral edema by multiple-dose mannitol. J Neurosurg 1992; 77:584–589.
103. Marschall LF, Smith RW, Rauscher LA, Shapiro HM: Mannitol dose requirements in brain injured patients. J Neurosurg 1978; 48:169-172.
104. Horgan KJ, Ottaviano YL, Watson AJ: Acute renal failure due to mannitol intoxication. Am J Nephrol 1989; 9:106–109.
105. Dorman HR, Sondheimer JH, Cadnapaphornchai P: Mannitol-induced acute renal failure. Medicine 1990; 69:153–159.
106. Rabetoy GM, Fredericks MR, Hostettler CF: Where the kidney is concerned, how much mannitol is too much? Ann Pharmacother 1993; 27:25–28.
107. Cottrell J, Robustelli A, Post K, Turndorf H: Furosemide and mannitol-induced changes in intracranial pressure and serum osmolality and electrolytes. Anesthesiology 1977; 47:28–30.
108. Melby J, Miner L, Reed D: Effect of acetazolamide and furosemide on the production and composition of cerebrospinal fluid from the cat choroid plexus. Can J Physiol Pharmacol 1982; 60:405–409.
109. Pollay M, Fullenwider C, Roberts P, Stevens F: Effect of mannitol and furosemide on blood-brain osmotic gradient and intracranial pressure. J Neurosurg 1983; 59:945–950.
110. Wilkinson H, Rosenfield S: Furosemide and mannitol in the treatment of acute experimental intracranial hypertension. Neurosurgery 1983; 12:405–410.
111. Albright A, Latchaw R, Robinson A: Intracranial and systemic effects of osmotic and oncotic therapy in experimental cerebral edema. J Neurosurg 1984; 60:481–489.
112. Wilkinson HA, Rosenfeld SR: Furosemide and mannitol in the treatment of acute experimental intracranial hypertension. Neurosurgery 1983; 12:405–410.
113. Cottrell JE, Robustelli A, Post K, Turndorf H: Furosemide- and mannitol-induced changes in intracranial pressure and serum osmolality and electrolytes. Anesthesiology 1977; 47:28–30.

114. Cottrell JE, Marlin AE: Furosemide and human head injury. J Trauma 1981; 21:805–806.
115. Roberts PA, Pollay M, Engles C et al: Effect on intracranial pressure of furosemide combined with varying doses and administration rates of mannitol. J Neurosurg 1987; 66:440–446.
116. Morse M, Milstein J, Haas J, Taylor E: Effect of hydration on experimentally induced cerebral edema. Crit Care Med 1985; 13:563- 565.
117. Clifton G, Allen S, Barrodale P et al: A Phase II study of moderate hypothermia in severe brain injury. J Neurotrauma 1993; 10: 263–271.
118. Marion D, Obrist W, Carlier P et al: The use of moderate therapeutic hypothermia for patients with severe head injuries: a preliminary report. J Neurosurg 1993; 79:354–362.
119. Shiozaki T, Sugimoto H, Taneda M et al: Effect of mild hypothermia on uncontrollable intracranial hypertension after severe head injury. J Neurosurg 1993; 79:363–368.
120. Muizelaar J: Editorial comment. J Neurotrauma 1993; 10:273.
121. Papo I, Caruselli G, Luongo A: CSF withdrawal for the treatment of intracranial hypertension in acute head injuries. Acta Neurochir 1981; 56:191–199.
122. Temkin NR, Dikmen SS, Wilensky AJ et al: A randomized, double-blind study of phenytoin for the prevention of post-traumatic seizures. N Engl J Med 1990; 323:497–502.
123. Eisenberg HM, Frankowski RF, Contant CF et al: High-dose barbiturate control of elevated intracranial pressure in patients with severe head injury. J Neurosurg 1988; 69:15–23.
124. Cold GE: Measurements of CO_2 reactivity and barbiturate reactivity in patients with severe head injury. Acta Neurochir 1989; 98: 153–163.
125. Jennett B, Bond M: Assessment of outcome after severe brain damage. Lancet 1975; 1:480–484.
126. Ward JD, Becker DP, Miller JD et al: Failure of prophylactic barbiturate coma in the treatment of severe head injury. J Neurosurg 1985; 62:383–388.
127. Schwartz ML, Tator CH, Rowed DW et al: The University of Toronto Head Injury Treatment Study: a prospective, randomized comparison of pentobarbital and mannitol. Can J Neurol Sci 1984; 11:434–440.
128. Neuwelt E, Kikuchi K, Hill S et al: Barbiturate inhibition of lymphocyte function: differing effects of various barbiturates used to induce coma. J. Neurosurg 1982; 56:254–259.
129. Sawada Y, Sugimoto H, Kobayashi H et al: Acute tolerance to high-dose barbiturate treatment in patients with severe head injuries. Anesthesiology 1982; 56:53–54.
130. Goldman K, Jacobs A: Anterior and posterior pituitary failure after head injury. Br Med J 1990; 2:1924.
131. Hall J, Robertsons C: Diabetes insipidus. In: Hall JB, Schmidt GA, Wood LD, eds: Principles of critical care. New York, McGraw-Hill, 1992; pp. 1946–1953.
132. Weisman S: Edema and congestion of the lungs resulting from intracranial hemorrhage. Surgery 1939; 6:722.
133. Simmmons R, Martin A, Heisterkamp C et al.: Respiratory insufficiency in combat casualties (pulmonary edema following head injury). Ann Surg 1969; 170:39.
134. Singbarth G, Cunitz G, Hamroundi H: Disturbed pulmonary gas exchange in patients with cerebral trauma. Anesthetist 1982; 31:228.

135. Theodore J, Robin E: Speculations on neurogenic pulmonary edema. Am Rev Respir Dis 1976; 113:405.
136. Demling R, Riessen R: Pulmonary dysfunction after cerebral injury. Crit Care Med 1990; 18:768–774.
137. Minnear F, Barie P, Malik A: Effect of large transient increases in pulmonary vascular pressures on lung fluid balance. J Appl Physiol 1983; 55:983–990.
138. Wohns R, Taman L, Pierce K et al.: Chlorpromazine treatment for neurogenic pulmonary edema. Crit Care Med 1985; 13:210–211.
139. Harrier H: Use of labetalol in trauma. Crit Care Med 1988; 16: 1159–1160.
140. Helling T, Evans L, Fowler D et al: Infectious complications in patients with severe head injury. J Trauma 1988; 28:1575–1577.
141. Hsieh AH, Bishop MJ, Kubilis PS et al: Pneumonia following closed-Head injury. Am Rev Respir Dis 1992; 146:290–294.
142. Goodpasture H, Romig D, Woth D et al.: A Prospective study of tracheobronchial bacterial flora in acutely brain injured patients with and without antibiotic prophylaxis. J Neurosurg 1979; 51:307–315.
143. Haider W, Lackner F, Schlick W et al: Metabolic changes in the course of severe acute brain damage. Eur J Intensive Care Med 1975; 1: 19–26.
144. Long CL, Shafferffer N, Geiger JW, et al: Metabolic response to injury and illness: estimation of energy and protein needs from indirect calorimetry and nitrogen balance. JPEN J Parenter Enteral Nutr 1975; 3: 452–456.
145. Chifton GL, Robertson LS, Grossman RG et al: The metabolic response to severe head injury. J Neurosurg 1984; 60:687–696.
146. Robertson CS, Clifton GL, Grossman RC: Oxygen utilization and cardiovascular function after severe head injury. Neurosurgery 1984; 15:307–314.
147. Young B, Ott L, Norton J et al: Metabolic and nutritional sequela in non-steroid treated head injury patients. Neurosurgery 1985; 17: 784–790.
148. Robertson CS, Goodman JC, Grossman RC: Blood flow and metabolic therapy in CNS injury. J Neurotrauma 1992; 9:S579-S594.
149. Myers R, Yamaguchi S: Nervous system effects of cardiac arrest in monkeys: preservation of vision. Arch Neurol 1977; 34:65.
150. Warner D, Smith M, Siesjo B: Ischemia in normo- and hyperglycemic rats: effects on brain water and electrolytes. Stroke 1987; 18: 464–471.
151. Young B, Ott L, Dempsy R et al: Relationship between admission hyperglycemia and neurological outcome of severely brain injured patients. Arch Surg 1989; 210:466–472.
152. Lam MM, Winn HR, Cullen BF, Sundling N: Hyperglycemia and neurological outcomes in patients with head injury. J Neurosurg 1991; 75:545–551.
153. Rapp RP, Young B, Twyman D et al: The favorable effect of early parenteral feeding on survival in head-injured patients. J Neurosurg 1983; 58:906–912.
154. Young B, Ott L, Twyman D et al: The effect of nutritional support on outcome from severe head injury. J Neurosurg 1987; 67:668–676.
155. Hadley MN, Graham TW, Harrington T et al: Nutritional support and neurotrauma: a critical review of early nutrition in 45 acute head injury patients. Neurosurgery 1986; 19:367–373.

156. Torner JC: Outcome evaluation in acute neurological injury. Curr Opin Neurol Neurosurg 1992; 5:831–839.
157. Marschall L, Gautille T, Klauber M et al: The outcome of severe closed head injury. J Neurosurg 1991; 75:S28-S36.
158. Choi S, Narayan R, Anderson R, Ward J: Enhanced specificity of prognosis in severe head injury. J Neurosurg 1988; 69:381–385.
159. Vollmer D, Torner J, Jane J et al: Age and outcome following traumatic coma: why do older patients fare worse? J Neurosurg 1991; 75:S37-S49.
160. Marmarou A, Anderson R, Ward J et al: Impact of ICP instability and hypotension on outcome in patients with severe head trauma. J Neurosurg 1991; 75:S59-S66.
161. Marshall L, Marshall S, Klauber M et al: A new classification of head injury based on computerized tomography. J Neurosurg 1991; 75: S14-S20.
162. Sazbon L, Groswasser Z: Outcome in 134 patients with prolonged posttraumatic unawareness. Part 1: Parameters determining late recovery of consciousness. J Neurosurg 1990; 72:75–80.
163. Landlow L, Lee P: Current trends in neurosurgical critical care medicine. J Neurosurg Anesthesiol 1989; 1:307–315.

CHAPTER 14

The Obtunded Patient

Scott B. Groudine
Philip D. Lumb

Case Report

A 78-year-old white man was admitted to the hospital through the emergency room. The chief complaint was lower gastrointestinal (GI) bleeding. Bright red rectal blood had been noticed. He had been cared for in a nursing home and had not eaten for 3 days before hospital admission. Apparently, some intravenous fluids had been administered in the nursing home.

Admission laboratory values included the following: blood urea nitrogen (BUN), 86 mg; creatinine, 2.8 mg; sodium, 121 mEq/L; potassium, 2.9 mEq/L; chloride, 85 mEq/L; carbon dioxide, 20 mEq/L; hematocrit and hemoglobin, 21% and 7.8. Vital signs were: blood pressure, 85/70 mm Hg; heart rate, 110/min; respirations, 22/min and regular.

An infusion of Ringer's lactate was started, the patient was eventually taken to the operating room for the removal of a large, fungating rectal tumor. In the operating room, the patient received 3 mg midazolam. Anesthesia for the 2.5-hour operation consisted primarily of fentanyl, at 150 μg/hr. The patient also received 120 mg ketamine. Fluid resuscitation was continued with Ringer's lactate solution.

Following the procedure, the patient was brought to the intensive care unit (ICU) in stable condition. He was left intubated because he was not awake at the end of the procedure. Three hours after ICU admission, the patient was still not awake and did not respond to commands, but only to painful stimuli. During examination, the left pupil was noted to be slightly larger than the right. However, no preoperative pupillary examination had been done. Postoperative laboratory values were as follows: sodium, 124 mEq/L; potassium, 3.1 mEq/L; chloride, 88 mEq/L; carbon dioxide, 21; BUN, 80 mg; creatinine, 2.7 mg; and blood glucose, 230 mg/dl. Other pertinent laboratory data included a phosphorus level of 1.8 mEq/L.

Therapy at that time included 0.4 mg naloxone; the patient did not respond. Flumazenil was also administered in a 2-mg dose. Failure of those two agents prompted the use of 2.0 mg physostigmine. The patient was taken for a computed tomographic (CT) scan, which revealed no abnormalities such as edema or any fluid shift. The pulse oximeter indicated 97%, and blood gas values were also normal.

The presence of altered mental status in the postoperative patient may be an expected result of the anesthesia or surgery. However, it can also signal a neurologic crisis that must be identified and treated early to minimize the potential for severe and permanent injury. The obtunded or comatose patient must be examined thoroughly before a significant mental status change can be attributed to anesthesia.

The obtunded critically ill patient is a diagnostic dilemma in whom a cause for the stupor or coma must be found. Treatment and prognosis are radically different and depend on the underlying cause.

EXAMINATION OF THE PATIENT

The exact nature of the physical, metabolic, pharmacologic, psychiatric, or endocrine problem must be sought (Table 14–1). A decrease in the level of consciousness needs to be quantified as terms such as obtunded, stuporous, semicomatose, clouded, blunted, and lethargic do not transmit enough information to allow an accurate assessment of improvement or deterioration in mental status. Description of the physical examination is more useful than compression of data into labels. Similarly, a detailed neurologic evaluation of these patients is mandatory.

Subsequent examinations need to be repeated frequently and are usually not as detailed. This has given rise to the widespread use of the Glasgow coma scale (GCS). The GCS is used widely because its ability to quantify a physical examination makes significant changes in neurologic status readily apparent (Table 14–2). The scores range from a perfect 15 to a low of 3. The term coma can be used to describe a score of less than 8.[1] As one third of the scoring comes from verbal ability, the GCS cannot be used unaltered in aphasic or intubated patients. However, it still may prove useful to score these patients with regards to motor ability and eye opening.

• *A diagnosis of coma is consistent with a Glasgow coma score of less than 8.*

The assessment of the obtunded patient must be enacted in a logical and systematic fashion (Table 14–3). One approach follows.

Verification that the patient is well oxygenated and vital signs are stable means a neurologic examination may be initiated. If this is not the case immediate life support must be initiated or continued. Blood pressure and oxygenation should be maintained by whatever means are necessary. Treatment of reversible causes of stupor and

Table 14–1.
Causes of Altered Mental Status

Cause	Examples
Structural	
Vascular disorders	Intracranial bleeding, epidural hematoma, subarachnoid hemorrhage, cerebral vasculitis, dural sinus thrombosis, air emboli, and thromboemboli
Trauma	Contusion, vascular trauma, fat embolism, concussion
Degenerative disorders	Primary brain, metastatic, and hematopoietic
Epilepsy	Senility, Alzheimer's disease, multiple sclerosis, amyotrophic lateral sclerosis
Infectious	Bacteria, viruses, slow viruses, fungi, protozoa
Metabolic	
Endocrine disorders	Diabetes, adrenal, parathyroid, thyroid, and pituitary disorders, chronic pancreatitis* (exocrine function)
Hepatic disorders	
Uremia	
Hypoglycemia	
Nutrition	Low thiamine, niacin, vitamin B_{12}, folate, and pyridoxine
Environment	Hypo- and hyperthermia, poisons, drugs
Cerebral hypoxia	Circulatory or pulmonary causes
Electrolytes	Abnormalities of Na, Ca, PO_4, Mg, hyper- and hypoosmolality
Hypercarbia	
Psychiatric	
Catatonia	
Hysteria	Conversion reactions
Malingering	

* Data from Sjnastad O, Gjessig L, Ritland S, et al: Chronic relapsing pancreatitis, encephalopathy, with disturbance of consciousness and SCF aberration. J Neurol 1970; 220:83–94.

Table 14–2.
Glasgow Coma Scale (GCS)

Response	Score
Motor (1–6 score available)	
Following commands	6
Localizing to stimulus	5
Flexion/withdrawal	4
Flexion only	3
Extension	2
No tone	1
Verbal (1–5 score available)	
Oriented and appropriate	5
Confused	4
Able to speak words	3
Moaning	2
Nothing	1
Ocular (1–4 score available)	
Opening spontaneously	4
Opening to voice	3
Opening to pain	2
No response	1
Score total of three categories:	
Maximum score:	15
Coma:	<8
Minimum:	3

Table 14–3.
Rostral-Caudal Spread of Brain Dysfunction

Level Involved	Pupils	Respiratory Pattern	Response to Pain	Glasgow Coma Score
None	Equal and reactive	Normal	Normal	15
Cerebral	Normal or small but reactive	Normal or Cheyne-Stokes	Normal or decorticate posturing	5–14
Midbrain + upper pons involving oculomotor complex	Midposition, 3–4 mm, and nonreactive	Central neurogenic hyperventilation (CNH)	Decerebrate	4
Medulla	Midposition and fixed or dilated (terminal)	Ataxic	None	3

coma should be administered. This will include thiamine 100 mg intramuscularly or intravenously, as empiric treatment for Wernicke's encephalopathy, which is observed more frequently in people with an alcohol dependency, and 50 ml 50% dextrose for the treatment of undiagnosed hypoglycemia. Both of these actions may prevent occurrence of further cerebral injury, and neither hurts patients suffering from other causes of obtundation.

When appropriate, the first to establish is the patient's level of consciousness. It will soon be evident whether or not the patient is arousable. If this is the case, the examiner immediately knows the functional status of the reticular activating system, the hypothalamus, and the pons. If the patient goes on to demonstrate purposeful and deliberate interaction with the environment, some cerebral function is intact. An arousable patient who remains unaware is considered in a persistent vegetative state. The term stupor describes a patient who can be aroused by strong stimuli but is generally unarousable to mild stimuli, such as vocal cues or light touch. Coma is the state of being unarousable and unaware, irrespective of the stimuli.

If the level of consciousness is compatible with verbal ability, this can now be checked. Speech indicates some intact cerebral function, whether it is oriented (GCS verbal score of 5) or moans (GCS verbal score of 2).

A brief physical examination of the patient's head should be performed to ensure that no unrecognized trauma occurred during transportation. Head injuries from monitors, pumps, and bed rails are possible and must be sought.

Respiration

The next part of the examination should concern itself with the patient's respiratory pattern. The cerebral cortex exhibits inhibitory control over the pontine respiratory control centers. In the absence of cerebral respiratory control, pontine hyperventilation ensues. When low enough levels of $PaCO_2$ are reached, the cerebral centers will again start to inhibit respiration. This pattern of breathing, Cheyne-Stokes, is an early sign of bilateral cerebral or diencephalonic dysfunction and may proceed to coma in the obtunded patient. It can also herald impending transtentorial herniation, and thus a cause for this pattern of respiration should be sought.[2]

A more ominous respiratory pattern is central neurogenic hyperventilation (CNH). This is seen in decerebrate animals and is caused by an uninhibited pons causing hyperventilation. This is occasionally the pattern seen in deep coma.[3] It differs from hyperventilation secondary to acidosis in that CNH is rapid but shallow, whereas respiratory compensation for metabolic acidosis includes rapid and deep breathing.

- *Cerebral cortex dysfunction can result in pontine control of respiration. This causes the so-called syndrome of central hyperventilation.*

As involvement proceeds more caudally, apneustic breathing can be seen. This presents with prolonged end-expiratory or inspiratory pauses. It is clinically seen in basilar artery occlusions and other conditions that affect the pons.

- *Basilar artery occlusion can cause apneustic breathing patterns.*

Finally, when dysfunction starts to include the medulla, ataxic breathing develops. As its name suggests, this is characterized by breathing that is highly variable in rate and depth. It is a harbinger of the apnea and death that are soon to follow.

Pupils

The pupils are an important component of any neurologic examination. Their examination does not require patient cooperation. Since pupillary pathways are resistant to metabolic insults, they are an important aid to differentiate metabolic, psychiatric, and structural causes of obtundation.

Constriction of the pupil is parasympathetically mediated. The oculomotor complex (Edinger-Westphal nucleus) arises in the midbrain and travels with the third cranial nerve. The sympathetic fibers that dilate the pupil arise in the hypothalamus and travel via the brain stem to the cervical sympathetic chain ganglion, from which they enter the eye. Thus, an isolated cerebral insult will be accompanied by normal size and reactive pupils. As damage proceeds caudad, the pupils become small and constricted due to hypothalamic compromise. They will still react to light under close examination. The addition of a Horner's syndrome presents a clinical picture consistent with a space-occupying lesion above the tentorium or other abnormality that would result in increased pressure or direct injury to the hypothalamus. Midbrain involvement causes the pupils to lose their parasympathetic tone and to approach midsize. Reactivity to light will be lost with the destruction of the oculomotor complex. If the insult continues to progress beyond this point, coma is irreversible, with the destruction of the midbrain (see Table 14–3). In the premorbid state, the pupils become fully dilated, the constrictor muscle of the pupil relaxes, and there is agonal release of norepinephrine.[3] Pupils also may dilate abruptly from uncal compression of the third cranial nerves.

- *Hypothalamic injury causes constricted pupils. Horner's syndrome develops with injury or increased pressure on the hypothalamus. Oculomotor injury or destruction causes pupillary loss of reactivity to light. Abrupt dilation of the pupils follows uncal compression of the third cranial nerve.*

• *Pontine injury results in pinpoint pupils that are reactive to light. Midsize or large pupils that respond to light may develop in metabolic coma.*

Isolated injuries can cause unilateral pupillary abnormalities or specific changes. A pontine lesion interrupts sympathetic fibers but leaves the parasympathetic fibers intact, with resultant pinpoint pupils reactive to light. Unilateral pupillary dilation suggests impingement of the ocular motor nerve on the ipsilateral side. This may also be accompanied by an elliptically shaped pupil, which also develops with brain stem compression. Pupil size consistent with parasympathetic destruction (midsized or large) but with the preservation of light reactivity suggests a metabolic cause for the coma. Light reflexes are usually preserved in metabolic coma. Hippus, which is rhythmic dilation and constriction of the iris after exposure to light, can be a normal occurrence, but its incidence is higher in the presence of multiple sclerosis or barbiturate exposure, which is a real possibility in the immediate postoperative patient.[4]

Other Ocular and Corneal Signs

• *Downward ocular bobbing indicates a pontine lesion. Upward bobbing develops with metabolic derangement. Deviated eyes can indicate drug overdosage or hypoxia.*

Many obtunded or comatose patients appear to be asleep, with eyes closed. A comatose patient's eyelid will stay closed due to the resting tone of the orbicularis oculi muscle. When opened, the eyelid will close slowly and continuously. This action is never voluntary and thus eliminates hysterical illness from the differential diagnosis. In addition, when the eyelid is opened, the eyes may appear to rove. Another pattern seen in the comatose patient is ocular bobbing[5] (rapid downward motion of the pupil followed by a slow return). This is often indicative of a pontine lesion. Reverse bobbing (rapid upward motion followed by a slow downward return) is seen in cases of metabolic derangement. Eyes that are deviated inferiorly and nasally are also present in metabolic coma or thalamic dysfunction. Upwardly deviated eyes develop frequently in certain drug overdoses, seizures, and hypoxic states.[6]

• *In a comatose patient, the doll's eye maneuver causes the eyes to attempt to stay focused in the original position.*

If the patient's neck can be rotated safely, evaluation of the ocular-vestibular reflexes can add significant information about the integrity of specific areas of the brain. They will also help ascertain whether the extraocular muscles are fully functional in the stuporous or comatose patient. The doll's eye maneuver is performed when the examiner quickly moves the patient's head in the vertical or horizontal plane. The eyes in a truly comatose patient will attempt to stay focused in the original position. Thus a head turn to the right will move the pupils to the left. This tests the right medial rectus muscle and the left lateral rectus muscle, as well as the vestibular portion of the eighth cranial nerve. This reflex can be imitated in noncomatose patients if the subject makes an effort to stay focused on a fixed object. This test cannot rule out hysterical illness. The normal awake subject refixes his or her gaze on head turning to an object in front, and doll's eyes are not seen.

• *Cold caloric stimulation in an aware patient initiates nystagmus with a slow component to the irrigated ear and a fast component away. In metabolic coma, the patient may not respond to cold caloric stimulation.*

Cold caloric stimulation can help differentiate metabolic, psychiatric, and structural abnormalities. After an ear examination to ensure a clear ear canal, the head of the bed is raised 30°, and ice water is slowly injected into the ear canal. A response is generally elicited before 120 ml water is injected. In the aware patient cold water will start a nystagmus with the slow component to the irrigated ear and the fast component away. As obtundation and coma approach, the fast phase fades away, and only tonic deviation of the eyes to the irrigated side occurs. The appearance of nystagmus after cold water calorics in an acutely unconscious patient may signify a psychiatric cause. In the persistent vegetative state (alert but not aware), the patient regains the nystagmus that was lost during the acute comatose phase of the illness. Patients in a metabolic coma may demonstrate no response to cold calorics (also seen in brain death and when wax persists in the ear canal). Drugs such as aminoglycosides, tricyclic antidepressants, phenytoin, barbiturates, and, of course, muscle relaxants may also have this effect.

Corneal reflexes should be checked to verify the functions of cranial nerves V and VII.

Motor Response

The patient's ability to move and the motor response to pain are important to track the course of cerebral dysfunction. The Glasgow coma scale weighs motor response most heavily, with 6 of the 15 scored alone from this category. If a patient follows commands, there is no reason to elicit a motor reflex to pain. The stuporous patient may need a painful stimulus to demonstrate motor ability. The type of response is indicative of the degree of rostral-caudal spread of brain dysfunction. If the cerebral cortex is impaired but the diencephalon is intact, a decorticate posture will result from painful stimulation. This may present as flexion of the upper extremities and extension of the lower extremities, with an incomplete effort to withdraw from the pain (flexion-withdrawal) or with no effort to withdrawal from the painful stimuli (flexion).

- *An impaired cerebral cortex results in decorticate posturing. This includes flexion of the upper extremities and an extension of the lower extremities. The patient makes no effort to withdraw from painful stimuli.*

If a decerebrate posture is seen (extension of both upper and lower extremities), midbrain involvement is suspected, and the patient is considered to be in deep coma. Further spread to the pons will result in flaccid quadriplegia and death will soon ensue.

- *Decerebrate posturing reflects midbrain injury. This involves extension of upper and lower extremities.*

Motor response must be gauged against deep pain. If no response is seen, consideration must be given to the depth of the noxious stimuli. Many use pressure on the nail beds or on the inferior border of the supraorbital ridge to generate deep pain.

Abnormal muscle activity such as asterixis, tremor, opthistonus, seizures, and myoclonus should be noted as this may help to determine the cause and treatment of the stupor.

In summary, an important aspect of the initial physical examination is to adequately define the degree of neurologic impairment, so that improvement or deterioration in function is quickly recognized. The Glasgow coma scale can prove useful when doing this. In addition, after a physical examination the reason for the obtunded mental status should be clearer. Psychiatric disorders will not present with abnormal calorics, structural lesions will proceed orderly in a rostral-caudal direction and may be asymmetric, and metabolic or drug-induced problems will present with disorders that cannot be explained anatomically and are usually bilateral, as characterized by a flaccid motor examination with pupils that react to light. Obviously, this section has focused on the examination of the central nervous system (CNS). However, in early assessment, examination of the abdomen and extremities must not be overlooked.

HISTORY

The obtunded perioperative patient's history is invaluable in determining cause. Most perioperative patients have a recent history of anesthesia and other pharmacologic interventions. Many also have a medical history that can provide important insight into neurologic dysfunction. A review of the medical record and information from available family members and the patient's prior medical history should help. Specific emphasis should be placed on prescription medications, illicit drug use, psychiatric history, liver and renal disease, diabetes and other endocrine disorders, recent trauma, hypertension, and neurologic symptoms.

An understanding of the surgical procedure, medication record, and anesthetic management must be sought, as obtundation and coma can result from these interventions. A clouded or dulled sensorium is an expected early result of anesthetic management. If there is any doubt, consultation with the anesthesiologist who provided the intraoperative care of the patient should be sought.

ANESTHETIC EFFECT ON LEVEL OF CONSCIOUSNESS

One of the purposes of a general anesthetic is to render the patient unaware and insensible to pain. It is not surprising that some of these effects may continue into the postoperative period and cause a decrease in the patient's level of consciousness when compared to his or her preoperative state. These are the anesthetic's expected effects. However, while the patient is unconscious, events may occur that alter brain function and lead to an abnormal neurologic recovery from anesthesia. The differentiation between normal and abnormal neurologic recovery is critical as the treatment and prognosis vary with the cause.

NEUROLOGIC EFFECTS OF ANESTHETICS

Drugs used for the induction of anesthesia can have a long and profound effect on the level of consciousness. Diazepam can impair reaction times in healthy individuals for up to 12 hours.[7] Barbiturates can reversibly depress activity in all nervous tissue. This usually is confined to the CNS, but in large doses, they can produce serious cardiovascular effects. The most commonly used barbiturate is thiopental. A 3- to 6-mg/kg dose of thiopental will rapidly cause loss of consciousness (one arm to brain circulation time) and has this effect for approximately 10 minutes. As thiopental is redistributed, awakening occurs. Thiopental is cleared slowly by the liver and is highly bound to albumin, so that lower doses are needed in hypoalbuminemic states. The elimination half-life is 5 to 12 hours.[8] Following normal induction doses, patients are not able to drive safely for 24 hours.[7] The amount of drug effect is proportional to the total amount of redistributed thiopental. Thus, a very high total dose of the drug can result in somnolence, stupor, and even prolonged coma. In fact, this is one of the drugs utilized to institute a barbiturate coma. The total barbiturate dose received by a stuporous patient should be available from the anesthesia record, as will be the notation of other CNS depressants.

• *Ordinarily, patients awaken rapidly following thiopental administration. However, doses higher than 500 mg can prolong loss of consciousness.*

Benzodiazepines are also used as induction agents. Midazolam, lorazepam, and diazepam belong in this group. These drugs produce amnesia, hypnosis, muscle relaxation, and, in larger doses, anesthesia. Midazolam is used most frequently in anesthesia because of its water solubility, faster onset time to loss of consciousness (less than 3 minutes), and a clearance that is 10 times faster than that of diazepam. Clearance is by the liver, and 95% of midazolam is protein bound.

Benzodiazepines exert a clinical effect for a longer time than thiopental. Diazepam's elimination half-life is 20 to 40 hours. Unlike with thiopental, the clinician has the ability to specifically reverse the CNS effects of the benzodiazepines with flumazenil, a new, specific benzodiazepine receptor antagonist. Flumazenil will partially antagonize the effects of benzodiazepines with a dose of 0.1 to 0.2 mg and totally reverse the effects of benzodiazepines in the dosage range of 0.4 to 1.0 mg. The reversal effect can be seen in under 3 minutes. The terminal half-life of this drug is shorter than that of most benzodiazepines (41 to 79 minutes); therefore, it is prudent to watch the patient closely for signs of recurrence of sedation for 2 hours after the last dose of flumazenil. Thus, if physical examination and review of the perioperative medications suggest the possibility of a benzodiazepine stupor, flumazenil can confirm this diagnosis and reverse the process.

• *The half-life of flumazenil, a benzodiazepine antagonist, is shorter than the half-life of most benzodiazepines.*

Ketamine, an agent related to phencyclidine (PCP), is also used to induce anesthesia. It may be used in trauma surgery or severe hemorrhage when the sympathetic stimulation often seen with this drug is desirable. The anesthetic state produced by this drug is called "dissociative anesthesia" because the patient feels removed from his or her surroundings. Patients will be sedated, analgesic, and still. Most will experience nystagmus, dreams, and occasionally, myoclonic movements. Salivary secretions are stimulated, and this drug is often co-administered with an anticholinergic agent. Perioperative emergence reactions are common after the use of ketamine (5 to 30%).[9] Emergence often takes hours, and patients may complain of hallucinations or bad dreams. These can recur weeks later.[10] Studies have shown a decrease in the incidence of these effects if a benzodiazepine is used intraoperatively. Respiratory depression with the drug is dose dependent, but normal carbon dioxide re-

• *Ketamine can produce pulmonary complications secondary to increased secretions.*

sponses can be seen even with anesthetic doses. Therefore, an extubated perioperative patient could still be under the influence of ketamine. In a patient with nystagmus, myoclonic movements, and intermittent delirium, a history of ketamine use should be sought.

Propofol is an increasingly popular induction agent due to its fast recovery time. Its elimination half-life is 55 minutes. However, patients awaken rapidly after an infusion is stopped. Because of the drug's high clearance and elimination, there is little drug accumulation even after prolonged use. Propofol has recently been approved for ICU use to provide short periods of anesthesia or, by constant infusion, to provide sedation.[11]

Occasional reports of propofol withdrawal syndromes have been described in adult and pediatric patients who have received prolonged dosing.[12,13] One such report noted an organic delusional state for 7 days after the abrupt discontinuation of propofol. Children have suffered various withdrawal symptoms, ranging from myoclonic movements to functional blindness,[14–16] all of which eventually resolved. These complications suggest that weaning patients from propofol may be more appropriate then abrupt cessation.

Reports of opisthotonus, decerebrate rigidity, and hyperreflexia are starting to appear after brief exposures to propofol.[13,17,18] These conditions are self-limiting, but provide a scare to both patient and physician. Additionally, propofol has been implicated in rare cases of reinducing an unconscious state in the awake perioperative patient.[17] Although rare, an unusual neurologic reaction to propofol should be considered in patients who previously received the drug and on examination have had a change in mental status. Additional propofol should probably not be given to these patients for sedation.

• *Etomidate has actions similar to those of thiopental but does not cause significant hypotension, particularly in hypovolemic patients.*

Etomidate is a commonly used induction agent in seriously ill patients due to its minimal effects on the cardiovascular system. Besides unconsciousness, it can produce vigorous myotonic activity during induction of anesthesia thought to be the result of subcortical disinhibition and may be confused with a seizure. Premedication with narcotics can reduce the incidence of this frequent occurrence. Of more concern to the critical care practitioner is that prolonged infusions of etomidate can suppress adrenal steroidogenesis and may result in addisonian symptomatology.[19] This may occur more frequently in patients with cirrhosis as they will experience an increase in elimination half-life secondary to this drug's hepatic metabolism.[20]

MUSCLE RELAXANTS

Muscle relaxants are commonly used in the operative period to facilitate intubation and surgery. Their effects may persist into the postoperative period. Residual paralysis will result in an abnormal neurologic examination. Patients may range in symptoms from diplopia (weakness of the extraocular muscles) to flaccid paralysis. Usually, the postoperative, fully paralyzed patient is brought to the ICU intubated and the reason for the paralysis is known. Occasionally, a patient will be extubated before the effects of the neuromuscular blocking agent have been dissipated or fully antagonized. The patient will have difficulty breathing with discordant muscle movements and difficult airway maintenance. Generalized muscle weakness is present, and the patient has slurred speech. In addition, they are incapable of airway protection, and the risk of aspiration increases. Patients lose facial wrinkles and may appear younger than their stated age. Attempted muscle activity in the face of neuromuscular blockade can look like agitation and can lead to an erroneous diagnosis. A nerve stimulator will aid in making the appropriate diagnosis. A situation may occur following administration of muscle relaxants and reversal agents in which the patient develops recurrent signs of relaxant-induced weakness. This "re-curarization" is a product of the different half-lives of the relaxant and reversal agents. Although not seen frequently, this phenomenon must enter the differential diagnosis of persistent or recurring postoperative muscle weakness. Excessive doses of reversal agents (neostigmine, pyridostigmine, and edrophonium) will paradoxically block the neuromuscular junction and act as a neuromuscular blocker in patients given multiple doses of reversal agents.

- *Excessive doses of neuromuscular blocker reversal agents can themselves block the neuromuscular junction and prolong blockade.*

Other medications can potentiate the effect of neuromuscular blocking agents and result in total or partial paralysis. These include some antibiotics (gentamicin, clindamycin, and tetracycline, to name the most common), local anesthetics (lidocaine), quinidine, trimethaphan, furosemide, and magnesium.

Recurrent paralysis occasionally gives the appearance of altered mental status and can lead to carbon dioxide narcosis with obtundation. This can develop either in patients extubated or those who receive partial ventilatory support such as intermittent mandatory ventilation.

ADJUVANT DRUGS

Narcotics are used in the perioperative period and can contribute to the appearance of stupor. Narcotized patients exhibit small pupils and have slow, deep respirations. Narcotic respiratory depression can lead to carbon dioxide narcosis and death. If narcotics are suspected as contributors to the patient's obtundation, a specific narcotic antagonist (naloxone) can be administered and subsequent effects noted. When the situation is not an emergency, naloxone can be slowly titrated in 0.05-mg increments until the desired respiratory results are seen. With careful naloxone administration, it may be possible to maintain the analgesic effect of the narcotic coupled with reversal of most of the respiratory depression. As the half-lives of most of the narcotics are longer than naloxone and the other narcotic antagonists, the potential for recurrent narcosis is real and should be expected. If narcosis again ensues, continuous infusion of naloxone can be titrated to minimize respiratory depression.

- *Narcotic depression is characterized by constricted pupils and a slow respiratory rate.*

Droperidol is commonly used as an adjunct in anesthesia because of its dual role as an antiemetic and as a component of neuroleptanesthesia when combined with fentanyl. Droperidol is a butyrophenone derivative, and its ability to produce a blunted affect is expected. In addition, extrapyramidal muscle movements, that is, dystonia, akathisia, and oculogyric crisis, occur in approximately 1% of patients and may present up to 12 hours after surgery.[10] Atropine and other anti-Parkinson drugs can usually successfully control these symptoms. This effect is seen more commonly in patients with Parkinson's disease, in whom droperidol is best avoided.

When neurolept anesthesia has been used, the prolonged action of droperidol (3 to 6 hours) relative to the fentanyl (30 minutes) must be recognized. If patients are given narcotics in the postoperative period, a neuroleptic state may develop again, and the patient will become obtunded. Once this is recognized as the cause of the mental status change, supportive treatment can be provided, and fears of a pathologic process extinguished.

Anticholinergics are a group of drugs frequently used by anesthesiologists that can also result in obtundation in the perioperative patient. The most commonly used drugs in this class are glycopyrrolate, atropine, and scopolamine. Glycopyrrolate contains a highly polar quaternary ammonium group that limits its access across the blood-brain barrier and thus, CNS toxicity is rare with this drug. Atropine and scopolamine are nonpolar tertiary amines and readily cross into the brain and cause a multitude of neurologic symptoms. Atropine does not depress the brain as much as scopolamine. When CNS depression is desired, as in premedication for surgery, scopolamine often is preferred.

Scopolamine can cause somnolence and fatigue and is a component in over-the-counter sleep medications. Antihistamines also block acetylcholine transmission in the brain and can have similar effects on sleep induction.

Large doses of atropine can cause a central anticholinergic syndrome. The CNS symptoms consist of somnolence, confusion, hallucinations, delirium, stupor, and coma. Peripherally, one sees dry mouth and skin that is warm, facial flushing, fever, hallucinations, mydriasis, tachycardia, and difficulty voiding. Other drugs with anticholinergic activity can cause this syndrome. They include phenothiazines, tricyclic antidepressants, butyrophenones, benzodiazepines, opioids, inhalational anesthetics, nitrous oxide, antihistamines, etomidate, and ketamine.[21,22] Case reports of this syndrome which demonstrate it can occur following sedation during regional anesthesia have been published.[23] It has also been described in patients who received sedation during ventilatory management.[22]

• *Symptoms of atropine overdose include fever, facial flushing, hallucinations, and tachycardia.*

A patient who has received drugs with anticholinergic effects and exhibits delirium, stupor, or other CNS changes may suffer from central anticholinergic syndrome (CAS). If peripheral signs are present and other causes have been eliminated, a trial of physostigmine may be warranted. Physostigmine is an anticholinesterase inhibitor that can cross the blood-brain barrier and reverse the effects of cholinergic blockade in the brain. Given slowly at a dose of 1 to 4 mg, physostigmine will rapidly return an obtunded patient to his or her prior neurologic status if the cause was CAS and this will

• *Physostigmine (1 to 4 mg) can reverse central nervous depression secondary to anticholinergic agents.*

help confirm the diagnosis. If the patient has a positive response to physostigmine, close observation will still be required as the drug is rapidly metabolized, and altered mental status may reappear in 1 to 2 hours. The use of glycopyrrolate as the anticholinergic agent may prevent the development of this syndrome.

OBTUNDATION ASSOCIATED WITH CERTAIN SURGICAL PROCEDURES

Carotid Endarterectomy

Patients who undergo carotid endarterectomy already have impaired cerebral blood flow, and many have presented for the operation with a history of stroke, transient ischemic attacks (TIAs), or reversible ischemic neurologic deficits (RINDS). The perioperative incidence of stroke ranges between 2 and 20%.[24–26] Dependent on the cause, a stroke can present at any time in the perioperative period. Cerebral injury that occurs as a result of hypoperfusion during carotid cross-clamping will present intraoperatively or in the immediate postoperative period. Protection of the patient from this complication has led to the use of shunts that allow flow to be maintained during most of the endarterectomy. However, these are not without risk. They can free plaque emboli or raise an intimal flap on insertion, release thromboemboli on removal, be difficult or impossible to place, and become kinked or dislodged during use.[27] Therefore, the use and indications for shunts are controversial among surgeons who perform carotid endarterectomies. Some never shunt, others always shunt or shunt selectively on the basis of preoperative anatomy from arteriography, or from information obtained by intraoperative monitors including electroencephalography, compressed spectral analysis, carotid stump pressure measurement, transcranial Doppler, and near infrared cerebral oximetry.[28] Other surgeons prefer to do this operation with the patient awake under a combination superficial and deep cervical plexus block. In this way, patients' neurologic status is constantly monitored, and the need to shunt is determined by a change in the level of consciousness. Patients may also suffer strokes when flow is reestablished in the repaired artery. Cerebral vessels in the previously ischemic areas can lose their ability to autoregulate. This dysfunction carries into the postoperative period, and sudden episodes of hypertension can be transmitted directly to the cerebral circulation, resulting in cerebral hemorrhage.[29] Pomposelli and associates reported 11 intracranial hemorrhages out of 1500 carotid endarterectomies performed over a 9-year period, making it a significant cause of perioperative stroke for this procedure.[30] In addition, air may be trapped in the carotid artery when it is opened, and this can be responsible for a cerebral air embolus. Good surgical technique minimizes this risk.

- *Hypertension following carotid artery surgery can lead to hyperemia and intracranial hemorrhage.*

- *Loss of consciousness following carotid endarterectomy requires reoperation to reestablish flow.*

Immediate evaluation of the patient who has undergone carotid endarterectomy and whose level of consciousness changes in the postoperative period is warranted. If Doppler flow studies of the operated carotid artery can be obtained quickly, they may help to determine whether the problem is surgically reversible (carotid occlusion from thrombus or intimal flap) or inoperable (embolus). If Doppler studies cannot be done promptly, immediate reexploration may be required as rapid repair of an occluded carotid artery will minimize the degree of permanent neurologic damage. Arteriography may delay the procedure inordinately.

Patients at higher risk to develop perioperative strokes during this procedure include those who are symptomatic, have multiple stenotic areas on arteriogram, and have significant bilateral disease.[31]

Cardiopulmonary Bypass

Shaw and colleagues have shown that 79% of patients who required cardiopulmonary bypass developed some degree of postbypass neuropsychologic dysfunction.[32] This can be moderate to severe in one quarter of all coronary artery bypass graft (CABG) patients studied.

The two mechanisms whereby cerebral dysfunction is thought to occur are hypoperfusion resulting in cerebral ischemia[33] and embolization.[34] Emboli can be formed from atheromatous plaques, gas-blood aggregates, fibrin, thrombus, and extrinsic material from the circuit or bypass machine. Hypoperfusion can result from incorrect setup of the bypass machine, low arterial pressures, and inadequate cardiac output.

• *Cerebral dysfunction following cardiopulmonary bypass usually results from ischemia or embolization.*

Current evidence and research seem to indicate that the majority of cerebral dysfunction from heart surgery is a result of microemboli. Slogoff and colleagues showed that perfusion pressures of less than 50 mm Hg are not associated with an increase in neuropsychologic dysfunction.[26] These and other researchers concluded that air or intrinsic particulate debris are the major cause of CNS difficulty in the postoperative cardiac patient. The use of transcranial Doppler monitoring has demonstrated that cerebral emboli occur commonly during aortic manipulation.[35]

• *Asymptomatic carotid disease does not increase the risk of central nervous system morbidity following cardiopulmonary bypass.*

Risk factors for neurologic complications after cardiopulmonary bypass include preexisting cerebral disease, age older than 60 years, prolonged bypass, and open cardiac chamber surgery.[36] Not all these risk factors are supported by all clinical studies. Recent studies show no difference in CNS morbidity in open or closed chamber surgeries.[37–39] Asymptomatic carotid disease has not been shown to increase a patients' risk of neurologic injury from bypass.[40,41]

Treatment of these patients is largely supportive, as little can be done once embolization has occurred. However, if air is seen in the venous cannula when on bypass or if other intraoperative events lead one to think that the cerebral insult is a result of air entrainment, then quick treatment in a hyperbaric oxygen chamber may be appropriate.[42] The ability to provide a hyperbaric environment is limited, as is clinical experience with this technique. It is therefore not considered standard of care but may be desirable on an individual basis.

Patients who have an adverse CNS outcome while on bypass

will present with these deficits when the effects of the anesthesia wear off. Patients who were neurologically intact postoperatively but then become confused or obtunded should have other causes of their cerebral dysfunction explored, such as new-onset atrial fibrillation, low cardiac output, and all other mechanisms that can result in obtundation.

TURP Syndrome

Transurethral resection of the prostate (TURP) is a surgical procedure usually performed on elderly men with urinary retention or cancer. During this procedure, large amounts of fluid are used to irrigate the prostate, and significant amounts are systematically absorbed. As hemostasis is obtained with electrocautery, it is important that the irrigation solution not conduct electricity well. This eliminates the use of balanced salt solutions as an irrigant. Water is hypotonic and causes hemolysis on absorption. Currently employed irrigants consist of sorbitol, glycine, urea, and mannitol added to the water to increase its osmolarity and minimize hemolysis.

The TURP syndrome includes CNS and cardiac dysfunction seen following significant absorption of the irrigant through open prostatic vessels. This occurs when the intravesical irrigant pressure is greater than the venous pressure. Its exact nature depends on the specific fluid used. CNS symptoms range from visual hallucinations to death. Henderson and Middleton reviewed 2000 patients undergoing this procedure and showed that 3.9% had hyponatremia and 0.7% were obtunded or comatose.[43] Following appropriate therapy, this change in neurologic status was corrected in all patients.

All irrigants are electrolyte free and on absorption decrease serum sodium. An abrupt serum sodium decrease to below 120 mEq/L can cause CNS dysfunction. Changes in osmolarity and tonicity can be important in the development of CNS symptoms. Although the calculated osmolarity will be low, the actual serum osmolarity will be higher due to the absorption of the irrigation solutes. This will often produce a calculated osmolal gap of greater than 10 mOsm/kg. The gap may get very large in renal failure patients due to the predominant renal excretion of most of the solutes.[44] Mannitol and sorbitol will increase the extracellular fluid more than intracellular volume, and this may lead to cerebral edema and cardiovascular overload. This is not true with glycine and urea. Glycine, however, when absorbed and metabolized, produces ammonia as a byproduct. Hyperammonemia alone may cause obtundation and coma. Glycine metabolism to ammonia may explain why obtundation sometimes develops hours after TURP when 1.5% glycine is used as the irrigant. High ammonia levels are seen more frequently in those individuals with liver disease because ammonia is converted by the liver to urea via the urea cycle.

- *Rapid sodium depletion (less than 6 hours) to levels lower than 120 mEq/L causes neurologic dysfunction.*

When TURP syndrome is suspected, electrolytes, osmolarity, ammonia, and glycine levels should be obtained to confirm the diagnosis. High ammonia and glycine levels are treated by supportive

• *Hyponatremia can be corrected with normal or 3% hypertonic saline. Sodium should be increased to levels above 124 mEq/L.*

measures. Symptomatic hyponatremia must be treated urgently, because this can cause permanent neurologic injury. Serum sodium should be aggressively increased if the level is below 120 mEq/L. Treatment is with hypertonic saline, 3 or 5%, 100 to 200 ml at a time given over 1 to 2 hours and repeated as needed to raise the serum sodium level above 124 mEq/L. Further normalization of the sodium can be obtained by water restriction, diuretic administration, and normal saline infusion. Aggressive treatment of chronic hyponatremia is associated with cerebral demyelination and abrupt decreases in cerebral volume. However, these complications of hypertonic saline treatment are rare in acute cases such as in the TURP syndrome.

In an effort to monitor CNS changes, most TURPs are done under regional anesthesia, so an intraoperative change in mental status can be identified quickly. Some centers have added ethanol to the irrigant and estimate fluid absorption by continuous breath analysis for exhaled ethanol with some success.[45–47]

Review of the medical record of a patient with suspected TURP syndrome should emphasize the amount and type of intravenous fluid, total resection time, and the fluid used for irrigation. Ideally, all fluids administered should be isotonic, and resection time should be less than 1 hour. Furthermore, the height of irrigant bags should be lowered to that compatible with good resection conditions and no higher. This will minimize passive fluid absorption. The type of solute in the irrigant can alert the physician to special problems that can occur with excessive absorption.

DELAYED ANESTHETIC EMERGENCE

Occasionally, a patient will have delayed emergence from anesthesia or just not appear to awaken as expected. Careful review of the perioperative medications and type of surgery may suggest no reason for this delay. It must be remembered, however, that the response to anesthetic agents is highly variable. Studies have shown that between 3 and 9% of patients are unarousable for prolonged periods (up to 1.5 hours) after uncomplicated anesthetics. Because neurologic events during anesthesia are relatively infrequent (0.04%),[48] delayed emergence from anesthesia is likely to be just that, rather than a catastrophic neurologic event.[49,50] Barnes and Havill reviewed anesthesia complications requiring ICU admission and found that only 2 of 110 complications were primarily neurologic.[51] Most neurologic sequelae were cardiac in origin.

METABOLIC CAUSES OF OBTUNDATION

It is important to identify metabolic causes of obtundation quickly (Table 14–4). After detailed physical examination (see the discussion earlier in this chapter), distinctions between metabolic and

Table 14–4.
Blood Studies Indicated in a Stuporous Patient

Glucose
Electrolytes (Na, K, Ca, Mg, PO_4, and Cl)
Blood, urea, nitrogen, and creatinine
Serum osmolarity
Arterial blood gas and ammonia
Endocrine test (thyroid and adrenal function)
Complete blood count
Cultures if indicated

other causes of decreased consciousness should be apparent. Metabolic derangements often present as bilateral deficits and, if the patient can communicate, are often heralded by changes in awareness. Delirium will often precede obtundation, and snouting and grasping reflexes may develop.

Pupillary responses to light are usually well preserved, even in deep coma of metabolic origins.[6] The absence of pupillary responses when a history of eyedrop or systemic anticholinergic use is absent usually indicates an anatomic problem. Respiratory patterns supported by blood gas analysis can be very informative. Severe acidosis with attempted respiratory compensation should be followed by investigations into the cause of the acidosis. Diabetic ketoacidosis, renal failure, lactic acidosis, and poisoning all cause metabolic acidosis with attempted respiratory compensation. Hepatic coma, salicylate overdose, sepsis, pneumonia, and psychiatric disorders (hyperventilation syndrome) cause a respiratory alkalosis. Hypoventilation without a metabolic alkalosis does not help discern metabolic versus anatomic injury. Inadequate reversal of neuromuscular blocking agents, anesthetics, narcotics, and brain stem injury all can result in this respiratory pattern.

Motor disturbances commonly develop during metabolic derangement. Tremors are bilateral and are often seen as a side effect of drug use or in alcohol withdrawal syndrome (delirium tremens). Asterixis is associated with hepatic dysfunction, but unilateral asterixis can be structural in origin. Diffuse myoclonus suggests uremia or another metabolic encephalopathy.[52]

In summary, metabolic derangement should be suspected when there is partial impairment of multiple brain areas while simultaneously other functions that originate from the same levels remain intact. Rostral-caudal spread and focal deficits suggest an intracranial pathologic process. Unresponsiveness with normal reflexes implies a psychologic cause for the obtundation.

- *Metaboic derangements often cause partial impairment of multiple brain areas.*

The most frequent cause of perioperative cerebral dysfunction is impaired oxygen delivery to the brain secondary to hypoxemia or cardiac problems. Hypoxia can occur at anytime in the perioperative period. If inadequate cerebral blood oxygen exists, then autoregulation can increase cerebral blood flow up to 200%. When this is inadequate, signs of cerebral hypoxia can develop.[53] Mental acuity and visual problems may develop early, followed by a decreased level of consciousness and then coma and death.

Decreased cerebral blood flow also results in global cerebral ischemia. When the normal cerebral blood flow of 50 ml/100 g brain/min is halved, the level of consciousness decreases. Levels below 20 ml/100 mg/min cause coma. If hypoperfusion persists or worsens, cerebral infarction can occur.[54]

Cardiac arrest is the most dramatic cause of cerebral dysfunction in the perioperative patient. Following cardiac arrest, patients tend to have patterns of neurologic injury, depending on the length of ischemia time.[55] Patients comatose following a short period of cardiopulmonary arrest have a rapid return of neurologic function within 12 hours.[56] Coma lasting 2 days after cardiac arrest has a variable outcome.[57] Synder and colleagues reported a 28% incidence of neurologic recovery.[58] Seizures and myoclonus were associated with a poorer outcome.[59] The majority had permanent focal neurologic defects. Intraoperative cardiac arrest may be associated with better neurologic outcome due to the protective cerebral effects of anesthetics and the rapid institution of cardiopulmonary resuscitation with high levels of oxygen. However, at least one study indicated that when coma developed as a result of intraoperative cardiac arrest, outcome was no different than when it occurred in the general hospital ward or in the ICU.[60] Unlike the study by Synder and associates, this study was unable to demonstrate that seizure were a negative prognostic sign once coma developed.

• *The degree of neurologic impairment following cardiac arrest does not always coincide with the duration of the arrest.*

Care for these patients consists of the immediate establishment of effective cardiopulmonary activity. Hyperglycemia should be avoided as this can encourage production of lactic acid under anaerobic conditions (anoxia) and may result in irreversible cerebral damage. Calcium channel blockers, free radical scavengers, and excitatory neurotransmitter blocking agents may have some cerebral protective effects in the postarrest patient. All are currently undergoing clinical and laboratory trials.

Less dramatic than cardiac arrest is decreased cardiac output. Cardiac arrhythmias, myocardial ischemia, and infarction can all result in hypoperfusion of the brain.

Following recovery from the original hypoxic insult, the patient may still develop a rare sequela called delayed postanoxic encephalopathy. Such patients initially appear to make a prompt and full recovery with no neurologic deficits. One to 3 weeks later, they abruptly have a new onset of neurologic symptoms that include spasticity, change in affect, coma, or death.[61] Autopsy results show prominent demyelination and diffuse bilateral cerebral leukoencephalopathy. There is no apparent treatment.

Lance-Adams syndrome (postanoxic myoclonus) can also occur after ischemic injury. In this syndrome, voluntary movements are accompanied by myoclonus. Otherwise, these patients are neurologically intact, with well-preserved intelligence. Satisfactory treatment of this has been reported with sodium valproate[62,63] and clonazepam.[64,65]

Hypoglycemia

The brain requires glucose for cerebral function. Hypo- and hyperglycemia can cause severe cerebral dysfunction. Hypoglycemia occurs in diabetics who use insulin or oral hypoglycemic agents. However, it can be seen in insulinoma or following abrupt discontinuation of hyperalimentation, or in alcoholics. Patients who take insulin or oral hypoglycemics and are allowed nothing by mouth preparatory to diagnostic testing or surgery can frequently become hypoglycemic. Hyperalimentation may be discontinued to start blood or give medications. The high circulating level of insulin with no continuing source of substrate causes hypoglycemia. Because of premedications or anesthesia, many of the initial symptoms of hypoglycemia will be missed.

• *Abrupt discontinuation of hyperalimentation or other nutritional support may result in hypoglycemia due to high circulating insulin levels.*

Symptoms in the hypoglycemic patient are related to the release of epinephrine to counter the effects of a low blood sugar. Patients complain of tachycardia, tremor, sweating, confusion, hunger, dizziness, and visual disturbances. They may proceed to develop seizures or lose consciousness.

Obtunded patients with hypoglycemia often have seizures and may have focal neurologic deficits suggestive of a nonmetabolic cause of the altered mental status.[66] Importantly, pupillary reflexes are usually spared. Irreversible neurologic injury can develop from hypoglycemia, and it must be treated early. All patients with unexplained obtundation should have an immediate blood glucose level obtained and should be administered 50 ml of a dextrose 50% solution. In most cases, if hypoglycemia is the cause, the clinical picture will immediately improve. Some patients may have already suffered some cerebral injury, and there may be no change in their level of consciousness.

• *Hypoglycemia may result in obtundation with intact pupillary reflexes.*

It should be emphasized that hypoglycemia cannot be ruled out as a cause of obtundation by history or physical examination, and empiric treatment is warranted pending confirmatory laboratory studies.

Hyperglycemia

Hyperosmolar, hyperglycemic, nonketotic syndrome (HHNS) usually develops from dehydration secondary to sustained glycosuria. This can exist with or without ketosis.[67] It develops when fluid intake does not balance the high urinary losses. Predisposing factors include decreased oral intake from debilitation, high carbohydrate or protein intake, peritoneal or hemodialysis, and the use of osmotic agents such as mannitol. Medications including steroids, diuretics, beta blockers, and phenytoin increase the risk of the syndrome.[68] It is hypothesized that insulin levels are sufficient to inhibit the hepatic carnitine acyltransferase system and thus prevent development of ketoacidosis. Thus, in hyperosmolar crisis, hyperglycemia is more common in the adult-onset variety of diabetes, but ketosis usually accompanies juvenile-onset diabetes.

Patients present with a depressed level of consciousness, extreme hyperglycemia, and hyperosmolarity. Thrombosis may occur due to increased blood viscosity secondary to severe dehydration. Blood glucose levels are in the range of 1000 mg/dl, and mortality exceeds 50%.[69]

Primary treatment is directed at the severe dehydration. Intravenous fluids, insulin, and potassium are the mainstays of treatment. Urine output and central venous pressure measurements are helpful for fluid management.[70] The average deficit is approximately 10 L. While free water is required, the patient is also sodium depleted. The initial fluid expansion is done with normal saline. Fluid administration should be fairly rapid and 2 to 4 L are given in the first 2 hours. After restoration of hemodynamic stability, half-normal saline can be used. When the glucose level falls to 200 to 300 mg/dl, many physicians initiate D5W to increase the amount of free water and to help prevent insulin-induced hypoglycemia. HHNS can occur in the nondiabetic hospitalized patient as a result of parental hyperalimentation, hemoperitoneal dialysis, and severe burns.

- *Patients with hyperglycemia and hyperosmolar nonketotic syndrome have large free water deficits. Blood glucose levels almost always exceed 700 mg/dl. This syndrome requires a continuous insulin infusion to correct blood glucose levels adequately.*

Diabetic ketoacidosis with hyperosmolar coma occurs most commonly as the presenting symptom in new-onset juvenile diabetes, a result of discontinuation of exogenous insulin, or increased insulin resistance seen with stress and surgery. Stress and surgery increase epinephrine secretions, which stimulate gluconeogenesis and antagonize the action of insulin. Glucosuria and dehydration develop. Free fatty acids are liberated by insulin deficiency, the hepatic carnitine acyltransferase system is activated, and accelerated ketone body production results.[69]

The ketosis will bring these patients to medical attention earlier than the nonketotic hyperosmolar state. The blood glucose will remain in the range of 250 to 700 mg/dl, substantially less than in HHNS. Patients complain of anorexia, nausea, and vomiting. Examination may show Kussmaul breathing, the spoiled-fruit odor of ketones on the breath, and an altered level of consciousness. There will be a significant metabolic acidosis and an anion gap made up almost entirely of acetoacetate and β-hydroxybutyrate. The acidosis maintains normal serum potassium values in spite of significant depletion. Because of the increase in free fatty acid metabolism, hypertriglyceridemia is common, and thus serum sodium levels may appear to be spuriously low.

In most cases, the major cause of coma and death is the hyperosmolar state, not the acidosis.[71] It is not surprising, then, that the treatment is essentially the same as for HHNS. Insulin therapy should continue in this group of patients even after the glucose has been normalized. The end point for insulin therapy should be resolution of the ketotic state. Mortality from this syndrome approaches 10%.

Hyponatremia

Hyponatremia or water intoxication occurs when sodium levels are low relative to body water. This can happen in hypo-, hyper-, and euvolemia. Causes in the hospitalized or surgical patient are multiple. They include the TURP syndrome (described earlier), sodium loss secondary to excessive gastric and bowel output, magnesium-containing antacids and antibiotics, diarrhea from magnesium containing-antacids or antibiotics, and inappropriate intravenous fluid replacement.[72]

In addition, intracranial surgery and some medications can lead to the syndrome of inappropriate antidiuretic hormone secretion (SIADH). The increase in vasopressin results in hyponatremia from water retention and an excess of total body water. Other brain disorders, such as stroke, subarachnoid hemorrhage, and meningitis, can lead to a cerebral salt-wasting syndrome which is excessive natriuresis in the face of low or normal vasopressin levels.[73,74] A causative role for inappropriate secretion of atrial natriuretic factor has not been conclusively demonstrated in this syndrome, although there may be cerebral production of atrial natriuretic factor.[75]

The treatment of hyponatremia is similar to that described for TURP syndrome. Asymptomatic patients can be corrected slowly sometimes with only water restriction. Symptomatic patients with sodium values less than 120 mEq/100 ml should be corrected to a level of 125 mEq/dl more urgently.[76] In addition, the cause of the hyponatremia should be sought and corrected, to prevent a relapse.

Clinically, symptomatic patients can be confused or obtunded. They may demonstrate asterixis and multifocal myoclonus. Seizures and coma occur late and are associated with poor outcomes. Diagnosis must be made by laboratory evaluation of the serum sodium level.

Hypernatremia

Hypernatremia is a rarer disorder that also exists in hypo-, hyper-, and euvolemic patients. It is the result of excess free water loss or increased solute load. Serum sodium levels of 150 mEq/L are well tolerated. Lethargy develops at 160 mEq/L and stupor can result at 180 mEq/L. Hospital-induced causes of this problem include tube feedings of concentrated solutions, dehydration, untreated diabetes insipidus, and hypothalamic or psychologic lack of thirst. A new cause involves the use of hypertonic salt solutions for fluid resuscitation. Large volumes or rapid infusion rates can cause hypernatremia.

- *Hypernatremia causes central nervous system symptoms when sodium levels exceed 160 mEq/L.*

Treatment is based on the cause of the disorder. If the cause is fluid administration, fluids should be stopped and hypotonic solutions begun. Diabetes insipidus can be treated with pitressin (5 U IV) for short-term therapy or DDAVP for long-term use. Attempts to replace urine at the same rate as loss causes only larger urine outputs and results in the administration of even more fluids. Instead, the replacement should be at a rate of 0.5 to 0.75 ml for every milliliter of urine. The free water defecit can be calculated from the total body water, which is 60% of body weight. Sodium equilibrates across all water-containing compartments. Replacement should be phased, with the first 25% in 2 to 4 hours and the remainder over the next 12 to 24 hours.

Hypocalcemia and Hypercalcemia

Hypocalcemia can rarely cause obtundation.[77] Most of the clinically apparent signs and symptoms reflect an increase in neuromuscular irritability. Hypomagnesemia is often seen with hypocalcemia and may be responsible for a functional hypoparathyroidism that will correct with magnesium replacement. Hypocalcemia is associated with seizures, and the postictal state could be mistaken for obtundation.

• *Hypercalcemia, unlike hypocalcemia, can cause mental obtundation.*

Hypercalcemia is more likely to cause obtundation than hypocalcemia. CNS symptoms range from mild changes in personality to psychosis and coma. The most common cause of clinically significant hypercalcemia is malignancy. Other causes include parathyroid hormone-secreting secreting tumors, hyperparathyroidism, immobilization of bone, post-transplant hypercalcemia,[77] and sarcoid. Certain drugs, such as lithium[78] and thiazides,[78,79] can also increase serum calcium levels. A serum calcium level is useful in all patients with unexplained decreases in mental status and is mandatory in any patient who also has a predisposing condition.

Along with CNS problems, high calcium levels may cause specific cardiac effects that can aid in the diagnosis, such as shortening of the QT interval,[80] renal stones, bone pain from reabsorption, duodenal ulcers (10 to 20% of patients),[81] constipation, nausea, and vomiting. Treatment should begin if serum levels are above 12 mg/dl and consists of encouraging diuresis by administering normal saline. Rates of 500 ml/hr may be required. Furosemide or other loop diuretics will help excrete the saline load and inhibit distal tubular reabsorption of calcium. During vigorous diuresis, potassium and magnesium replacements are also necessary. Other treatments include mithramycin, in doses of 25 μg/kg in D5W given over 4 hours which will lower calcium over several days. However, the drug is toxic with multiple side effects. Phosphate will lower calcium but could trigger widespread metastatic calcifications. Steroids such as hydrocortisone, at 5 mg/kg/day, can inhibit calcium absorption from the intestine and bone,[82] but it can aggravate the peptic ulcer disease often seen in these patients. Calcitonin, at 4 MRC U/kg intravenously followed by a similar subcutaneous dose in 12 hours, can lower calcium in the hypercalcemic patient.

Hypophosphatemia

Hypophosphatemia is a common problem in the surgical patient. Approximately 30% of postoperative patients may have serum phosphate levels below 2.4 mg/dl.[83] Other predisposing factors include alcoholism, burns, intravenous hyperalimentation, and aluminum-containing antacids.[84]

Hypophosphatemia can often be seen in ICU patients not receiving adequate replacement for phosphate loss while they are unable to take anything by mouth (NPO) (Table 14–5). In addition to cardiac and renal problems, hypophosphatemia can cause confusion, obtundation, and a variety of abnormal physical findings such

Table 14–5.
Causes of Hypophosphatemia

Reduce absorption and increased gastrointestinal loss
Phosphorus-poor feedings
Decreased intake
Vomiting
Antacid use
Vitamin D deficiency
Diarrhea and malabsorption syndrome
Increased renal loss
Acidosis (diabetic ketoacidosis, gout, and lactic acid)
Hyperparathyroidism
Renal tubular dysfunction
Alcohol
Diuretic use
Hemodynamics
Burns (renal phosphate wasting may develop)
Intracellular shift from extracellular fluid
High carbohydrate load
Alkalosis
Androgens and corticosteroid use

as peripheral neuropathy, unequal pupils, nystagmus, and ataxia. Muscle strength is severely limited, and problems with speech, swallowing, and breathing occur.[85] At this stage, phosphate levels are usually less than 1 mg/dl. Treatment of severe hypophosphatemia is with potassium phosphate or sodium phosphate for patients in renal failure. The administration of intravenous phosphate is not without risk. Development of hypotension, metastatic soft tissue calcifications, renal failure, hypocalcemia, and hypomagnesemia are possible. Slow infusion will minimize their likelihood. It is usually not necessary to give over 18 mmol of phosphorus per day to raise the serum phosphate safely to an adequate level.[86]

• *Hypophosphatemia can cause mental confusion or obtundation.*

TEMPERATURE

Patients who return from the operating room or have extensive intravenous therapy with room-temperature fluids may develop hypothermia. A temperature below 32.2°C is usually accompanied by a depressed level of consciousness.[87] In addition to many drugs, alcohol use, myxedema, and neurologic disorders can predispose a patient to hypothermia. Hypothermic patients will awaken from anesthetics more slowly and remain paralyzed longer.[88] Physical examination may show a pale, cold patient. Temperature in all patients should be measured, and if the temperature is too low to register, a thermometer with a lower range must be found. If the patient is not in danger, passive rewarming is safe, cheap, and effective. If shivering develops, supplemental oxygen should be provided as this will significantly increase oxygen utilization. If hypothermia is causing cardiac problems, the patient should be actively rewarmed. Heated intravenous fluids, warmed humidified oxygen,

• *Temperatures below 32.2°C depress the level of consciousness.*

peritoneal and gastric lavage with 40°C saline, and cardiopulmonary bypass with rewarming have all been used successfully. Rapid rewarming will decrease a high peripheral vascular resistance often seen in hypothermia and could result in hypotension. High levels of lactic acid are often released during active rewarming. Although rarely the sole reason for obtundation, hypothermia may play a contributing part in the depression of the perioperative patient's sensorium.

- *Temperatures must exceed 42 to 43°C to cause mental obtundation. The most important disorders found with malignant hyperthermia are cardiac and electrolyte disturbances, not temperature elevation.*

Hyperthermia significant enough to cause obtundation (42 to 43°C) occurs in heat stroke, which is rarely seen in hospitalized patients, or with malignant hyperthermia. Malignant hyperthermia is a genetic disorder in which certain anesthesia-triggering agents promote a hypermetabolic state. Extreme hyperthermia is a late development of this syndrome. Cardiac and electrolyte disruption predominate early in this syndrome and overshadow the CNS effects. Specific treatment is with dantrolene, 1 to 10 mg/kg intravenously titrated to effect, discontinuation of the trigger agents, and active cooling for hyperthermia.[89] Cardiac arrhythmias and hyperkalemia are treated if they develop. Anesthetic trigger agents are to be avoided for life.

MALIGNANT NEUROLEPTIC SYNDROME

Psychotropic drugs can produce a neuroleptic malignant syndrome that is characterized by hyperthermia, muscle rigidity, and autonomic dysfunction.[90] The incidence is 0.2% of patients treated with neuroleptic agents. The mechanism appears to be related to a decrease in function of dopamine-containing neurons. Treatment consists of immediate discontinuation of the triggering neuroleptic agent, temperature reduction, and administration of bromocriptine and dantrolene. A prior episode of neuroleptic malignant syndrome is a risk factor for its recurrence, but it is not an absolute contraindication to the continued use of neuroleptic drugs.[91]

UREMIA

Uremic encephalopathy can occur in acute or chronic renal failure. Neurologic symptoms tend to develop more quickly in patients with acute renal failure than in those with chronic renal failure.

The CNS symptoms in uremia are nonspecific. Dulled consciousness, confusion, seizures, and coma can all be presenting complaints. Hyperpnea is often seen, as well as muscular disorders. These patients are weak and exhibit tremors, myoclonus, and asterixis. Fifty percent of these patients have dysarthria and cannot stick out their tongues past their lips.[92]

Physical examination shows a weak, hyperreflexic patient with signs of peripheral neuropathy that may present with a "restless leg syndrome", in which uremic patients constantly move their legs due to a vague discomfort in their feet.[93]

Uremic encephalopathy is a misnomer. Urea infusions do not produce this syndrome in patients who are not in renal failure. High levels of parathyroid hormone have been implicated as one cause of this syndrome, and parathyroidectomy has resulted in improvement of neurologic symptoms in some patients.[94] Other toxins may be important. Although urea makes up 80% of the nitrogen waste of protein metabolism, many other products including aliphatic amines, creatinine, and guanidinosuccinic acid are created and accumulated. BUN values are useful in detecting a uremic state, but they do not correlate well with the cerebral effects.

With progressive renal impairment, acid secretion falls and metabolic acidosis develops. The combination of metabolic acidosis with compensatory hyperventilation, obtundation, and the muscle dysfunctions described previously suggest encephalopathy secondary to renal disease. Laboratory confirmation of azotemia can help with the diagnosis. Patients in renal failure often have low sodium levels, which, combined with hypo-osmolality, may be contributory to the depressed level of consciousness. The treatment for both of these conditions is dialysis. Improvement is usually rapid, but neurologic deficits can take days to reverse following initiation of dialysis.

- *Dialysis to correct hyponatremia and hypo-osmolality can improve the encephalopathy associated with renal failure.*

Dialysis can often produce its own CNS complications. Dialysis dysequilibrium syndrome is a diagnosis of exclusion used to describe a variety of CNS complaints that patients have after dialysis. These include headache, nausea and vomiting, fatigue, and muscle cramping. CNS symptoms occur in the more severe form of this syndrome and include syncopy, seizures, and confusion. This syndrome is most common in younger patients. It is thought to develop secondary to a rapid decrease of blood urea that is not followed by as rapid a decrease in cerebral urea, which then causes absorption of fluid into the brain. Improved dialysis techniques have reduced the frequency of this syndrome.[92]

- *Dialysis disequilibrium syndrome results from a reduction of blood urea, with a consequent shift of fluid into the brain with higher urea levels than the vascular compartment.*

Dialysis dementia or progressive dialysis encephalopathy occurs most frequently in patients on chronic dialysis for a period of years who then develop neurologic changes. Earliest symptoms involve difficulty with speech such as stammering. This progresses to somnolence that is worse immediately after dialysis. As the disease progresses, symptoms persist longer until they are constant. Seizures, stupor, and coma can develop. Death usually comes within the year.[95] Alfrey and colleagues have implicated aluminum as the source of this syndrome.[96] Efforts to remove aluminum from dialysate by using deionized water have met with some success.[97] Campistol and associates reported a case of acute aluminum encephalopathy in a patient in renal failure who was receiving aluminum hydroxide and sucralfate (160 mg elemental aluminum/g) that appeared similar to dialysis dementia.[98]

Treatment of these patients is supportive. It probably would be prudent to remove sources of aluminum contamination from these patients. This would include aluminum-containing antacids and sucralfate.[98] As with dialysis dysequilibrium, this is a diagnosis of exclusion, and treatable causes for a change in mental status should be sought before labeling the patient with a dialysis-induced encephalopathy.

HEPATIC DYSFUNCTION

Acute and chronic liver disease, as well as portal systemic shunts, can result in the development of perioperative encephalopathy. This can develop without the stress of the perioperative period but is often triggered or aggravated by certain drugs (sedatives, diuretics),[99] sepsis, GI bleeding, constipation, hypokalemia, and increased nitrogen load from high-protein diets (Table 14–6).

The patient may at first appear confused, with blunted affect. Patients often complain of night sleep disturbances and start to sleep for increasing periods of time during the day. This can progress to somnolence, disorientation, and stupor. Other physical findings include a liver flap or asterixis that involves the hands, feet, and tongue. Fetor hepaticus, thought to be due to sulfur compounds that can be detected on the breath of some patients, and hyperventilation may develop. Other signs of liver disease should be sought such as jaundice, spider angiomata, and abnormal liver enzymes and coagulation studies.

Special laboratory studies can help diagnose the cause of the worsening mental status. Elevated arterial ammonia levels can help point to the liver as a source of the obtundation, but generally are not well correlated with the severity of the encephalopathy or its prognosis. Arterial levels are chosen as they provide a more consistent level due to the peripheral muscles' ability to convert ammonia to glutamine.[100] Low glucose levels may also be a confounding problem in that hepatic disease will often result in decreased glycogen storage. Gastric and stool guaiac tests can point to occult GI bleeding; electrolytes can elucidate a low potassium level, and an elevated white blood cell count may indicate sepsis. Arterial blood gases are helpful and will typically show a metabolic acidosis overcorrected by hyperventilation and resultant alkalosis. Cerebral spinal fluid levels of glutamine and alpha-ketoglutaramate do corre-

Table 14–6.
Causes of Worsening Hepatic Encephalopathy

Portosystemic shunting
Low glucose, K, Na
Hypoxemia
Infection
Constipation
Gastrointestinal bleeding
Renal dysfunction
Diuretic use
Benzodiazepine and sedative use
Hyperventilation
High nitrogen load

late with encephalopathy and should be assessed if a spinal tap is done to rule out meningitis.[101]

There appears to be multiple hypotheses to explain the development of encephalopathy in the presence of liver impairment. Arguments for or against all theories of hepatic encephalopathy have been forthcoming. The leading hypothesis deals with ammonia as a neurotoxin and increased gamma-aminobutyric acid (GABA) transmission.

The etiologic role of ammonia seems to be the basis of one of the older hypotheses of hepatic encephalopathy. In the intestines, protein is degraded by glutaminase and by the urease of intestinal microorganisms with the ultimate production of ammonia. The liver converts ammonia to urea or glutamine before it reaches the systemic circulation in significant amounts. Support for the ammonia hypothesis is largely circumstantial. Ammonia is present in other forms of cerebral dysfunction such as Reye's syndrome, TURP syndrome, and sodium valproate toxicity. Mechanisms to reduce ammonia production at the bowel level are often successful in reversing the symptoms of hepatic encephalopathy. An argument against the ammonia hypothesis is the poor correlation between serum ammonia levels and the severity of symptoms. The clinical picture of ammonia toxicity is very different than the appearance of hepatic encephalopathy. Ammonia toxicity will commonly present with seizures, but this is rare in hepatic encephalopathy.[101]

- *Serum ammonia levels correlate poorly with the encephalopathy of hepatic disease.*

The GABA neurotransmission theory or benzodiazepine receptor concept suggests that liver failure will result in the accumulation of endogenous benzodiazepine ligands that bind to the GABA-benzodiazepine receptor complex. This allows the GABA-mediated facilitation of chloride ion entry into the cell resulting in hyperpolarization and neuroinhibition. If, in fact, the hepatic encephalopathy is a result of an accumulation of benzodiazepine ligands, then one might expect to see some clinical improvement with a benzodiazepine antagonist. Flumazenil will antagonize the effects of benzodiazepines at the GABA-benzodiazepine receptor. Studies have demonstrated this effect.[102–104]

- *Flumazenil antagonism of the GABA-benzodiazepine receptor complex indicates a role for benzodiazepine ligands in hepatic encephalopathy.*

Ferenci and Grimm studied 20 episodes of hepatic encephalopathy.[105] After receiving 15 mg flumazenil over 3 hours, 12 of the 20 cases improved rapidly. Of the 8 episodes that did not improve, 5 were also associated with increased intracranial pressure. Of those that improved, two thirds deteriorated to preflumazenil states within 4 hours of drug discontinuation. Animal studies have also demonstrated an improvement in neurologic function after flumazenil therapy.[106] That not all animals or patients improved with flumazenil suggests that other toxins, such as ammonia, octopamine, methanethiol, and fatty acids, may also play a role in the development of hepatic encephalopathy.[107–109]

The benzodiazepine ligand hypothesis awaits the isolation of these chemicals in the CNS and demonstration that they can induce encephalopathy in healthy animals. Moreoever, larger controlled studies of the effect of flumazenil on hepatic encephalopathy would be helpful.

Therapy for hepatic encephalopathy is directed at correction of the precipating factors discussed previously. The nitrogen load is decreased by restriction of protein intake to that required for basic nutrition. Vegetable-derived proteins are preferable due to their decreased ammoniagenesis. The use of branched-chain amino acid protein formulas has shown no consistency in prevention of hepatic encephalopathy. One prospective study of 56 cirrhotic patients showed no perioperative benefit in the use of branched-chained amino acids.[110] Use of this expensive formulation is best reserved only for the most protein-intolerant patients as consistent evidence for its benefit is lacking.

- *Branched-chain amino acid therapy has not consistently improved hepatic encephalopathy.*

The production of nitrogenous toxins from the gut can be decreased by antibiotics and reduced bowel absorption. Lactulose, a disaccharide, is metabolized by anaerobic bacteria to lactic acid in the colon and will favor the passage of ammonia back into the intestine and inhibit some fatty acid production. Lactulose also acts as a cathartic. Lactulose is given orally at a dose of 15 to 30 ml, up to four times per day. Improvement takes 2 to 3 days. Lactulose may also be administered as an enema in comatose patients; 300 ml/L has slightly faster results. A new disaccharide, Lactitol, has a faster onset of activity.

- *Lactulose can improve neurologic status in patients with hepatic encephalopathy.*

Antibiotics that reduce the amount of urease-splitting bacteria in the colon can have beneficial results. Neomycin, at 2 to 8 g/day, can be given to patients with normal renal function. Renal toxicity and ototoxicity can develop. If renal function contraindicates the use of neomycin, metronidazole, 250 mg twice a day, or vancomycin, 500 mg four times daily, is an alternative with good activity against urease-splitting bacteria.

Other therapies that may have some activity but are treatments of last resort include occlusion of a portocaval shunt and colectomy. Bromocriptine, a dopamine agonist, can counteract the effects of "weak neurotransmitters" produced in the intestines such as octopamine. Once in the systemic circulation, they interfere with dopamine and norepinephrine function.

NEW POSTOPERATIVE NEUROLOGIC IMPAIRMENT THAT RESULTS IN OBTUNDATION

In a large, prospective, multicentered study, the incidence of stroke was only 7 in 17,201 patients following noncardiac or carotid surgery.[111] A more recent retrospective study showed almost identical numbers, with 19 of 24,641 (0.08%) patients experiencing a postoperative stroke.[112]

Although strokes are infrequent, their effects are devastating to the patient and family. Perioperative strokes are associated with a 16 to 50% mortality.[29] Asymptomatic carotid bruits are not predictive of perioperative stroke. Twenty percent of patients undergoing peripheral vascular surgery have carotid bruits, but postoperative stroke remains rare in this segment of the patient population.[111] No

- *Asymptomatic carotid bruits do not predict perioperative stroke.*

contemporary study supports asymptomatic carotid bruits as a risk factor for stroke.[113] Studies are equivocal about the predictive effect on perioperative stroke rate of TIAs or amaurosis fugax.[38]

Intraoperative hypotension, often thought as a cause of stroke, has not been documented to be a risk factor.[114] Most patients who suffer a perioperative stroke experience it postoperatively. This makes it difficult to ascribe an intraoperative risk factor to this deficit. Most intraoperative untoward events such as hypotension and dysrhythmias are transient and quickly diagnosed because of monitoring in the operating room. In addition, almost all general anesthetics decrease the cerebral metabolic rate and may have cerebral protective effects.

The number one cause of perioperative stroke is cardiogenic embolism. This accounted for 42% of the postoperative strokes in one study.[115] Atrial fibrillation was a finding in one third of the patients studied, and myocardial infarction preceded the stroke in 17% of the patients. This study is dramatic evidence of the value of a cardiac examination in the obtunded patient. Almost half of the strokes were due to cardiac events. These findings are supported by a more recent study by Parikh and Cohen, who reviewed their 5-year experience with perioperative stroke in the general surgical patient.[112] Out of 19 patients diagnosed with stroke, only 1 patient had an intraoperative stroke thought to be due to hypotension, and 1 had a hemorrhagic cause; 32% (6 patients) had atrial fibrillation. Two developed this arrhythmia in the postoperative period. This percentage is almost identical to that reported by Hart and Hindman over a decade earlier.[115] Parikh and Cohen found a 37% incidence of previous neurologic symptoms in their stroke patients.[112] Histories of carotid bruits, heart disease not affecting rhythm, diabetes, and intraoperative blood loss were all unassociated with increased stroke risk. Only prior neurologic problems, abnormal cardiac rhythm, hypertension, and smoking were associated with the development of perioperative stroke.

- *Most perioperative strokes result from cardiogenic embolism such as atrial fibrillation.*

It may be reasonable to consider anticoagulation in perioperative patients with atrial fibrillation, especially those with prior neurologic disorders. Obviously, anticoagulants must not be a surgical contraindication. Warfarin is often used in medical patients with atrial fibrillation and has a significant effect in preventing thromboembolic disease.[116]

Air embolism most often causes cardiovascular compromise rather than neurologic problems. However, following a surgical procedure in which air entrapment is possible, this must be part of the differential diagnosis of a patient who fails to awaken from anesthesia. Air entrapment into the circulation occurs not only during craniotomies in the sitting position, but also in any procedure in which a vein is held open by bone, tissue, or retraction and has contact with ambient air pressure. This can occur during pelvic surgery performed with the patient in the Trendelenberg position and bone surgery when the patient has a low venous pressure or the bone is held above the patient's heart. An example of the latter is the report by Liu and colleagues of a patient who failed to awaken

- *Air embolism can cause both cardiovascular and neurologic deficits.*

from anesthesia after hip surgery.[117] No signs of cardiovascular instability were seen intraoperatively. CT scanning of the head showed a defect in the area of the brain supplied by the left middle cerebral artery. The patient died, and at autopsy, a patent foramen ovale and air in the left internal carotid artery were discovered. It is unusual for venous air embolism to be present with only cerebral symptoms. Usually, the first symptoms are cardiac. Treatment in the postoperative period is supportive. If a hyperbaric oxygen chamber is available, its use might be considered.

Another cause of perioperative obtundation can be primary neurologic disease that becomes unmasked by general anesthesia and surgery. A space-occupying lesion such as a fibroma or meningoma might be well tolerated until the patient undergoes surgery.[118] Head-down positioning, episodes of hypertension above the range of cerebral autoregulation, and carbon dioxide retention secondary to sedatives and narcotics can all lead to an increase in intracranial pressure in the patient with a noncompliant brain. Intracranial tumors occur with an incidence of 12.5 in 100,000,[119] so although rare, in an otherwise healthy person delayed awakening may be a sign of increased intracranial pressure and should be considered in patients with postoperative obtundation.

NEUROLOGIC TRAUMA

Patients when rendered unconscious for anesthesia may experience head trauma while being transported or in the operating or recovery room. Narcotized patients can forcefully bump their heads and not be aware of the extent of their resultant head injuries. Trauma patients may be taken to the operating room without an adequate neurologic examination because of serious and obvious torso injuries and no known history of head trauma. In addition, alcoholics and patients on anticoagulants can have chronic subdural hematomas that become symptomatic intra- or postoperatively due to the stress of acute illness and maneuvers that might increase intracranial pressure intraoperatively.

The hallmark of subdural hematoma, headache, occurs in over 80% of patients.[120] If a patient has received sedatives and narcotics, this symptom may be lacking or unappreciated. Symptoms then appear focal in origin. Hemiparesis develops in approximately 40% of patients while only 5% will have a dilated pupil.[121] Diagnosis will be made by a CT scan. Treatment is usually drainage of the clot.

Hypertension intraoperatively or secondary to postoperative pain may induce an intracerebral hemorrhage. Onset appears abruptly in one third of patients and progresses steadily in the rest.[122] A mental status change from alert to stuporous that occurs over a matter of minutes in a hypertensive patient is highly suggestive of intracranial bleeding. Subarchanoid hemorrhage will present very similarly to intracerebral bleeding. Headache is followed by a decrease in the level of consciousness. The diagnosis is made by CT scan. Lumbar puncture should be undertaken with great caution in these patients because cerebrospinal fluid pressures can be as high as 1000 cm H_2O.[122]

Medical management of this condition requires control of hypertension and bedrest. Valsalva maneuvers, such as straining to stool, are discouraged. Seizures are anticipated and are treated prophylactically with antiepileptics. Nimodipine, a calcium channel blocker, is indicated to prevent the cerebral vasospasm that occurs in 50% of the survivors. It develops approximately 4 to 14 days after the original hemorrhage. This drug should be given within 4 days of the subarchanoid hemorrhage, at a dose of 60 mg by mouth or nasogastric tube every 4 hours for 3 weeks.

Many critically ill patients are septic and under go multiple procedures including lumbar puncture for diagnostic and anesthetic reasons. The presence of meningitis should be ruled out in any patient who exhibits nuchal rigidity, fever, and headache. A history of lumbar puncture, prolonged nasotracheal intubation (sinusitis), or systemic sepsis should increase the index of suspicion. Spinal fluid analysis is probably warranted in the stuporous patient with these symptoms after increased intracranial pressure has been ruled out. Elderly patients may present only with stupor and coma and may not have headache or meningism. In these cases, if a diagnosis of stroke cannot be confirmed by CT scan, a lumbar puncture is indicated to help rule in or out stroke, hemorrhage, or infection.

- *Once a CT scan has ruled out elevated intracranial pressure in a stuporous patient, spinal fluid analysis should be done.*

ENDOCRINE DISORDERS

Diabetes is discussed earlier in this chapter as a cause of obtundation. Patients with thyroid disorders can also present with stupor or coma, but this is rare. Myxedema coma can be triggered in the severely hypothyroid patient by infection, trauma, or general anesthesia and surgery.

These patients, in addition to altered mental status, have the clinical picture of hypothyroidism. Hypothermia, high serum creatinine phosphokinase levels, and bradycardia are present. Treatment is with sodium levothyroxine, at 400 μg, followed by 100 to 200 μg per day, or 20 to 40 μg T_3 intravenously.[123]

The profound hypermetabolism of thyroid storm is rarely a diagnostic dilemma. Hyperthermia, tachycardia, and stupor can comprise the clinical presentation. Occasionally, hyperthyroidism can be subtle and present, especially in the elderly, with atrial fibrillation, weight loss, and proximal myopathy. If not diagnosed and treated with antithyroid medications or radiation, this syndrome can progress to produce cerebral depression.[124,125]

Adrenal dysfunction may produce cerebral impairment secondary to electrolyte disturbances. Full-blown Addison's or Cushing's disease is often diagnosed before cerebral symptoms predominate. If a patient has an electrolyte disturbance that results in cerebral effect, a cause of the electrolyte disturbance should be sought.

ILLICIT DRUG USE

Illicit drug use is quite prevalent in modern society. Such agents can contribute to the depressed mental status of an obtunded patient. A urine drug screen by immunoassay techniques can detect cocaine, marijuana, opiates, amphetamines, barbiturates, benzodiazepines, and hallucinogens.[126] With current technology, it is possible to get qualitative results about the presence of these compounds in less than 1 hour. Ethanol can also produce a depression on the CNS, and blood or breath alcohol samples should be obtained. The patient's mental status may be due to the drug directly or to side effects such as hypertension followed by cerebral bleeding.

- *All newly admitted patients with abnormal mental status should have a drug screen.*

CONCLUSION

In summary, a variety of medical and surgical problems can contribute to the development of perioperative obtundation. General anesthesia's main purpose is to depress or alter the CNS. Some surgical procedures such as carotid endarterectomy, TURP, and cardiopulmonary bypass are more prone to cause neurologic dysfunction. Liver and kidney impairments are often made worse or develop during the stress of critical illness and surgery. They can cause metabolic stupor or coma. Cardiac arrest can result in global cerebral ischemia. Cardiac arrhythmias are sources of thromboembolism and are a risk factor for perioperative stroke. Illness can cause changes in thyroid, adrenal, and pancreatic endocrine function. Diabetics can be obtunded from hypo- and hyperglycemia. Hyperalimentation can result in electrolyte disturbances and hyperosmolality. Trauma frequently results from the use of alcohol and illicit drugs. Thermoregulation is altered in some postoperative patients. All operative patients may experience unrecognized head trauma. In addition, a preexistent neurologic condition can be exacerbated by anesthesia and surgery. The stress of illness can bring out psychiatric disorders and may complicate a patient's hospitalization.

Such a large variety of causes for perioperative obtundation makes the diagnosis challenging. The first step is to classify the disorder into one of four groups: (1) structural; (2) metabolic; (3) infectious; or (4) psychiatric.

Structural lesions are suggested by focal cerebral deficits that are asymmetric. These deficits can usually be localized to a particular area of the brain and worsen in a rostral-to-caudal direction. CT scans and magnetic resonance imaging can localize structural deficits and confirm the clinical diagnosis. Electrocardiography can allow one to confirm the rhythm and suggest a cause for defects secondary to thromboembolism.

Metabolic deficits are symmetric (both sides of the brain are exposed to the same toxins). Importantly, the pupils' response to light is usually well preserved, and abnormal muscle activity, such as asterixis and tremors, is common. As this involves brain function rather than structure, the electroencephalogram is more likely to be helpful than other cerebral studies. In addition, because most causes of metabolic encephalopathy are carried to the brain by blood, laboratory tests can help in their diagnosis. Arterial blood gases, electrolytes, glucose, serum osmolality, liver function tests, coagulation parameters, arterial ammonia, thyroid, thyroid-stimulating hormone levels, adrenal function studies, and toxicology screen can all indicate the source of the central depression.

Infective causes can behave like metabolic (encephalitis or meningitis) or structural (abscess) problems. Their hallmark is a fever and leukocytosis. Lumbar puncture with cerebrospinal fluid analysis will make the diagnosis in all but a few infectious conditions (viral and fungal) that are uncommon in the perioperative period. When possible, CT scanning should precede lumbar puncture to minimize the risk of brain herniation.

Psychiatric stupor should be a diagnosis of exclusion as even patients with a history of catatonia can develop organic disease. Hysterical coma can be excluded by demonstration of reflexes that cannot be voluntarily controlled and do not exist in the comatose state, such as by cold caloric testing.

Once the cause of the cerebral dysfunction is recognized, appropriate treatment can be instituted, guaranteeing the patient the best hope of recovery.

REFERENCES

1. Allen S: Advanced neurological life support. In: Hoyt JW, Tonnesen AS, Allen SJ, eds: Critical care practice. Philadelphia, WB Saunders, 1991; pp. 104–119.
2. Cheiniack NS, von Euler C, Humma I et al: Experimentally induced Cheyne-Stokes breathing. Respir Physiol 1979; 37:185–200.
3. Wolf JK: Practical clinical neurology. Garden City, NY, Medical Examination Publishing, 1980; pp. 159–178.
4. Gilroy J, Holiday PL: Basic neurology. New York, MacMillan, 1982; pp. 48–55.
5. Fischer CM: Ocular bobbing. Arch Neurol 1964; 11:543–546.
6. Plum F, Posner JB: The diagnosis of stupor and coma. Philadelphia, FA Davis, 1980; pp. 30–70.
7. Korttila K, Linnoila M, Ertama P et al: Recovery and simulated driving after intravenous anesthesia with thiopental, methohexital, propanidid, or alphadione. Anesthesiology 1975; 43:291–299.
8. Way W, Trevor A: Pharmacology of intravenous non-narcotic anesthetic. In: Miller RD, ed: Anesthesia, 2nd ed. New York, Churchill Livingstone, 1986; pp. 799–824.
9. White PF, Way WL, Trevor AJ: Ketamine: its pharmacology and therapeutic uses. Anesthesiology 1982; 56:119–136.
10. Marshall BE, Longnecker DE: General Anesthetics. In: Goodman LS, Gilman A, ed: Goodman and Gilman's the pharmacological basis of therapeutics, 8th ed. New York, Pergamon Press, 1990; pp. 285–310.
11. Silbergeld DL, Mueller WM, Colley PS et al: Use of propofol (Diprivan) for awake craniotomies: technical note. Surg Neurol 1992; 38: 271–272.
12. Au J, Walker WS, Scott DHT: Withdrawal syndrome after propofol infusion. Anaesthesia 1990; 45:741–742.

13. Trotter C, Serpell MG: Neurological sequelae in children after prolonged propofol infusion. Anaesthesia 1992; 47:340–342.
14. Macrae D, James IG: Propofol sedation of children (letter). Anaesthesia 1992; 47:811.
15. Schaffer HG, Marsh SLU: Am I blind? The fear of a 4-year old boy after total intravenous anesthesia with propofol. Pediatr Anesth 1991; 1:53–55.
16. Lanigan C, Sury M, Bingham R et al: Neurological sequelae in chidren after prolonged infusion. Anaesthesia 1992; 47:810–811.
17. Saunders PRI, Harris MNE: Opisthotonus and other unusual neurological sequelae after outpatient anesthesia. Anaesthesia 1990; 45: 552–557.
18. Laycock GJA: Opisthotonus and propofol: a possible association (letter). Anaesthesia 1988; 43:257.
19. Wagner RL, White PF, Kan PB et al: Inhibition of adrenal steroidogenesis by the anesthetic etomidate. N Engl J Med 1984; 310:1415–1421.
20. van Beem H, Manger FW, Van Boxtel C et al: Etomidate anesthesia in patients with cirrhosis of the liver. Anaesthesia 1982; 38(suppl): 61–62.
21. Rupreht J, Dworacek B: Central anticholinergic syndrome during postoperative period. Ann Fr Anesth Reanim 1990; 9:295–304.
22. Schneck HJ, Rupreht J: Central anticholinergic syndrome (CAS) in anesthesia and intensive care. Acta Anaesthesiol Belg 1989; 40: 219–228.
23. Carras PM, Mion G, Pats B: A postoperative syndrome of confusion and stupor or a central anticholinergic syndrome? Cah Anesthesiol 1992; 40:212–213.
24. Fode NC, Sundt TM Jr, Robertson JT et al: Multicenter retrospective review of results and complications of carotid endarterectomy in 1981. Stroke 1986; 17:370–376.
25. Toronto cerebrovascular study group: Risks of carotid endarterectomy. Stroke 1986; 17:848–852.
26. Slogoff S, Girgis KZ, Keats AS: Etiologic factors in neuropsychiatric complications associated with cardiopulmonary bypass. Anesth Analg 1982; 61:903–911.
27. Halsey JH: Risks and benefits of shunting in carotid endarterectomy: the International Transcranial Doppler Collaborators. Stroke 1992; 23:1583–1587.
28. Williams I, McCollum C: Cerebral oximetry in carotid endarterectomy and acute stroke. In: Greenhalgh RM, Hollier LH, ed: Surgery for stroke. London, WB Saunders, 1993; pp. 129–137.
29. Hindman BJ: Perioperative stroke: the non-cardiac surgery patient. In: Hindman BJ, ed: Neurological and psychological complications of surgery and anesthesia. Int Anesthesiol Clin 1986; 24:101–124.
30. Pomposelli FB, Lamparello PJ, Riles TS et al: Intracranial hemorrhage after carotid endarterectomy. J Vasc Surg 1988; 7:248–255.
31. Skillman JJ: Neurological complications of cardiovascular surgery: procedures involving the carotid arteries and abdominal aorta. In: Hindman BJ, ed: Neurological and psychological complications of surgery and anesthesia. Int Anesthesiol Clin 1986; pp. 135–152.
32. Shaw PG, Bates D, Cartlidge NEF et al: Early neurological complications of cardiopulmonary bypass surgery. Br Med J 1985; 291: 1384–1387.
33. Kuroda Y, Uchimoto R, Kaieda R et al: Central nervous system complications after cardiac surgery: a comparison between coronary artery bypass grafting and valve surgery. Anesth Analg 1992; 76: 222–227.

34. Solin RT, Noon GP, Beall AC et al: Particulate microembolism during cardiac surgery. Ann Thorac Surg 1974; 17:332–344.
35. Padayachee TS, Parsons S, Theobod R et al: The effect of arterial filtration on reduction of gaseous microemboli in the middle cerebral artery during cardiopulmonary bypass. Ann Thorac Surg 1988; 45: 647–649.
36. Murkin JM: Neurologic dysfunction after CAB or valvular surgery: is the medium the miscreant? (editorial). Anesth Analg 1993; 76: 213–214.
37. Townes BD, Bashican G, Hornbein TF et al: Neurobehavioral outcomes in cardiac operations. J Thorac Cardiovasc Surg 1987; 98: 744–782.
38. Crosby G: Impaired central nervous system function. In: Benomof JL, Saidman LJ, eds: Anesthesia and perioperative complications. St. Louis: CV Mosby, 1991; pp. 356–370.
39. Nussmeier NA, Arlund C, Slogoff S: Neuropsychiatric complications after cardiopulmonary bypass: cerebral protection by a barbiturate. Anesthesiology 1986; 64:165–170.
40. Corman LC: Strokes and the carotid: myths and realities. Geriatrics 1990; 45:28–32.
41. Harrison MJG, Schneidar A, Ho R et al: Cerebravascular disease and functional outcome after coronary artery bypass surgery. Stroke 1989; 20:235–237.
42. Winter PM, Alvis HG, Gage AA: Hyperbaric treatment of cerebral air embolism during cardiopulmonary bypass. JAMA 1971; 215: 1786–1788.
43. Henderson DJ, Middleton RG: Coma from hyponatremia following transurethral resection of the prostate. Urology 1980; 15:267–271.
44. Jensen V: The TURP syndrome. Can J Anaesth 1991; 38:90–96.
45. Hjertberg H, Jorfeldt L, Schelin S: Use of ethanol as a marker substance to increase patient safety during transurethral prostatic resection: screening investigation of irrigating fluid absorption in four hospitals and comparison of experienced and inexperienced urologists. Urology 1991; 38:423–428.
46. Hahn RG: Monitoring of TURP with ethanol (letter). Lancet 1991; 338:1602.
47. Hahn RG: Blood ammonia concentrations resulting from absorption of irrigating fluid containing glycine and ethanol during transurethral resection of the prostate. Scand J Urol Nephrol 1991; 25:115–119.
48. Forrest JB, Calahan MK, Rehder K et al: Multicenter study of general anesthesia. II. Results. Anesthesiology 1990; 72:262–267.
49. Zelcer J, Wells DG: Anaesthetic related recovery room complications. Anesth Intensive Care 1987; 15:168–174.
50. Rosenberg H, Clofine R, Bialik O: Neurologic changes during awakening from anesthesia. Anesthesiology 1981; 54:125–130.
51. Barnes PJ, Havill JH: Anesthetic complications requiring intensive care: five year review. Anesth Intensive Care 1980; 8:404–409.
52. Tarsy D, Lieberman B, Chirico-Post J et al: Unilateral asterixis associated with a mesencephalic syndrome. Arch Neurol 1977; 34: 446–447.
53. Gilroy J, Holiday PL: Basic neurology. New York, MacMillan, 1982; pp. 259–261.
54. Morawetz RB, Crowell RH, DeGirolami U et al: Regional cerebral blood flow thresholds during cerebral ischemia. Fed Proc 1979; 38: 2493–2494.

55. Caronna JJ, Finklestein S: Neurological syndromes after cardiac arrest. Stroke 1978; 9:517–520.
56. Maiese K, Caronna JJ: Coma after cardiac arrest: clinical features, prognosis and management. In: Ropper AH, ed: Neurological and neurosurgical intensive care. Rockville, MD, Aspen Publishers, 1988; pp. 233–246.
57. Koehler RC, Michael JR: Cardiopulmonary resuscitation, brain blood flow, and neurological recovery. In: Rogers MC, Traystman RJ, ed: Crit Care Clin 1985; 1:205–222.
58. Synder BD, Lowenson RB, Gurnnit RJ et al: Neurological prognosis after cardiopulmonary arrest. II. Level of consciousness. Neurology 1980; 30:52–58.
59. Snyder BD, Hauser WA, Loewenson RB et al: Neurological prognosis after cardiopulmonary arrest: III. Seizure activity. Neurology 1980; 30:1292–1295.
60. Levy DE, Caronna JJ, Singer BH et al: Predicting outcome from hypoxic-ischemic coma. JAMA 1985; 253:1420–1426.
61. Plum F, Posner JB, Hain RF: Delayed neurological deterioration after anoxia. Arch Intern Med 1962; 110:18–25.
62. Rollinson RD, Gilligan BS: Postanoxic action myoclonus (Lance-Adams syndrome) responding to valproate. Arch Neurol 1979, 6: 44–45.
63. Fahn S: Post-anoxic action myoclonus: improvement with valproic acid. N Engl J Med 1978; 299:313–314.
64. Harper SJ and Wilkes RG: Posthypoxic myoclonus (the Lance-Adams syndrome) in the intensive care unit. Anaesthesia 1991; 46:199–201.
65. Goldberg MA, Dorman JD: Intention myoclonus: successful treatment with clonazepam. Neurology 1976; 26:24–26.
66. Montgomery BM and Pinner CA: Transient hypoglycemic hemiplegia. Arch Intern Med 1964; 114:680–684.
67. Gordon EE, Kibadi UM: The hyperglycemic, hyperosmolar syndrome. Am J Med Sci 1976; 271:252–268.
68. Levine SN, Sanson TH: Treatment of hyperglycaemic hyperosmolar non-ketotic syndrome. Drugs 1989; 38:462–472.
69. Foster DW: Diabetes mellitus. In: Braunwald E, Isselbacher KJ, Petersdorf RG et al, ed: Harrison's principles of internal medicine, 11th ed. New York, McGraw-Hill, 1987; pp. 1778–1796.
70. Pope DW, Dansky D: Hyperosmolar hyperglycemic nonketotic coma. Emerg Med Clin North Am 1989; 7:849–857.
71. Siperstein MD: Diabetic ketoacidosis and hyperosmolar coma. Endocrinol Metab Clin North Am 1992; 21:415–432.
72. Kennedy PG, Mitchell DM, Hoffbrand BI: Severe hyponatremia in hospital inpatients. Br Med J 1978; 2:1251–1253.
73. Diringer M, Ladenson PW, Borel C et al: Sodium and water regulation in a patient with cerebral salt wasting. Arch Neurol 1989; 46: 928–930.
74. Kroll M, Juhler M, Lindholm J: Hyponatraemia in acute brain disease. J Intern Med 1992; 232:291–297.
75. Wijdicks EF, Ropper AH, Hunnicutt EJ et al: Atrial natriuretic factor and salt wasting after aneurysmal subarachnoid hemorrhage. Stroke 1991; 22:1519–1524.
76. Arieff AI, Llach F, Massry SG: Neurological manifestations and morbidity of hyponatremia: correlation with brain water and electrolytes. Medicine 1976; 55:121–129.
77. David DS, Sakai S, Brennan BL et al: Hypocalcemia after renal trans-

plantation: long-term follow-up data. N Engl J Med 1973; 289: 398–401.
78. Gammon GD, Docherty JP: Thiazide-induced hypercalcemia in a manic-depressive patient. Am J Psychiatry 1980; 137:1453–1455.
79. Koppel MH, Massry SG, Shinaberger JH et al: Thiazide-induced rise in serum calcium and magnesium in patients on maintenance hemodialysis. Ann Intern Med 1970; 72:895–901.
80. Nierenberg DW, Ransil BJ: Q-aTc interval as a clinical indicator of hypercalcemia. Am J Cardiol 1979; 44:243–248.
81. Hellstrom J: Hyperparathyroidism and gastroduodenal ulcer. Acta Chir Scand 1959; 116:207–221.
82. Strumpf M, Kowalski MA, Mundy GR: Effects of glucocorticoids on osteoclast-activating factor. J Lab Clin Med 1978; 92:772–778.
83. Swaminathan R, Bradley P, Morgan DB et al: Hypophosphatemia in surgical patients. Surg Gynecol Obstet 1979; 148:448–454.
84. Spencer H, Kramer L, Norris C et al: Effect of small doses of aluminum-containing antacids on calcium and phosphorus metabolism. Am J Clin Nutr 1982; 36:32–40.
85. Newman JH, Neff TA, Ziporin P: Acute respiratory failure associated with hypophosphatemia. N Engl J Med 1977; 296:1101–1103.
86. Vannatta JB, Whang R, Papper S: Efficacy of intravenous phosphorus therapy in the severely hypophosphatemic patient. Arch Intern Med 1981; 141:885–887.
87. Plum F, Posner JB: The diagnosis of stupor and coma. Philadelphia, FA Davis, 1980; p. 259.
88. Herr RD, White GL Jr: Hypothermia: threat to military operations. Mil Med 1991; 156:140–144.
89. Gronert GA: Malignant hyperthermia. In: Miller RD, ed: Anesthesia, 2nd ed. New York, Churchill Livingstone, 1986; pp. 1971–1994.
90. Byrd C: Neuroleptic malignant syndrome: a dangerous complication of neuroleptic therapy. J Neurosci Nurs 1993; 25:62–65.
91. Caroff SM, Mann SC: Neuroleptic malignant syndrome. Med Clin North Am 1993; 77:185–202.
92. Fraser CL, Arieff AI: Metabolic encephalopathy associated with water, electrolyte, and acid-base disorders. In: Maxwell MH, Kleeman CR, Narins RG, eds: Clinical disorders of fluid and electrolyte metabolism, 4th ed. New York, McGraw-Hill, 1987; pp. 1153–1165.
93. Brenner BM, Lazarus JM: Chronic renal failure: pathophysiologic and clinical considerations. In: Braunwald E, Isselbacher KJ, Petersdorf RG et al, eds: Harrison's principles of internal medicine, 11th ed. New York, McGraw-Hill, 1987; pp. 1155–1161.
94. Goldstein DA, Feinstein EI, Chui LA et al: The relationship between the abnormalities in electroencephalogram and blood levels of parathyroid hormone in dialysis patients. J Clin Endocrinol Metab 1980; 51:130–134.
95. Dunea G, Mahurkar SD, Mamdani B et al: Role of aluminum in dialysis dementia. Ann Intern Med 1978; 88:502–504.
96. Alfrey AC, LeGendre GR, Kaehny WD: The dialysis encephalopathy syndrome: possible aluminum intoxication. N Engl J Med 1976; 294: 184–188.
97. Dialysis dementia in Europe. Report from the Registration Committee of the European Dialysis and Transplant Association. Lancet 1980; 2:190–192.
98. Campistol JM, Cases A, Botey A et al: Acute aluminum encephalopathy in an uremic patient. Nephron 1989; 51:103–106.

99. Posner JB, Plum F: The toxic effects of carbon dioxide and acetazolamide in hepatic encephalopathy. J Clin Invest 1960; 39:1246–1258.
100. Blei AT: Hepatic encephalopathy. In: Kaplowitz N, ed: Liver and bilary diseases. Baltimore, Williams & Wilkins, 1992; pp. 552–565.
101. Plum F, Posner JB: The diagnosis of stupor and coma. Philadelphia, FA Davis, 1980; pp. 222–225.
102. Butterworth RF, Layrargues GP: Benzodiazepine receptors and hepatic encephalopathy. Hepatology 1990; 11:499–501.
103. Rothstein JD and Olasmaa M: Endogenous GABAergic modulators in the pathogenesis of hepatic encephalopathy. Neurochem Res 1990; 15:193–197.
104. Ritz R, Zuber M, Elsasser S et al: Use of flumazenil in intoxicated patients with coma: a double-blind placebo-controlled study in ICU. Intensive Care Med 1990; 16:242–247.
105. Ferenci P, Grimm G: Benzodiazepine antagonist in the treatment of human hepatic encephalopathy. Adv Exp Med Biol 1990; 272: 255–265.
106. Gammal SH, Basile AS, Geller D et al: Reversal of the behavioral and electrophysiological abnormalities of an animal model of hepatic encephalopathy by benzodiazepine receptor ligands. Hepatology 1990; 11:371–378.
107. Blom HJ, Ferenci P, Grimm G et al: The role of methanethiol in the pathogenesis of hepatic encephalopathy. Hepatology 1991; 13: 445–454.
108. Farmer PM, Mulakkan T: The pathogenesis of hepatic encephalopathy. Ann Clin Lab Sci 1990; 20:91–97.
109. Maddison JE: Hepatic encephalopathy: current concepts of the pathogenesis. J Vet Intern Med 1992; 6:341–353.
110. Kanematsu T, Koyanagi N, Matsumata T et al: Lack of preventive effect of branched-chain amino acid solution on postoperative hepatic encephalopathy in patients with cirrhosis: a randomized, prospective trial. Surgery 1988; 104:482–488.
111. Forrest JB, Cahalan MK, Rehderk et al: Multicenter study of general anesthesia. II. Results. Anesthesiology 1990; 72:262–268.
112. Parikh S, Cohen JR: Perioperative stroke following general surgical procedures. NY State J Med 1993; 93:162–165.
113. Hertzer NR, Beven EG, Young JR et al: Incidental asymptomatic bruits in patients scheduled for peripheral vascular reconstruction: results of cerebral and coronary angiography. Surgery 1984; 96: 535–544.
114. Carney WI, Stewart WB, DePinto DJ et al: Carotid bruit as a risk factor in aorticoiliac reconstruction. Surgery 1977; 81:567–570.
115. Hart R, Hindman B: Mechanisms of perioperative cerebral infarction. Stroke 1982; 13:766–773.
116. Laupacis A, Albers G, Dunn M et al: Antithrombotic therapy in atrial fibrillation. Chest 1992; 102:426S-433S.
117. Liu S, Holley HS, Stulberg SD et al: Failure to awaken after general anaesthesia secondary to paradoxical venous embolus. Can J Anaesth 1991; 38:335–337.
118. Fraser ACL, Goat VA: Unrecognised presentation of a meningioma: delayed recovery after general anaesthesia presenting as a sign of intracranial patholoy. Anaesthesia 1983; 38:128–131.
119. Percy AK, Elverback LR, Okazaki H et al: Neoplasms of the central nervous system: epidemiologic considerations. Neurology 1972; 22: 40–48.

120. Plum F, Posner JB: The diagnosis of stupor and coma. Philadelphia, FA Davis, 1980; pp. 123–127.
121. Cameron MM: Chronic subdural hematoma: a review of 114 cases. J Neurol Neurosurg Psychiatry 1978; 41:834–839.
122. Kistler JP, Ropper AH, Martin JB: Cerebrovascular diseases. In: Braunwald E, Isselbacher KJ, Petersdorf RG et al, eds: Harrison's principles of internal medicine, 11th ed. New York, McGraw-Hill, 1987; pp. 1930–1960.
123. Burger AG, Philippe J: Thyroid emergencies. Baillieres Clin Endocrinol Metab 1992; 6:77–93.
124. Howton JC: Thyroid storm presenting as coma. Ann Emerg Med 1988; 17:343–345.
125. Gilbert RE, Thomas GW, Hope RN et al: Coma and thyroid dysfunction. Anaesth Intensive Care 1992; 20:86–87.
126. Holbrook JM, McCurdy HH: Drug screening. In: Bennett G, Woolf D, eds: Substance abuse: pharmacologic, developmental, and clinical perspective. Albany, NY, Delmar Publisher, 1991; pp. 93–100.

CHAPTER 15

Acute Renal Insufficiency

Steven R. Ford
Donald S. Prough

Case Report

A 68-year-old, 84-kg, white male was scheduled for removal of an infected aortobifemoral graft. In preparation for surgery, ureteral splints were placed to aid in identification of the ureters.

At surgery, the distal portion of the graft was removed. An axillary femoral-femoral graft was then placed. The patient spent 2 days in the intensive care unit (ICU) without any specific problems. He made an uneventful recovery and was discharged to the surgical ward. Two days later he was noted to have a urinary output decrease to 20 ml/hr. His fluids were then increased from 125 to 175 ml/hr. There was no apparent improvement in urinary output. The next day, the patient was noted to be febrile to 38.9°C. His blood pressure had dropped to 70 mm Hg, and his heart rate was 130/min. He also had no urine output. He was rapidly transferred to the ICU with a diagnosis of septic shock.

In the ICU, he required emergency intubation and institution of mechanical ventilatory support. After blood, urine, and sputum cultures were drawn, the patient was placed on antibiotic therapy. Initially, this consisted of vancomycin, metronidazole, and ceftazidime. Initially, fluids were given in the form of normal saline both to increase blood pressure and to restore urine output. A pulmonary artery catheter was placed to guide fluid management. Normal saline was infused to increase pulmonary capillary wedge pressure to 19 to 20 mm Hg. Albumin was noted to be 1.6 mg. Fluid resuscitation was then changed to colloid-containing solutions. His initial cardiac output was 7 L/min. Dopamine was then added, 12 μg/kg/min, both to increase blood pressure and, it was hoped, to improve urine output. Electrocardiogram revealed sinus tachycardia with ST-T-wave depression. His heart rate was slowed with diltiazem, and the ST segments returned toward normal. With dopamine, his cardiac output increased to 10 L/min. However, there was no urine output.

Furosemide was administered in increasing doses up to 300 mg without any response. Abdominal ultrasound revealed some hydronephrosis on the right kidney. It was thought the ureteral stent may have become occluded. The patient was given local anesthesia, and the stent was removed through a fiberoptic scope. Unfortunately, this did not result in any urine flow. Another 300 mg of furosemide was given, and the patient was then started on a furosemide-mannitol infusion. After 3 hours, the infusion was stopped; again, the patient had no urine output.

By the next morning, despite attempts to limit fluid, the wedge pressure had increased to 23 mm Hg. The chest radiograph showed signs of fluid overload. Dopamine was still necessary to support blood pressure. Because of the patient's recent surgical procedures, only one vessel was believed to be potentially available to cannulate for continuous arterial venous hemofiltration (CAVH). Therefore, it was elected first to attempt hemodialysis because it would require only one double-lumen catheter in a large vein. Following initiation of hemodialysis, the patient had an immediate drop in systolic blood pressure to 76 mm Hg. Despite large-dose epinephrine, his blood pressure only increased to 80 mm Hg. Hemodialysis was then discontinued. The catheter was wired for a single-lumen catheter, and the axillary artery on the left was cannulated in preparation for CAVH. This commenced with a plan to remove 100 ml fluid per hour. The patient suffered no decrease in blood pressure, and over the next 48 hours, 5.3 L fluid were successfully removed.

By this time, the patient had become afebrile, and urine output actually began to increase. The initial volume of 20 ml/hr increased over the next 3 days. Ultimately, his blood urea nitrogen (BUN) peaked at approximately 90 mg/dl, and his creatinine at 3.9 mg/dl.

After discontinuation of CAVH, the patient appeared to stabilize and urine output continued to increase. Over the next 9 days, his urine volume, BUN, and creatinine returned to normal values. He was extubated on the seventh day. He made a complete recovery and was ultimately discharged from the ICU.

INCIDENCE

Acute renal insufficiency (ARI) and acute renal failure (ARF) are common complications of critical surgical illness. Acute elevations of BUN and serum creatinine (SCr) occur in approximately 5% of all general hospital admissions and in up to 20% of critically ill patients. Perioperative ARF accounts for half of all patients who require acute dialysis.[1] Despite the development over the past 25 years of sophisticated techniques to supplement renal function, ARF still has an associated mortality in excess of 50%.[2–4] Even intensive dialytic therapy, once thought to improve outcome in comparison with less aggressive dialysis,[5] appears to produce no additional reduction of mortality.[6] Recent reports do suggest that continuous renal replacement modes of therapy may improve outcome in comparison with conventional dialysis.[7–9]

• *Acute renal failure still is associated with a mortality rate of 50%. Fifty percent of all patients who acutely require dialysis have had or will have a surgical procedure.*

Mild to moderate ARI develops surprisingly often after surgery. Charlson and associates studied renal function in 278 patients after nonemergency general, vascular, or gynecologic surgery: 76% had hypertension and 38% had diabetes.[10] Within the first 6 postoperative days, 65 of 278 patients demonstrated an increase in Cr greater than or equal to 20%. In 32 of 78 patients, the increases were sustained for at least 48 hours. For half those patients, by the time of discharge, creatinine clearance (CCr) had not returned to baseline levels. In 9 of 32 patients, renal function continued to deteriorate, although only 2 developed frank ARF. The risk of a 20% increase in Cr was greatest on the first postoperative day. Risk then rapidly declined (Fig. 15–1).[10] Novis and associates reviewed previous studies and concluded that perioperative renal dysfunction, cardiac dysfunction, and advanced age were, in descending order, most often associated with postoperative renal failure.[11]

The incidence of severe ARF varies widely, depending on the patient population. It ranges from as low as 0.01% in trauma patients and 2.7% in cardiac surgery patients to as high as 16% in medical ICU patients and 38% in liver transplant patients.[12–15] Cardiovascular surgery (valvular heart surgery, coronary artery bypass grafting, and aortic aneurysm repair) represents the most common cause of postoperative ARF.[16] Vascular surgical procedures threaten renal perfusion. This results from extensive tissue manipulation, loss of plasma volume into the interstitium, and sometimes massive hemorrhage. Aortic and renal vascular procedures, because of the suprarenal cross-clamp or temporary renal artery occlusion, also reduce renal perfusion. Even infrarenal cross-clamping reduces renal blood flow.[17,18]

• *Cardiovascular and aortic surgery are the most common procedures associated with postoperative renal failure. Renal failure can even develop in patients following infrarenal aortic cross-clamping.*

In patients who have the thoracic aorta cross-clamped, the incidence of ARF varies between 2.7 and 13.8%.[19–21] Less severe ARI occurs in 50% of patients.[20] Following an infrarenal aortic cross-clamp, 15% of patients develop an increase in Cr greater than or equal to 0.5 mg/dl.[22] Of 47 patients who developed ARF after aortic aneurysm surgery, 79% died, 15% regained renal function, and the remainder required long-term hemodialysis.[16] Following repair of ruptured abdominal aortic aneurysms, aggressive management of ARF has improved survival in only one small series.[23] Larger studies report a high mortality,[24] resulting from infection.

• *Renal insufficiency occurs in 50% of patients whose thoracic aorta has been cross-clamped.*

ARF also complicates extensive nonvascular abdominal procedures,[25] as well as hepatic insufficiency, sepsis, and volume depletion. McMurray and associates reported that gastrointestinal surgery caused 32% of postoperative ARF.[24] Ten to 50% of critically

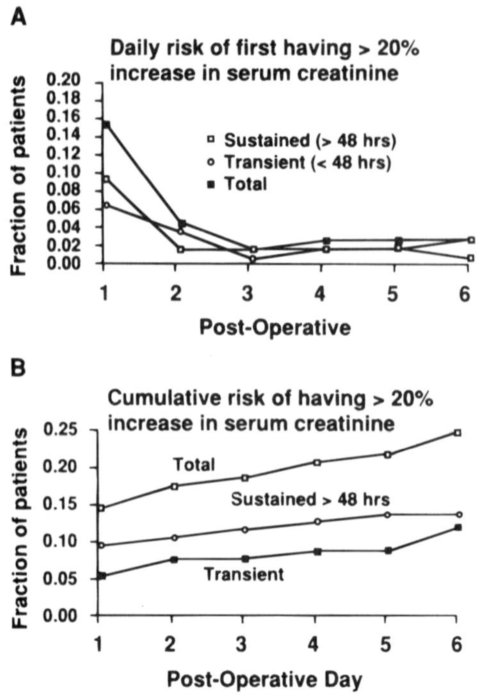

Figure 15–1.
Postoperative risk of development of increased serum creatinine higher than 20%. Daily risk (A) and cumulative risk (B). Overall, 65 of 278 patients in this study developed such an increase. (From Charlson ME, MacKenzie CR, Gold JP, Shires GT: Postoperative changes in serum creatinine: when do they occur and how much is important? Ann Surg 1989; 209:328–333.)

• *Despite the availability of dialysis, the mortality rate in critically ill patients with acute renal failure probably exceeds 50%.*

ill patients with respiratory failure, sepsis, or hepatic failure will develop ARF. The majority will succumb. Despite sophisticated support systems, the survival rate of those patients who require dialysis remains extremely low. Mortality in one study of critically ill patients with ARF was 88%. The need for ventilatory support increases the predicted mortality to 100% (89 to 100%; 95% confidence limits).[26]

PATHOPHYSIOLOGY

ARF commonly develops without antecedent oliguria (Fig. 15–2). However, in patients at risk for ARF, the occurrence of intraoperative oliguria continues to represent an ominous sign. We define oliguria in acutely stressed patients as a urinary output of less than 0.5 ml/kg/hr. This urinary volume (30 ml/hr on the average) exceeds that which defines oliguria in unstressed patients, 17 ml/hr. The higher limit is necessary in acutely stressed patients because many such patients are unable to maximally concentrate urine. Oliguric states are conventionally defined as prerenal, renal, and postrenal. Prerenal oliguria occurs as a consequence of acutely decreased renal perfusion. It is usually accompanied by hormonal (i.e., aldosterone

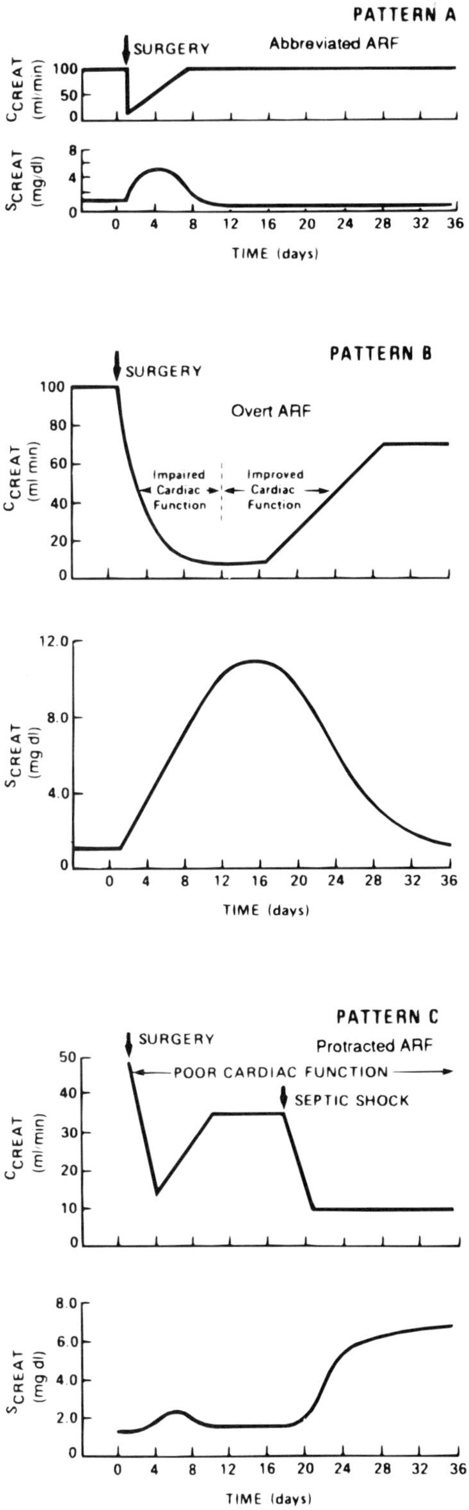

Figure 15–2.
Three patterns of hemodynamically mediated acute renal failure (ARF) that follow major vascular surgery. Pattern A (abbreviated ARF) consists of acute reduction in creatinine clearance (CCr) with prompt recovery. Serum creatinine (SCr) may still be increased even as CCr recovers. Pattern B (overt ARF) consists of concurrent, mirror-image decreases in CCr and increases in SCr. These usually occur in association with compromised cardiac function followed by recovery. Pattern C (protracted ARF) develops as a consequence of prolonged hemodynamic compromise, often complicated by systemic sepsis. (From Myers BD, Moran SM: Hemodynamically mediated acute renal failure. N Engl J Med 1986; 314:97–105.)

and antidiuretic hormone—ADH) stimuli for sodium and water conservation. Based on a more recent study,[27] ADH may be increased despite apparently adequate extracellular volume. Renal refers to parenchymal disease; postrenal denotes obstructive oliguria.

Prerenal Oliguria

• Renal hypoperfusion causes a decrease in GFR and increases salt and water reabsorption.

The conditions that produce this state primarily cause acute renal hypoperfusion. They lead to an acute reduction in glomerular filtration rate (GFR) and an acute increase in the tubular reabsorption of salt and water. Physiologic factors that can decrease urine ouput include increased circulating levels of exogenous or endogenous alpha-adrenergic agonists as well as decreased release of atrial natriuretic peptide. Also common are increased concentrations of ADH and aldosterone. The production of severe prerenal oliguria does not require frank hypotension. If not treated promptly, prerenal oliguria may progress to parenchymal renal failure.

Experience with military trauma convincingly demonstrates the crucial link between the severity (i.e., magnitude and duration) of prerenal insults and the subsequent development of parenchymal renal failure. In World War II, the overall incidence of ARF was 5% in all wounded combatants and 42% in those with severe wounds. During the Korean conflict, the overall incidence declined to 35% of severely wounded soldiers.[25,28] The incidence further declined in the Vietnam War to 0.17% of those severely wounded,[25,28] presumably because of rapid, effective resuscitation and evacuation.

Oliguria Associated With Excess ADH

Perioperative oliguria associated with excess ADH develops with no evidence of renal hypoperfusion.[27] This normovolemic form of oliguria, associated with the release of excess ADH due to pain and surgical trauma, differs from prerenal oliguria secondary to hypoperfusion. The latter is due to a combination of renal blood flow and atrial natriuretic peptide release, as well as increased ADH and aldosterone secretion. Unlike prerenal oliguria, this type of oliguria is associated with lower serum sodium and osmolality and higher urinary sodium and fractional excretion of sodium.

• Excessive ADH secretion following trauma or pain can produce normovolemic oliguria.

Renal Oliguria

ARF, alternatively termed acute tubular necrosis, may be produced by a variety of factors that interfere with glomerular filtration and tubular reabsorption. The pathogenesis of ARF includes initiation, maintenance (Table 15–1), and a recovery period.[29]

• In surgical patients, hypovolemia or low cardiac output causes the majority of cases of acute renal failure.

Renal hypoperfusion, nephrotoxic insults, or both may initiate ARF. In surgical patients, hypoperfusion, produced either by external or by internal fluid loss or sepsis, constitutes a frequent cause. Experimental renal hypoperfusion, whether induced by hemorrhagic shock or by intrarenal norepinephrine infusion at supraphysi-

Table 15–1.
Pathogenesis of Acute Renal Failure

Initiation	Maintenance
Renal hypoperfusion	Tubular dysfunction
Hemodynamic factors	Tubular obstruction
Nephrotoxins	Decreased glomerular filtration
	Decreased renal blood flow

ologic doses, impairs renal function in proportion to the depletion of high-energy phosphates.[30,31] One hypothesis states that when total renal blood flow is reduced, the disproportionately low baseline flow to the renal medulla places it at risk.[32]

The initiating insult ultimately culminates in the development of one or more of the factors (e.g., decreased tubular function, tubular obstruction, decreased glomerular filtration, and decreased renal blood flow) that reduce urinary flow and osmolar excretion. Decreased renal blood flow characterizes both the initiation and the maintenance phases. However, once the maintenance phase begins, pharmacologic improvement in renal blood flow will not reverse ARF. In contrast, the hemodynamic factors that initiate perioperative ARF and ARI often prove amenable to acute therapeutic intervention.

- *In ARF, after initiation of the so-called maintenance phase, any improvement of blood flow will not reverse renal failure.*

In general, improved management of acute prerenal oliguria has decreased the incidence of ARF. It has also increased the proportion of patients with ARF who remain nonoliguric.[33] Myers and Moran proposed a practical, clinical classification of hemodynamically mediated ARF.[33] These investigators divided it into abbreviated, overt, and protracted ARF. This was based on the pattern of CCr reduction and the increase in SCr (Fig. 15–2). The categories emphasize the frequency of nonoliguric ARF and provide a useful framework in which to group patients. This classification is clinically pertinent because it emphasizes the role of secondary insults, such as sepsis. Sepsis often complicates the course of patients with protracted critical illness.[33,34]

Nonoliguric Renal Insufficiency

Critically ill patients often have urinary outputs that exceed the oliguric threshold despite the development of ARI. Without support of renal perfusion during such intervals, patients may later develop oliguria and more severe renal insufficiency (Fig. 15–3).

Situations that lead to impaired tubular reabsorption of filtrate, despite markedly decreased glomerular filtration, cause nonoliguria. The normal kidney reabsorbs 98 to 99% of the filtrate and excretes only 1 to 2%. An injured kidney will not reabsorb filtrate this efficiently. This can lead to a "normal" urinary output, that is, nonoliguria, despite a markedly reduced GFR. If tubular dysfunction causes filtrate reabsorption to decrease from 99 to 90%, filtrate

- *Impaired tubular reabsorption results in nonoliguric renal failure. This often occurs with aminoglycoside therapy or sepsis.*

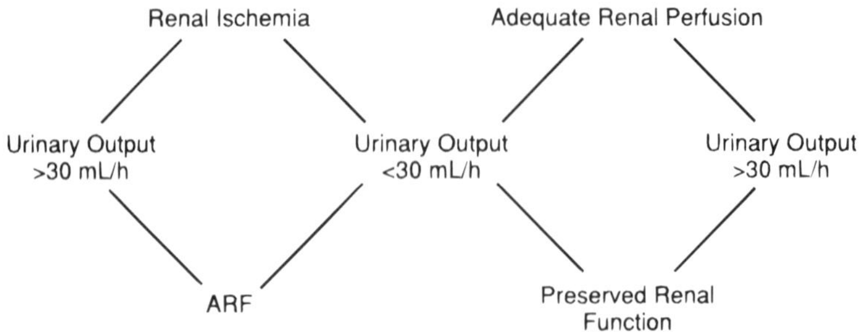

Figure 15–3.
Prevention of acute renal failure (ARF) may be difficult because of an inability to recogize inadequate renal perfusion. Oliguria, the most easily recognized sign of acute renal ischemia, can also occur with adequate renal perfusion. This is especially so when salt and water conservation are maximal. Conversely, urinary output may exceed 30 ml/hr (or 0.5 ml/kg/hr) during both adequate renal perfusion and renal ischemia. Thus, ARF may follow oliguria, or it may occur unexpectedly without sentinel oliguria. Satisfactory renal function may follow acceptable urinary output or oliguria. (From Prough DS, Bauman LA: Protecting the kidney during vascular surgery. In: Kaplan JA, ed: Vascular anesthesia. New York, Churchill Livingstone, 1991; p. 522.)

excretion would increase from 1 to 10%. If simultaneously, the GFR fell to 10 ml/min, the urinary output would remain normal despite an extremely low GFR. Situations that cause renal tubular cell dysfunction, decreased renal tubular permeability or inhibited filtrate reabsorption, can lead to nonoliguria. Specific disorders include anoxia, aminoglycoside toxicity (altered cell function), sepsis, diabetes insipidus (abnormal permeability of the collecting ducts), and diuretic toxicity (inhibit tubular reabsorption).

Experimental Versus Clinical ARF

Many therapeutic approaches to ARF have their origins in animal models that differ substantially from clinical ARF. The development of clinical ARF involves moderate to severe prerenal hemodynamic insults, often in combination with nephrotoxic factors. Following exhaustion of compensatory mechanisms, these progress over a highly variable period of time to acute parenchymal injury (Fig 15–4). In contrast, very severe insults over a short period of time generate experimental renal failure. Table 15–2 summarizes the differences between typical clinical and experimental ARF.

• *The reversibility of renal failure relates to the total ischemic time.*

At present, the most widely used experimental models of ARF employ a 40- to 60-minute interval of complete renal ischemia. This produces a lesion physiologically and prognostically (in terms of reversibility) similar to human ARF. Ischemia of shorter duration does not cause reproducible ARF. More prolonged ischemia produces irreversible injury.[35] The majority of interventions shown to alleviate experimental ARF must be administered before or immediately after an ischemic insult. The clinical setting, unlike the laboratory, does provide an opportunity to limit the magnitude and duration of the initiating insult. This includes prompt, adequate hemodynamic resuscitation. Table 15–3 lists potential therapeutic

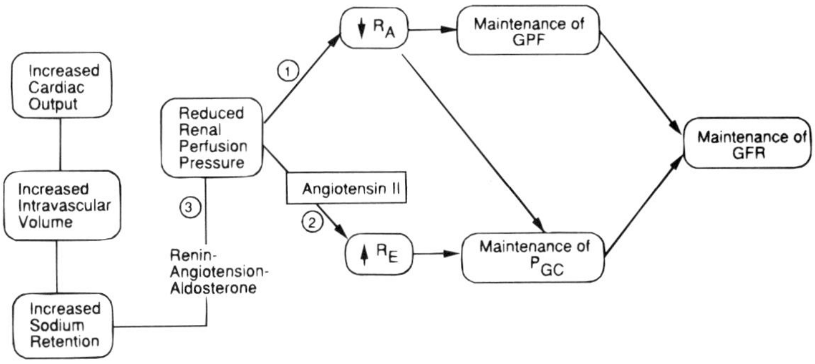

Figure 15–4.
In response to hypotension are highly efficient homeostatic mechanisms to maintain the glomerular filtration rate (GFR). These include (1) a marked reduction in afferent arteriolar resistance (R_A), and (2) an increase in efferent arteriolar resistance (R_E) because of locally released angiotensin II. Maintenance of the glomerular plasma flow rate (GPF) and of glomerular capillary hydraulic pressure (P_{GC}) preserves the GFR. Concomitantly, increased release of renin (3) initiates the renin-angiotensin-aldosterone sequence. This results in sodium retention and increased intravascular volume. (Modified from Badr KF, Ichikawa I: Prerenal failure: a deleterious shift from renal compensation to decompensation. N Engl J Med 1988; 319:623–629.)

approaches to treat fixed experimental versus variable clinical renal insults. The potential management options are similar except for the critical role of effective hemodynamic management.

Most clinical approaches aimed at the reduction of the incidence and severity of perioperative ARF and ARI rely on inferences from animal models of acute, norepinephrine-induced renal ischemia.[36] Mannitol, dopamine, and furosemide promote urinary flow. As such, these agents should reduce the renal damage produced by experimental renal ischemia.[37–47] Mannitol improves renal cortical blood flow and may exert a renal cellular protective effect.[38–40] The high tubular flow that results may decrease the incidence and severity of ARF secondary to contrast media or pigmenturia. However, in dogs, mannitol does not reverse the profound reduction in

• *Mannitol, dopamine, and furosemide all promote renal blood flow. The agents cannot reverse the injury that follows protracted aortic cross-clamping.*

Table 15–2.
Comparison of Clinical and Experimental Renal Ischemia

Fixed Insult	Variable Insult
Animal Models	Animal Models
Complete renal ischemia	Profound hemorrhagic shock
Intrarenal norepinephrine	
Renal artery occlusion	
Nephrotoxin	
Uranyl nitrate	
Clinical Models	Clinical Models
Complete surgical ischemia	Shock
Suprarenal aortic cross-clamp	Sepsis
	Multifactorial cause (often including nephrotoxic antibiotics)

Table 15–3.
Treatment Strategies for Acute Renal Insults

Fixed Experimental Insult	Variable Clinical Insult
Increase solute excretion	Limit magnitude and duration
Mannitol[38–40]	Hemodynamic support
Furosemide[39,40]	Increase renal blood flow
Dopamine[42,43]	Dopamine
Increase renal blood flow	Mannitol
Mannitol[38–40]	Furosemide
Furosemide[39,40]	Increase solute excretion
Dopamine[42,43]	Dopamine
Decrease substrate consumption	Mannitol
Hypothermia[69]	Furosemide
Antagonize calcium entry	Decrease substrate consumption
Calcium entry blockers[57,70–72]	Hypothermia
	Enhance cellular metabolism
Antagonize free radicals[77,78]	ATP-$MgCl_2$
Vasodilatory prostaglandins	
PGI_2[83]	
PGE_1[81,82]	
PGE_2[79,80]	
Antagonize vasoconstrictor prostaglandins[55]	
Antagonize leukotrienes[55]	
Antagonize endothelin[55]	
Enhance cellular metabolism	
ATP-$MgCl_2$[67,68]	
5′nucleotidase[157]	
Fructose-1,6-diphosphate[158]	
Thyroxine[159]	
Enhance tubular regeneration	
Growth factors[53,56,58,60,61]	
Atrial natriuretic peptide[54,56,58]	

GFR and renal blood flow induced by 60 minutes of a suprarenal aortic cross-clamp.[41] Dopamine, like mannitol, does not reliably reverse the renal injury produced by a thoracic aortic cross-clamp.[41] Dopamine, in doses of 1 to 3 μg/kg/min, increases renal cortical blood flow with minimal systemic effects.[42] It also induces natriuresis, increases GFR, and improves urinary flow.[42,43] Dopamine can be a useful adjunct to treat oliguria. Dopamine may work by inhibition of aldosterone secretion.[48] Fenoldopam, a novel dopamine-1 receptor agonist, substantially enhances urinary flow, sodium excretion, and CCr. Moreover, fenoldopam simultaneously reduces systemic vascular resistance.[49–52] Although fenoldopam will likely become a valuable perioperative adjunct, its precise role remains to be demonstrated.

Furosemide is helpful in experimental models of complete renal ischemia.[39,40] Generally, it is less effective than mannitol. Clinicians often use furosemide in an attempt to convert established oliguric ARF to nonoliguric ARF. However, this practice does not uniformly improve outcome or reduce the frequency of dialysis.[44,47] The combination of dopamine and furosemide may be beneficial. Lindner and colleagues infused both dopamine and furosemide in a canine model of nephrotoxic canine ARF. They demonstrated a synergistic renal protective effect.[45] Subsequently, in an uncontrolled trial in a small group of patients who had oliguric ARF, this combination resulted in a brisk diuresis and stabilization of renal function.[46] However, this has not been duplicated in a controlled, randomized trial. A variety of other agents have demonstrated efficacy in experimental models of ARF.[53–88] Perhaps effective pharmacologic therapy will be available within the decade. Numerous reviews address potential mechanisms that may lead to therapeutic progress.[36,89–94]

Renal hypoperfusion reduces renal concentrations of high-energy phosphate.[31] The thick ascending limb of Henle's loop may be most vulnerable to such changes.[32,64–66] Infusion of adenine nucleotides in combination with magnesium chloride can preserve experimental postischemic renal function.[67,68] Presumably, the renal protective effects of hypothermia are also dependent upon preservation of high-energy phosphate.[69]

Depletion of high-energy phosphates initiates a pathophysiologic sequence that involves a variety of potentially toxic biochemical intermediates. In the kidneys, as in other organs, ischemia causes an increase in intracellular calcium ions. Pretreatment with calcium entry blockers limits the renal injury produced by experimental, complete renal ischemia.[57,70–72] However, we still require additional clinical evidence before calcium entry blockers can be added to the management of those patients who undergo complete renal ischemia.[73] In partial renal ischemia, calcium entry blockers may produce salutary or deleterious effects. The results depend on the magnitude of drug-induced blood pressure decline and the etiology of the renal hypoperfusion.[74–76]

• *Renal injury when due to renal ischemia can be experimentally minimized by pretreatment with calcium channel blockers.*

Oxygen-derived free radicals, arachidonate metabolites, leukotrienes, neutrophils, and endothelin have also been implicated in ischemic renal damage. Following renal ischemia, oxygen free radicals appear to be produced in large quantities.[77] This may explain why pretreatment with superoxide dismutase or allopurinol reduces experimental renal ischemic injury.[78] Renal vascular tone depends in part on the balance between the vasodilator prostaglandin (PGI_2) and the vasoconstrictor thromboxane (TxA_2). That balance may be disrupted by ischemic renal injury. The administration of exogenous vasodilator prostaglandins such as PGE_2,[79,80] PGE_1,[81,82] and PGI_2[83] reduces experimental renal injury. Leukotrienes, presumably derived from neutrophils, appear to partially mediate ischemic renal injury.[55] Neutrophil depletion improves postischemic renal function.[84] In rats, inhibition of TxA_2 synthesis protects against tubular necrosis which follows experimental ischemia.[85] Surprisingly, oxygen-derived free radical scavengers also inhibit synthesis of TxA_2 and improve renal outcome.[86] Antagonism of endothelin, another potent renal vasoconstrictor, also ameliorates ischemic renal damage.[55]

• *Experimentally, oxygen radical scavengers and prostaglandins appear to limit renal injury following ischemia. The clinical role remains clouded.*

Although a variety of agents appear to offer promise for amelioration of ARF, clinical application requires careful clinical testing. Clinical ARF is more heterogeneous than experimental ARF. It frequently occurs in elderly patients with reduced renal reserve and highly variable degrees of renal ischemia. Two experimental studies particularly emphasize the extent to which small differences in preischemic status could affect the subsequent course of ARF. Rats maintained in the weeks before renal ischemia on no-protein or low-protein diets survived. Those maintained on normal or high-protein diets before ischemia had a much higher mortality.[87] Postischemic protein ingestion did not affect recovery. Seguro and colleagues demonstrated that preischemic potassium depletion markedly accentuated renal injury secondary to ischemia.[88]

Research has emphasized the potential influence of interventions that improve the rate of tubular regeneration. After acute renal injury, several growth factors including epidermal growth factor, transforming growth factor α, and insulin-like growth factor have improved the rate of cellular recovery.[53,56,58,60,61] Atrial natriuretic peptide, in addition to its renal vasodilating properties, also appears to enhance tubular recovery.[54,56,58]

• *Potential therapies derived from animal studies may not apply to the human situation. Often, the mechanism of in vivo kidney injury differs from experimental studies.*

The clinician should be skeptical of the uncritical application of results from animal studies of ARF to the clinical setting. Experimental data that demonstrate the protective effects of dopamine, mannitol, and furosemide may not apply to clinical acute oliguria with a typical cause of hypovolemia. Diuresis produced by any of these agents, singly or in combination, may further complicate hemodynamic management. Theoretically, these agents may increase the magnitude and duration of the prerenal insult.[95] However, one can reasonably conclude from experimental and clinical data that dopamine, mannitol, or furosemide, coupled with appropriate hemodynamic support and monitoring, may limit renal injury more than hemodynamic management alone. The experimental demonstration of the renal protective effects of various pharmacologic interventions holds promise. However, the reduction in blood pressure associated with many potential interventions, such as calcium entry blockers, suggests that their clinical application may be limited to hemodynamically stable patients.

DIAGNOSTIC TESTS

Clinical investigators have expended considerable effort to develop tools and tests to clearly differentiate prerenal from renal oliguria, to predict the outcome of acute oliguric states, and to direct therapy intended to prevent ARF. Unfortunately, none is sufficiently sensitive or specific or able to predict which patients will or will not respond to therapy. Consequently, the physician usually must treat the acutely oliguric patient without accurate information on the presence of or potential to develop ARF.

Table 15–4 compares typical laboratory findings in patients with prerenal oliguria, secondary to hypoperfusion or ADH excess

Table 15–4.
Diagnostic Tests in Acute Oliguria

Test	Prerenal Hypo-perfusion	Prerenal ADH-Excess	Renal
Urinary osmolality (mOsm/kg)	>400	>400	<400
Urine/plasma osmolality	>1.3	>1.8	<1.1
Urinary sodium (mEq/L)	<20	>40	>40
Urine/plasma creatinine	>40	>40	<20
FENa (%)*	<1	>1	>2

* FENa = fractional excretion of sodium, calculated as:

$$\frac{U/P_{Na}}{U/P_{Cr}} \times 100$$

where U = urinary concentration, P = plasma concentration, Na = sodium, and Cr = creatinine

to those with renal oliguria. Prerenal oliguria is associated with physiologic mechanisms that conserve salt and water. This results in excretion of waste products and minimal urine volume. Such patients with prerenal oliguria classically produce urine with high osmolality and low sodium. Patients with a long-term reduction in concentrating ability owing to preexisting renal disease cannot achieve prerenal values of urinary sodium and osmolality. In addition, diuretics increase urinary sodium and decrease urinary osmolality.

The fractional excretion of sodium (FENa) is a laboratory guide that can more accurately differentiate prerenal from renal oliguria. The FENa is calculated as follows:

- *FENa can help differentiate prerenal from renal failure. The test becomes inaccurate following diuretic therapy.*

$$\text{FENa} = \frac{U_{Na}/P_{Na}}{U_{Cr}/P_{Cr}} \times 100$$

Where U = urine; Na = sodium; P = plasma; and Cr = creatinine. Values less than 1% suggest prerenal azotemia. However, in critically ill postoperative patients,the test has limited diagnostic and prognostic use.[96,97] When hemodynamically mediated prerenal factors are still reversible, the FENa may suggest established parenchymal ARF. Moreover, these tests are unreliable in patients with liver failure, nephrotic syndrome, and cirrhosis. In those, urinary sodium may be low despite inexorably progressive renal failure.[98]

Zaloga and Hughes reported that postoperative oliguria could result from avid water conservation in the absence of sodium conservation (Table 15–4).[27] Of 100 prospectively studied patients admitted to a surgical ICU, 7 developed oliguria associated with increased urinary osmolality, low urinary sodium, and an FENa well below 1.0%. These data are consistent with the conventional description of the prerenal oliguric state. Eleven patients, in contrast, developed oliguria with high urinary osmolality similar to prerenal oliguria, (i.e., > 500 mOsm/kg). However, the urinary sodium generally was higher than 60 mEq/L, instead of the less than 20 mEq/L normally seen in prerenal oliguria.[27] In these patients, calculated FENa averaged 1.15 ± 0.2.[27]

• Urine output is not a sensitive or specific indicator of the status of renal function.

Urinary output assessment is the diagnostic test that responds most quickly to changes in renal perfusion. However, it is neither specific nor sensitive.[99,100] Postoperative patients can have normal urinary outputs with clinically significant renal insufficiency, that is, artificial nonoliguria. They can also demonstrate abnormally low urinary outputs with no primary renal injury, that is, excess ADH oliguria. In critically ill patients at risk for ARI, not only should GFR be known, but also whether it continues to improve or deteriorate. Clinically, this can best be evaluated using serial evaluations of CCr. It requires collection periods as short as 1 and 2 hours (Fig. 15–5).[101,102] However, short-term CCr may overestimate GFR when compared with measurements using inulin.[103] In several studies in critically ill patients, CCr seems to be superior to other diagnostic tests (i.e., SCr, BUN, free water clearance, FENa, urinary volume, or 24-hour CCr). Specifically, SCr may not change significantly during the first 24 postoperative hours of ARI. This results from the dilutional effects of aggressive fluid administration. Measurement of serial 2-hour CCr will improve renal function monitoring.

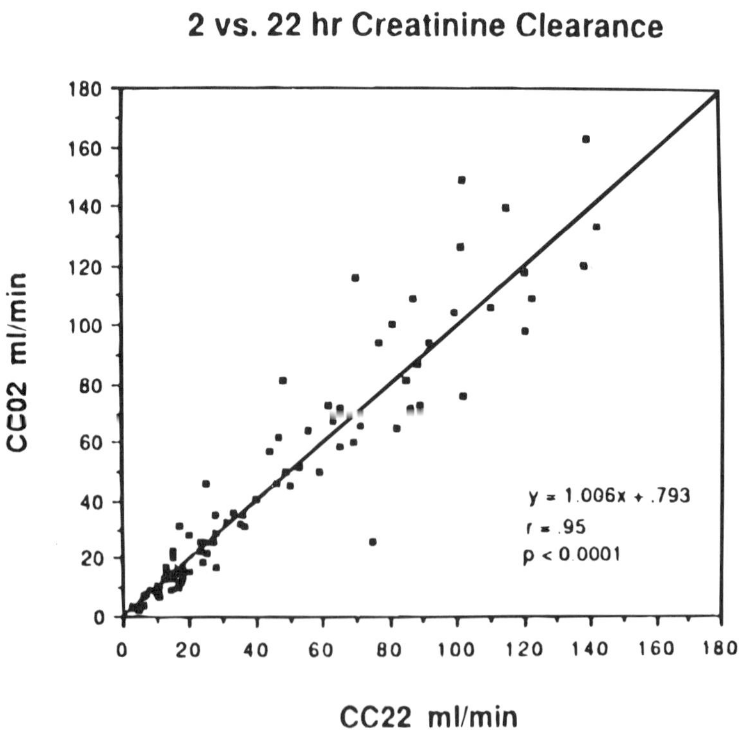

Figure 15–5.
Correlation between the 2-hour creatinine clearance (CC02) and 22-hour creatinine clearance (CC22). (From Sladen RN, Endo E, Harrison T: Two-hour versus 22-hour creatinine clearance in critically ill patients. Anesthesiology 1987; 67:1013–1016.)

SUGGESTED MANAGEMENT TO PREVENT ARI AND ARF

No specific guidelines exist that routinely and simultaneously produce the least compromise to the kidneys, lungs, and heart. Instead, therapy needs to be individualized, based on the apparent risk to each system. Lacking an easy cookbook approach to prevent the progression from acute prerenal oliguria to ARF, the following generalizations form the basis of a logical approach:

1. Renal hypoperfusion most commonly causes ARF.
2. The duration and magnitude of the initial renal insult determine the severity of ARF.
3. The prevention of ARF reduces mortality more effectively than does dialytic therapy.

Based on the foregoing generalizations, the following strategies can be applied, as described in the following sections.

Identification of Perioperative Patients at Risk

Patients at particular risk include those with preexisting renal dysfunction, left ventricular dysfunction, and advanced age.[11] Other such patients include those who receive nephrotoxic antibiotics or undergo angiography, especially if they are diabetic. It is important to note the limitations of routine laboratory tests used to identify preoperative renal dysfunction (Table 15–5).

Table 15–5.
Preoperative Assessment of Renal Function

Test	Normal Range	Limitations
BUN	8–20 mg/dl	Dehydration Variable protein intake Gastrointestinal bleeding Catabolism
SCr	0.5–1.2 mg/dl	Advanced age Muscle mass Catabolic state
CCr (estimated)*	120 ml/min	Advanced age Muscle mass Catabolic state
CCr (measured)†	120 ml/min	Weight-dependency Inaccurate urine volume measurement

* Using the formula:

$$CCr = \frac{(140 - age)\ wt\ (kg)}{72 \times SCr}$$

† Using the formula:

$$CCr = \frac{UV}{P}$$

where BUN = blood urea nitrogen, SCr = serum creatinine, CCr = creatinine clearance, U = urinary creatinine concentration, V = urinary volume, and P = plasma creatinine concentration

Limitation of the Magnitude and Duration of Renal Ischemic Insults

This constitutes the key strategy. In the majority of patients, oliguria signals inadequate systemic perfusion. This warrants carefully monitored efforts to improve perfusion. Efforts should include volume expansion, pulmonary artery catheterization, inotropic support (ideally with dopamine), and, occasionally, vasodilation.

However, oliguria and other monitors of intraoperative renal function are insufficiently sensitive and specific to always detect hypoperfusion.[99,100] High-risk patients, such as those who require aggressive volume and blood product administration, may benefit from serial evaluation of CCr to detect renal insufficiency. This should be considered despite satisfactory urinary output, blood pressure, heart rate, and cardiac output. A 2-hour CCr test is an accurate and effective early marker of renal disturbance.[101,102]

• *Serial creatinine clearance measurements are the most sensitive indicators of renal function.*

Several studies of high-risk surgical patients suggest that certain postoperative surgical complications, such as renal failure, hepatic failure, and sepsis, may result from unrecognized, subclinical tissue hypoperfusion during the immediate perioperative period.[104–106] Average cardiac output and systemic oxygen transport (DO_2) (cardiac output × arterial oxygen content) are greater in high-risk surviving surgical patients than in those who succumb.[104,105] Therefore, Shoemaker and associates adjusted hemodynamic therapy to achieve the higher values for cardiac output and DO_2 previously associated with improved survival.[106] In the first of two studies, the protocol group had as goals for therapy, hemodynamic values titrated to the levels of previous survivors. In this group, cardiac output and DO_2 were elevated. Survival was improved and complications were reduced.[106] These data suggest that so-called supranormal support may prevent clinically inapparent hypoperfusion. As a consequence, it may limit the mortality and morbidity secondary to that process. It is worth noting that the target for oxygen delivery (600 ml/min/m^2) used by Shoemaker and associates[106] is equivalent to a normal cardiac index (3.0 L/min/m) multiplied by a normal oxygen content (20 ml/min/m). Additional clinical investigations in high-risk critically ill patients,[107] and in septic patients, show support for the association of supranormal oxygen transport with improved outcome.[108] Figure 15–6 summarizes three possible approaches to prevention of ARF.

Promotion of Solute Excretion

When aggressive attempts to restore perfusion have failed to establish adequate urinary output, dopamine, mannitol, and/or furosemide should be added. Earlier use, although theoretically attractive, will further compromise the value of urinary output as a monitor of the adequacy of resuscitation. No evidence exists that small test doses of diuretics decrease either morbidity or mortality in patients with uncertain volume status. At best, there will be no effect. At worst, production of short-term increases in urinary output will

• *When urine does not flow following restoration of intravascular volume, dopamine, mannitol, or furosemide should be used to promote renal blood flow.*

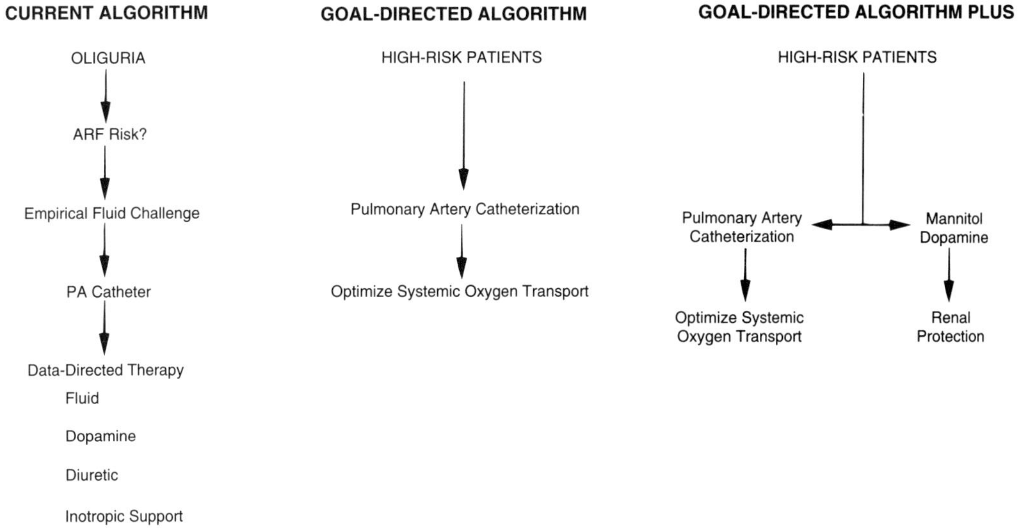

Figure 15–6.
Three possible approaches to prevention of acute renal failure (ARF). The left-hand algorithm reflects the approach used by many clinicians. Following recognition of oliguria, the diagnostic and therapeutic approach consists of empiric volume expansion, supplemented if necessary by pulmonary artery (PA) catheterization. Subsequent data-directed therapy consists of fluid, dopamine, inotropic support, mannitol, or furosemide. In contrast, the goal-directed algorithm has been developed for high-risk patients. Such patients require pulmonary artery catheterization with subsequent support of systemic oxygen transport (cardiac output × arterial oxygen content) at levels previously associated with improved survival in high-risk surgical patients. The right-hand figure combines goal-oriented therapy with early pharmacologic support. This assumes that the earlier the pharmacologic intervention, the greater its effectiveness will be. Induced diuresis may perpetuate hypovolemia and may interfere with monitoring of urinary output. (From Prough DS, Foreman AS: Anesthesia and the renal system. In Barash PG, Cullen BF, Stoelting RK, eds: Clinical anesthesia, 2nd ed. Philadelphia, J.B. Lippincott, 1992; p. 1125–1155.)

delay effective therapy and potentiate the development of volume deficits.[95] However, in the special circumstance of rhabdomyolysis-induced pigmenturia, early high-volume diuresis may limit the incidence of ARF.[109] The use of diuretics earlier in the course of prerenal oliguria would be easier to defend if an appropriate monitor of renal function were available to permit rapid assessment of changes in renal function.

Need for Cautious Consideration of Diagnostic Data

Urinary output, although an extremely crude estimate of renal function, offers the most consistently useful diagnostic information. Hemodynamic data prove useful in situations where empiric volume expansion does not restore urinary flow. Such data can be used to prevent clinically inapparent tissue hypoperfusion.[106] In acute illness, most therapeutic decisions should not rely on urinary sediment, electrolytes, osmolality, or complex formulas derived from urinary and plasma sodium and creatinine measurements. The discriminatory value of these measurements is too limited for application in the perioperative setting. Unfortunately, the readily available tests are insufficiently sensitive and specific, require excessive time, and provide little information. All acutely oliguric patients at risk

• *Therapeutic decisions should not rely on urinary sediment, electrolytes, osmolality, and other formulas.*

for ARF should receive fluids and should undergo monitoring and hemodynamic support in the same fashion. All should be treated to the same end points, regardless of the test results. The resuscitation of patients with perioperative oliguria should be sufficiently aggressive and continues until oliguria persists despite a pulmonary capillary wedge pressure of 15 mm Hg or higher, a systemic oxygen delivery of more than 550 ml/min/m^2, and the administration of dopamine and diuretics.

Excessive reliance on the determination of urinary electrolytes, osmolality, or specialized indices may lead to the delay, interruption, or premature termination of appropriate, timely therapy. It increases the chance that a patient will suffer the high morbidity and mortality of ARF.

SPECIAL CONSIDERATIONS

Sepsis

Several points are of special concern to prevent sepsis-associated ARI or ARF. Maintenance of renal perfusion remains paramount. Both cardiac output and perfusion pressure must be monitored. Systemic oxygen delivery should be addressed with aggressive volume expansion. If cardiac index does not improve to a normal or supranormal level, inotropic agents should be added. Commonly, in severe sepsis and septic shock, despite a markedly increased cardiac index, renal perfusion pressure (mean arterial pressure – central venous pressure) remains low (i.e., below the renal autoregulatory threshold of 50 mm Hg). When cardiac index is adequate but systemic vascular resistance and perfusion pressure are abnormally low, several animal and human studies have shown norepinephrine to have beneficial effects.[110–113] Even when patients were refractory to high dopamine doses ($\geq$ 80 μg/kg/min), some of these studies have shown improvement in perfusion pressure and urinary flow.

- *Septic patients may require high perfusion pressures to maintain renal blood flow. These pressures can be accomplished with alpha-adrenergic agents.*

Norepinephrine used in this manner improves urinary output without a decrease in renal blood flow. When used in combination with low-dose dopamine, that is renal-dose dopamine, norepinephrine significantly increases renal blood flow, relative to baseline values. It will increase the fraction of cardiac output that perfuses the kidneys and lowers renal vascular resistance.[113] Norepinephrine should be infused only at a rate to restore the severely reduced perfusion pressure to a level that improves renal perfusion. Norepinephrine-induced renal ischemia has been used as a model of ARF in animals. Many clinicians are reluctant to use this agent since they fear it may precipitate ARF in patients already at high risk for renal damage. However, in these studies, the doses far exceed those used in the clinical setting.

Mechanical Ventilation

Several studies have shown that positive pressure ventilation decreases GFR, urinary output, and urinary sodium excretion. Positive end-expiratory pressure (PEEP) further reduces this diuresis and natriuresis.[114,115] These changes result from decreased secretion of atrial natriuretic peptide and increased plasma renin activity. Aggressive volume expansion will reverse their effects.[116,117] Normally, these are appropriate compensatory mechanisms to offset the decreased atrial transmural pressure and atrial dimensions produced by positive intrathoracic pressure. Mechanically ventilated patients require more aggressive hydration than spontaneously breathing patients.

Therapeutic Conflicts in the Management of Acute Oliguria

Effective treatment of oliguria requires not only an understanding of the effects of various therapeutic interventions on the kidney, but also knowledge of their effects on the lungs and the heart.

Kidney-Lung Therapeutic Conflicts

Aggressive expansion of intravascular volume can potentially lead to pulmonary edema. In a healthy person, clinical pulmonary edema will occur at a pulmonary microvascular pressure higher than or equal to 25 mm Hg. However, in patients with decreased serum oncotic pressure or increased pulmonary capillary permeability, pulmonary edema may occur at much lower pulmonary microvascular pressures.[118] Consequently, clinicians who treat prerenal oliguria frequently confront the dilemma that treatment of ARF causes acute respiratory failure.[119] Approximately 40% of patients with ARF develop pulmonary complications.[119–121] Conversely, more than 50% of patients with the adult respiratory distress syndrome (ARDS) develop ARF.[122] In a broader cross-section of patients with respiratory failure, 11 to 33% developed ARF.[123,124]

In general, the argument to sacrifice pulmonary function to save renal function rests on the ease with which mechanical ventilation can support the patient with deteriorating pulmonary function. One can further defend this position because the known mortality from ARF ranges from 50 to 70%.[2,119] The counterargument, less often heard, states that renal function can be sacrificed because dialysis or continuous hemofiltration or hemodiafiltration can effectively support patients with acute ARF. Proponents of this approach indicate that ARDS has a mortality rate of 50 to 70%.[125]

- *In acute renal failure, volume expansion should be carried out to the point of early pulmonary edema. The resulting pulmonary dysfunction can be treated with greater ease than can renal failure.*

Certainly, in the provision of hemodynamic support for the oliguric patient, one should avoid the two extremes of frank hypovolemia and inappropriate overhydration. However, the practical definition of these two terms presents a problem. In everyday terms, the pulmonary capillary wedge pressure, though imperfect, may be the best single estimate. The use of this parameter in conjunction with measurements of flow (i.e., cardiac index or stroke volume index) can establish a ventricular performance curve for each patient. This will decrease the likelihood of excessively high or low filling pressures. The lower the wedge pressure limit, the greater the chance of inadequate resuscitation and the more frequent the need for inotropic support. The higher the pressure, the greater the risk of pulmonary edema. Nevertheless, pulmonary edema does not occur simply because of fluid administration. For example, Shin and associates reported that post-traumatic respiratory failure occurred less often in patients who received a greater amount of fluid and less frequent diuretics.[126] More thorough shock resuscitation may limit the release of systemic mediators that produce pulmonary capillary leakage.

Kidney-Heart Therapeutic Conflicts

• High intracardiac filling pressures can decrease ventricular perfusion pressure gradients.

Aggressive volume expansion may worsen pulmonary edema and may also lead to increased left ventricular end-diastolic pressure and wall tension. Myocardial oxygen consumption will increase. Left ventricular end-diastolic pressure limits left ventricular subendocardial perfusion. Therefore, increases in filling pressure may also limit myocardial oxygen availability. The production of myocardial ischemia secondary to aggressive volume loading represents a more subtle, less easily appreciated complication of volume resuscitation. However, limitation of volume expansion to a lower limit of pulmonary capillary wedge pressure and earlier use of positive inotropic agents or vasodilators does not necessarily reduce the cardiac risk. Rather, inotropes that increase heart rate and myocardial contractility may also increase myocardial oxygen consumption. Vasodilators, particularly if used in hypovolemic patients, may precipitate sudden hypotension and myocardial ischemia. However, when used with careful augmentation of intravascular volume, vasodilators such as nitroprusside can substantially improve both hemodynamic and renal function.[127]

Comparison of Oliguric and Nonoliguric ARF

Nonoliguric ARF, once uncommon, now occurs frequently. In contrast to oliguric ARF, nonoliguric ARF is somewhat easier to manage. It requires less scrupulous control of fluid and electrolyte intake. The first extensive clinical description of nonoliguric ARF stressed its lower mortality rate.[128] In that study, a larger percentage of patients with nonoliguric ARF had a nephrotoxic injury. The oliguric patients developed ARF in association with surgery, prolonged volume depletion, or impaired cardiac output. Therefore, it appears that nonoliguric ARF that occurs spontaneously has a lower associated mortality. Nonoliguric ARF that follows as a complication of trauma may also carry a better prognosis than oliguric ARF. Shin and associates reported on two consecutive groups (A and B) of trauma patients.[126] In group B, more liberal fluid administration and less frequent diuretic administration compared with group A increased the incidence of nonoliguric ARF and decreased that of oliguric ARF. Group A received less fluid and more diuretics. Group B had lower mortality and morbidity.[126]

ARF represents a syndrome that includes both oliguric patients and a heterogeneous group of nonoliguric patients. Accurate characterization and classification of clinical ARF should improve prognosis and treatment. Myers and colleagues extensively studied hemodynamically mediated ARF in surgical patients. They used a combination of clinical variables and creatinine kinetic modeling to describe the key pathogenetic features of three types of ARF (see Fig. 15–2).[33,129–133] Protracted ARF, the third type, represents the net effects of multiple episodes of renal injury. Prognostically, one can anticipate a low mortality in patients with abbreviated ARF and a high mortality when protracted ARF exists.[33]

The reported improved mortality and morbidity in patients with nonoliguric ARF has caused several investigators to attempt to convert established oliguric ARF. Generally, these investigators have used diuretics, with or without dopamine. Uncontrolled series emphasize the efficacy of induced diuresis.[46,134] However, controlled randomized trials have failed to demonstrate that conversion of oliguric ARF to nonoliguric ARF improves mortality, morbidity, the duration of renal failure, or the number of necessary dialyses.[44,47] In addition, direct intrarenal administration of furosemide (275 mg over 30 minutes) failed to improve renal function or renal blood flow in patients with ARF.[135] The aforementioned data support the conclusion that early, aggressive hemodynamic support of the patient with prerenal oliguria may produce a better outcome, even if nonoliguric ARF develops. Conversely, the chemical conversion of oliguric to nonoliguric ARF has no effect on outcome.

MANAGEMENT OF ARF

Despite the fact that outcome may not change, we believe that nonoliguric renal failure can be more easily managed than oliguric renal failure. The continued urine flow makes fluid management and nutritional support easier. Moreover, if invasive lines for dialysis are not needed, the likelihood of infection also decreases. Therefore, once we have restored adequate volume replacement and cardiac output, high-dose diuretic therapy (e.g., 200 to 400 mg furosemide) is employed. Obviously, we always use low-dose dopamine (3 to 4 μg/kg/min). When all other measures have failed, a combination infusion of furosemide and mannitol (500 mg furosemide in 500 ml 20% mannitol at 20 to 40 ml/hr) will often produce adequate urine.

- *Furosemide-mannitol infusions can often restore urine output when all other measures fail.*

Despite intensive efforts to prevent or manage ARF, renal replacement therapy may become necessary. Several aspects of care deserve special consideration. The choice of optimal therapy can prove controversial. Consideration must be given to: (1) the timing and selection of renal replacement techniques; (2) current pharmacologic management; (3) fluid and electrolyte therapy; and (4) nutritional support. The likelihood of infection will also increase.

Timing and Renal Replacement Therapy Techniques

After establishment of the diagnosis of ARF, the timing of renal replacement therapy becomes important. Additionally, the appropriate modality must be chosen. Many clinicians now prefer continuous modalities.[136–141] Many of these patients will have undergone extensive fluid resuscitation for the management of traumatic, surgical, or septic sequestration of sodium and water. Therefore, aggressive attempts are often used to remove fluid. Unfortunately, the processes that caused the initial fluid sequestration frequently still exist. Aggressive attempts to remove sodium and water with hemodialysis, peritoneal dialysis, or continuous methods will frequently result in intravascular volume depletion. Rather than persist, the dialytic therapy should be refocused on the basic goals of such therapy: (1) intravascular volume overload; (2) azotemia; (3) hyperkalemia; and (4) severe acid-base disturbances. Dialysis can also facilitate improvement of both white cell function, enhance neurologic function, and permit more aggressive nutritional support.[142,143]

For patients in acute renal and hepatic failure, improved cardiovascular stability can sometimes be achieved with a continuous technique of renal replacement therapy compared with intermittent machine hemofiltration.[136] Many clinicians believe that continuous therapies, such as continuous arteriovenous hemofiltration (CAVH), continuous arteriovenous hemodiafiltration (CAVHD), and continuous venovenous hemodiafiltration (CVVHD) offer important clinical advantages.[136–141,144]

As expected, each has specific advantages and disadvantages. Hemodialysis requires only one double-lumen catheter placed in a central vein. It can easily remove fluid and improve electrolytes as well as BUN and SCr. It also only requires 3 to 4 hours at most per day. However, hemodynamically unstable patients do not usually tolerate hemodialysis. Hypotension readily develops and can further damage the kidney. Despite attempts to minimize the required heparin, coagulopathies can develop.

• *Hemodialysis often causes hypotension, particularly in patients already on vasopressors.*

Peritoneal dialysis requires continuous exchange of fluids via the peritoneal catheters. The slow process provides good hemodynamic stability. However, it cannot be safely used in patients with abdominal sepsis. Many surgeons are reluctant to use peritoneal dialysis following major intra-abdominal procedures. BUN and SCr are reduced slowly. The brain probably has less exposure to significant fluid shifts.

CAVH requires two catheters, one in a large central vein and one usually in the femoral vein (Fig. 15–7). The system can be run at the bedside and does not require a dialysis team. The process, as the name implies, goes on continuously. Since no pumps are employed, the patient's own systemic blood pressure drives all flow. Hypotension rarely develops. The method ordinarily can remove significant amounts of water. The amount of fluid lost per hour can be controlled in one of two ways. The usual method simply replaces all the fluid lost during the previous hour minus the desired volume to be removed. The composition can be based on close monitoring of serum electrolytes, including calcium. We now connect the collection limb of the filter through a standard infusion pump and then into the collection bag. The volume of fluid lost during each hour then becomes equal to the rate set on the pump.

• *Continuous arteriovenous hemofiltration allows easy control of fluid loss.*

CAVH requires heparinization to prevent the filter from clotting.

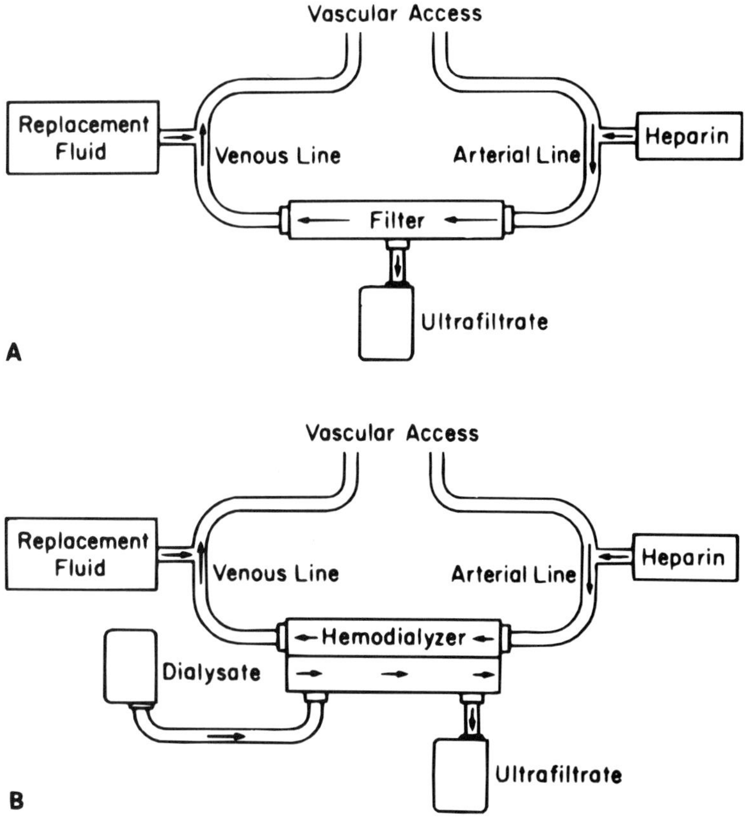

Figure 15–7.
Schematic representation of (A) continuous arteriovenous hemofiltration (CAVH) and (B) continuous arteriovenous hemodialysis (CAVHD). (From Nahman NS Jr, Middendorf DF: Continuous arteriovenous hemofiltration. Med Clin North Am 1990; 74:975–984.)

Hypotension and a low flow rate can also cause clotting. While the system can easily removc water, it does not predictably correct electrolyte abnormalities or significantly reduce BUN or SCr. It primarily removes excess fluid. The filter usually requires replacement every third day.

In general, CAVHD works like CAVH. However, the different type of filter permits gentle, continuous dialysis. CAVHD may be best suited to the hemodynamically unstable patient who would likely become hypotensive during hemodialysis.

- *Continuous arteriovenous hemodiafiltration is the preferred method of dialysis in hemodynamically unstable patients.*

Pharmacologic Therapy

The kidney excretes a large number of drugs. Some can be removed by dialytic therapy or continuous methods. At the time of initiation of renal replacement therapy, the clinician should review all pharmacologic therapy. Doses should be adjusted to reflect the change in the patient's renal status. Dosages of antibiotics, particularly aminoglycosides, require alteration.[145]

Patients with ARF have a high incidence of stress gastritis. Most will require some form of stress ulcer prophylaxis. Three different regimens are aggressive antacid titration,[146] H_2 receptor antagonists, and sucralfate.[147,148] Antacids have been the gold standard for prophylaxis.[146] However, they frequently require large quantities. H_2 receptor antagonists appear most effective in patients with few risk factors for stress gastritis. These agents work less well in patients with renal failure.[148–150] Sucralfate, originally used for the management of duodenal ulceration, compares favorably in the prevention of gastrointestinal bleeding with either antacids or cimetidine.[147,148]

Fluid and Electrolyte Management

Patients with ARF cannot compensate for excessive intravascular volume expansion. For hemodynamically stable patients, fluids can be restricted to that necessary to provide adequate nutrition. Despite the cessation of renal function, patients with sepsis or multiple system failure often require continued sodium and water administration. Serum potassium, calcium, magnesium, and phosphate levels should be monitored carefully. In general, potassium excretion reflects urinary flow rate rather than GFR. Magnesium may accumulate in patients who receive magnesium-containing antacids. Hyperphosphatemia results from excretory failure. Conversely, hypophosphatemia may develop because of aggressive nutritional support and phosphate-binding antacids. Dialysis best manages metabolic acidosis. Patients with nonoliguric renal failure develop a hyperchloremic acidosis. Sodium bicarbonate, usually on a continuous basis, will correct the situation.

• *Despite renal failure, if renal output remains adequate, hyperkalemia will usually not develop.*

Nutritional Support

The recovery of patients with ARF may depend, in part, on the adequacy of their nutritional support. Specialized formulas do not appear to have any impact on outcome. Limitation of amino acids to 1 g/kg/day helps to control BUN. Inadequate nutrition results in muscle wasting and immune compromise. Renal replacement therapy should remove sufficient excess fluid to permit administration of adequate calories and protein.

Infection Surveillance

Infection remains the most common cause of death in patients with ARF. Additionally, ARF constitutes one of the earliest manifestations of multiple system organ failure.[151–153] The control of overt infection, the search for occult sepsis, and vigilance in regard to new infectious complications must be intensive and persistent. The clinician must recognize that ARF may be followed by other organ system failures.

Hemodynamic and Renal Monitoring

The indications for pulmonary artery catheterization in patients with ARF resemble those indications in other critically ill patients. Hemodynamic monitoring proves especially useful when the need for aggressive dialytic removal of sodium and water remains unclear. The estimation of pulmonary capillary wedge pressure before and during dialysis may assist in fluid removal during dialysis. It may also help one to determine appropriate therapy for hypotension.

We cannot yet determine the rate of recovery of renal function in patients with ARF. The inability to estimate renal blood flow and GFR accurately means that dialysis will frequently continue for an unnecessarily long period of time. Myers and Moran have suggested that a limitation on the number of dialyses, with their attendant risk of hypotension, would in some patients, hasten recovery from renal failure.[33]

In summary, prevention of ARF remains a high priority in the management of surgical patients. Although several promising interventions are undergoing evaluation, the most effective remains aggressive hemodynamic support. For patients who develop ARF, continuous modes of renal replacement therapy offer substantial advantages over conventional dialysis. Careful attention to the details of medical management may limit morbidity.

REFERENCES

1. Kasiske BL, Kjellstrand CM: Perioperative management of patients with chronic renal failure and postoperative acute renal failure. Urol Clin North Am 1983; 10:35–50.
2. Abreo K, Moorthy AV, Osborne M: Changing patterns and outcome of acute renal failure requiring hemodialysis. Arch Intern Med 1986; 146:1338–1341.
3. Lordon RE, Burton JR: Post-traumatic renal failure in military personnel in Southeast Asia: experience at Clark USAF Hospital, Republic of the Philippines. Am J Med 1972; 53:137–147.
4. Hou SH, Bushinsky DA, Wish JB, Cohen JJ, Harrington JT: Hospital-acquired renal insufficiency: a prospective study. Am J Med 1983; 74:243–248.
5. Conger JD: A controlled evaluation of prophylactic dialysis in post-traumatic acute renal failure. J Trauma 1975; 15:1056–1063.
6. Gillum DM, Dixon BS, Yanover MJ et al: The role of intensive dialysis in acute renal failure. Clin Nephrol 1986; 25:249–255.
7. Bellomo R, Boyce N: Continuous venovenous hemodiafiltration compared with conventional dialysis in critically ill patients with acute renal failure. ASAIO J 1993; 39:M794-M797.
8. Kruczynski K, Irvine-Bird K, Toffelmire EB, Morton AR: A comparison of continuous arteriovenous hemofiltration and intermittent hemodialysis in acute renal failure patients in the intensive care unit. ASAIO J 1993; 39:M778-M781.
9. Alarabi AA, Danielson BG, Wikstrom B: Continuous arteriovenous

hemodialysis: outcome in intensive care acute renal failure patients. Nephron 1993; 64:58–62.

10. Charlson ME, MacKenzie CR, Gold JP, Shires GT: Postoperative changes in serum creatinine: when do they occur and how much is important? Ann Surg 1989; 209:328–333.
11. Novis BK, Roizen MF, Aronson S, Thisted RA: Association of preoperative risk factors with postoperative acute renal failure. Anesth Analg 1994; 78:143–149.
12. Morris JA Jr, Mucha P Jr, Ross SE et al: Acute posttraumatic renal failure: a multicenter perspective. J Trauma 1991; 31:1584–1590.
13. Schmitt H, Riehl J, Boseila A et al: Acute renal failure following cardiac surgery: pre- and perioperative clinical features. Contrib Nephrol 1991; 93:98–104.
14. Groenveld ABJ, Tran DD, van der Meulen J et al: Acute renal failure in the medical intensive care unit: predisposing, complicating factors and outcome. Nephron 1991; 59:602–610.
15. Pascual E, Gómez-Arnau J, Pensado A et al: Incidence and risk factors of early acute renal failure in liver transplant patients. Transplant Proc 1993; 25:1837.
16. Gornick CC Jr, Kjellstrand CM: Acute renal failure complicating aortic aneurysm surgery. Nephron 1983; 35:145–157.
17. Gamulin Z, Forster A, Morel D et al: Effects of infrarenal aortic cross-clamping on renal hemodynamics in humans. Anesthesiology 1984; 61:394–399.
18. Gamulin Z, Forster A, Simonet F et al: Effects of renal sympathetic blockade on renal hemodynamics in patients undergoing major aortic abdominal surgery. Anesthesiology 1986; 65:688–692.
19. Crawford ES, Walker HS III, Salch SA, Normann NA: Graft replacement of aneurysm in descending thoracic aorta: results without bypass or shunting. Surgery 1981; 89:73–85.
20. Carlson DE, Karp RB, Kouchoukos NT: Surgical treatment of aneurysms of the descending thoracic aorta: an analysis of 85 patients. Ann Thorac Surg 1983; 35:58–69.
21. Najafi H, Javid H, Hunter J et al: Descending aortic aneurysmectomy without adjuncts to avoid ischemia. Ann Thorac Surg 1980; 30: 326–335.
22. Alpert RA, Roizen MF, Hamilton WK et al: Intraoperative urinary output does not predict postoperative renal function in patients undergoing abdominal aortic revascularization. Surgery 1984; 95: 707–711.
23. Sinicrope RA, Serra RM, Engle JE et al: Mortality of acute renal failure after rupture of abdominal aortic aneurysms. Am J Surg 1981; 141:240–242.
24. McMurray SD, Luft FC, Maxwell DR et al: Prevailing patterns and predictor variables in patients with acute tubular necrosis. Arch Intern Med 1978; 138:950–955.
25. Schrier RW: Acute renal failure. JAMA 1982; 247:2518–2525.
26. Spiegel DM, Ullian ME, Zerbe GO, Berl T: Determinants of survival and recovery in acute renal failure patients dialyzed in intensive-care units. Am J Nephrol 1991; 11:44–47.
27. Zaloga GP, Hughes SS: Oliguria in patients with normal renal function. Anesthesiology 1990; 72:598–602.
28. Tilney NL, Lazarus JM: Acute renal failure in surgical patients: causes, clinical patterns, and care. Surg Clin North Am 1983; 63: 357–377.

29. Wilkes BM, Mailloux LU: Acute renal failure: pathogenesis and prevention. Am J Med 1986; 80:1129–1136.
30. Sinsteden TD, O'Neil TJ, Hill S et al: The role of high-energy phosphate in norepinephrine-induced acute renal failure in the dog. Circ Res 1986; 49:93–104.
31. Ratcliffe PJ, Moonen CTW, Holloway PAH et al: Acute renal failure in hemorrhagic hypotension: cellular energetics and renal function. Kidney Int 1986; 30:355–360.
32. Brezis M, Rosen S, Silva P, Epstein FH: Renal ischemia: a new perspective. Kidney Int 1984; 26:375–383.
33. Myers BD, Moran SM: Hemodynamically mediated acute renal failure. N Engl J Med 1986; 314:97–105.
34. Wardle N: Acute renal failure in the 1980s: the importance of septic shock and of endotoxaemia. Nephron 1982; 30:193–200.
35. Cronin RE, Erickson AM, de Torrente A et al: Norepinephrine-induced acute renal failure: a reversible ischemic model of acute renal failure. Kidney Int 1978; 14:187–190.
36. Finn WF: Diagnosis and management of acute tubular necrosis. Med Clin North Am 1990; 74:873–891.
37. Cronin RE, de Torrente A, Miller PD et al: Pathogenic mechanisms in early norepinephrine-induced acute renal failure: functional and histological correlates of protection. Kidney Int 1978; 14:115–125.
38. Burke TJ, Cronin RE, Duchin KL et al: Ischemia and tubule obstruction during acute renal failure in dogs: mannitol in protection. Am J Physiol 1980; 238:F305-F314.
39. Patak RV, Fadem SZ, Lifschitz MD, Stein JH: Study of factors which modify the development of norepinephrine-induced acute renal failure in the dog. Kidney Int 1979; 15:227–237.
40. Hanley MJ, Davidson K: Prior mannitol and furosemide infusion in a model of ischemic acute renal failure. Am J Physiol 1981; 241:F556-F564.
41. Pass LJ, Eberhart RC, Brown JC et al: The effect of mannitol and dopamine on the renal response to thoracic aortic cross-clamping. J Thorac Cardiovasc Surg 1988; 95:608–612.
42. Henderson IS, Beattie TJ, Kennedy AC: Dopamine hydrochloride in oliguric states. Lancet 1980; 2:827–828.
43. Schwartz LB, Gewertz BL: The renal response to low dose dopamine. J Surg Res 1988; 45:574–588.
44. Kleinknecht D, Ganeval D, Gonzales-Duque LA, Fermanian J: Furosemide in acute oliguric renal failure: a controlled trial. Nephron 1976; 17:51–58.
45. Lindner A, Cutler RE, Goodman WG: Synergism of dopamine plus furosemide in preventing acute renal failure in the dog. Kidney Int 1979; 16:158–166.
46. Lindner A: Synergism of dopamine and furosemide in diuretic-resistant, oliguric acute renal failure. Nephron 1983; 33:121–126.
47. Brown CB, Ogg CS, Cameron JS: High dose furosemide in acute renal failure: a controlled trial. Clin Nephrol 1981; 15:90–96.
48. Dick M, Dasta J, Choban P et al: Urine output (UO) and serum aldosterone (ALDO) concentrations in oliguric ICU patients (PTS) receiving low dose dopamine. Crit Care Med 1993; 21:S177 (abstract).
49. Elliott WJ, Weber RR, Nelson KS et al: Renal and hemodynamic effects of intravenous fenoldopam versus nitroprusside in severe hypertension. Circulation 1990; 81:970–977.

50. Allison NL, Dubbs JW, Ziemniak JA et al: The effect of fenoldopam, a dopaminergic agonist, on renal hemodynamics. Clin Pharmacol Ther 1987; 41:282–288.
51. Murphy MB, McCoy CE, Weber RR et al: Augmentation of renal blood flow and sodium excretion in hypertensive patients during blood pressure reduction by intravenous administration of the dopamine-1 agonist, fenoldopam. Circulation 1987; 76:1312–1318.
52. Hughes JM, Ragsdale NV, Felder RA et al: Diuresis and natriuresis during continuous dopamine-1 receptor stimulation. Hypertension 1988; 11:I69-I74.
53. Nouwen EJ, Verstrepen WA, De Broe ME: Epidermal growth factor in acute renal failure. Ren Fail 1994; 16:49–60.
54. Pollock DM, Opgenorth TJ: Atrial natriuretic peptides in the treatment of acute renal failure. Ren Fail 1993; 15:439–449.
55. Badr KF: Novel mediators of sepsis-associated renal failure. Semin Nephrol 1994; 14:3–7.
56. Lake EW, Humes HD: Acute renal failure: directed therapy to enhanced renal tubular regeneration. Semin Nephrol 1994; 14:83–97.
57. Epstein M: Calcium antagonists and the kidney: future therapeutic perspectives. Am J Kidney Dis 1993; 21:16–25.
58. Eliahou HE, Ben-David A, Blau A: Recovery can be enhanced in acute renal failure of multisystem organ failure. Contrib Nephrol 1994; 106:59–62.
59. Agmon Y, Brezis M: Acute renal failure: a multifactorial syndrome. Contrib Nephrol 1993; 102:23–26.
60. Safirstein R: Gene expression in nephrotoxic and ischemic acute renal failure. J Am Soc Nephrol 1994; 4:1387–1395.
61. Humes HD: Potential molecular therapy for acute renal failure. Cleve Clin J Med 1993; 60:166–168.
62. Brezis M, Epstein FH: Cellular mechanisms of acute ischemic injury in the kidney. Annu Rev Med 1993; 44:27–37.
63. Goligorsky MS, Lieberthal W, Racusen L, Simon EE: Integrin receptors in renal tubular epithelium: new insights into pathophysiology of acute renal failure. Am J Physiol 1993; 264:F1-F8.
64. Vetterlein F, Petho A, Schmidt G: Distribution of capillary blood flow in rat kidney during postischemic renal failure. Am J Physiol 1986; 251:H510-H519.
65. Ratcliffe PJ, Endre ZH, Tange JD, Ledingham JGG: Ischaemic acute renal failure: why does it occur? Nephron 1989; 52:1–5.
66. Mason J, Torhorst J, Welsch J: Role of the medullary perfusion defect in the pathogenesis of ischemic renal failure. Kidney Int 1984; 26: 283–293.
67. Hirasawa H, Odaka M, Soeda K et al: Experimental and clinical study on ATP-MgCl2 administration for postischemic acute renal failure. Clin Exp Dial Apheresis 1983; 7:37–47.
68. Siegel NJ, Glazier WB, Chaudrey IH et al: Enhanced recovery from acute renal failure by the postischemic infusion of adenine nucleotides and magnesium chloride in rats. Kidney Int 1980; 17:338–349.
69. Zager RA, Gmur DJ, Bredl CR, Eng MJ: Degree and time sequence of hypothermic protection against experimental ischemic acute renal failure. Circ Res 1989; 65:1263–1269.
70. Wait RB, White G, Davis JH: Beneficial effects of verapamil on postischemic renal failure. Surgery 1983; 94:276–282.
71. Goldfarb D, Iaina A, Serban I et al: Beneficial effect of verapamil in

ischemic acute renal failure in the rat. Proc Soc Exp Biol Med 1983; 172:389–392.
72. Silverman M, Rose H, Puschett JB: Modification in proximal tubular function induced by nitrendipine in a rat model of acute ischemic renal failure. J Cardiovasc Pharmacol 1989; 14:799–802.
73. Russell JD, Churchill DN: Calcium antagonists and acute renal failure. Am J Med 1989; 87:306–315.
74. Leahy AL, Galla J, Fitzpatrick JM, Wait RB: The canine kidney in haemorrhagic shock: effect of verapamil. Eur Urol 1987; 13: 401–406.
75. Loutzenhiser RD, Epstein M: Renal hemodynamic effects of calcium antagonists. Am J Med 1987; 82:23–28.
76. Diamond JR, Cheung JY, Fang LST: Nifedipine-induced renal dysfunction: alterations in renal hemodynamics. Am J Med 1984; 77: 905–909.
77. Canavese C, Stratta P, Vercellone A: The case for oxygen free radicals in the pathogenesis of ischemic acute renal failure. Nephron 1988; 49:9–15.
78. Ratych RE, Bulkley GB: Free-radical-mediated postischemic reperfusion injury in the kidney. J Free Radicals Biol Med 1986; 2:311–319.
79. Mauk RH, Patak RV, Fadem SZ et al: Effect of prostaglandin E administration in a nephrotoxic and a vasoconstrictor model of acute renal failure. Kidney Int 1977; 12:122–130.
80. Mandal AK, Miller J: Protection against ischemic acute renal failure by prostaglandin infusion. Prostaglandins Leukot Med 1982; 8: 361–373.
81. Tobimatsu M, Konomi K, Saito S, Tsumagari T: Protective effect of prostaglandin E1 on ischemia-induced acute renal failure in dogs. Surgery 1985; 98:45–52.
82. Torsello G, Schror K, Szabo Z et al: Effects of prostaglandin E1 (PGE1) on experimental renal ishaemia. Eur J Vasc Surg 1989; 3: 5–13.
83. Lifschitz MD, Barnes JL: Prostaglandin I2 attenuates ischemic acute renal failure in the rat. Am J Physiol 1984; 247:F714-F717.
84. Klausner JM, Paterson IS, Goldman G et al: Postischemic renal injury is mediated by neutrophils and leukotrienes. Am J Physiol 1989; 256: F794-F802.
85. Lelcuk S, Alexander F, Kobzik L et al: Prostacyclin and thromboxane A2 moderate postischemic renal failure. Surgery 1985; 98:207–212.
86. Kaufman RP Jr, Klausner JM, Anner H et al: Inhibition of thromboxane (Tx) synthesis by free radical scavengers. J Trauma 1988; 28: 458–464.
87. Andrews PM, Bates SB: Dietary protein prior to renal ischemia dramatically affects postischemic kidney function. Kidney Int 1986; 30: 299–303.
88. Seguro AC, Shimizu MHM, Monteiro JL, Rocha AS: Effect of potassium depletion on ischemic renal failure. Nephron 1989; 51:350–354.
89. Bonventre JV: Mediators of ischemic renal injury. Annu Rev Med 1988; 39:531–544.
90. Corwin HL, Bonventre JV: Acute renal failure. Med Clin North Am 1986; 70:1037–1054.
91. Cronin RE: Drug therapy in the management of acute renal failure. Am J Med Sci 1986; 292:112–119.
92. Corwin HL, Bonventre JV: Acute renal failure in the intensive care unit. Part 2. Intensive Care Med 1988; 14:86–96.

93. Epstein FH, Brown RS: Acute renal failure: a collection of paradoxes. Hosp Pract 1988; 23:171–194.
94. Mandal AK, Lightfoot BO, Treat RC: Mechanisms of protection in acute renal failure. Circ Shock 1983; 11:245–253.
95. Lucas CE, Zito JG, Carter KM et al: Questionable value of furosemide in preventing renal failure. Surgery 1977; 82:314–320.
96. Oken DE: On the differential diagnosis of acute renal failure. Am J Med 1981; 71:916–920.
97. Pru C, Kjellstrand CM: The FE_{Na} test is of no prognostic value in acute renal failure. Nephron 1984; 36:20–23.
98. Diamond JR, Yoburn DC: Nonoliguric acute renal failure associated with a low fractional excretion of sodium. Ann Intern Med 1982; 96:597–600.
99. Prough DS, Zaloga GP: Monitoring renal function. Crit Care Clin 1988; 4:573–589.
100. Kellen M, Aronson S, Roizen MF et al: Predictive and diagnostic tests of renal failure: a review. Anesth Analg 1994; 78:134–142.
101. Shin B, Mackenzie CF, Helrich M: Creatinine clearance for early detection of posttraumatic renal dysfunction. Anesthesiology 1986; 64: 605–609.
102. Sladen RN, Endo E, Harrison T: Two-hour versus 22-hour creatinine clearance in critically ill patients. Anesthesiology 1987; 67: 1013–1016.
103. Kim K, Onesti G, Ramirez O et al: Creatinine clearance in renal disease: a reappraisal. Br Med J 1969; 4:11.
104. Bland RD, Shoemaker WC, Abraham E, Cobo JC: Hemodynamic and oxygen transport patterns in surviving and nonsurviving postoperative patients. Crit Care Med 1985; 13:85–90.
105. Bland RD, Shoemaker WC: Probability of survival as a prognostic and severity of illness score in critically ill surgical patients. Crit Care Med 1985; 13:91–95.
106. Shoemaker WC, Appel PL, Kram HB et al: Prospective trial of supranormal values of survivors as therapeutic goals in high-risk surgical patients. Chest 1988; 94:1176–1186.
107. Yu M, Levy MM, Smith P et al: Effect of maximizing oxygen delivery on morbidity and mortality rates in critically ill patients: a prospective, randomized, controlled study. Crit Care Med 1993; 21: 830–838.
108. Tuchschmidt J, Fried J, Astiz M, Rackow E: Elevation of cardiac output and oxygen delivery improves outcome in septic shock. Chest 1992; 102:216–220.
109. Honda N: Acute renal failure and rhabdomyolysis. Kidney Int 1983; 23:888–898.
110. Desjars P, Pinaud M, Potel G et al: A reappraisal of norepinephrine therapy in human septic shock. Crit Care Med 1987; 15:134–137.
111. Meadows D, Edwards JD, Wilkins RG, Nightingale P: Reversal of intractable septic shock with norepinephrine therapy. Crit Care Med 1988; 16:663–666.
112. Martin C, Papazian L, Perrin G et al: Norepinephrine or dopamine for the treatment of hyperdynamic septic shock? Chest 1993; 103: 1826–1831.
113. Schaer GL, Fink MP, Parrillo JE: Norepinephrine alone versus norepinephrine plus low-dose dopamine: enhanced renal blood flow with combination pressor therapy. Crit Care Med 1985; 13:492–496.
114. Ramamoorthy C, Rooney MW, Dries DJ, Mathru M: Aggressive hy-

dration during continuous positive-pressure ventilation restores atrial transmural pressure, plasma atrial natriuretic peptide concentrations, and renal function. Crit Care Med 1992; 20:1014–1019.
115. Andrivet P, Adnot S, Sanker S et al: Hormonal interactions and renal function during mechanical ventilation and ANF infusion in humans. J Appl Physiol 1991; 70:287–292.
116. Christensen G, Bugge JF, Ostensen J, Kiil F: Atrial natriuretic factor and renal sodium excretion during ventilation with PEEP in hypervolemic dogs. J Appl Physiol 1992; 72:993–997.
117. Rossaint R, Jörres D, Nienhaus M et al: Positive end-expiratory pressure reduces renal excretion without hormonal activation after volume expansion in dogs. Anesthesiology 1992; 77:700–708.
118. Prewitt RM, Matthay MA, Ghignone M: Hemodynamic management in the adult respiratory distress syndrome. Clin Chest Med 1983; 4: 251–268.
119. Miller SB, Anderson RJ: The kidney in acute respiratory failure. J Crit Care 1987; 2:45–48.
120. Frankel MC, Weinstein AM, Stenzel KH: Prognostic patterns in acute renal failure: the New York Hospital, 1981–1982. Clin Exp Dialysis Apheresis 1983; 7:145–167.
121. Bullock ML, Umen AJ, Finkelstein M, Keane WF: The assessment of risk factors in 462 patients with acute renal failure. Am J Kidney Dis 1985; 5:97–103.
122. Bell RC, Coalson JJ, Smith JD, Johanson WG Jr: Multiple organ system failure and infection in adult respiratory distress syndrome. Ann Intern Med 1983; 99:293–298.
123. Bartlett RH, Morris AH, Fairley HB et al: A prospective study of acute hypoxic respiratory failure. Chest 1986; 89:684–689.
124. Kraman S, Khan F, Patel S, Seriff N: Renal failure in the respiratory intensive care unit. Crit Care Med 1979; 7:263–266.
125. Montgomery AB, Stager MA, Carrico CJ, Hudson LD: Causes of mortality in patients with the adult respiratory distress syndrome. Am Rev Respir Dis 1985; 132:485–489.
126. Shin B, Mackenzie CF, McAslan TC et al: Postoperative renal failure in trauma patients. Anesthesiology 1979; 51:218–221.
127. Maseda J, Hilberman M, Derby GC et al: The renal effects of sodium nitroprusside in postoperative cardiac surgical patients. Anesthesiology 1981; 54:284–288.
128. Anderson RJ, Linas SL, Berns AS et al: Non-oliguric acute renal failure. N Engl J Med 1977; 296:1134–1138.
129. Moran SM, Myers BD: Pathophysiology of protracted acute renal failure in man. J Clin Invest 1985; 76:1440–1448.
130. Hilberman M, Derby GC, Spencer RJ, Stinson EB: Sequential pathophysiological changes characterizing the progression from renal dysfunction to acute renal failure following cardiac operation. J Thorac Cardiovasc Surg 1980; 79:838–844.
131. Hilberman M, Myers BD, Carrie BJ et al: Acute renal failure following cardiac surgery. J Thorac Cardiovasc Surgery 1979; 77:880–888.
132. Moran SM, Myers BD: Course of acute renal failure studied by a model of creatinine kinetics. Kidney Int 1985; 27:928–937.
133. Myers BD, Miller DC, Mehigan JT et al: Nature of the renal injury following total renal ischemia in man. J Clin Invest 1984; 73: 329–341.
134. Krasna MJ, Scott GE, Scholz PM et al: Postoperative enhancement

of urinary output in patients with acute renal failure using continuous furosemide therapy. Chest 1986; 89:294–295.
135. Epstein M, Schneider NS, Befeler B: Effect of intrarenal furosemide on renal function and intrarenal hemodynamics in acute renal failure. Am J Med 1975; 58:510–516.
136. Davenport A, Will EJ, Davidson AM: Improved cardiovascular stability during continuous modes of renal replacement therapy in critically ill patients with acute hepatic and renal failure. Crit Care Med 1993; 21:328–338.
137. Bellomo R, Tipping P, Boyce N: Continuous veno-venous hemofiltration with dialysis removes cytokines from the circulation of septic patients. Crit Care Med 1993; 21:522–526.
138. Monaghan R, Watters JM, Clancey SM et al: Uptake of glucose during continuous arteriovenous hemofiltration. Crit Care Med 1993; 21:1159–1163.
139. Pichette V, Leblanc M, Bonnardeaux A et al: High dialysate flow rate continuous arteriovenous hemodialysis: a new approach for the treatment of acute renal failure and tumor lysis syndrome. Am J Kidney Dis 1994; 23:591–596.
140. Bonnardeaux A, Pichette V, Ouimet D et al: Solute clearances with high dialysate flow rates and glucose absorption from the dialysate in continuous arteriovenous hemodialysis. Am J Kidney Dis 1992; 19:31–38.
141. Bellomo R, Boyce N: Acute continuous hemodiafiltration: a prospective study of 110 patients and a review of the literature. Am J Kidney Dis 1993; 21:508–518.
142. Prough DS, Adams PL, Hamilton RW: Complications of renal replacement therapy. In: Lumb PD, Bryan-Brown CW, eds: Complications in critical care medicine. Chicago, Year Book, 1988; pp. 145–160.
143. Gotloib L, Barzilay E, Shustak A, Lev A: Sequential hemofiltration in nonoliguric high capillary permeability pulmonary edema of severe sepsis: preliminary report. Crit Care Med 1984; 12:997–1000.
144. Nahman NS Jr, Middendorf DF: Continuous arteriovenous hemofiltration. Med Clin North Am 1990; 74:975–984.
145. Bernstein JM, Erk SD: Choice of antibiotics, pharmacokinetics, and dose adjustments in acute and chronic renal failure. Med Clin North Am 1990; 74:1059–1076.
146. Hastings PR, Skillman JJ, Bushnell LS, Silen W: Antacid titration in the prevention of acute gastrointestinal bleeding: a controlled, randomized trial of 100 critically ill patients. N Engl J Med 1978; 298: 1041–1045.
147. Borrero E, Bank S, Margolis I et al: Comparison of antacid and sucralfate in the prevention of gastrointestinal bleeding in patients who are critically ill. Am J Med 1985; 79:62–64.
148. Tryba M, Zevounou F, Torok M, Zenz M: Prevention of acute stress bleeding with sucralfate, antacids, or cimetidine: a controlled study with pirenzepine as a basic medication. Am J Med 1985; 79:55–61.
149. Priebe HJ, Skillman JJ, Bushnell LS et al: Antacid versus cimetidine in preventing acute gastrointestinal bleeding: a randomized trial in 75 critically ill patients. N Engl J Med 1980; 302:426–430.
150. Zinner MJ, Zuidema GD, Smith PL, Mignosa M: The prevention of upper gastrointestinal tract bleeding in patients in an intensive care unit. Surg Gynecol Obstet 1981; 153:214–220.

151. Tilney NL, Bailey GL, Morgan AP: Sequential system failure after rupture of abdominal aortic aneurysms: an unsolved problem in postoperative care. Ann Surg 1973; 178:117–122.
152. Fry DE, Pearlstein L, Fulton RL, Polk HC Jr: Multiple system organ failure. The role of uncontrolled infection. Arch Surg 1980; 115: 136–140.
153. Knaus WA, Draper EA, Wagner DP, Zimmerman JE: Prognosis in acute organ-system failure. Ann Surg 1985; 202:685–693.
154. Prough DS, Bauman LA: Protecting the kidney during vascular surgery. In: Kaplan JA, ed: Vascular anesthesia. New York, Churchill Livingstone, 1991; p. 522.
155. Badr KF, Ichikawa I: Prerenal failure: a deleterious shift from renal compensation to decompensation. N Engl J Med 1988; 319:623–629.
156. Prough DS, Foreman AS: Anesthesia and the renal system. In: Barash PG, Cullen BF, Stoelting RK, eds: Clinical anesthesia. Philadelphia, JB Lippincott, 1992; pp. 1125–1155.

CHAPTER 16

Postoperative Bleeding

Craig S. Kitchens

Case Reports

Case 1

A 36-year-old, post-traumatic paraplegic woman developed a huge decubitus ulcer over her right hip extending into the ischial region. The ulcer was infected. The patient had occasionally manifested signs of septicemia. Minor surgical approaches to the skin ulcer had proven futile. Accordingly, she was scheduled for a more aggressive and definitive surgical procedure. She had no history of bleeding despite minor procedures and the previous surgical attempts to correct the ulcer. Her preoperative complete blood count (CBC), prothrombin time (PT), partial thromboplastin time (PTT), thrombin time (TT), and platelet count were all normal.

The wound was aggressively debrided, followed by attempts to close the ulcer, which was accomplished without any evidence of hemostatic failure. Upon return to the recovery room she began to bleed excessively, but only from the operative site. There were no signs of bleeding from any of the vascular accesses nor was there any bloody drainage through the urinary catheter. Repeat coagulation studies were normal. Despite that, over the next 48 hours she received 64 units of packed red cells, 40 units of platelets, 19 units of fresh frozen plasma, and 20 units of cryoprecipitate. Hematology consultation was subsequently requested in order to find an alleged coagulopathy. Because of her clinical presentation, the hematologists suggested that her bleeding was from a structural site. She underwent reexploration of the wound without finding a site of bleeding. Following the second operation, she continued to bleed bright red blood. She then underwent arteriography, which disclosed a lacerated right internal pudendal artery. Embolization returned hemostasis to normal.

Case 2

A robust, 26-year-old Marine sought removal of four wisdom teeth. His hemostatic past history had been entirely normal. He had not experienced bruising, epistaxis, or other evidence of bleeding, despite his occupation. Four wisdom teeth were removed without difficulty with normal hemostasis, according to the oral surgeon. The patient was prescribed an aspirin-containing medicine. The following day he began bleeding from all four operative sites. His bleeding was enough to require multiple returns to the oral surgeon, who attempted to repack and resuture the surgical area, but to no avail. Hematology consultation was obtained. His CBC, platelet count, and PT were normal. His PTT was prolonged by 2 seconds. He vaguely recalled that his mother's brother had experienced excessive bleeding after prostate surgery. Evaluation of prolonged PTT indicated that the factor VIII coagulant level was 8% of normal. Accordingly, he was diagnosed as having mild hemophilia A, which was manifested at 26 years of age following a surgical procedure for which an aspirin-containing medicine was prescribed. His bleeding promptly ceased after the administration of factor VIII.

• *Most postoperative bleeding is surgical.*

Operative and postoperative hemostasis are of great concern for the surgeon and those taking care of such patients. Loss of hemostatic control obscures not only the operative field, making the mission of the surgical procedure more difficult, but also leads to blood loss, which, if severe enough, can result in decreased intravascular volume. Loss of hemostatic control may also potentiate other postoperative complications such as wound infection or failure to achieve desired cosmetic results. In modern medicine, only rarely does bleeding, in and of itself, lead to the death of a patient. Although operative and postoperative hemostasis is of concern, when viewed from the proper perspective, bleeding causes less morbidity and far less mortality than postoperative thrombosis.[1] The foregoing case reports illustrate important features of postoperative bleeding.

CLINICAL FEATURES

The two cases at the beginning of this chapter represent features of postoperative bleeding that are due to structural (surgical) defects (Case 1) or to hemostatic failure (Case 2). Clinical features that favor each situation are presented in Table 16–1. The vast majority (80 to 90%) of patients who experience postoperative bleeding do so because of structural defects.[2,3] These structural defects include failure to ligate vessels or unappreciated nicks or tears in adjacent vessels or organs. Most structural bleeding is associated with a bleeding site that is readily identified after the operator exposes and observes the operative area. These sites can be readily identified and individually approached with either ligature, cautery, or other surgical maneuver. Most structural bleeding comes from vessels that

Table 16–1.
Clinical Features of Hemorrhage

Clinical features favoring structural or technical defects
Bleeding from a single site while other candidate sites are not bleeding
Sudden onset of massive and/or rapid bleeding
Bright red or pulsatile bleeding from an identifiable source
Clinical features favoring hemostatic defect
Multiple simultaneous bleeding sites:
Surgical incision
Vascular access sites
Mucosal membranes
Skin
Hematuria
Hemoglobinuria or hemoglobinemia
Slow persistent ooze of blood from a nonidentifiable source
Delayed hemorrhage following adequate hemostasis

are large enough to be seen and range from major named vessels to small arterioles and occasionally venules. On the other hand, hemostatic failure is a microvascular (capillary) event. Failure of the hemostatic system, whether due to inadequate platelets or inadequate coagulation factors, is almost always associated with microvascular bleeding.[4] Accordingly, the operator is not readily able to identify a particular site and therefore cannot cauterize or ligate a vessel in patients who hemorrhage due to hematologic reasons. Rather, an entire surface may simply seem to ooze or weep blood without any clearly identifiable point of bleeding.

While patients with structural bleeding may dramatically bleed from a single site, other candidate bleeding sites, such as vascular access sites, urinary bladder, gums, or even other surgical sites (such as vein donation sites, stab wounds for chest tubes and like) do not bleed. Because bleeding is often arterial, the blood may be quite red in its appearance and bleeding may be brisk. Occasionally, it is even pulsatile. Such bleeding often is sudden and massive, as presented in Case 1.

Patients suffering hemostatic failure are more notorious for the slow persistence rather than their volume of bleeding. Bleeding may occur in all candidate sites and even uninvolved skin may show signs of hemostatic perturbations by the appearance of petechiae or ecchymosis. Such bleeding is quite troublesome. Several spectacular reports exist of surgeons having inadvertently operated on patients not known to be hemophiliacs.[5–8] Bleeding is often delayed, occurring after hemostasis was initially achieved. The explanation for this observation is that acute, major disruption of tissue during the surgical procedure generates thromboplastic forces (tissue factor) in quantities sufficient to serve hemostasis adequately for the first 6 to 36 hours. As these tissue thromboplastins cease further generation, hemostasis then must rely on the integrity of the clot. As the fibrinolytic system is then physiologically called into play, structurally imperfect clots weaken, and delayed postoperative bleeding begins.

Because postoperative bleeding may mean multiple things to different surgeons, even a working definition is difficult to establish. Several situations may be encountered. One is sudden, massive bleeding at the time of surgery due to inadvertent interruption of a major artery. Such bleeding is extremely brisk and alarming, but clearly does not involve hemostatic failure. Another example involves a surgeon who may state that the bleeding is much more profuse than he or she has previously experienced. The surgeon may cite hundreds of similar cases without such hemorrhage. Other situations involve true delayed postoperative bleeding, as represented in Case 2. Accordingly, evaluation of the patient should not be limited to "postoperative bleeding," but must take into account the nature, quantity, location, and timing of the hemorrhage. These are all important variables and have enormous diagnostic and therapeutic implications.

These differences notwithstanding, the prevalence of postoperative bleeding, as defined by many large series and reviews of series,[9–11] appears to be rather constant at approximately 2 to 4% of all operations. This seems intuitively correct as one would think that such events should fit a gaussian distribution. Data regarding mortality due to bleeding itself are not available, but clearly death is a rare event. When it does occur, it is nearly always associated with a structural lesion of a major vessel such as a ruptured aorta or an esophageal variceal hemorrhage.

Table 16–2 lists several conditions, including some not thought to be associated with excessive bleeding, some that may be associated with excessive bleeding, and others that clearly appear to be associated with excessive bleeding. Table 16–2 is not meant to be absolutely definitive, but serves as a guideline.

Heparin, administered in doses of 5000 U subcutaneously every

Table 16–2.
Factors that Affect Postoperative Hemorrhage

Do Not Affect
Low-dose heparin prophylaxis
Low-dose warfarin prophylaxis
Osler-Weber-Rendu syndrome
Mild thrombocytopenia ($\geq$ 60–80 K/mm^3)
Occasionally Affect
Aspirin or ketorolac administration
Adjusted-dose heparin prophylaxis
Poor metabolic/nutrition states*
Moderate thrombocytopenia (50–60 K/mm^3)
Frequently Affect
Ticlopidine
Platelet defects, especially with concomitant aspirin or ketorolac administration
Factor VIII or IX levels $<$ 30% of normal
Fibrinogen $<$ 60 mg/dl
Multiorgan failure
Severe thrombocytopenia ($\leq$ 40–80/mm^3)

* Prolonged use of glucocorticosteroids, malnutrition, inanition, bedridden state from chronic illness, septicemia, and chronic renal or hepatic failure

12 hours commencing 2 hours before surgery as prophylaxis against thrombosis (low-dose heparin), has been proved not to be associated with excessive bleeding.[11,12] Similarly, warfarin, administered in doses to maintain an international normalized ratio (INR) of 1.8 ± 0.2 is not associated with abnormal hemostasis in controlled studies, even with aggressive surgery.[9] Some underlying diseases associated with excessive bleeding are not associated with abnormal surgical hemostasis. These include vascular processes such as Ehlers-Danlos syndrome or Osler-Weber-Rendu syndrome (hereditary hemorrhagic telangiectasia). Mild thrombocytopenia (60,000 to 100,000/mm^3) is not thought, in and of itself, to be associated with abnormal surgical bleeding.[13]

• *Prophylactic low-dose heparin administration, even started preoperatively, does not contribute to postoperative bleeding.*

Situations possibly associated with abnormal bleeding include the perioperative administration of aspirin. Aspirin administration commonly occurs in patients with ischemic heart disease, including those who undergo coronary artery bypass grafting (CABG). In a double-blind study,[14] patients who underwent CABG and who had been on an aspirin regimen bled more than those who had not. These studies were reproduced in the Veterans Administration multicenter study.[15] Such bleeding, although statistically significant, is not of clinical significance in the average patient. Hypothermia during cardiopulmonary bypass surgery has also been associated with mild excessive bleeding. It appears to be acutely reversed by rewarming the patient. This event is associated with the release of new hemostatically competent platelets into the circulation.[16] Patients at very high risk for postoperative vein thrombosis and pulmonary embolus undergo effective prophylaxis with heparin, administered in doses larger than the usual 5000 U twice a day. Heparin in these patients is usually administered in doses sufficient to slightly prolong the PTT. While this dosage will effectively prevent thrombosis in these high-risk patients, the risk of hemorrhage may be slightly increased.[11] Similarly, patients who have platelet counts in the range of 50,000 to 60,000/mm^3 may be at slight extra risk during surgical procedures. Patients who are chronically and critically ill will have poor wound healing and excessive blood loss. These include bedridden patients, as well as those infected, malnourished, or on long-term glucocorticosteroid therapy.

• *Patients on heparin therapy and with platelet counts of less than 60,000 mm^3 may have an increased risk for postoperative bleeding.*

A variety of situations are associated with excess bleeding at the time of surgical procedures. Patients who receive ticlopidine, an antiplatelet agent,[17] and patients with significant acquired platelet defects, such as in uremia, frequently experience abnormal hemostasis. Aspirin administration is notoriously incriminated in patients who additionally have mild, subtle platelet defects or even von Willebrand's disease. These patients may make up as much as 1% of the population.[18,19] These patients have normal hemostasis in the absence of aspirin, but will bleed excessively following aspirin administration. Ketorolac is increasingly being implicated as a cause of such bleeding. Patients with multiorgan failure are also at risk, not only for hemostatic failure but development of acute gastrointestinal hemorrhage. This high incidence of abnormal hemostasis actually helps define the syndrome of multiorgan failure.[20]

• *Aspirin or ketorolac in patients with even mild or subtle platelet defects may cause excessive bleeding.*

EFFECTS OF SURGERY ON HEMOSTASIS

Surgery disrupts normal tissue and vascular planes placing enormous challenges on the hemostatic system.[9] Such trauma initiates the coagulation, fibrinolytic, kallikrein, and complement systems simultaneously.[21] When these multiple systems are called into play, the final clinical expression may be hemorrhage, thrombosis, or occasionally both. Particularly disruptive is trauma, especially trauma to the central nervous system.[22,23] Cardiopulmonary bypass surgery is associated with activation of platelets,[24,25] as well as with a transient acquired platelet dysfunction. Cardiopulmonary bypass also greatly increases circulating levels of endothelial-derived tissue plasminogen activator (tPA).[26–30] Attempts to pharmacologically negate these perturbations have led to the use of DDAVP (desmopressin; 1-desamino-8-D-arginine vasopressin), an agent that enhances the interaction of platelets and subendothelial tissues.[31] Despite its attractiveness, DDAVP, when administered prophylactically to unselected patients undergoing cardiopulmonary bypass, has not consistently caused a decrease in blood loss.[9] On the other hand, DDAVP administration does decrease blood loss in patients who experience excessive hemorrhage during cardiopulmonary bypass surgery.[14,32] Accordingly, DDAVP should not be advocated as prophylaxis, but used for those few patients who develop abnormal hemostasis following cardiopulmonary bypass. Others have used antifibrinolytic agents to negate the high levels of circulating endogenous tPA. One agent, aprotinin (Trasylol),[33] has been particularly useful. The use of aprotinin in unselected patients undergoing CABG has been consistently associated with dramatic decreases both in blood loss and in blood transfusion.[9] Aprotinin has also been equally hemostatically effective as a hemostatic agent during orthotopic liver transplantation.[9,34,35]

• *Abnormal hemostasis during or following cardiopulmonary bypass may be due to increased levels of endothelial-derived tissue plasminogen activator. DDAVP may enhance platelet function during such situations.*

Surgical procedures can be safely performed in patients known to have congenital hemostatic defects such as hemophilia A or B. This requires adequate accurate preoperative diagnosis, as well as aggressive replacement treatment therapy both pre- and postoperatively.[36,37] Although hemophilia is not the subject of this text, these patients should undergo aggressive or urgent surgery using the same operative indications as other patients without hemophilia enjoy. Such surgery now has an acceptable hemorrhagic morbidity (18%) and mortality (0.2%).[9]

ROLES OF LABORATORY TESTS AND HISTORY

It is perhaps the success of operations on patients with hemophilia that has led to a subliminal overreliance on hemostatic screening. In fact, most patients who suffer from classic, severe hemophilia A or B are diagnosed by both clinical and laboratory means during their first year of life. This is usually well before most operative procedures. Because these patients do have clearly abnormal screening tests (such as PTTs), the notion has developed that a prolonged PTT should similarly identify all patients who are subject to bleed, and conversely, normal preoperative screening tests should imply normal hemostasis at the time of surgery. However, such has not proved to be the case. There are several reasons why this notion is incorrect. These include:

• A prolonged PTT does not adequately serve as a screening test for abnormal postoperative bleeding.

1. The most notorious of hemostatic defects, namely, the hereditary deficiency of either factor VIII (hemophilia A) or factor IX (hemophilia B), are readily diagnosed because of the patients' lifelong pattern of bleeding. Because these diseases are already diagnosed, screening for hemostatic defects with the PTT is not necessary because the patients are already known to suffer hemophilia.
2. Since 80 to 90% of postoperative bleeding is not due to hemostatic failure, but is due to surgical and structural problems, preoperative screening cannot identify those who will suffer postoperative bleeding.
3. The sensitivity and specificity of hemostatic screening tests were designed primarily to detect severe hemophilia and related syndromes, and therefore are not well designed to detect milder defects.
4. Because many cases of intraoperative hemostatic failure are due to a suddenly acquired hemostatic abnormality, such as disseminated intravascular coagulation (DIC), septicemia, or transfusion mismatch, preoperative screening cannot detect those events prior to surgery.
5. The PT and PTT tests will result in abnormalities 2 to 3% of the time. The diseases intended to be screened, namely, undetected (mild or moderate) hemophilia A and B, have a prevalence of only 1:40,000. Therefore, the ratio of true positives to false positives with such tests is on the order of 1:1000.[38] Multiple studies have proven that hemostatic screening tests in patients without a previous history of abnormal hemostasis result in more false positives than true positives.

One review indicated that the positive predictive value of these tests (3%) is essentially the same as the bleeding prevalence (2%).[9] This means that the prevalence of not bleeding is 98%, precisely the negative predictive value of these tests. Accordingly, there is no rationale for performing screening tests for patients who have no history of bleeding. Persons with a history of post-traumatic or postoperative bleeding should be screened. On the other hand, patients who do have mild, undetected hemophilia (Case 2) do suffer extensive hemorrhage when they sustain trauma or undergo surgical procedures. Three papers have addressed the nature and clinical presentation of mild hemophilia not appreciated before the challenge of surgical procedures.[39–41] These reviews indicate that a history of abnormal hemostasis is still by far the rule rather than the exception. Twenty-five of 26 patients who had had dental extractions experienced abnormal bleeding following the procedure; 16 of 18 who had

• Patients without a history of bleeding do not require a screening test before surgery.

undergone tonsillectomies bled abnormally at operation. In fact, all patients who had had either a tonsillectomy or a dental extraction had bled abnormally following at least one of those procedures. Accordingly, the predictive value of routine screening tests is very high and very acceptable in those patients who have a history of abnormal bleeding. On the other hand, no battery of screening tests is more likely than the history to detect underlying hemostatic deficiencies.

The history of abnormal bleeding cannot consist of merely "Have you experienced abnormal bleeding?" Rather, the following questions comprise a more definitive approach:

1. Have you or has anyone in your family ever been labeled a "bleeder"?
2. Have you ever bled after surgery or childbirth? Negative responses are also important, namely those who have undergone several surgical procedures and have not bled are very unlikely to experience abnormal hemorrhage.
3. Have you ever had to be returned to an operating suite to control bleeding following a surgical procedure?
4. Are your menstrual periods excessive? How many pads or tampons are needed each day? Have your periods ever required iron supplementation?
5. Do you bruise excessively? Are these bruises multiple? Are these bruises ever palpable (i.e., are they true hematomas as opposed to ecchymoses)?
6. Have you ever had spontaneous nosebleeds?
7. Have you ever required transfusion of blood or blood products and, if so, why?
8. Have you developed hematomas as a result of trauma, accidents, athletic events, altercations, or other acts of physical violence?

EVALUATION

The evaluation of the postoperatively hemorrhaging patient requires an inquisitive and broad-based point of view. One must guard against jumping to conclusions and diagnoses. Although the vast majority of postoperative bleeding will be proven to be due to structural and technical problems, the evaluation must proceed with openmindedness.

One of the first actions requires a fresh sample of blood for a prompt TT, PT, PTT, and blood smear (Table 16–3). This should be the initial part of the consultation as these can be carried out by laboratory staff while the clinician performs the bedside evaluation. Of prime importance is a blood sample worthy of underpinning one's diagnostic thoughts and opinion. A poor sample frequently gives disinformation. Adequate evaluation *requires* fresh blood drawn from a fresh venipuncture. One of the most common causes of false abnormal tests from an intensive care unit (ICU) or recovery

Table 16–3.
Evaluation of Postoperative Hemorrhage

Obtain fresh venipuncture sample of blood for:
Thrombin time
Prothrombin time
Partial thromboplastin time
1:1 Mix with normal plasma of the above if any are abnormal
Blood smear for schistocytes
Signs of sepsis such as leftward shift, toxic granulation, or vacuolization of granulocytes
Note features of bleeding (see text)
Repeat directed history and physical examination
Review patient's chart:
Were liver and renal tests normal?
Were coagulation screening tests normal?
Was aspirin administered?
Is the patient septic?
Was the patient transfused? With what? When?
Was bovine thrombin used as hemostatic agent?
What surgical procedure was performed?
Was anesthesia time prolonged?
Note type and rate of bleeding
Estimate consequences of continued bleeding

room is an inadequate sample of blood which has been drawn through some type of vascular access line.[42] The heparin frequently used in such lines to prevent clotting will result in false-positive tests.[1,42,43] Ellis demonstrated that, when blood samples were carefully procured through a heparinized line in hemostatically normal patients, 52% of the PTTs were falsely abnormal, as were 44% of the PTs.[44] Of all patients, 68% had at least one falsely abnormal test. Additionally, among patients who had true abnormal tests due to either administration of heparin or warfarin, or congenital coagulopathies, when samples were drawn through an intravascular line, the test used for monitoring those patients was grossly abnormal, probably due to overanticoagulation with heparin or warfarin. This paper also examined attempts to neutralize the heparin in the sample with small amounts of protamine added to the blood specimen tube. While this action decreased the rate of false-abnormal results from 68 to 16%, the rate is still clinically unacceptable. Accordingly, I recommend that fresh samples be obtained from a new venipuncture.[42] Should the TT, PT, or PTT be prolonged, the sample should be retested following 1:1 mixture of the patient's plasma with normal plasma. This will distinguish between an inhibitor (failure to correct the test) and a deficiency state (total correction of the test). The sample can also be held by the laboratory for any further indicated tests.

- *Blood drawn through heparinized arterial lines, even if first cleared, is highly susceptible to inaccurate test results.*

Review of the blood smear may yield valuable information. The presence of schistocytes supports microangiopathic hemolysis, as may be seen in DIC. Toxic granulation with or without vacuolization of the polymorphonuclear leukocytes supports a diagnosis of septicemia. Platelet estimates can rapidly be made by examination of the smear.

While the laboratory examines the blood sample, the physician should again inquire of the patient, or family members, about any history of abnormal hemostasis. Frequently, this will result in positive responses to questions that were previously answered as negative in the initial, frequently more cursory, preoperative situation. Questions should include those mentioned in the section on history. A directed physical examination can assess evidence of bleeding as well as comorbid processes. Evidence of hemorrhage includes the presence of petechiae, ecchymoses, gum bleeding, hematuria, bleeding from vascular access sites, and bleeding at other operative sites. If bleeding develops from multiple incisions, a bleeding time is not indicated as this situation, by definition, indicates a long bleeding time. The physical examination should seek underlying disease. Signs of systemic illness such as liver disease might not have been appreciated by the original physicians. Findings include palmar erythema, jaundice, and vascular spiders. One must then determine whether aspirin or other antiplatelet agents had been administered before the operation. Review of the medical record should include liver and renal function tests. Despite the previous comments regarding preoperative screening coagulation tests, occasionally these tests have been ordered yielding overt abnormalities that were neither appreciated nor acted on.[45,46]

One should ascertain the number and type of transfusions administered during the operation. The possibility of transfusion mismatch with subsequent DIC is always present, especially when bleeding is profuse and free hemoglobin is present in urine and plasma. Septicemia frequently causes DIC and can follow operations for empyemas, abscesses, and obstructions. It is important to know what procedures were done and whether an abnormal length of time was required for the operation. Several cases of acquired antibodies against either thrombin or factor V following the administration of bovine thrombin as a hemostatic agent have now been described. This hemorrhagic condition occurs 1 to 2 weeks postoperatively and can cause significant systemic bleeding.[47,48]

• *Septicemia can often cause disseminated intravascular coagulation, particularly following operation for drainage of a septic site.*

As demonstrated by Case 1, the bleeding rate can aid in the differential diagnosis. Sudden, massive bleeding more typically develops because of surgical bleeding, rather than from a true hematologic defect. The tempo of the workup is often based on the consequence of the bleeding. A small amount of central nervous system bleeding may be much more worrisome than a large amount in the thigh. One must also estimate the consequences of the bleeding versus those of therapy.

The timing of bleeding in relation to the surgical procedure can aid in formation of the differential diagnosis (Table 16–4). Bleeding that occurs during the operation typically results from a structural lesion, DIC, inadvertent heparin overdosage, or hyperfibrinolysis. Bleeding that begins late in the operation or up to 24 hours later still represents most often a structural or technical problem. Bleeding due to thrombocytopenia and/or qualitative platelet disorders

• *Bleeding due to thrombocytopenia usually begins within the first 24 hours following surgery. If due to massive transfusion, it may develop during the operative procedure itself.*

Table 16–4.
Causes of Postoperative Hemorrhage

Intraoperative hemorrhage
Structural/technical defects
Disseminated intravascular coagulation
Heparin overdosage
Hyperfibrinolysis
Postoperative days 0 to 2
Structural/technical defects
Thrombocytopenia
Qualitative platelet disorders
Mild/moderate hereditary coagulative disorder
Delayed postoperative bleeding, days 2 to 7
Thrombocytopenia
Aspirin or ketorolac administration
Vitamin K deficiency
Multiorgan failure
Antibodies to factors II or V following use of bovine thrombin

most frequently occurs in the first 24 postoperative hours. Platelets are involved in the more immediate stages of hemostasis. Occasionally, mild to moderate hereditary coagulation problems also show up at this time.

Bleeding between postoperative days 2 and 7 may be due to sudden-onset thrombocytopenia. This can be seen in drug-induced thrombocytopenia. It is also the time of inadvertent aspirin or ketorolac administration.[36] The first postoperative week is also the time to manifest a vitamin K deficiency, particularly in poorly nourished or catabolic patients.[49] Multiorgan failure may occur at this time, and hemorrhage may be a major manifestation. Although rare, acquired antibodies to thrombin and/or factor V as a result of bovine thrombin use as a hemostatic agent may also occur at this time.[47,48]

• *Thrombocytopenia that appears 2 to 7 days following surgery may be drug-induced.*

The interpretation of laboratory tests has great importance. Concomitant abnormalities of the TT, PT, and PTT, especially when they fail to correct with 1:1 mixing with normal plasma, are extremely strong but circumstantial evidence for DIC. The prompt and total correction of a prolonged TT, PT, PTT, or any combination of these tests following the 1:1 mixture of the patient's plasma with normal plasma implies a deficiency of some coagulation factor or factors as seen in hemophilia, liver disease, or warfarin administration. On the other hand, failure to correct implies the presence of an inhibitor, most commonly heparin or fibrin degradation products. This suspicion can be quickly abetted by the presence of thrombocytopenia and hypofibrinogenemia. Severe, significant DIC is usually accompanied by platelet counts lower than 100,000/mm^3 and fibrinogen concentrations of less than 60 mg/dl.[50] Should DIC be implicated, survival depends upon correction of the underlying cause of DIC. Causes include sepsis, shock, multiple trauma, or the presence of dead or dying tissue, such as with a tumor, abruptio placentae, or placenta previa. A TT proportionately much more prolonged than the PTT and PT most commonly is associated with

• *Heparin will disproportionally prolong the TT compared to the PTT and PT.*

heparin. This can be a contaminant in the vascular access or as therapeutic agent. Accordingly, if heparin has been therapeutically administered one must ascertain that a mathematical error in dosage calculation has not occurred. This represents a frequent cause of significant heparin overdosage.

Other causes of a prolonged TT include severe hypofibrinogenemia (which can result from DIC, administration of thrombolytic agents, or severe liver disease) or the presence of fibrin degradation products. The presence of fibrin degradation products is synonymous with activation of the fibrinolytic system through DIC, pharmacologic agents, or endogenous release of tPA, as may happen with CABG or orthotopic liver transplantation.

- *An isolated prolonged PT usually represents liver disease or vitamin K deficiency.*

An isolated prolonged PT usually indicates previously unknown liver disease or vitamin K deficiency. Vitamin K deficiency develops in patients who have not eaten for several days preoperatively and are administered antibiotics. Approximately half of the required vitamin K is produced by normal gut flora. Catabolic events such as renal failure, burns, and extensive surgery accelerate vitamin K deficency.[49]

- *An isolated prolonged PTT may be due to heparin administration.*

An isolated abnormality of the PTT can frequently be explained by heparin administration, the presence of fibrin split products, liver disease, or, rarely, a previously unappreciated hemophilic state. The presence of liver disease can be defined by additional liver function tests. The inherited deficiency of factor VIII, IX, or XI is best inferred by the correction of the isolated abnormal PTT by 1:1 mix testing. If no liver disease exists, then analysis for specific levels of factors VIII, IX, and XI should be requested along with hematologic consultation.

Thrombocytopenia can be caused by a variety of conditions.[51] One of the more common includes unappreciated bone marrow failure. This can develop either because of nutritional anemias (vitamin B_{12} and folate deficiency), infiltrative processes (such as cancer, to include leukemia and lymphoma), or bone marrow aplasia. A verified platelet count below 50,000/mm^3 is probably significant and should result in hematologic consultation. A bone marrow examination may be indicated.

Other frequent causes of thrombocytopenia in the postoperative situation include DIC and drug-induced thrombocytopenia. Nearly all drugs are suspect; some of the more common being antibiotics, antiarrhythmics, diuretics, and, especially, heparin. If the patient has received heparin, or even if vascular access lines are flushed with heparin, thrombocytopenia can develop. All exposure to the heparin should cease.[52] Hematologic consultation should be undertaken. Thrombocytopenia is also an extremely sensitive marker of endotoxemia or other infectious processes.

When all the foregoing laboratory tests are negative, the evidence supports structural hemorrhage. At that time, reconsultation with surgical colleagues becomes mandatory in order to further explore those possibilities.

TREATMENT

During the initial evaluation and laboratory testing, careful use of volume expanders and red cell transfusion may be indicated for acute resuscitation (Table 16–5). If the initial evaluation shows that hematologic reasons are unlikely to account for the ensuing hemorrhage, surgical reexploration of the wound is highly recommended. This approach may be bolstered by preoperative studies such as angiography. Angiography can be therapeutic if embolization of the hemorrhaging artery is feasible. Reexploration of the wound usually documents a bleeding site and, once ligated or cauterized as deemed appropriate, promptly brings the hemorrhage to a close.

In the event that hematologic problems are thought to be causative, several treatment modalities are possible. Those which are not advocated are the unjudicial and blind "shotgun" use of hemostatic agents. The indiscriminate use of blood products, as portrayed in Case 1, illustrates this point. The injudicious use of platelet transfusion therapy,[13] fresh frozen plasma,[53] and red cells[54] has been repeatedly documented as too common and unwise. The use of fresh frozen plasma to correct, in a nonspecific manner, prolonged PT and PTT is also inappropriate.[55] One randomized, prospective, double-blind study documented that the prophylactic administration of platelet transfusions following massive ($\geq$ 12 units) red cell transfusions is not indicated.[56]

If a patient is thrombocytopenic, questions of etiology need to be addressed. Bone marrow examination may be indicated to differentiate states of low production versus increased destruction of platelets. In situations of increased destruction, platelet transfusion is not warranted. Rather, attention needs to be directed to drug-induced thrombocytopenia, with particular reference to heparin. Shortened survival of platelets may be due to septicemia and other causes of DIC. Platelet transfusions may be indicated in hemorrhaging patients with platelet counts less than 50,000/mm^3 and without evidence of increased destruction.

- *Massive bleeding in intra- and postoperative periods results in thrombocytopenia and depletion of factors V and VIII. Replacement therapy should be guided by the platelet count, as well as by PT and PTT. Cryoprecipitate contains more factor VIII than fresh frozen plasma.*

In DIC, the only known effective treatment is directed toward reduction, reversal, or elimination of the cause.[50] This involves treatment of sepsis, treatment of mismatched transfusion reactions,

Table 16–5.
Therapeutic Options in Postoperative Hemorrhage

Acute volume and red cell administration as indicated
Angiography with or without arterial embolization
Watchful waiting
Reexploration of bleeding site
Limited use of fresh frozen plasma, cryoprecipitate, and platelet transfusion, except for precise diagnoses and indications
Desmopressin (DDAVP)
Antifibrinolytic agents

reversal of shock, and other measures directed at reversal of the cause, rather than the symptoms or laboratory manifestations. Hyperfibrinolysis accounts for most abnormal bleeding associated with cardiopulmonary bypass and orthotopic liver transplantation. As previously mentioned, the role of antifibrinolytic agents, particularly aprotinin, is well documented. Aprotinin or other antifibrinolytic agents, such as epsilon-aminocaproic acid (EACA, Amicar), should be used only after consultation. In the face of adequate hepatic function and good perfusion, hyperfibrinolysis will often correct itself in 6 to 8 hours. A conservative stance should be taken on heparin overdosage. Mild overheparinization is best corrected simply by allowing it to clear, as it has a half-life of 50 to 60 minutes. In the rare cases of massive (i.e., 10- to 100-fold) heparin overdosage, protamine administration, although fraught with its own difficulties, may be indicated.

- *In most cases, heparin overdosage can be treated by simply letting the clotting abnormality self-correct over time.*

Qualitative platelet disorders are frequently encountered. The most common cause still appears to be the inadvertent or even surreptitious administration of aspirin or other antiplatelet agents. Rather than platelet transfusions, this malady best responds to DDAVP administration. DDAVP is also the treatment of choice for most cases of von Willebrand's disease. Vitamin K deficiency requires vitamin K_1 administration by a 30-minute intravenous infusion.[49,57] This method represents a cheaper, safer, more direct, and faster way than administration of fresh frozen plasma. It is far safer than the use of factor concentrates, which are not indicated and not approved for this usage. Vitamin K_1 administration in the face of adequate perfusion of a patient with normal liver function requires approximately 4 to 8 hours to completely correct either vitamin K deficiency or reversal of warfarin's effects. The correction of the abnormal coagulation tests following vitamin K administration also confirms the diagnosis.

- *DDAVP administration best corrects drug-induced platelet deficiencies.*

Multiorgan failure is a very difficult problem and its treatment is beyond the scope of this review. Patients who are identified to have congenital hemostatic defects, such as deficiency of factor VIII, IX, or XI, are best treated by aggressive replacement of the missing factors in concert with hematology consultation. Once those factors have been replaced to hemostatic levels, normal hemostasis promptly returns.

REFERENCES

1. Kitchens CS: Hypercoagulability and the pathophysiology of thrombosis in the critically ill patient In: Rippe JM, Irwin RS, Fink MP, Cerra FB, eds: Intensive care medicine, 3rd ed. Boston, Little, Brown, 1995.
2. Woodman RC, Harker LA: Bleeding complications associated with cardiopulmonary bypass. Blood 1990; 76:1680–1687.
3. Grant PJ, Prentice CR: Haemorrhagic and thromboembolic complications associated with surgery. Br Med Bull 1988; 44:453–474.
4. Kitchens CS: The anatomic basis of purpura. Prog Hemost Thromb 1980; 5:211–244.

5. Edmonds AR: Death from respiratory obstruction in haemophilia. Med J Aust 1951; 1:227–228.
6. MacDonald AC, Robson JB, Waapshaw: Haemophilia with respiratory obstruction. Br Med J 1953; 1:1144–1146.
7. Pappas AM, Barr JS, Salzman EW et al. The problem of unrecognized "mild hemophilia". JAMA 1964; 187:772–774.
8. Coy J, Bivins BA, Belin RP: Surgical procedures in unsuspected hemophilia. Arch Surg 1974; 109:835–836.
9. Kitchens CS: Surgery and hemostasis. In: Ratnoff OD, Forbes CD, eds: Disorders of hemostasis, 3rd ed. Orlando, FL, Grune & Stratton, 1995.
10. Collins R, Scrimgeour A, Yusuf S et al: Reduction in fatal pulmonary embolism and venous thrombosis by perioperative administration of subcutaneous heparin: overview of results of randomized trials in general, orthopedic, and urologic surgery. N Engl J Med 1988; 318: 1162–1173.
11. Levine MN, Hirsh J, Landefeld S, Raskob G: Hemorrhagic complications of anticoagulant treatment. Chest 1992; 102(suppl):352S-363S.
12. Clagett GP, Anderson FA Jr, Levine MN et al: Prevention of venous thromboembolism. Chest 1992; 102(suppl):391S-407S.
13. NIH Consensus Conference: Platelet transfusion therapy. JAMA 1987; 257:1777–1780.
14. Gratz I, Koehler J, Olsen D et al: The effect of desmopressin acetate on postoperative hemorrhage in patients receiving aspirin therapy before coronary artery bypass operations. J Thorac Cardiovasc Surg 1992; 104:1417–1422.
15. Sethi GK, Copeland JG, Goldman S et al: Implications of preoperative administration of aspirin in patients undergoing coronary artery bypass grafting: Department of Veterans Affairs Cooperative Study on Antiplatelet Therapy. J Am Coll Cardiol 1990; 15:15–20.
16. Khuri SF, Wolfe JA, Josa M et al: Hematologic changes during and after cardiopulmonary bypass and their relationship to the bleeding time and nonsurgical blood loss. J Thorac Cardiovasc Surg 1992; 104: 94–107.
17. Nevelsteen A, Mortelmans L, Van de Cruys A et al: Effect of ticlopidine on blood loss, platelet turnover and platelet deposition on prosthetic surfaces in patients undergoing aorto-femoral bypass grafting. Thromb Res 1991; 64:363–369.
18. Czapek EE, Deykin D, Salzman E et al: Intermediate syndrome of platelet dysfunction. Blood 1978; 52:103–113.
19. Werner EJ, Broxson EH, Tucker EL et al: Prevalence of von Willebrand disease in children: a multiethnic study. J Pediatr 1993; 123:893–898.
20. Bumaschny E, Doglio G, Pusajo J et al: Postoperative acute gastrointestinal tract hemorrhage and multiple-organ failure. Arch Surg 1988; 123:722–726.
21. Blomback M, Eklund J, Hellgren M et al: Blood coagulation and fibrinolytic factors as well as their inhibitors in trauma. Scand J Clin Lab Invest 1985; 178(suppl):15–23.
22. Goodnight SH, Kenoyer G, Rapaport SI et al: Defibrination after brain-tissue destruction: a serious complication of head injury. N Engl J Med 1974; 290:1043–1047.
23. Enderson GL, Chen JP, Robinson R et al: Fibrinolysis in multisystem trauma patients. J Trauma 1991; 31:1240–1246.
24. Harker L, Malpass TW, Branson HE et al: Mechanism of abnormal bleeding in patients undergoing cardiopulmonary bypass: acquired

transient platelet dysfunction associated with selective α-granule release. Blood 1980; 56:824–834.

25. Mammen EF, Koets MH, Washington BC et al: Hemostatic changes during cardiopulmonary bypass. Semin Thromb Hemost 1985; 11: 281–292.
26. Tanaka K, Tako M, Yada I et al: Alterations in coagulation and fibrinolysis associated with cardiopulmonary bypass during open heart surgery. J Cardiothor Anesth 1989; 3:181–188.
27. Lu H, Soria C, Commin P-L et al: Hemostasis in patients undergoing extracorporeal circulation: the effect of aprotinin (Trasylol). Thromb Haemost 1991; 66:633–637.
28. Paramo JA, Rifon J, Llorens R et al: Intra- and postoperative fibrinolysis in patients undergoing cardiopulmonary bypass surgery. Haemostasis 1991; 21:58–64.
29. Gram J, Janetzko T, Jespersen J et al: Enhanced effective fibrinolysis following neutralization of heparin in open heart surgery increases the risk of post-surgical bleeding. Thromb Haemost 1990; 63:241–245.
30. Holloway DS, Summaria L, Sandesara J et al: Decreased platelet number and function and increased fibrinolysis contribute to postoperative bleeding in cardiopulmonary bypass patients. Thromb Haemost 1988; 59:62–67.
31. Richardson CS, Robinson AG: Desmopressin. Ann Intern Med 1985; 103:228–239.
32. Czer LSC, Bateman TM, Gray RJ et al: Treatment of severe platelet dysfunction and hemorrhage after cardiopulmonary bypass: reduction in blood product usage with desmopressin. J Am Coll Cardiol 1987; 9:1139–1147.
33. Royston D: The serine antiprotease aprotinin (Trayslol): a novel approach to reducing postoperative bleeding. Blood Coagul Fibrinolysis 1009; 1:55–60.
34. Havel M, Owen AN, Simon P et al: Decreasing use of donated blood and reduction of bleeding after orthotopic heart transplantation by use of aprotinin. J Heart Lung Transplant 1992; 11:348–349.
35. Himmelreich G, Muser M, Neuhaus P et al: Different aprotinin applications influencing hemostatic changes in orthotopic liver transplantation. Transplantation 1992; 53:132–136.
36. Kitchens CS: Surgery in hemophilia and related disorders: a prospective study of 100 consecutive procedures. Medicine 1986; 65:34–45.
37. Kasper CK, Boylen AL, Ewing NP et al: Hematologic management of hemophilia after surgery. JAMA 1985; 253:1279–1283.
38. Clarke JR, Eisenberg JM: A theoretical assessment of the value of the PTT as a preoperative screening test in adults. Med Decis Making 1981; 1:40–43.
39. Aggeler PM, Hoag MS, Wallerstein RO et al: The mild hemophilias: occult deficiencies of AHG, PTC and PTA frequently responsible for unexpected surgical bleeding. Am J Med 1961; 30:84–94.
40. Bachmann F: Diagnostic approach to mild bleeding disorders. Semin Haematol 1980; 17:292–305.
41. Kitchens CS: Occult hemophilia. Johns Hopkins Med J 1980; 146: 255–259.
42. Kitchens CS: The prolonged partial thromboplastin time: a prospective study of 100 consecutive cases sent for consultation. Am J Hematol 1988; 27:38–45.
43. Czapek E: Iatrogenic prolonged PTT: a nondisease state. JAMA 1974; 227:1304.

44. Ellis RE: Coagulopathy screening in children with heparinized central venous catheters. Pediatrics 1993; 91:1147–1150.
45. Golub R, Cantu R, Sorrento JJ et al: Efficacy of preadmission testing in ambulatory surgical patients. Am J Surg 1992; 163:565–571.
46. Kaplan EB, Sheiner LB, Boeckmann AJ et al: The usefulness of preoperative laboratory screening. JAMA 1985; 253:3576–3581.
47. Spero JA: Bovine thrombin-induced inhibitor of factor V and bleeding risk in postoperative neurosurgical patients: report of three cases. J Neurosurg 1993; 78:817–820.
48. Rapaport SI, Zivelin A, Minow RA et al: Clinical significance of antibodies to bovine and human thrombin and factor V after surgical use of bovine thrombin. Am J Clin Pathol 1992; 97:84–91.
49. Alperin JB: Coagulopathy caused by vitamin K deficiency in critically ill, hospitalized patients. JAMA 1987; 258:1916–1919.
50. Mant MJ, King EG: Severe, acute disseminated intravascular coagulation: a reappraisal of its pathophysiology, clinical significance and therapy based on 47 patients. Am J Med 1979; 67:557–563.
51. Kitchens CS: Diagnostic aspects of the platelet count. Mil Med 1985; 150:555–558.
52. Markentin TE, Kelton JG: Heparin-induced thrombocytopenia. Prog Hemost Thromb 1991; 11:1–34.
53. NIH Consensus Conference: Fresh frozen plasma: indications and risks. JAMA 1985; 253:551–553.
54. NIH Consensus Conference: Perioperative red cell transfusion. JAMA 1988; 260:2700–2703.
55. Gazzard BG, Henderson JM, Williams R: The use of fresh frozen plasma or a concentrate of factor IX as replacement therapy before liver biopsy. Gut 1975; 16:621–625.
56. Reed RL, Heinbach DM, Counts RB et al: Prophylactic platelet administration during massive transfusion. Ann Surg 1986; 203:40–48.
57. Shetty HGM, Backhouse G, Bentley DP et al: Effective reversal of warfarin-induced excessive anticoagulation with low dose vitamin K. Thromb Haemost 1992; 67:13–15.

CHAPTER 17

Deep Vein Thrombosis—Pulmonary Embolism

Frederick R. Bode
R. Phillip Dellinger

Case Report

A 49-year-old, 80-kg woman had been in the intensive care unit (ICU) for 7 days following an aneurysm rupture and successful clipping. However, she had failed to awaken sufficiently from her semicomatose state and still required mechanical ventilatory support. She was arousable but did not follow commands. These changes were thought due to postoperative vasospasm. The chest radiograph on day 7 revealed the presence of a right lower lobe infiltrate. It was unclear if this represented a new pneumonia or aspiration syndrome. She was afebrile with a normal white blood cell count. Antibiotics had not been started.

Ventilatory support included the following: positive end-expiratory pressure (PEEP), 8 cm H_2O; pressure support, 15 cm H_2O; intermittent mandatory ventilation (IMV), 4/min; F_IO_2, 0.4. Blood gas values were: PO_2, 96 mm Hg; PCO_2, 39 mm Hg; pH, 7.38; pulse oximetry, 99%.

At 2:30 in the morning, the patient was turned so the sheets could be changed. The nursing staff noted an increase in the spontaneous respiratory rate to 36/min. The pulse oximeter decreased to 87%. Blood gases were analyzed, and simultaneously the F_IO_2 was increased to 100%. The increased F_IO_2 ultimately resulted in an oxygen saturation of 95%. The blood gas analysis revealed: PO_2, 66 mm Hg; PCO_2, 37 mm Hg, and pH 7.38. The chest radiograph showed no changes. Some distant wheezes were noted on chest auscultation. There was no change in size of the lower extremities, and no venous cords were present. A ventilation-perfusion (V/Q) scan was performed, which showed a low probability for pulmonary embolism. A flow Doppler study of the lower extremities was also normal.

INCIDENCE

Every postoperative patient enters the ICU at significant risk for acute deep venous thrombosis (DVT) and subsequent pulmonary thromboembolism (PE). The ICU patient should always be assessed for the risk of DVT. For years, we have known that 80% or more of patients with PE have thrombi that originate in the lower extremities.

Venous thromboembolism is difficult to diagnose and expensive to treat.[1] Clinical signs of DVT are often absent, and PE has many clinical pictures. Therefore, major efforts should be made to prevent these problems in high-risk groups. Adequate prophylaxis should be considered. The critically ill patient often has multiple risk factors for DVT. These are described in Table 17–1.[2,3] Less important factors, such as age over 50, obesity, cancer, and the use of estrogen-containing compounds, are additive.

Until recently, no reliable data existed about the frequency of DVT in an ICU patient.[4] We are now able to identify the patients at highest risk, such as those with hip surgery. Barnes and associates studied 78 patients with total hip or knee arthroplasty.[5] The preoperative prevalence and postoperative incidence of major DVT were 2.5% and 14.1% of patients, respectively, despite intensive mechanical and pharmacologic prophylaxis.

• *Thrombosis may occur with catheterization of the femoral or subclavian systems.*

A study by Trottier and colleagues found acute DVT in 25% of patients with femoral vein catheters.[6] Horattas and co-workers reviewed the literature on DVT of the upper extremity.[7] They found that in 28% of all subclavian catheterizations, venous thrombosis developed, often subclinically. In their series and in their literature review, the incidence of PE was 12%, and PE often occurred even during anticoagulant therapy.

Flinn and associates, in a prospective surveillance program of 361 major neurosurgical procedures in which the patients received

Table 17–1.
Risk Factors for Deep Vein Thrombosis

Trauma or surgery of pelvis or lower extremities
Indwelling vascular catheters
General anesthesia for more than 30 minutes
Right ventricular failure
Prolonged immobility
Hypercoagulable state

standard DVT prophylaxis, still found 17 cases of perioperative DVT (4.7%).[8]

In summary, this information from ICU and surgical reviews supports the concept that all seriously ill patients in an ICU are at high risk for the development of DVT and PE. Prophylaxis against venous thrombosis must be strongly considered in every ICU patient.

PREVENTION

In the awake and cooperative patient, there are general measures that help to avoid venous stasis. Patients should exercise their legs by repeatedly flexing their ankles and feet. These exercises empty the veins of the lower leg. The knees should also be frequently flexed and extended. These exercises should be explained to the patient before the period of extended immobility.

Properly fitted, carefully applied elastic stockings that provide graded compression from ankle to thigh decrease venous stasis and reduce the incidence of DVT.[9] Such stockings need not be custom-made and are safe and effective if properly fitted and applied preoperatively. Studies of their use have mainly involved patients undergoing major surgery. They are inexpensive and, in many situations in the ICU, may be the most cost-effective prophylactic measure.

There are precise guidelines on specific preventive therapy for venous thromboembolism. In 1986, the American College of Chest Physicians and the National Heart and Lung and Blood Institute first made recommendations at the National Conference on Antithrombotic Therapy.[10] These were updated in 1989 and most recently in 1992.[11] We summarize these recommendations pertinent to surgical critical care as follows:

1. No specific prophylaxis other than early ambulation is recommended for patients less than age 40, undergoing minor operation and having no other significant risk factors.
2. Aspirin is *not* recommended for prophylaxis in general surgery patients.
3. Elastic stockings, low-dose heparin given every 12 hours, or intermittent pneumatic compression should be used for patients over age 40 and moderate-risk general surgery patients undergoing major operations.
4. Use intermittent low-dose heparin or low-molecular-weight heparin in higher risk general surgery patients. If they are prone to wound hematomas, dextran or intermittent pneumatic compression would be good alternative choices.
5. In selected patients, intermittent pneumatic compression may be combined with low-dose heparin, low-molecular-weight heparin, or dextran.
6. Use perioperative warfarin for selected high-risk general surgery patients.

7. Warfarin, low-molecular-weight heparin, and heparin in adjusted doses are the most effective prophylaxis in patients undergoing total hip replacement. Warfarin and low-molecular-weight heparin may also be used for patients with hip fracture.
8. Use intermittent pneumatic compression in patients undergoing knee surgery.
9. Prophylactic inferior vena cava filters are recommended for high-risk orthopedic and multiple trauma patients in whom other forms of therapy would be contraindicated or ineffective.
10. Use intermittent pneumatic compression, warfarin, or low-molecular-weight heparin when feasible in multiple trauma patients.
11. Use intermittent pneumatic compression with or without elastic stockings in patients undergoing intracranial neurosurgery.
12. Adjusted-dose heparin or low-molecular-weight heparin is recommended for prophylaxis of paralyzed patients with acute spinal cord injury.
13. Low dose-heparin and low-molecular-weight heparin are effective in patients with ischemic stroke and lower extremity paralysis.
14. Warfarin, 1 mg daily, is recommended in patients with long-term indwelling central vein catheters to prevent axillary-subclavian venous thrombosis.

These proven prophylactic measures are still underused. Prophylaxis with adjusted-dose heparin should prolong the activated partial thromboplastin time to a value in the upper half of the normal range. Use moderate-dose warfarin, to prolong the prothrombin time to 1.2 to 1.5 times the control value. The World Health Organization introduced a system for international standardization of the prothrombin time, using a unit called the international normalized ratio (INR).[12] (This topic is further discussed in the section of this chapter on warfarin therapy.) For elective hip surgery, the recommended INR is 2.0 to 3.0.

Low-molecular-weight heparin (roughly 2000 to 7000 daltons) is also being evaluated for prophylaxis. It has been recently approved in the United States, and the results of an increasing number of clinical trials are encouraging.[11,13]

• *A newly admitted patient to the ICU should either have thrombosis prophylaxis continued or anticoagulation considered.*

For all new ICU admissions, we recommend that patients already on preventive measures be continued on the therapy previously started if the measure is appropriate for that patient. A coagulation profile which includes a complete blood count, partial thromboplastin time, prothrombin time, and a standardized bleeding time, should be assessed. If there has been no previous therapy, anticoagulation should be considered. Relative contradictions to anticoagulation include a history of abnormal bleeding, recent bleeding from a peptic ulcer or the esophagus, corticosteroid therapy, recent intraocular or intracranial bleeding, or recent pericarditis.

The anticipated therapeutic course should be assessed and appropriate prophylaxis considered. The reader should be aware of how routine prophylaxis is carried out in his or her ICU. What goes on in that unit is more important specifically than are general textbook guidelines. Orabella and associates studied this question in a prospective study of 96 consecutive patients.[14] These investigatores found that only 38% of patients received adequate prophylaxis for DVT and PE prevention.

DIAGNOSIS

Pulmonary embolism can at times be difficult to diagnose in critically ill ICU patients. However, the initial screening tests are straightforward and include arterial blood gases, chest roentgenogram, electrocardiogram, complete blood count, and stool and gastric occult blood (Hemoccult). In patients with new or worsening hypoxemia, the diagnosis of PE should move to the head of a list of differential diagnoses to explain deterioration of vital signs, coupled with increased dyspnea and worsened oxygenation in the absence of newly recognized atelectasis, pneumonia, pneumothorax, or endotracheal tube malposition. Moreover, evidence of an acute myocardial infarction or acute blood loss must be eliminated. The astute clinician always considers PE, although this disorder is more frequently seen in the autopsy room and missed in the clinical setting.

- *Pulmonary embolism should always be considered with new-onset or worsening hypoxemia. All other causes of hypoxemia must be eliminated.*

The most common presentation of PE consists of sudden-onset dyspnea, tachycardia, tachypnea, or low-grade fever (Table 17–2). Leeper and associates found dyspnea or tachypnea in 96% of their patients.[15] Absence of either finding argues strongly against PE. However, they may be very transient in appearance. Apprehension, cough, fatigue, and oppressive chest discomfort are other presenting complaints. The lung examination usually remains unremarkable; focal wheezing may be noted.[16] Pleuritic chest pain commonly develops following acute PE.[17]

- *Pulmonary embolism most often clinically presents with sudden onset of tachypnea, dyspnea, or tachycardia.*

Presenting symptoms of the syndrome of pulmonary infarction are dyspnea, hemoptysis, and pleuritic chest pain. This constellation of clinical features, although more specific, only develops in up to 25% of patients with PE.[15,18,19] Temperatures that exceed 39.0°C do not typically develop in patients with PE unless bacterial superinfection has complicated the pulmonary infarction. A pleural-based rub frequently appears early in the course of pulmonary infarction.

- *Hemoptysis and pleuritic chest pain often accompany pulmonary infarction. However, this is a rare occurrence in most patients.*

Table 17–2.
Signs and Symptoms of Pulmonary Embolism

Dyspnea
Substernal pain
Cyanosis
Hypotension
Right ventricular failure

Table 17–3.
Signs of Acute Cor Pulmonale

Right ventricular tap
Augmented split pulmonic closure sound
Right ventricular S_3 gallop
Distended neck veins
Pulsus paradoxus
Kussmaul's sign

Sudden syncope in a hospitalized patient should also alert the clinician to this diagnosis and will require differentiation from acute massive myocardial infarction. The signs of acute cor pulmonale associated with massive acute PE are listed in Table 17–3. Kussmaul's sign is paradoxic distention of the neck veins during inspiration. Signs of shock and sustained hypotension signify life-threatening PE.[20]

Acute cor pulmonale from massive PE must be differentiated from right ventricular infarction or acute cardiac tamponade. Patients with right ventricular infarction do not have intensified heart sounds. In fact, they may be muffled. Pericardial tamponade presents with a silent precordium and muffled heart sounds. Tachycardia and a narrow pulse pressure may also indicate tamponade.[21]

Benotti and Dalen have described subtle manifestations of PE in ICU patients:[22]

1. Spontaneously ventilating patients develop worsening arterial hypoxemia and respiratory alkalosis.
2. Patients with chronic lung disease and known carbon dioxide retention will have a reduction in arterial carbon dioxide values and persistent dyspnea and hypoxemia, despite bronchodilator therapy.
3. Unexplained fever, atelectasis, or pleural-based pulmonary infiltrate can occur.
4. A hemodynamically stable and monitored patient will have a sudden outset of pulmonary hypertension.
5. Sudden elevation of central venous pressure often develops.
6. Unexplained tachycardia and tachypnea are common.
7. A sedated patient who requires controlled mechanical ventilation will develop worsening hypoxemia, hypercapnia, and respiratory acidosis.

• *Signs of pulmonary embolism in the critically ill patient may include unexplained deterioration in pulmonary status and pulmonary hypertension.*

The critically ill patient does not usually present with the straightforward and classic history and physical findings of PE. However, the usual ICU-based monitors may demonstrate variable signs of PE. An unexplained increase in minute ventilation should prompt consideration of PE. Pulmonary embolism leads to an increase in dead space and causes a detectable fall in end-tidal (ET) carbon dioxide. $PaCO_2$ rises after extensive PE. In the paralyzed patient, who is unable to increase minute ventilation in response to increased dead space, there are other causes for a rising carbon dioxide but an elevated $PaCO_2$ should increase suspicion of a possible PE. Occasionally, a pulmonary artery catheter may demonstrate an elevation of right atrial, right ventricular, and pulmonary artery pressures. Cardiac output may fall. Whereas the normal relationship of end-diastolic pulmonary artery pressure and pulmonary artery occlusive pressure (PAOP) agrees within 5 mm Hg, a greater difference may suggest pulmonary artery obstruction due to PE. Echocardiographic findings typical of PE include a dilated, thin-walled, poorly contracting right ventricle. Also present is displacement of the interventricular septum to the left. All these findings are compatible with acute increases in pulmonary artery pressure.[23] Thus, the wealth of information available in the ICU setting may point to PE and provide the clinician with the confidence to proceed with more specific diagnostic studies.

With any of the foregoing suggestive findings, there are definitive diagnostic paths to follow. These are shown in Figure 17–1 and will be discussed in detail.

Some physicians may believe that a sudden change in clinical status in a patient that is "classic for PE" warrants proceeding directly to a full course of anticoagulant therapy. In some cases, we would agree if one more positive diagnostic study were added. This could be either a positive duplex scan confirming DVT or a high-probability V/Q scan. When manifestations suggestive of PE develop, several generalizations about the next steps can be made. Stein and colleagues published a most interesting finding.[24] On the basis of bedside examination, blood gas levels, chest radiograph, and electrocardiogram, if physicians were confident that PE was

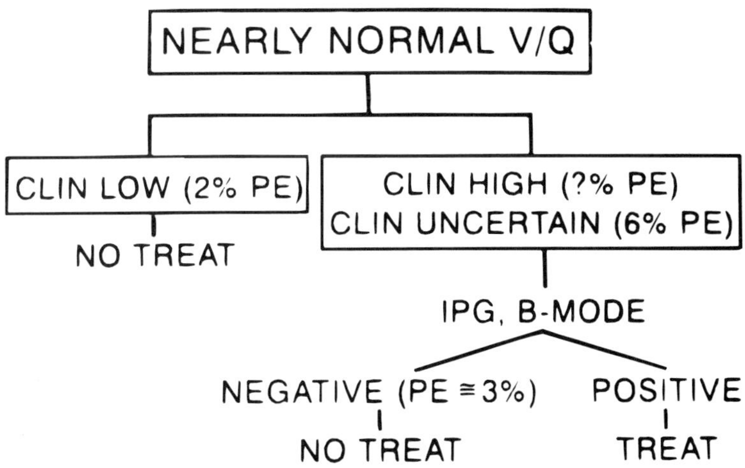

Figure 17–1.
Strategy for diagnosis of patients with a nearly normal ventilation-perfusion (V/Q) scan: algorithm for the patient with a normal or near-normal V/Q scan. Combined with a low clinical index of suspicion (left), no treatment is recommended. On the right, with a higher index of suspicion, no treatment is indicated unless additional noninvasive studies are positive. Clin, Clinical; IPG, impedance plethysmography; treat, treatment; B-mode, B-mode ultrasound. (From Stein PD, Hull RD, Saltzman HA et al: Strategy for diagnosis of patients with suspected acute pulmonary embolism. Chest 1993; 103:1553–1559.)

• Studies suggest that clinical data can rule out pulmonary embolism. However, the same data cannot confirm the diagnosis.

absent, they were correct 91% of the time. When they were confident that PE was present, this was confirmed correct in 68 to 78% of the patients. If they were uncertain, which was a large percentage of the time, PE was present in 30 to 58%.[24] These findings support the need for additional diagnostic tests.

• In patients with undiagnosed pulmonary embolism, the mortality rate approaches 30%.

Some clinicians may prefer no further diagnostic studies and simply hope that the clinical situation is not PE. This is risky and radical. Overall, 70% of PE go undiagnosed. It has been estimated that a 30% death rate exists from untreated PE compared to 8% in treated cases.[25] Critically ill patients are likely to have limited cardiopulmonary reserve, so PE may be particularly lethal. Have the resolve to pursue diagnostic studies, even in the complicated setting of the ICU.

Duplex Ultrasound

• If duplex ultrasound confirms deep vein thrombosis of the lower extremities, and if clinical signs and symptoms of pulmonary embolism are present, this is often sufficient to begin definitive therapy.

In the ICU, we believe that duplex ultrasound represents the diagnostic test of choice to detect DVT. It will not diagnose PE, but given a positive test in the clinical setting of PE, the physician may choose to then proceed with therapy since treatment of DVT also treats PE. Stein and Hull and associates introduced the concept that it may be sufficient to diagnose and treat DVT as an alternate to proving the presence of PE.[24] This approach may avoid hard-to-interpret tests, such as a V/Q scan in a patient with chronic obstructive lung disease or atelectasis. It may also avoid more invasive studies, such as the pulmonary angiogram.

At the Lahey Clinic in Boston, all patients who undergo major orthopedic surgery and surgical patients with multiple risk factors are entered into a well-established venous monitoring program.[26] The physician can then recommend therapy on the basis of a change in the results of the noninvasive study. Other authors have recommended that duplex ultrasound be done at regular intervals in the ICU to detect new DVT.[5,8]

Real-time ultrasonic evaluation of the deep veins is truly a revolutionary imaging modality.[27] The equipment can be moved to the bedside, and the study requires minimal patient cooperation. For patients who are confined in an ICU or who are restrained by orthopedic devices, bedside study is a major advantage. A lower extremity study costs significantly less than that of lower extremity venography, and takes only 15 to 30 minutes to perform a complete examination of both legs. In contrast to impedance plethysmography, this modality provides direct anatomic visualization of the venous system.[28]

The results of recent studies that have evaluated the diagnostic value of real-time ultrasound suggest that is has a very high sensitivity and specificity for proximal DVT. Lensing and associates reported a sensitivity of 100% and a specificity of 99%.[29] In their study, no patient had an inconclusive ultrasound study. Venography was found to be inconclusive in up to 22% of patients.[29] After all studies were pooled, the sensitivity of duplex ultrasound for proximal deep vein thrombi reached 95% and the specificity 99%.[28]

Table 17–4.
Duplex Ultrasound Characteristic of Deep Vein Thrombosis

Visualization of thrombi
Doppler absence of spontaneous flow
Absence of phasicity during respiration
Incompressibility of vein

Compressive duplex ultrasound images veins as nonechogenic structures, either in the longitudinal or the transverse plane. Duplex ultrasound refers to the combined use of high-resolution, high-frequency ultrasound transducers. The high-frequency transducers and pulse-gated Doppler technology permit assessment of the venous system. Table 17–4 lists the criteria for demonstration of DVT. Diagnosis of DVT requires assessment of all the factors, not isolation of one or two.

Vein compressibility has been heavily emphasized by some investigators. We caution against this. Assessment is difficult in the abdomen and pelvis. It is often not possible to compress veins because of overlying structures or bowel gas. Usually, in normal controls the superficial femoral vein cannot be compressed at its entry into the abductor canal.[30]

In a study by Killewich and colleagues,[31] the Doppler criteria, which included the absence of spontaneous flow and the phasicity of flow with respiration, remained the most reliable criteria for diagnosing DVT. The most effective use of the duplex scanner may be utilization of ultrasonography for vein location followed by Doppler determination of the presence of thrombosis.

Duplex ultrasound can differentiate acute and chronic thrombus formation. Fronek reported the differential criteria.[32] However, duplex ultrasound has a serious limitation in resolution of recurrent DVT. The changes are not readily separable from those associated with acute DVT. Therefore, it is recommended that follow-up baseline ultrasonography be performed 1 to 2 years after the diagnosis of acute DVT. This will identify those with completely resolved clot. Through follow-up studies, laboratories have now become more confident in their ability to differentiate between acute and chronic DVT.[26]

- *Duplex ultrasound usually diagnoses acute and chronic thrombosis formation, but not recurrent deep vein thrombosis.*

For above-the-knee veins, false-negative studies with duplex ultrasound are almost nonexistent. False-positive studies are extremely unusual, but calf veins are not adequately screened. Ultrasound has the ability to detect Baker's cysts and calf hematomas. Duplex scanning cannot readily detect common iliac thrombi. However, such thrombi are rare.[33]

Color flow imaging may improve the ability of duplex ultrasound to document recanalization in a nonoccluded thrombus. The Doppler signal from erythrocytes can generate a color image. Blood that moves toward the transducer has one color, and blood that moves in the opposite direction has a different color. Flow velocity determines color intensity.[34]

Duplex ultrasound more reliably detects proximal vein thrombosis than does impedance plethysmography. We think that this technique will supplant venography for the initial evaluation of suspected acute DVT. A European study suggested that contrast venography had moved from gold standard to "golden backup" in clinically suspected DVT. The authors recommended duplex ultrasound.[35]

Hillner and colleagues evaluated the optimal management of suspected lower extremity DVT with cost assessment of 24 management strategies.[36] Their analysis revealed that the optimal approach was to perform real-time ultrasonography followed by anticoagulation therapy if DVT is found. If the initial study was negative, serial studies saved additional lives but were costly. They concluded that venography should play a limited role in the contemporary evaluation of patients suspected to have DVT.

Perfusion-Ventilation Lung Scans

• *In critically ill patients, ventilation-perfusion scans may be limited to perfusion scans only. This results because of difficulty in performing xenon studies in intubated, ventilated patients.*

Pulmonary scanning was developed by Taplin and associates in the early 1960s and remains the best noninvasive means to establish or exclude the diagnosis of PE.[37] The perfusion lung scan characterizes the regional distribution of pulmonary arterial blood flow. Interpretation presumes that a number of abnormalities, including PE, can alter pulmonary blood flow and produce abnormal scans. The perfusion scan involves intravenous injection of small particulate aggregates of albumin or microspheres labeled with a suitable radionuclide (e.g., ^{99m}technetium). The distribution of the particles trapped in the pulmonary capillary bed reflects the relative distribution of pulmonary blood flow.

Ventilation scanning, often done with xenon, adds specificity to the perfusion scan, but does not increase sensitivity. It may be performed before or shortly after the perfusion scan.[38] We prefer the perfusion scan be done first. A normal scan nullifies the need for the ventilation study.

A perfusion scan that demonstrates subsegmental defects only or perfusion defect(s) with corresponding radiographic infiltrate(s) equal to or greater in size will not be further helped by the ventilation study. The patient will usually require pulmonary angiography.

The combination of a ventilation scan and perfusion scan presumes that an embolic vascular obstruction causes a perfusion defect without interruption of ventilation (i.e., V/Q mismatch). The alternative includes a ventilation defect smaller than the perfusion defect. Most other processes that cause perfusion defects also cause ventilation abnormalities These are likely equal to or larger than the perfusion defect.

The Prospective Investigation of Pulmonary Embolism Diagnosis (PIOPED) was a multicenter study of more than 900 patients. It attempted to clarify the role of ventilation and perfusion scanning in the diagnosis of PE (Table 17–5).[39] The sensitivity and specificity of V/Q scanning were determined by pulmonary arteriography. Scans were classified as normal or as indicating a high, intermediate,

Table 17–5.
Prospective Investigation of Pulmonary Embolism Diagnosis (PIOPED) Central Scan Interpretation Categories and Criteria

High probability
≥ 2 Large (> 75% of a segment) segmental perfusion defects without corresponding ventilation or roentgenographic abnormalities or substantially larger than either matching ventilation or chest roentgenogram abnormalities
≥ 2 Moderate segmental (≥ 25% and ≤ 75% of a segment) perfusion defects without matching ventilation or chest roentgenogram abnormalities and 1 large mismatched segmental defect
≥ 4 Moderate segmental perfusion defects without ventilation or chest roentgenogram abnormalities
Intermediate probability (indeterminate)
Not falling into normal, very low-, low-, or high-probability categories
Borderline high or borderline low
Difficult to categorize as low or high
Low probability
Nonsegmental perfusion defects (e.g., very small effusion causing blunting of the costophrenic angle, cardiomegaly, enlarged aorta, hila, and mediastinum, and elevated diaphragm)
Single moderate mismatched segmental perfusion defect with normal chest roentgenogram
Any perfusion defect with a substantially *larger* chest roentgenogram abnormality
Large or moderate segmental perfusion defects involving no more than 4 segments in 1 lung and no more than 3 segments in 1 lung region with *matching* ventilation defects either equal to or larger in size and chest roentgenogram either normal or with abnormalities substantially smaller than perfusion defects
> 3 Small segmental perfusion defects (< 25% of a segment) with a normal chest roentgenogram
Very low probability
≤ 3 Small segmental perfusion defects with a normal chest roentgenogram
Normal
No perfusion defects present
Perfusion outlines exactly the shape of the lungs as seen on the chest roentgenogram (hilar and aortic impressions may be seen; chest roentgenogram and/or ventilation study may be abnormal)

(From the PIOPED Investigators: value of the ventilation/perfusion scan in acute pulmonary embolism. JAMA 1990; 263:2753.)

low, or very low probability of PE. Most patients with acute PE had abnormal scans (i.e., high, intermediate, or low probability), but so did most patients without emboli. Thus, the sensitivity of the scan was high (98%), but the specificity was low (10%). Normal perfusion scans almost always indicated the absence of pulmonary emboli. Therefore, with high clinical suspicion but a normal perfusion scan, angiography will rarely be indicated. A high-probability scan was associated with PE in 88% of the cases in the PIOPED study. However, fewer than half of those with PE had high-probability scans (i.e., sensitivity, 41%; specificity, 97%). Thirty-three percent of those with intermediate-probability scans and 12% of those with low-probability scans had PE.[39]

• *A low-probability ventilation-perfusion scan rules out pulmonary embolism. Less than half of all patients with documented pulmonary embolism have high-probability scans.*

We need to reiterate what others have previously stated. A high-probability scan may be used as an indication to treat. An intermediate- or low-probability scan indicates a need for further studies.

What is the role of duplex ultrasound in the decision to proceed with pulmonary angiography? A positive duplex ultrasound is an indication for treatment. Some would use the low-probability scan to justify discontinuation of the workup. A negative duplex ultrasound study plus a low-probability V/Q scan supports close follow-up but no specific therapy. A negative duplex ultrasound and an intermediate-probability V/Q scan necessitates pulmonary arteriography. Pulmonary angiography should be performed when a V/Q scan is not practical (unavailable or patient too ill), is not likely to be helpful (adult respiratory distress syndrome, chronic obstructive pulmonary disease, asthma), or has not aided the physician (intermediate- or low-probability scan).

• *Despite other studies, an intermediate-probability ventilation-perfusion scan indicates the need for a pulmonary angiogram.*

Strategy for diagnosis of patients with suspected acute PE was presented by Stein and associates in 1993 (Figs. 17–1 to 17–3).[24] It is based on both the PIOPED and Canadian study groups. In this strategy, one third of patients still require pulmonary angiography. Stein and Hull and associates have proposed serial studies for proximal DVT for physicians who do not have access to pulmonary angiography when the patient has a V/Q scan that does not indicate a high probability of PE.[24] Further prospective studies are needed in this area.

The various strategies in the diagnostic management of PE require cost-effectiveness analysis.[40] At present, the definitive diagnos-

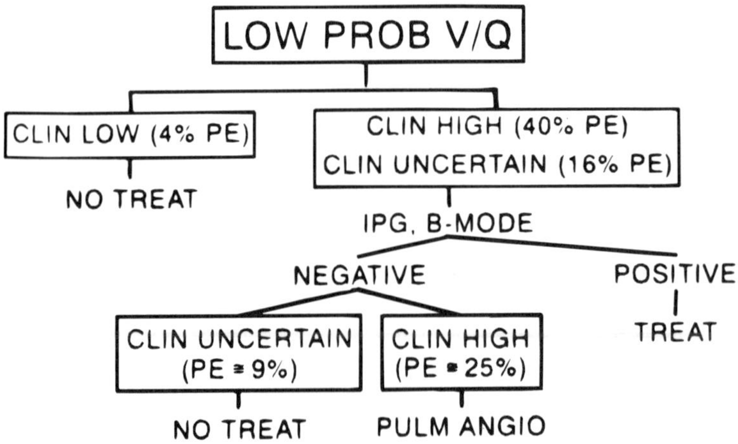

Figure 17–2.
Strategy for diagnosis of patients with a low-probability (prob) ventilation-perfusion (V/Q) scan: similar algorithm for the patient with a V/Q scan read as "low probability for pulmonary embolus." Only if your clinical suspicion is very low should you elect to stop the workup and not treat the patient (left). In all other instances, with a 16 to 40% chance that the patient has had a pulmonary embolism, further noninvasive studies or a pulmonary angiogram are indicated to confirm or more confidently to exclude the diagnosis. Pulm Angio, Pulmonary angiogram; Clin, clinical; IPG, impedance plethysmography; treat, treatment; B-mode, B-mode ultrasound. (From Stein PD, Hull RD, Saltzman HA et al: Strategy for diagnosis of patients with suspected acute pulmonary embolism. Chest 1993; 103:1553–1559.)

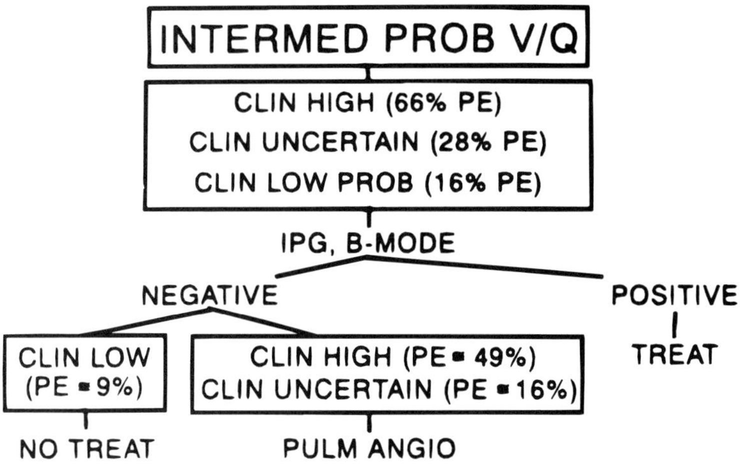

Figure 17–3.
Strategy for diagnosis of patients with an intermediate-probability (Intermed Prob) ventilation-perfusion (V/Q) scan: algorithm for the patient with an "intermediate probability for pulmonary embolus" as the interpretation of the V/Q scan. With a 16 to 66% possibility that this still represents a pulmonary embolism, further diagnostic studies are indicated. In contrast to the algorithm in the circumstance of low clinical suspicion and negative impedance plethysmography (IPG), we would still recommend angiography or at a minimum follow with serial IPGs.(From Stein PD, Hull RD, Saltzman HA et al: Strategy for diagnosis of patients with suspected acute pulmonary embolism. Chest 1993; 103:1553–1559.)

tic management strategy includes pulmonary angiography. Use of duplex ultrasound and perfusion ventilation lung scans can result in a 40 to 50% reduction in the number of patients who will require pulmonary angiography. This can be cost effective.

Pulmonary Angiogram

Pulmonary angiography is the gold standard for the diagnosis of PE. Table 17–6 lists the indications. This invasive test does have risks. Morbidity ranges from 1 to 4%. This includes arrhythmias, acute right-sided heart failure, and right ventricular perforation.[41] The mortality risk in experienced hands approximates 0.3%.[42] Safe-

- *All patients requiring pulmonary angiography should have a physician available at the bedside to monitor and treat as necessary.*

Table 17–6.
Indications for Pulmonary Angiography

Nondiagnostic ventilation-perfusion scan and noninvasive venous studies for deep vein thrombosis are nondiagnostic, especially in patients with preexisting cardiopulmonary disease
Patients at high risk for anticoagulation (e.g., recent stroke, bleeding disorders)
Anticipated thrombolytic therapy
Anticipated embolectomy
Anticipated inferior vena cava filter placement for recurrent pulmonary embolism

guards for a proper study include detailed precatheterization evaluation, oxygen administration, limitation of total contrast medium volume, and availability of complete emergency resuscitative capabilities.

Specific angiographic findings for PE include a filling defect and abrupt cut-off of a vessel. Oligemia, lower zone delayed filling, asymmetric filling, and prolonged arterial phase all suggest PE.[42,43] Cut-off of a vessel to a lung zone that appeared normal on the perfusion scan should raise the question of artifact.

Angiography must be properly performed. In many hospitals, pulmonary angiography consists of injection in the main pulmonary artery and films in the anteroposterior projection only. These studies can exclude large central emboli, but they are inadequate for the exclusion of most peripheral emboli.

• *In order to visualize successfully the clot in the pulmonary system, angiograms may require multiple films in various projections.*

Many investigators are concerned that small microemboli may cause false-negative arteriograms.[44,45] A lung scan has greater sensitivity and can detect these emboli.[46] A small number of false-negative angiograms have been reported in the National Cooperative and other studies.[47,48]

What happens to patients with a negative angiogram, but a clinical high suspicion of PE and high-possibility lung scan? Should these patients be treated anyway? These questions were addressed by Novelline and colleagues.[49] They studied 167 consecutive patients (minimum follow-up, 6 months) with suspected PE and negative angiograms. None of the 167 untreated patients died as a result of thromboembolic disease during this period. Twenty people died of unrelated causes. None of the 147 survivors suffered a recurrent embolism during the follow-up.

Patients with a high risk for complications during pulmonary angiography include those with recent myocardial infarction, arrhythmias, or severe pulmonary hypertension (right ventricular end-diastolic pressure > 20 mm Hg). However, the procedure can be performed even in patients with severe pulmonary hypertension.[50] Selective lobar or segmental injections can enhance the safety of pulmonary angiography.[51]

DVT Related To Central Vein Access

In 1958, an autopsy study of patients who had received femoral intravascular catheters revealed a DVT incidence of 46%.[52] A 1986 autopsy study demonstrated a 34% incidence of mural thrombi secondary to central venous catheterization.[48] Advances in DVT prophylaxis, catheter composition, and insertion technique have led to reevaluation of this issue. Clinical signs remain totally unreliable, but with duplex ultrasound, diagnosis improves. A study that utilized V/Q scans documented that PE occurred in 15% of patients with central lines who had an upper extremity positive venogram.[53]

Trottier and colleagues used duplex ultrasound and serial examinations to monitor prospectively for the development of DVT in 45 patients in a medical-surgical ICU who required central venous access.[6] None of the 21 patients with upper access sites developed DVT; 6 of 24 patients (25%) randomized to the femoral access site developed lower extremity DVT. Each patient had received standard DVT prophylaxis. In each case, the DVT was diagnosed at the time of catheter removal, and none had clinical evidence of DVT or PE. They concluded that the femoral vein remains an important emergency venous access route. However, because of the high risk, the physician should consider performing lower extremity duplex ultrasound upon removal of femoral vein catheters.

- *Femoral vein catheterization significantly increases the likelihood of development of deep vein thrombosis.*

Bern and associates found that, in cancer patients with central venous catheters, very low doses of warfarin, 1 mg per day, could prevent thrombosis.[54] Four of 42 patients on warfarin had venogram-proved thrombosis; 15 of 40 patients who did not receive warfarin had venogram-proved thrombosis.

THERAPY

Morbidity and mortality from PE are more closely related to cardiovascular compromise than to respiratory failure. Circulatory failure due to right heart ischemia (acute cor pulmonale) usually causes death that follows PE. Further embolic events and potential death from the current event dictate therapeutic choices and actions.

The primary goal of therapy is to prevent reembolization. The hypoxemia responds well to oxygen therapy. Following these supportive measures, we move directly to specific therapy. Unless there are contraindications, heparin should be initiated as soon as the diagnosis is seriously considered.

Vena Cava Filters

Table 17–7 lists the indications for vena cava filter placement. Placement of vena cava filters by interventional radiologists usually presents little difficulty and maintains caval patency.[55] Alexander and colleagues suggested that insertion of a vena cava filter should be considered before the second event in all patients with PE who have DVT of sufficient extent to be detected by noninvasive studies.[56] We recommend the consideration of filter placement, especially in patients with tenuous cardiopulmonary reserve.

- *Heparin therapy immediately exerts an antithrombotic effect. However, it has minimal effect on clots already present in the pulmonary circulation.*

Heparin

Heparin is the most efficacious therapy available because it exerts an immediate and sustained antithrombotic effect. Therapy should begin with an initial loading dose of 5000 to 10,000 U of heparin,

Table 17–7.
Indications for Vena Cava Filter Placement

Contraindication to anticoagulation
Hemorrhage following anticoagulation
Failure of anticoagulation to prevent recurrent pulmonary embolism
Prophylaxis for extremely high-risk patients

administered as a bolus. Thereafter, most patients require about 1000 U/hr. The exact effective dosage varies with the patient's weight and other factors. Heparin requirements are highest during the first 3 days of therapy. Circadian variations in the effect of heparin on the activated partial thromboplastin time, thrombin time, and factor Xa inhibition assay have been described. Maximal anticoagulation activity has been observed at night and minimal activity occurs in the morning.[57] The activated partial thromboplastin time best monitors the effects of heparin. The end-point prolongation should be 1.5 to 2.0 times the control value. Excellent results have also been obtained by utilization of the whole-blood activated coagulation time.[58] Following 7 to 10 days of heparin therapy and while in the general hospital, the patient is then switched to warfarin. We recommend that the patient remain on heparin while in the ICU.

Heparin action can be terminated almost immediately, if necessary, by the intravenous injection of protamine sulfate. The usual dosage is 1 mg of protamine for every 100 U of heparin. Protamine should be administered by slow intravenous injection over 1 to 3 minutes.

Table 17–8 lists the adverse reactions to protamine. They are more common in diabetic patients who have received protamine insulin and have developed antiprotamine antibodies.[59]

- *Heparin-induced thrombocytopenia may develop in as many as one third of all treated patients.*

Heparin-induced thrombocytopenia develops in 3 to 30% of patients. A complement-mediated mechanism may be responsible.[60,61] Thrombocytopenia occurs usually 2 days after therapy is begun and promptly reverses, often within a day, following drug discontinuation. The platelet count occasionally falls below 50,000/mm^3. Dangerous hemorrhagic and arterial thrombotic complications may develop. Platelet counts should be monitored daily. Heparin-dependent immune injury to endothelial cells may play a role in the thrombocytopenia and arterial thromboses.[62]

Hunter and associates described three surgical patients with the white clot syndrome, a complication of heparin-induced thrombocytopenia.[63] The syndrome is idiosyncratic, immune mediated, and not dose dependent. It is equally likely to occur with prophylactic and therapeutic heparin dosage regimens. Patients who have been exposed to heparin even through line flushes are at risk. Prior sensitization may result in the rapid onset of complications.

The thromboses consist mainly of platelets and a few red cells that have not become enmeshed within them by fibrin. These thromboses occur in up to 20% of patients with heparin-induced throm-

Table 17–8.
Adverse Reactions to Protamine

Rash
Urticaria
Bronchospasm
Pulmonary hypertension
Hypotension

bocytopenia and present life-threatening complications.[64] Thrombotic events include myocardial infarction, thrombotic stroke, and mesenteric thrombosis. Clots can also develop in the renal, adrenal, and spinal arteries. Since they are not associated with atherosclerotic lesions, such thrombi are frequently amenable to removal with an embolectomy catheter. If the anticoagulant indications remain, heparin should be discontinued and replaced by oral anticoagulation. Alternatively, low-molecular-weight heparin may be tried, but cross-reactions occur in one third of cases.

Rare, serious complications of heparin therapy include anaphylaxis, hyperkalemia, and vertebral fractures secondary to osteoporosis following prolonged administration. Necrosis of the skin and subcutaneous tissue has been attributed to the use of heparin and warfarin.[65,66] "Purple toe syndrome" follows cholesterol microembolization. Although it has been associated with the use of anticoagulants, it is usually caused by arterial invasive procedures.[67]

Heparin may elevate the serum aminotransferase levels. These tend to peak after 7 days and may decline despite continuous treatment.[68] Therapeutic advances include enoxaparin (Lovenox), the first low-molecular-weight heparin to become commercially available in the United States. This drug was recently approved by the Food and Drug Administration for use in the prevention of DVT. Five other low-molecular-weight heparin products have been marketed in Europe. These preparations have a potential advantage over intravenous standard heparin because they can be administered subcutaneously as a fixed dose once or twice daily without the need for partial thromboplastin time monitoring. In two representative studies, Prandoni and colleagues found that fixed-dose subcutaneous low-molecular-weight heparin was as effective as adjusted-dose intravenous heparin for the prevention of recurrent PE or the development of new PE in patients with DVT. There was no greater risk of bleeding.[69] Hull and colleagues, in a study reported in the *New England Journal of Medicine* in 1992, concluded that treatment of proximal vein thrombosis with low-molecular-weight heparin given once per day was as effective and safe as intravenous heparin therapy.[70]

• *When compared with standard heparin therapy, low-molecular-weight heparin administered intravenously at a standard dosage can adequately prevent recurrence or development of new pulmonary embolism.*

Low-molecular-weight heparin fragments have relatively more antifactor Xa activity than standard heparin, which could result in an increased antithrombotic effect. They cause less thrombin inactivation, less platelet inhibition, and less vascular permeability, all of which could lead to less bleeding.[13] Nurmohamed and associates reported a meta-analysis of studies done on low-molecular-weight heparin from 1984 to 1991.[71] They concluded that risks for DVT and PE were less using low-molecular-weight heparin than standard heparin. Risk reduction was greatest in patients having orthopedic hip surgery. The benefits in general surgery patients were less clear.[71]

• *Low-molecular-weight heparin more effectively reduces the risk of deep vein thrombosis and pulmonary embolism than does standard heparin.*

Warfarin

Warfarin causes the abnormal synthesis of a number of vitamin-K-dependent proteins, including coagulation factors II, VII, IX, and

X and proteins C and S. The drug does not act immediately, because time is required for the plasma clearance of normal factors already present. The time to maximal effect on all vitamin-K-dependent factors equals at least 4 to 5 days.[72,73] Protein C also has rapid clearance kinetics similar to factor VII.[74] This could cause a thrombotic tendency with a large loading dose. Warfarin should be administered without a loading dose or at no more than 10 mg daily on days 1 and 2.

The therapeutic range for the prothrombin time has been precisely defined for warfarin at 1.3 to 1.5 times the control value.[75–77] The prothrombin time performed with rabbit brain thromboplastin should be prolonged.

• *Maximum effect of warfarin therapy is not present until day 4 or 5. This drug should be started concurrently with heparin.*

Two well-controlled studies have shown that warfarin therapy can be started concurrently with heparin.[78,79] For critically ill postoperative patients with an increased bleeding risk, we hesitate to begin warfarin, because it is more difficult to quickly reverse its therapeutic effects.

• *Fresh frozen plasma and vitamin K promptly correct bleeding problems of patients receiving warfarin.*

A patient currently on warfarin may require prompt control of bleeding. Hemostatic concentrations of factors II, VII, IX, and X can usually be established by the rapid infusion of 500 to 600 ml of fresh frozen plasma, repeated every 6 hours. Vitamin K_1 can also be given, but it may not take effect for 24 hours. The usual dose is 10 mg. A period of resistance to warfarin develops after the administration of vitamin K_1. If fresh frozen plasma is administered, vitamin K_1 should be concurrently given with fresh frozen plasma.

Patients with continuing risk factors or recurrent DVT should be treated indefinitely. Symptomatic calf vein thrombosis should be treated with anticoagulation for 3 months.

Thrombolytic Therapy

Thrombolytic agents have become important in cardiology. However, no survival benefit has ever been demonstrated for thrombolytic treatment of venous thromboembolism.[80,81] More important, for postoperative patients a contraindication often exists to their use. Markel and colleagues prospectively studied patients with DVT documented by duplex scanning.[82] Only 15 (7%) of 209 patients with DVT exhibited no contraindications for thrombolytic treatment. Recent surgery was the most frequent factor that precluded therapy. It was present in 71 patients.

• *Thrombolytic therapy should be considered for patients with massive pulmonary embolism and hemodynamic compromise.*

The concept of thrombolytic agents that dissolve clots presents an attractive alternative to clinicians. The results and dangers of such therapy for PE must be weighed against the lungs' own intrinsic fibrinolytic mechanisms. The most striking advantage of thrombolytic agents appears to be in the setting of proved massive embolism and shock. In this situation, thrombolytic therapy is the therapy of choice.[83]

Table 17–9 lists the potential advantages of thrombolytic therapy over anticoagulation.[84,85] These potential benefits must be weighed against hemorrhagic complications, especially devastating intracranial hemorrhage.

Table 17–9.
Advantages of Thrombolytic Therapy over Anticoagulation

Removal of thrombotic source
Reduction of postphlebitic syndrome
More rapid restoration of circulation
Prevention of chronic pulmonary thromboembolism
Prevention of chronic pulmonary hypertension
More rapid clot lysis

Urokinase, streptokinase, and tissue plasminogen activator are all used to treat invasive venous thromboembolism.[85] Heparin should be discontinued before use of these agents. It can be restarted after completion of the thrombolytic agent infusion. Current ongoing studies will hopefully ultimately define the exact role for this promising therapeutic modality.

Pulmonary Embolectomy

Pulmonary embolectomy for acute massive PE is the last therapeutic option. Mattox and others reported a series of only 39 patients collected during 29 years.[86] These patients were in extremis. A successful outcome requires a prompt diagnosis and immediate availability of a portable cardiopulmonary bypass machine and operating room. With that equipment, obviously an expert surgical team must also be at hand. Preoperative angiography will better guide appropriate surgical management. In the Baylor series, angiography was performed in 57% of cases.[86] In another 10 patients suspected of having massive PE, angiography prevented unnecessary thoracotomy.

- *Pulmonary embolectomy rarely provides any benefit for patients with pulmonary embolism.*

Lund and associates reported excellent results with a more routine use of embolectomy in all patients with large PE, regardless of hemodynamic stability.[87] However, most physicians still consider surgical embolectomy a procedure only for patients with proven massive PE who are hemodynamically unstable and with contraindications for thrombolytic therapy.

Fluids and Inotropic-Vasoactive Drugs

Suggested methods to support the hemodynamic status of these patients have generated controversy. Volume administration to improve pulmonary blood flow may have a detrimental effect on hemodynamics.[88] We believe that volume administration should only be used when the patient clearly demonstrates hypovolemic symptoms. Fluid management should be guided by right ventricular pressures and changes noted by echocardiography.

Vasoconstrictor therapy assumes that right ventricular ischemia is the fundamental problem. Vasopressors will increase coronary arterial blood flow. Norepinephrine, infused at a rate sufficient to achieve a response, can be a good first choice. In animal models of sublethal PE, norepinephrine was superior to no therapy, to volume administration and to isoproterenol.[89]

• *Inotropic agents rather than fluids are usually more effective to improve hemodynamic instability in patients with pulmonary embolism.*

Inotropes such as dopamine and dobutamine can improve right ventricular function in some patients with pulmonary emboli and hypotension. Unfortunately, these agents also increase myocardial oxygen demand. Vasodilators have also been considered, but they risk reduction of systemic vascular resistance as well.

SPECIAL CONSIDERATIONS

A history of recurrent venous thromboembolism, particularly venous thrombosis in unusual sites, prompts consideration of an occult malignancy. Moreoever, deficiencies of thrombin inhibitors may lead to a so-called hypercoagulable state.

Several circulating proteins function as inhibitors of thrombin and other coagulation factors. The most important is antithrombin III. Proteins C and S are naturally occurring anticoagulant proteins that are vitamin K dependent. Deficiencies of either protein can result in venous thrombosis.[90] Antibodies to certain phospholipids important to the coagulation cascade were first described in association with systemic lupus erythematosus (i.e., lupus anticoagulant).[91] These antibodies can exist in other disease states and in normal individuals.[92]

• *Patients with recurrent thromboembolism following discontinuation of anticoagulation therapy should be studied for occult malignancy.*

When should the physician screen for the hypercoagulable state? A history of recurrent venous thromboembolism after discontinuation of antithrombotic therapy requires further laboratory studies. Usually, the routine studies can identify those with leukemia, connective tissue, or inflammatory diseases. It is probably warranted to evaluate a sample of unanticoagulated blood for antithrombin activity, protein C and S activity, and the presence of antiphospholipid antibodies. This is especially true for women with a history of recurrent spontaneous abortions.

DVT and PE occur during pregnancy and present unique challenges. Radiation exposure for the fetus is the most obvious. Duplex ultrasound can still be utilized. Impedance plethysmography is less useful as pregnancy advances due to mechanical compression of the inferior vena cava by the enlarged uterus. Serial impedance plethysmography has been studied in pregnant patients with clinically suspected DVT.[93] Anticoagulant therapy was withheld in 139 patients with negative serial impedance plethysmography, and the patients followed long term. None of the 139 had symptomatic PE or recurrent DVT.

V/Q scans pose little risk to the fetus. Risk from a missed diagnosis overshadows the minimally increased radiation exposure.[94] To reduce radiation exposure in pregnant women who required a V/Q lung scan, the Ontario physicians used only 1 mCi instead of the usual 3 mCi.[95]

• *Warfarin crosses the placenta and should not be used for deep vein thrombosis during pregnancy.*

Anticoagulant therapy during pregnancy poses special problems. Warfarin crosses the placenta and should not be used.[96] Adjusted-dose heparin therapy is probably the preferred method of therapy.

Heparin does not cross the placenta and may offer other advantages. A retrospective study of heparin therapy in 77 women involving 98 pregnancies complicated by venous thromboembolism found that the rates of abortion, stillbirth, prematurity, neonatal death, and congenital abnormalities were similar to those in the general population. There were two bleeding episodes and no instances of thrombosis.[95]

Management of isolated deep calf vein thrombosis remains an area of controversy.[97] Usually, these thrombi present low embolic risk unless they propagate into the deep veins of the thigh. Symptomatic isolated calf vein thrombi are more likely to propagate proximally and embolize. These patients usually benefit from 3 months of oral anticoagulation.[98] Patients with asymptomatic calf vein thrombi can be anticoagulated or followed with a noninvasive leg test to identify the subgroup who do develop proximal vein thrombosis.

There are two situations of DVT that may require more than heparin therapy. The first is total iliofemoral occlusion of the left lower extremity. This may develop because the left common iliac vein is vulnerable to occluding pressure from the right iliac artery. Currently used approaches include emergency thrombectomy and low-dose thrombolytic therapy. Even with timely treatment, the patient often develops chronic venous occlusive disease. Half of the time the outcome includes development of the postphlebitic syndrome. Infection is common and requires vigorous antimicrobial therapy.[99]

The second problem is DVT discovered before or after major pulmonary thromboembolism in a patient with a cerebral neoplasm. The patient should be considered for placement of an inferior vena caval filter to prevent recurrence. However, Olin and colleagues treated half of a series of patients who had primary and metastatic brain tumors as well as DVT and PE with anticoagulants.[100] Only 2 of 24 anticoagulated patients had complications. These investigators concluded that patients who received anticoagulant therapy had no more significant central nervous system bleeding complications when compared to those who received Greenfield filters. Overall survival was identical in both groups.

• *Some studies suggest that anticoagulation therapy can be successfully instituted in patients with primary and metastatic brain tumors.*

Low-dose subcutaneous heparin has been used in the prevention of DVT and PE following acute stroke.[101] There was no increase in the number of hemorrhagic strokes.

Hyperalgesic pseudothrombophlebitis, a syndrome described in the AIDS patient, can closely mimic DVT.[102] Characteristics include pain and swelling of the lower extremity, associated with overlying erythema. Most often, this syndrome occurs in association with Kaposi's sarcoma. Phlebography is negative. The pathogenesis is unknown, but an association with humoral substances (e.g., bradykinin) has been postulated. Other conditions that mimic DVT include rupture of calf muscle fibers (e.g., in middle-aged athletes) and dissection or rupture of popliteal synovial cysts (e.g., knee arthropathy).[103]

FUTURE CONSIDERATIONS

Acute DVT should be prevented before it occurs or diagnosed and treated before PE develops. The axiom "prevention is better than cure" could not be truer than in the arena of DVT.

There remains the quest for better diagnostic studies. Duplex ultrasound has supplanted venography for DVT diagnosis. However, a substitute for pulmonary angiography has not yet been established. Novel tests, such as the measurement of free plasma DNA in patients with PE, are currently undergoing investigation.[104] Computed tomography has been investigated for the diagnosis of chronic PE.[105] The application of single photon emission computed tomography (SPECT) represents another promising development.[106]

Detection of DVT by magnetic resonance imaging (MRI) was reported by Spritzer and associates.[107] A prospective clinical experience in 216 consecutive patients concluded that MRI, which used gradient-recalled sonographic acquisition, can accurately diagnose acute DVT. MRI was 97% sensitive, 95% specific, and 96% accurate.

Thrombolytic therapy continues to undergo active investigation. In addition to previously cited references, Kessler reviewed the pharmacology of numerous thrombolytic agents and their clinical use in research studies intended to determine the safest and most efficacious regimens.[108]

Becker and associates reviewed the indications, safety, and effectiveness of inferior vena cava filters.[109] These investigators concluded that many questions remain about this method of PE prevention.

There remains much to learn about current and new diagnostic tests and strategies for DVT and PE. We need to know more about noninvasive, cost-effective tests for DVT that are applicable especially to calf thrombosis, as well as to chronic and recurrent DVT. We need to know more about the natural history and treatment of PE. The challenges for meaningful progress with DVT and PE prevention and treatment will persist for some time to come. However, with perseverance we will continue to improve our therapies and preventive measures for this devastating disease.

REFERENCES

1. Weinmann EE, Saleman EW: Deep vein thrombosis. N Engl J Med 1994; 331:1630–1641.
2. Coon WW: Venous thromboembolism: prevalence, risk factors and prevention. Clin Chest Med 1984; 5:391–401.
3. Coon WW: Risk factors in pulmonary embolism. Surg Gynecol Obstet 1976; 143:385–390.
4. Geerts WH, Code KI, Jay RM et al: A prospective study of thromboembolism after major trauma. N Engl J Med 1994; 331:1601–1606.
5. Barnes RW, Nix ML, Barnes CL et al: Perioperative asymptomatic venous thrombosis: role of duplex scanning versus venography. J Vasc Surg 1989; 9:251–260.

6. Trottier SJ, Hyers T, Auer AI et al: Femoral deep vein thrombosis associated with central venous catheterizations. Crit Care Med, in press.
7. Horattas MC, Wright DJ, Fenton AH: Changing concepts of deep venous thrombosis of the upper extremity: report of a series and reveiw of literature. Surgery 1988; 104:561–567.
8. Flinn WR, Sandager GP, Cerullo LJ et al: Duplex venous scanning for the prospective surveillance of perioperative venous thrombosis. Arch Surg 1989; 124:901–905.
9. Holford CP: Graded compression for preventing DVT. Br Med J 1976; 2:969–970.
10. Dalen JE, Hirsch J (co-chairmen): American College of Chest Physicians and the N.H.L.B.I. National Conference on Antithrombotic Therapy. Chest 1986; 89(suppl):1s.
11. Clagett GP, Anderson FA, Levine MN et al: Prevention of venous thromboembolism. 1992; 102:391S-407S.
12. Poller L: Therapeutic ranges in anticoagulant administration. Br Med J 1985; 290:1683–1686.
13. Enoxaparin: a low-molecular-weight heparin. Med Lett 1993; 35(903):75–76.
14. Orabella C, Mehra MR, Bode FR: A prospective study of DVT/PE prophylaxis in a community teaching hospital's medical intensive care unit (abstract). Paper presented at 1992 Ohio Chapter of American College of Physicians, Columbus, Ohio.
15. Leeper KV, Popovich J, Adams D, Stein PD: Clinical menifestations of acute PE: Henry Ford Hospital experience, a 5-year review. Henry Ford Hosp Med J 1988; 36:29–34.
16. Webster JR, Saadeh GB, Eggum PR, Suker JR: Wheezing due to pulmonary embolism: treatment with heparin. N Engl J Med 1966; 274: 931–933.
17. Bell WR, Simon TL: Current status of pulmonary thromboembolic disease: pathophysiology, diagnosis, prevention and atreatment. Am Heart J 1982; 103:239–262.
18. National Cooperative Study: The urokinase pulmonary embolism trial. Circulation 1973; 47(suppl 2):1–101.
19. Stein PD, Willis DW, De Meets DL: History and physical exam in acute PE in patients without preexisting cardiac or pulmonary disease. Am J Cardiol 1981; 47:218–223.
20. Perloff JK: Auscultatory and phonocardiographic manifestations of pulmonary hypertension. Prog Cardiovasc Dis 1967; 9:303–340.
21. Wenger NK, Stein PD, Willis DW: Massive acute PE, the deceivingly nonspecific manifestations. JAMA 1972; 220:843–844
22. Benotti JR, Dalen JE: Pulmonary embolism. In: Rippe JM et al, eds: Intensive care medicine. Boston, Little, Brown, 1985; p. 129.
23. Come PC: Echocardiographic evaluation of pulmonary embolism and its response to therapeutic interventions. Chest 1992; 101(suppl): 151S-162S.
24. Stein PD, Hull RD, Saltzman HA et al: Strategy for diagnosis of patients with suspected acute pulmonary embolism. Chest 1993; 103: 1553–1559.
25. Dalen JE, Alpert JS: Natural history of pulmonary embolism. Prog Cardiovasc Dis 1975; 17:259–270.
26. Persson AV, Davis RJ, Villavicencio JL: Deep venous thrombosis and pulmonary embolism. Surg Clin North Am 1991; 71:1195–1209.
27. Mehra MR and Bode FR: Acute deep venous thrombosis. In: Civetta

JM, Taylor RW, Kirby eds: Critical care. Philadelphia, JB Lippincott, 1992; pp. 1283–1291.

28. White RH, McGahan JP, Daschbach MM, Hartling RP: Diagnosis of deep vein thrombosis using duplex ultrasound. Ann Intern Med 1989; 111:297.
29. Lensing AW, Pradoni P, Brandjes D et al: Detection of deep vein thrombosis by real-time B-mode ultrasonography. N Engl J Med 1989; 320:342–345.
30. Wright DJ, Shepard AD, McPharlin M, Ernst CB: Pitfalls in lower extremity venous duplex scanning. J Vasc Surg 1990; 11:675–679.
31. Killewich LA, Bedford GR, Beach KW, Strandness DE: Diagnosis of deep venous thrombosis: a prospective study comparing duplex scanning to contrast venography. Circulation 1989; 79:810–814.
32. Fronek A: The venous system of the lower extremities. In: Fronek A, ed: Non-invasive diagnostics in vascular surgery. New York, McGraw-Hill, 1989.
33. Cronan JJ, Dorfman GS, Grusmark J: Lower-extremity deep venous thrombosis: further experience with and refinements of US assessment. Radiology 1988; 168:101–107.
34. Persson AF: Use of the Triplex scanner in diagnosis of deep venous thrombosis. Arch Surg 1989; 124:593–596.
35. DeValois JC, Van Schaik CC, Verzijlbergen F et al: Contrast venography: from gold standard to "golden backup" in clinically suspected deep vein thrombosis. Eur J Radiol 1990; 11:131–137.
36. Hillner BE, Philbrick JT, Becker DM: Optimal management of suspected lower-extremity deep vein thrombosis. Arch Intern Med 1992; 152:165–175.
37. Taplin GV, Johnson DE, Dore EK, Kaplin HS: Suspensions of radioalbumin aggregates for photoscanning of liver, spleen, lung and other organs. J Nucl Med 1964; 5:259–275.
38. Overton DT, Bocka JJ: The alveolar-arterial oxygen gradient in patients with documented pulmonary embolism. Arch Intern Med 1988; 148:1617–1619.
39. The PIOPED Investigators: Value of the ventilation/perfusion scan in acute pulmonary embolism. JAMA 1990; 263:2753.
40. Oudkerk M, Van Beek EJR, Van Putten WLJ, Büller HR: Cost-effectiveness analysis of various strategies in diagnostic management of pulmonary embolism. Arch Intern Med 1993; 153:947–954.
41. Kramer Fl, Teitelbaum G, Merli GJ: Panvenography and pulmonary angiography in the diagnosis of DVT and pulmonary thromboembolism. Radiol Clin North Am 1986; 24:397–418.
42. Sasahara AA, Stein M, Simon M, Littmann D: Pulmonary angiography in the diagnosis of thromboembolic disease. N Engl J Med 1964; 279:1075–1081.
43. Bettman MA: Pulmonary angiography. In: Hirsh J, ed: Venous thrombosis and pulmonary embolism: diagnostic methods. New York, Churchill Livingstone, 1987; pp. 150–160.
44. Dalen JE: Pulmonary angiography in pulmonary embolism. Bull Physiopathol Respir 1970; 6:45.
45. McIntyre KM, Sasahara AA, Sharmar GV: Pulmonary thromboembolism: current concepts. Adv Intern Med 1972; 18:199–218.
46. Mishkin FS, Johnson PM: The role of lung imaging in pulmonary embolism. Postgrad Med J 1973; 49:487–502.
47. National Cooperative Study: The urokinase pulmonary embolism trial. Circulation 1973; 47(suppl 2):1–101.

48. Wellman HN: Pulmonary thromboembolism: current status report on the role of nuclear medicine. Semin Nucl Med 1986; 16:236–274.
49. Novelline RA, Baltarowich OH, Athanasoulis CA et al: The clinical course of patients with suspected PE and a negative arteriogram. Radiology 1978; 126:561–567.
50. Nicod P, Peterson KL: Pulmonary angiography in severe chronic pulmonary HTN. Ann Intern Med 1987; 107:565–568.
51. Granger RA: The clinical and financial implications of low osmolar radiologic contrast media. Clin Radiol 1984; 35:251–252.
52. Bansmer G, Keith D, Tesluk H: Complications following use of indwelling catheters of the inferior vena cava. JAMA 1958; 167: 1606–1611.
53. Monreal M, Lafoz E, Ruiz J et al: Upper extremity deep vein thrombosis and pulmonary embolism. Chest 1991; 99:280–283.
54. Bern MM, Lokich JJ, Wallach SR: Very low doses of warfarin can prevent thrombosis in central venous catheters. Ann Intern Med 1990; 112:423–428.
55. Jones TK, Barnes RW, Greenfield LJ: Greenfield vena caval filters: rationale and current indications. Ann Thorac Surg 1986; 42(suppl): S48-S55.
56. Alexander JJ, Gewertz BL, Lu C, Zarins CK: New criteria for placement of a prophylactic vena cava filter. Surg Gynecol Obstet 1986; 163:405–409.
57. Decousus HA, Croze M, Levi FA et al: Circadian changes in anticoagulant effect of heparin infused at a constant rate. Br Med J 1985; 290:341–344.
58. Hattersley PG, Mitsuoka JC, King JH: Heparin therapy for thromboembolic disorders: a prospective evaluation of 134 cases monitored by the activated coagulation time. JAMA 1983; 250:1413–1416.
59. Weiss ME, Nyham D, Peng Z et al: Association of protamine IgE and IgG antibodies with life-threatening reactions to intravenous protamine. N Engl J Med 1989; 320:886–892.
60. Cines DB, Kaywin P, Bina M et al: Heparin-associated thrombocytopenia. N Engl J Med 1980; 303:788–795.
61. Bell WR, Rogall RM: Heparin-associated thrombocytopenia: a comparison of three heparin preparations. N Engl J Med 1980; 303: 902–907.
62. Cimo PL, Moake JL, Weinger RS et al: Heparin-induced thrombocytopenia: association with a platelet aggregating factor and arterial thromboses. Am J Hematol 1979; 6:125–133.
63. Hunter JB, Lonsdale RJ, Wenham PW et al: Heparin induced thrombosis: an important complication of heparin prophylaxis for thromembolic disease in surgery. Br Med J 1993; 307:53–55.
64. Warkentin TE, Kelton JG: Heparin and platelets. Hematol Oncol Clin North Am 1990; 4:243–264.
65. Deykin D: Current status of anticoagulant therapy. Am J Med 1982; 72:659–664.
66. Stricker H, Lämmle B, Furlan M, Sulzer I: Heparin-dependent in vitro aggregation of normal platelets by plasma of a patient with heparin-induced skin necrosis: specific diagnostic test for a rare side effect. Am J Med 1988; 85:721–724.
67. Colt HG, Begg RJ, Saporito JJ et al: Cholesterol emboli after cardiac catheterization. Medicine 1988; 67:389–400.
68. Dukes GE, Sanders SW, Russo J Jr et al: Transaminase elevations in

patients receiving bovine or procine heparin. Ann Intern Med 1984; 100:646–650.

69. Prandoni P, Lensing AW, Büller HR et al: Comparison of subcutaneous low-molecular-weight heparin with intravenous standard heparin in proximal deep-vein thrombosis. Lancet 1992; 339:441–445.
70. Hull RD, Raskob GE, Pineo GF et al: Subcutaneous low-molecular-weight heparin compared with continuous intravenous heparin in the treatment of proximal-vein thrombosis. N Engl J Med 1992; 326: 975–982.
71. Nurmohamed MT, Rosendaal FR, Büller HR et al: Low-molecular-weight heparin versus standard heparin in general and orthopedic surgery: a meta-analysis. Lancet 1992; 340:152–156.
72. O'Reilly RA, Aggler PM, Leong LS: Studies on coumarin anticoagulant drugs: pharmacodynamics of warfarin in man. J Clin Invest 1963; 42:1542–1551.
73. O'Reilly RA, Aggler PM: Studies on coumarin anticoagulant drugs: initiation of warfarin therapy without a loading dose. Circulation 1968; 38:169–177.
74. Viganò S, Mannucci PM, Solinas S et al: Decrease in protein C antigen and formation of an abnormal protein soon after starting oral anticoagulant therapy. Br J Haematol 1984; 57:213–220.
75. Hull RD, Delmore TJ, Genton E et al: Warfarin sodium versus low-dose heparin in the long-term treatment of venous thrombosis. N Engl J Med 1979; 301:855–858.
76. Hull RD, Delmore TJ, Carter C et al: Adjusted subcutaneous heparin versus warfarin sodium in the long-term treatment of venous thrombosis. N Engl J Med 1982; 306:189–194.
77. Hull RD, Hirsh J, Ray R et al: Different intensities of oral anticoagulant therapy in the treatment of proximal-vein thrombosis. N Engl J Med 1982; 307:1676–1681.
78. Gallus A, Jackaman J, Tillett J et al: Safety and efficacy of warfarin started early after submassive venous thrombosis or pulmonary embolism. Lancet 1986; 2:1293–1296.
79. Hull RD, Raskob GF, Rosenbloom D et al: Heparin for 5 days as compared with 10 days in the initial treatment of proximal venous thrombosis. N Engl J Med 1990; 322:1260–1264.
80. National Heart, Lung, and Blood Institute: Urokinase pulmonary embolism trial: phase one results. JAMA 1970; 214:2163–2172.
81. National Heart, Lung, and Blood Institute: Urokinase pulmonary embolism trial: phase 2 results. JAMA 1974; 229:1606–1613.
82. Markel A, Manzo RA, Strandners D Jr: The potential role of thrombolytic therapy in venous thrombosis. Arch Intern Med 1992; 152: 1265–1267.
83. Hirsh J, Hull RD: Treatment of venous thromboembolism. Chest 1986; 89(suppl):426S-433S.
84. Sharma GVRK, Burleson VA, Sasahara AA: Effect of thrombolytic therapy on pulmonary-capillary blood volume in patients with pulmonary embolism. N Engl J Med 1980; 303:842–845.
85. Come PC, Kim D, Parker JA et al: Early reversal of right ventricular dysfunction in patients with acute pulmonary embolism after treatment with intravenous tissue plasminogen activator. J Am Coll Cardiol 1987; 10:971–978.
86. Mattox KL, Feldtman RW, Beall AC Jr, DeBakey ME: Pulmonary embolectomy for acute massive pulmonary embolism. Ann Surg 1982; 195:726–731.

87. Lund O, Nielsen TT, Schifter S, Roenne K: Treatment of pulmonary embolism with full-dose heparin, streptokinase or embolectomy: results and indications. Thorac Cardiovasc Surg 1986; 34:240–246.
88. Belenkie I, Dani R, Smith ER, Tyberg JV: Effects of volume loading during experimental acute pulmonary embolism. Circulation 1989; 80:178–188.
89. Molloy WD, Lee KY, Girling L et al: Treatment of shock in a canine model of pulmonary embolism. Am Rev Respir Dis 1984; 130: 870–874.
90. McGehee WG, Klotz TA, Epstein DJ, Rapaport SI: Coumarin necrosis associated with hereditary protein C deficiency. Ann Intern Med 1984; 100:59–60.
91. Triplett DA, Brandt JT, Musgrave KA, Orr CA: The relationship between lupus anticoagulants and antibodies to phospholipid. JAMA 1988; 259:550–554.
92. Fields RA, Toubbeh H, Searles RP, Bankhurst AD: The prevalence of anticardiolipin antibodies in a healthy elderly population and its association with antinuclear antibodies. J Rheumatol 1989; 16: 623–625.
93. Hull RD, Raskob GE, Carter CJ: Serial impedence plethysmography in pregnant patients with clinically suspected deep-vein thrombosis. Ann Intern Med 1990; 112:663–667.
94. Kaunitz AM, Hughes JM, Grimes DA et al: Causes of maternal mortality in the United States. Obstet Gynecol 1985; 65; 605–612.
95. Ginsberg JS, Kowalchuk G, Hirsh J et al: Heparin therapy during pregnancy: risks to the fetus and mother. Arch Intern Med 1989; 149: 2233–2236.
96. Stevenson RE, Burton OM, Ferlauto GJ, Taylor HA: Hazards of oral anticoagulants during pregnancy. JAMA 1980; 243:1549–1551.
97. Moser KM, LeMoine JR: Is embolic risk conditioned by location of deep venous thrombosis? Ann Intern Med 1981; 94:439–444.
98. Lagerstedt CI, Olsson C-G, Fagher BO et al: Need for long-term anticoagulant treatment in symptomatic calf-vein thrombosis. Lancet 1985; 2:515–518.
99. Rubenstein E: XVIII thromboembolism. In: Scientific American medicine. New York, Scientific American, 1990; pp. 1–14.
100. Olin JW, Young JR, Graor RA et al: Treatment of deep vein thrombosis and pulmonary emboli in patients with primary and metastatic brain tumors. Arch Intern Med 1987; 147:2177–2179.
101. McCarthy ST, Turner J: How-dose subcutaneous heparin in the prevention of deep vein thrombosis and pulmonary emboli following acute stroke. Age Aging 1986; 15:84–88.
102. Abramson SB, Odajnyk CM, Grieco AJ et al: Hyperalgesic pseudothrombophlebitis. Am J Med 1985; 78:317–320.
103. Katz RS, Zizic TM, Arnold WP, Stevens MB: The pseudothrombophlebitis syndrome. Medicine (Baltimore) 1977; 56:151–164.
104. Goldhaber SZ, Hennekins CM, Markisz JA et al: Low sensitivity of plasma DNA in screening for PE. Am Rev Respir Dis 1982; 126: 360–361.
105. Kereiakes DJ, Herfkens RJ, Brundage BH et al: Computerized tomography in chronic thromboembolic pulmonary hypertension. Am Heart J 1983; 106:1432–1436.
106. Palla A, Tumeh SS, Nagel JS et al: Detection of pulmonary perfusion defects by single photon emission computed tomography (SPECT). J Nucl Med Allied Sci 1988; 32:27.

107. Spritzer CE, Norconk JJ, Sostman HD, Coleman RE: Detection of deep venous thrombosis by magnetic resonance imaging. Chest 1993; 104:54–60.
108. Kessler CM: Modern treatment of pulmonary embolism. Lung 1990; 168(suppl):841–848.
109. Becker DM, Philbrick MD, Selby B: Inferior vena cava filters. Arch Intern Med 1992; 152:1985–1994.

CHAPTER 18

Use of Neuromuscular Blockade in the Intensive Care Unit (Appropriate Use of Muscle Relaxants)

Philip G. Boysen

Case Report

A 48-year-old white male was admitted to the intensive care unit (ICU) from the operating room. Earlier that day, he had been injured in a high-speed automobile accident that resulted in bilateral pneumothoraces and lung contusions. Chest tubes had been placed in the emergency room. He also suffered intra-abdominal injuries including a lacerated liver and fractured femur. In the operating room, he initially had repair of the liver laceration and required 6 units of blood replacement. A splenic laceration could not be repaired, and his spleen had to be removed. During internal rodding of the femur, he lost an additional 3 units of blood. He was in the operating room a total of 6.5 hours.

On return to the ICU, his temperature was 34.8°C. A pulmonary artery catheter placed for management showed, among other things, an arterial venous oxygen content difference (Ca-vDO_2) of 6.8 ml/dl. This was coupled to a cardiac output of 6.8 ml/min. The patient was grossly shivering. During mechanical ventilation, the peak inflation pressures were 55 cm H_2O with a tidal volume of 700 ml. The patient weighed 80 kg. His spontaneous respiratory rate was 38/min. F_IO_2 was 0.5 and 12 cm H_2O positive end-expiratory pressure (PEEP). PaO_2 was 58 mm Hg.

Because of shivering, poor blood gases, high respiratory rate, and high inflation pressure, the patient was paralyzed. He was given an initial bolus of 10 mg of vecuronium. This was followed by a continuous infusion of 4 mg/hr. The train-of-four was then monitored with a nerve stimulator. Following the patient's initial paralysis, blood gases were repeated. PaO_2 was now 88 mm Hg, and $PaCO_2$ was 39 mm Hg. Temperature remained at 34.8°C. His Ca-vDO_2 had reduced to 4.2 ml/dl. Cardiac output remained unchanged. The patient required paralysis for the next 48 hours until his chest contusions began to resolve. At that point, vercuronium was discontinued, and the patient was easily able to assume spontaneous respirations. He was weaned and extubated on the fifth postinjury day.

The use of neuromuscular blockers in the ICU exemplifies pharmacotherapy originally utilized in the operating room, now extended into the critical care environment. Until the 1950s, most general anesthetics employed spontaneous breathing.[1] Agents such as ether supported ventilation and preserved cardiac output. Anesthetics were delivered through a breathing apparatus that volatilized the anesthetic and entrained room air. The introduction of paralytics, such as curare, facilitated certain surgical procedures. However, these agents required positive pressure mechanical ventilation. This coincided with the development of newer anesthetic agents, the halogenated hydrocarbons, which suppressed spontaneous ventilation. These agents also often depressed cardiac function. These drugs provided the ability to perform abdominal operative procedures with a more relaxed abdomen and led to their designation as muscle relaxants. Since these drugs induce temporary paralysis, we prefer the term "neuromuscular blocker," with its more descriptive definition of the intended pharmacologic effect.

• *For most critically ill patients, neuromuscular blockade should not be instituted unless the patient also receives adequate sedation and pain relief.*

For the critically ill, neuromuscular relaxants should be administered in three steps. First, the physician should determine the presence or absence of pain and whether any narcotic regimen has been employed to alleviate pain and discomfort.[2] Second, either in concert with narcosis or separately, the issue of anxiety and agitation must be addressed.[3] Although many narcotics have a sedative effect, it may be necessary to administer a sedative agent concomitantly with the use of neuromuscular blocking agents. The benzodiazepines have been widely employed for this purpose. Third, patient selection implies a benefit from the use of neuromuscular blockade. In certain patients, for example, such therapy may facilitate mechanical ventilation. The goals should be clear and well understood, and the duration of therapy should be minimized while still achieving specific other therapeutic goals.[4] The combination of improved mechanical ventilators, monitoring systems, and the specific neuromuscular blocking agents permits somewhat wider use of these drugs for critically ill patients.[5–10] Problems and complications with these agents persist due to their potency, the effects of long-term administration, and drug interactions.[11–12]

INDICATIONS

The indications for neuromuscular blockers vary by institution and practice patterns.[13] General indications have included the control of intracranial pressure, immobilization during patient transport such as for diagnostic studies, and mechanical ventilation of patients with severe respiratory insufficiency. Some patients with multiple organ failure also require paralysis. Other indications include post-anoxic injury, Reye's syndrome, and neuroleptic malignant syndrome (Table 18–1).

Critically ill patients often have combined impairment of both cardiac and pulmonary systems. As such, oxygen delivery may only marginally meet metabolic demands. Induction of paralysis can decrease total metabolic demands. At times, such as when a patient shivers or has rigor, the decrease in oxygen consumption can be dramatic. Monitors such as mixed venous oxygen saturation (SVO_2) can easily demonstrate these results with a rapid increase in SVO_2 following the onset of paralysis. Furthermore, the reduction of peripheral and respiratory muscle activity will divert nutritive flow to already hypoxic vital organs.

• *Specific indications for neuromuscular blockade include reduction of metabolic demands and improvement of ventilation and perfusion during mechanical ventilation.*

Other perioperative indications for neuromuscular blockers include wound stability, such as when a vascular anastomosis or a skin flap is at risk in the immediate postoperative period. Similarly, following wound dehiscence or closure of a distended, "tight" abdomen, paralysis may be necessary for several days.

The anxious, agitated patient, not able to synchronize with the ventilator, may benefit from a short period of neuromuscular blockade, which can aid in the achievement of hemodynamic stability. In such cases, the overactivity of the respiratory muscles will cause wide swings in intrapleural pressure. This will result in artifactual deviations of the intravascular pressure trace such as the pulmonary artery and pulmonary capillary wedge pressure (or any intravascular pressure measurement of vessels within the thorax). Neuromuscular blockade and the transition to controlled mechanical ventilation provide a clearer interpretation of the influence of positive airway

• *Paralysis can often aid in determination of pulmonary capillary wedge pressure in patients who otherwise breathe at a rapid spontaneous rate.*

Table 18–1.
Indications for Neuromuscular Blockade as Adjunct to Mechanical Ventilation

Common indications
Facilitate mechanical ventilation
Reduce intracranial pressure
Reduce oxygen delivery/demand
Eliminate postoperative shivering
Decrease agitation or "fighting the ventilator"
Transport
Immobilization for diagnostic studies
Less common indications
Supportive therapy for tetanus or neuroleptic malignant syndrome
Hemodynamic instability
Immobilization

pressure on intravascular pressures. This, in turn, improves the ability to choose an end point as a reference for measurement, such as at end-exhalation. This will significantly aid in the assessment of intravascular cardiac filling pressure.

PHARMACOKINETICS AND PHARMACODYNAMICS

For most drugs, we profile body distribution by measurement of plasma concentrations over time following administration of a single bolus dose.[13,14] For first-order kinetics drugs, the log of the plasma concentration plotted against time produces specific phases or slopes. The first, and usually steeper, slope is termed the alpha slope and corresponds to the initial distribution of the drug (Fig. 18–1). Following a transition, a second slope, termed beta, corresponds to the elimination of the drug from the body. To treat a critically ill patient, it is preferable to use an agent that has a smaller or at least a predictable volume of distribution as well as shorter elimination half-time. This allows more specific dosing at shorter intervals and lends itself to a continuous infusion.

• *Shorter acting agents allow better titration.*

Importantly, we assume that the plasma concentration of the drug relates to the desired pharmacologic effect. For example, with a bronchodilator, the plasma concentration should relate to the FEV_1 improvement. For a narcotic, the plasma concentration should correlate with pain relief. Similarly, for a neuromuscular blocker, the established and maintained plasma concentration should result in a specific decrease in spontaneous and voluntary muscle activity. As

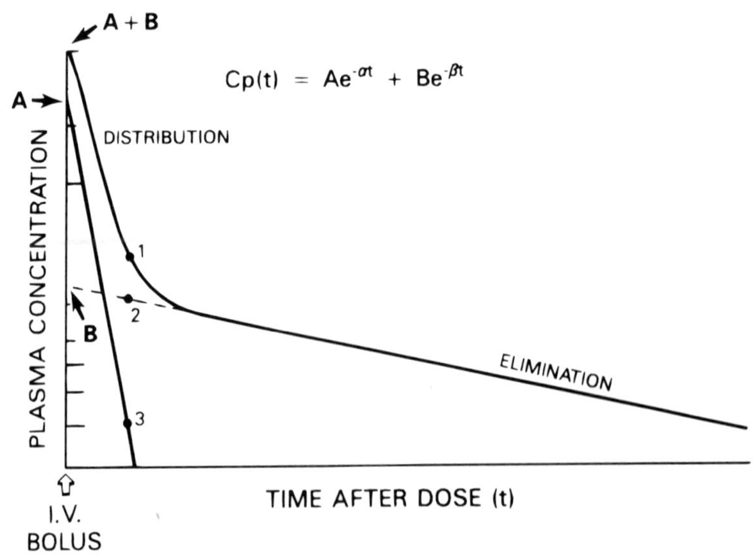

Figure 18–1.
Schematic illustration of plasma concentration over time after rapid intravenous injection of a drug. Arrow A points to the alpha slope and arrow B to the beta slope. The slopes of the two distinct phases are used to calculate the volume of distribution and the elimination half-time.

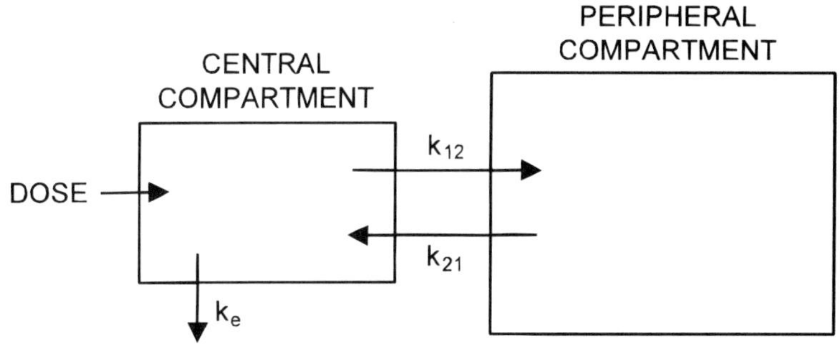

Figure 18–2.
The two-compartment biexponential model derived from the time concentration curve, with rate constants (K_{12} + K_{21}) indicating intercompartmental movement. A neuromuscular blocker or its metabolite that is widely redistributed must return to the central compartment from the peripheral site to be metabolized or eliminated. (From Stanski DR, Watkins WD: Drug disposition in anesthesia. New York, Grune & Stratton, 1982).

such, monitoring peripheral neuromuscular twitch is the preferred method of choice to maintain correct dosing in the operating room. Unfortunately, despite the effectiveness having been demonstrated in the surgical suite, it has not yet been widely adopted in the intensive care environment.

Other important considerations exist for these drugs (Fig. 18–2). First, we conceptualize that intravenous administration of a drug will result in its distribution within a central compartment.[15] Redistribution of the drug to another compartment (the so-called peripheral compartment) becomes problematic. When redistribution occurs, the pharmacologic effect usually disappears. Second, following redistribution, the agent obviously accumulates in the body, and elimination will take place at some later time. Last, a drug can only be metabolized or eliminated from the central compartment. Therefore, a widely distributed drug must at some point return to the central compartment to eventually be metabolized and eliminated. This also holds for active metabolites. The presence of an active metabolite coupled with its wide redistribution may prolong the effect of the drug beyond that anticipated by basic dosing regimens. Therefore, whatever the route of administration, whether repeated bolus doses or continuous infusion, drug accumulation may easily occur. Bedside monitoring can minimize or prevent such occurrences.

- *Drugs with active metabolites may make it difficult to judge the accuracy of response based on plasma concentration levels.*

- *When patients receive neuromuscular blocking agents, continuous bedside monitoring should be performed to prevent the effects of accumulation of active metabolites or reduced elimination.*

Once aware of the volume of distribution and the elimination half-time, we can derive a third variable, the infusion method. Most drug infusion regimens assume that the drug infusion rate matches the clearance or elimination rate. If the infusion rate exceeds the clearance, then drug accumulation begins. When the infusion rate does not match the clearance, the drug will dissipate. Although we do not calculate clearance in all clinical situations, monitoring a specific, definable, reproducible physiologic variable will directly affect dosing and therapy. Another important basic principle of drug infusion involves the rate at which plasma concentration develops

• *For most agents, it requires five multiples of the elimination half-time to reach a steady state.*

following initiation of the infusion. As a basic tenet, it takes approximately five multiples of the elimination half-time to reach a steady state in plasma. Therefore, assume an elimination half-time for a specific drug at between 4 and 6 hours. Following establishment of an infusion at a specific rate, it will require between 20 and 30 hours to establish a steady state. To shorten this time, a larger initial bolus dose will establish a plasma concentration within therapeutic range. It also follows that failure to obtain an adequate level of neuromuscular blockade requires not only that the infusion rate be increased, but a small bolus of the drug should be given to rapidly establish the desired therapeutic effect. This general rule also works in reverse. Following discontinuation, it will take approximately five multiples of the half-time for successful elimination.

MECHANISM OF ACTION

The standard interspecies operating mechanism of neuromuscular blockers have caused them to receive considerable attention over the years. Manipulation of the neuromuscular junction with neuromuscular blockers exemplifies the utilization of agonist-antagonist interactions and activation of receptor sites. The neuromuscular blocker receptor site consists of five proteins of specific size that float in the bilipid cytoplasmic membrane (Fig. 18–3).[16] Interestingly, they seem to be dispersed in random fashion until release of the agonist, acetylcholine, into the neuromuscular cleft. Following this, a specific conformational change aligns these five proteins into a rosette formation. Two of the proteins are of the same size and act as the active receptor sites. Acetylcholine occupies both of these receptor sites during depolarization. Once the receptor site becomes activated, the system functions as a channel that opens into the internal cellular milieu. This releases potassium from intracellular

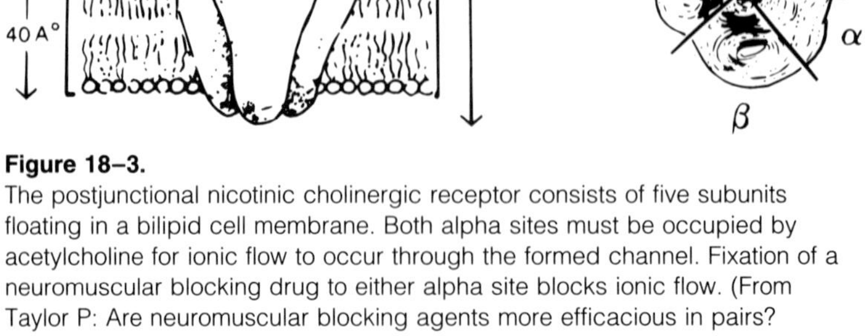

Figure 18–3.
The postjunctional nicotinic cholinergic receptor consists of five subunits floating in a bilipid cell membrane. Both alpha sites must be occupied by acetylcholine for ionic flow to occur through the formed channel. Fixation of a neuromuscular blocking drug to either alpha site blocks ionic flow. (From Taylor P: Are neuromuscular blocking agents more efficacious in pairs? Anesthesiology 1985; 63:1–3.)

stores and causes an influx of sodium and calcium. When a neuromuscular blocker occupies one or the other of these receptor sites, it makes no difference what occurs at the other receptor site.[17] This site is essentially blocked, and ionic flow, which ordinarily results in neuromuscular transmission, will not occur.

Specific dosing considerations may be problematic for critically ill patients. First, there may be alteration in the numbers, function, and structure of the receptor sites.[18] Small amounts of the drug may cause an effect greater than anticipated under other situations. Second, critically ill patients receive multiple drugs, many of which interfere with the activity, distribution, and elimination of the neuromuscular blockers.[12] A classic example is the aminoglycoside antibiotics, which can cause prolonged neuromuscular blockade following the concomitant use of both drugs. Additionally, there are situations in which the channel does not function properly for a variety of reasons.[19] We term this either closed or open channel blockade. There may be times which require an increased dose of neuromuscular blocker. These include an altered number of functional receptor sites as well as hypermetabolic states. However, in general, critically ill patients exhibit a tendency toward marked effects from small amounts of the neuromuscular blocker. In addition, drug accumulation and the possibility of prolonged blockade should always be kept in mind.

- *Agents such as aminoglycosides can enhance the effects of neuromuscular blockers. Hypermetabolic states and an increased volume of distribution may both require increased amounts of drug to provide adequate blockade.*

When agents are used to reverse the effects of neuromuscular blockers, an agonist-antagonist interaction takes place. For example, neostigmine interferes with the enzyme that metabolizes acetylcholine. At the neuromuscular junction, this effectively increases the concentration of the agonist at the neuromuscular junction. The sought after effect is an increased likelihood that both sites on the receptor will be occupied by an agonist molecule, as opposed to the still present neuromuscular blocker. It should be remembered that these so-called reversal agents also have their own volume of distribution and half-life. In some instances, administration of the reversal agent results in recovery of neuromuscular function, but only for a short time. If the reversal agent is eliminated faster than the neuromuscular blocker, receptor blockade will be reestablished.

- *Reversal agents principally interfere with the enzymes that metabolize acetylcholine. This results in increased acetylcholine concentrations, which will attempt to displace neuromuscular agents from the receptor sites.*

CHOICE OF AGENTS

The neuromuscular blockers currently in use can be divided according to several categories. One group consists of depolarizing or nondepolarizing agents (Table 18–2). Succinylcholine is a depolarizing agent. This means that when the drug interacts with the receptor sites, a generalized depolarization commences prior to paralysis. This mechanism explains the muscle fasciculation common before the onset of neuromuscular blockade. The other major class of agents is referred to as nondepolarizing neuromuscular blockers. Following administration of a nondepolarizing agent, patients exhibit no visible change in muscle activity.

The nondepolarizing drugs fall into two further categories, based

Table 18–2.
Nondepolarizing Neuromuscular Blockers: Use in the Intensive Care Unit

	Selected Agents for ICU Use					
	Tubocurarine (Curare)	**Metocurine (Metubine)**	**Atracurium (Tracrium)**	**Vecuronium (Norcuron)**	**Doxacurium (Nuromax)**	**Pancuronium (Pavulon)**
Introduced (yr)	1942	1952	1983	1984	1991	1972
ED_{95} dose (mg/kg)	0.51	0.3	0.25	0.05	0.025–0.030	0.07
"Initial" dose (mg/kg)*	0.2–0.3	0.3–0.35	0.4–0.5	0.1	up to 0.1	0.1
Duration (min)	80	70–90	25–35	35–45	120–150	90–100
Infusion described	?	?	Yes	Yes	No	Yes
Infusion dose (μg/kg/min)	—	—	4–12	1–2	Not routine	1–2
Recovery (min)	80–180	90–180	40–60	45–60	120–180	120–180
% Renal excretion	40–45	45–55	5–10	50	70	45–70
Δ Renal failure	↑	↑↑	No change	↑, especially metabolites	↑ to ↑↑	↑ to ↑↑, any metabolites
% Biliary excretion	10–40	2	Minimal	35–50	Unclear	10–15
Δ Hepatic failure	Minimal change to mild ↑	No change	Minimal to no change	Variable, mild increase	?	Mild ↑
Active metabolites	No	No	No, but ? laudanosine	Yes: 3-desacetyl-vecuronium	?	Yes: 3-OH and 17-OH-pancuronium
Histamine release hypotension	Marked	Moderate	Minimal, but dose-dependent	None	None	None
Vagal block tachycardia	Minimal	Minimal	No	No	No	Modest to marked
Ganglionic blockade hypotension	Marked	Modest	Minimal to none	No	No	No
Structure†	Bz-iso	Bz-iso	Bz-iso	Steroid	Bz-iso	Steroid
Prolonged ICU block	?	?	Rare	Yes	Too early to tell?	Yes
Estimated U.S. ICU use	Very rare	Rare	20%–25%	60%	Infrequent	15%
Cost ($)	Low	Low	High	High	High	Low

ED_{95}, effective dose 95; ↑, increased.

* The "initial" recommended dose may be significantly more or less than the ED_{95} dose, depending on autonomic and other expected hemodynamic side-effects, which practically limit the acceptable initial bolus dose of the drug.

† Benzyl isoquinolinium (Bz-iso) or steroid-based molecular structure.

(From Prielipp RC, Coursin DB: Pharmacology of neuromuscular blocking drugs. New Horizons 1994; 2:34–37.)

on chemical structures.[20] One class of drugs has a steroidal nucleus with a branched side chain that closely resembles acetylcholine. The agents pancuronium, vecuronium, rocuronium, and pipecuronium fall into this classification. The remainder of the agents are benzylisoquinolines. Benzylisoquinolines have a unique structure that results in the different method of metabolism. Drugs include tracrium, atracurium, mivacurium, and doxacurium.[21] With these agents there is a unique tendency for the molecule to "self-destruct" once it is introduced into the body. It cleaves into two inactive fragments. This type of elimination has been called Hoffman elimination. Since these compounds do not depend on organ function for either metabolism or elimination, the dissipation of their effects can be predicted. Furthermore, the shorter acting agents are well suited to infusion therapy. During long-term tracrium administration, a metabolite (laudanosine) accumulates, the significance of which is unknown.[22,23]

- *Agents such as tracrium, atracurium, mivacurium, and doxacurium all are eliminated by cleavage into two inactive fragments. They do not depend on organ function for metabolism or elimination.*

Whether these drugs are utilized to aid in tracheal intubation or for facilitation of continuous mechanical ventilation, each has its own difficulties and side effects. For aid in tracheal intubation, the newer agents are compared with succinylcholine, the benchmark.[24,25] In essence, succinylcholine administration will provide for complete flaccid paralysis within about 90 to 120 seconds following administration. It should be realized, however, that when used as an adjunct to intubation very large doses of succinylcholine are administered. It is a very forgiving drug. Despite a massive dose, the serum pseudocholinesterase enzyme system will still metabolize the drug within minutes. Therefore, not only does the agent demonstrate a very rapid and predictable onset but the duration of action lasts just minutes. Thus, during anesthesia induction, other anesthetic agents with an onset and duration that coincide with the succinylcholine profile are selected. Some of the newer agents such as rocuronium and mivacurium will approximate this profile. However, the use of large doses to induce paralysis may result in the prolongation of neuromuscular blockade. Intermediate-acting agents, such as vecuronium and atracurium, can also be used to facilitate intubation as well as maintain neuromuscular blockade during mechanical ventilation. Here again, the onset of neuromuscular blockade can be accelerated by administration of a larger dose, but unwanted side effects may result. A large vecuronium dose will indeed shorten the time to paralysis, but prolonged neuromuscular blockade may be the result.[26] For atracurium, larger doses are associated with histamine release, which may, in turn, cause hypotension.[27] In either case, it has been recommended that a very small dose, a so-called priming dose, be administered 5 to 7 minutes before administration of the remainder of the drug. This small dose will occupy some of the receptor sites such that a subsequent, more moderate dose will result in an acceptable onset of neuromuscular blockade. Response to the priming dose varies among patients. Therefore, it is imperative that monitoring be established, oxygenation maintained, and that direct visual observation of the patient continue. For atracurium, an alternative method involves adminis-

- *Succinylcholine effects are usually eliminated within minutes despite even large overdosage. The rapid return to function following succinylcholine makes it the ideal drug to use for tracheal intubation.*

tration of the total dose over a 45- to 60-second period. This will minimize histamine release and hypotension.

The goals for maintenance of neuromuscular blockade during mechanical ventilation differ from those outlined in the operating room.[28] Total, flaccid paralysis is generally not necessary. Instead, paralysis of the peripheral and respiratory muscles should enable easy delivery of synchronous positive pressure ventilation. The desired effect can be judged by visual observation and examination of the patient or by continued monitoring of the peripheral neuromuscular twitch.

• *Critically ill patients do not require total, flaccid paralysis during neuromuscular blockade.*

MONITORING

Monitoring of the peripheral neuromuscular twitch and hence the degree of neuromuscular blockade has been standardized.[29,30] Generally, four successive shocks are applied to a specified site, such as the ulnar nerve, and motion of the adductor pollicis is noted. The train-of-four means successive stimulative shocks are delivered at 0.5-second intervals (Fig. 18–4). Normally, each successive stimulus of the train-of-four occurs at the same amplitude. Following succinylcholine or depolarizing neuromuscular blocker administration, the amplitude of each beat remains the same throughout the train-of-four stimulus. With a nondepolarizing neuromuscular blocker, each successive beat has a lower amplitude, which results in a decrescendo response (Fig. 18–4). As the degree of blockade becomes established, the fourth stimulus in the train-of-four, followed by the third, and then the second, will be ablated. No elicited response indicates total paralysis.[31] Recovery rate will be predicted by the level of established blockade. In theory, then, if the train-of-four is not monitored, or if the patient has no response to these stimulations, he or she may be massively overdosed. In such a situation, one cannot anticipate timing of recovery.

• *The train-of-four probably provides the best method to monitor the degree of neuromuscular blockade. The fourth train-of-four response should be 25% of the amplitude of the first response.*

A rational approach to therapy therefore involves establishment of neuromuscular blockade with whatever agent seems appropriate. The infusion dose must then be continued or tapered until some response to the train-of-four becomes apparent. In general, when the fourth and third stimuli of the train-of-four are ablated but the first and second remain, mechanical ventilation will be facilitated, even if the disease state alters the drug response.[32]

Such monitoring is simple and easily performed by nursing personnel. In general, once or twice per shift will suffice. However, one should remember that these stimulative shocks may be painful. Therefore, attention to pain and anxiety remains of paramount importance. This is why we do not recommend monitoring post-tetanic facilitation. This test requires a maximal shock to assess response. This may not only be painful but also, in our view, does not afford any additional information than provided by the train-of-four.

Neurologic monitoring of the paralyzed patient cannot be readily accomplished. Once the patient is immobilized, it is nearly im-

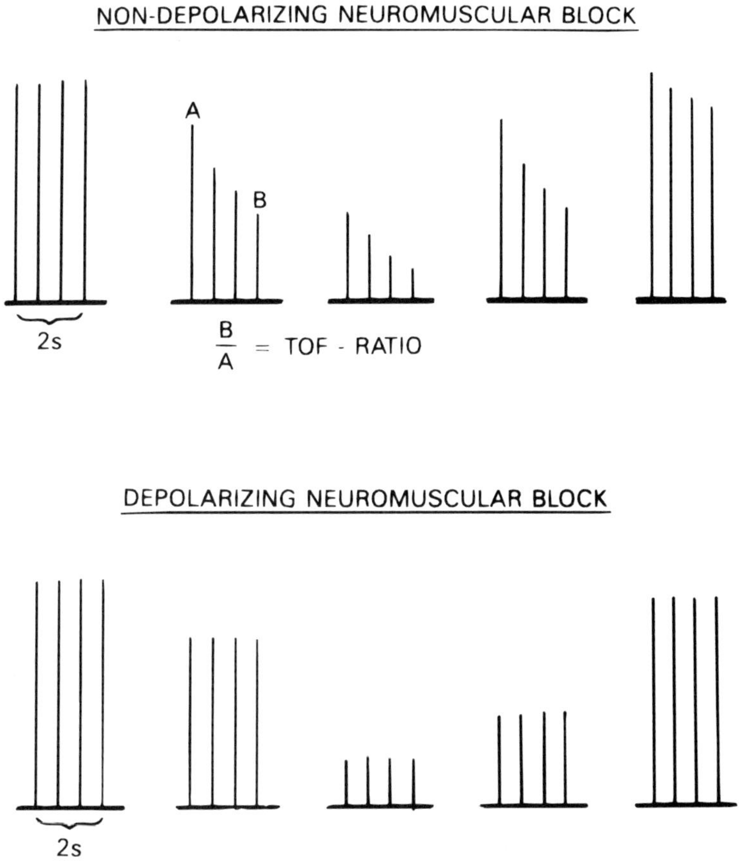

Figure 18–4.
Initial response and return of normal function when train-of-four is used to monitored nondepolarizing or depolarizing neuromuscular blockade. At the top, the nondepolarizing drug has a successively decreased amplitude with each stimulus. The amplitude of the fourth response (B) is compared with the amplitude of the first response (A). For depolarizing agents, all responses have the same decrease in amplitude. (From Viby-Magensen J: Clinical assessment of neuromuscular transmission. Br J Anaesth 1982; 54:203–209.)

possible to assess the sedation level or pain relief other than by nonspecific measures such as pulse rate and blood pressure. Electroencephalographic monitoring proves cumbersome and difficult to interpret. Signal processing and computer applications may provide important information in the ICU environment. However, they remain as yet untested.[33–35]

SIDE EFFECTS OF PROLONGED NEUROMUSCULAR BLOCKADE

As opposed to short-term institution of neuromuscular blockade in the operating room, there are some problems inherent in this therapy specific to prolonged use in the critically ill. The drugs with a steroi-

• *Neuromuscular blocking agents with a steroid nucleus, such as pancuronium and vecuronium, have been associated with prolonged neuromuscular blockade following use of the agents. These agents appear to cause direct injury to muscle fibers.*

dal nucleus may lead to prolonged neuromuscular blockade long after therapy has been discontinued. Although well described,[36–42] this problem remains rare. Most instances of prolonged neuromuscular blockade simply result from dosage and accumulation of the original drug or an active metabolite. However, complications may result from interaction with corticosteroids. Administration of these two compounds together, both of which have a steroidal nucleus, can result in a myopathy characterized by generalized weakness, as well as specific respiratory muscle weakness. This myopathic state can last for many months despite discontinuation of therapy. It is unclear whether the duration of simultaneous administration has any effect on the prolonged blockade. The myopathic state can be demonstrated by muscle biopsy, which often reveals marked atrophy of single fibers and small groups. It occurs in a variety of different types of patients with widely variant diagnoses.[43] These patients all have in common the simultaneous administration of these two drugs. Other diagnostic studies such as motor evoked response amplitudes may or may not show a latency. Similarly, motor conduction velocities may be normal or reduced.

• *Prolonged use of neuromuscular blockade can result in disuse atrophy. Clinically, the patient may appear as though he or she has a prolonged blockade.*

Although not described for nonsteroidal neuromuscular blockers, prolonged respiratory muscle weakness may occur when any of these drugs are given.[44–46] It may be a particular issue in those patients with neuromuscular weakness due to an underlying pathophysiologic state. Following discontinuation, there may be generalized muscle weakness or dyssynchronous breathing. In essence, disuse atrophy develops. This can prevent weaning of a patient from mechanical ventilation. Muscle retraining may enable these specific patients to achieve or renew strength and endurance. Ultimately, patients will recover to a level that will support weaning and extubation.

RECOVERY AND DISCONTINUATION OF THERAPY

When adequate monitoring of peripheral neuromuscular blockade has been instituted, more precise dosing becomes possible. The aim is to position the patient just on the fringe of recovery. Following discontinuation of therapy, return to normal function will be facilitated. Additionally, adjunctive bedside testing can be helpful (Table 18–3). It must be remembered that administration of these drugs causes respiratory muscle paralysis and induced neuromuscular re-

Table 18–3.
Indication of Recovery from Neuromuscular Blockade

Return of peripheral neuromuscular twitch
Sustained 5-second head lift
Vital capacity > 15 ml/kg
Maximum inspiratory force > 25 cm H_2O
Minute ventilation ≤ 10 L/min *and* synchronous breathing pattern

spiratory failure. The ability of the patient to sustain a headlift for 5 seconds from the supine position provides an easy method to ensure an intact neuromuscular respiratory system. Such a patient should be able to maintain a patent airway. Adequacy of respiratory muscle strength can be tested by the peak negative pressure against an occluded airway developed by the patient. The negative pressure drop should exceed -25 cm H_2O. A further useful parameter measures the ability to maintain a vital capacity of approximately 15 ml/kg. In addition, such bedside observations as breathing patterns and synchronous muscle function can be helpful. With activation of higher neural centers, the patient should be able to simultaneously maintain a patent airway and activate chest wall muscles while the diaphragm descends. Dyssynchronous breathing implies respiratory muscle fatigue, disuse atrophy, or upper airway malfunction. Simultaneous measurement of minute ventilation can also help. The patient with dyssynchronous breathing may also have increased dead space ventilation. This condition will result in an elevated respiratory rate. The minute ventilation will usually exceed 10 L/min in those patients unable to be weaned. The accumulated clinical indicators of return of neuromuscular function, in combination with assessment of peripheral neuromuscular twitch, usually provide the necessary information to ascertain recovery from neuromuscular blockade.

• *Clinical tests such as the ability to raise one's head off the bed can judge the accuracy of muscle strength. A vital capacity of 15 ml/kg also indicates adequate short-term muscle strength. Neither tests muscle endurance.*

For a variety of reasons, we do not recommend reversal agents for the critically ill. The accumulation of the neuromuscular blocker, as well as of the active metabolites, increases the tendency toward recurrent paralysis following a single dose of a reversal agent. The administration of an acetylcholinesterase inhibitor can cause additional problems. It may stimulate other muscarinic sites and cause intense bradycardia and hypotension. Fixed combinations have been recommended for reversal therapy. This may be an erroneous judgment for the patient in the ICU. It is therefore preferable to permit the neuromuscular blocker to dissipate naturally and then assess recovery as previously noted.

In conclusion, neuromuscular blockers are required for a small minority of critically ill patients. However, this use can dramatically improve certain clinical situations. Safe usage requires experience, a thorough knowledge of their pharmacology and pharmokinetics, as well as close monitoring.

REFERENCES

1. Topulos GP: Neuromusclar blockade in adult intensive care. New Horizons 1993; 1:447–462.
2. Hansen-Flaschen JH, Brazinsky S, Basile C et al: Use of sedating drugs and neuromuscular blocking agents in patients requiring mechanical ventilation for respiratory failure. JAMA 1991; 266:2870–2876.
3. Durbin CG Jr: Neuromuscular blocking agents and sedative drugs: clinical uses and toxic effects in the critical care unit. Crit Care Clin 1991; 7:489–506.

4. Loper KA, Butler S, Nessly M, et al: Paralyzed with pain: the need for education. Pain 1989; 37:315–317.
5. Sharpe MD: The use of muscle relaxants in the intensive care unit. Can J Anaesth 1992; 39:949–962.
6. Isenstein DA, Venner DS, Duggan J: Neuromuscular blockade in the intensive care unit. Chest 1992; 102:1259–1266.
7. Coursin DB, Kelly JS, Prielipp RC: Muscle relaxants in critical care. Curr Opin Anaesthesiol 1993; 6:341–365.
8. O'Conner MF, Roizen MF: Use of muscle relaxants in the intensive care unit. J Intensive Care Med 1993; 8:34–46.
9. Agoston S, Seyr M, Khuenl-Brady K et al: Use of neuromuscular blocking agents in the intensive care unit. Anesth Clin North Am 1993; 11: 345–360.
10. Fiamengo SA, Savarese JJ: Use of muscle relaxants in intensive care units. Crit Care Med 1991; 19:1547–1559.
11. Hansen-Flaschen J, Cowan J, Raps EC: Neuromuscular blockade in the ICU: more than we bargained for. Am Rev Respir Dis 1993; 147: 234–237.
12. Erkola O: Complications of neuromuscular blockers: interaction with concurrent medications and other neuromuscular blockers. Anesth Clin North Am 1993; 11:427–444.
13. Klessig HT, Geiger HJ, Murray MJ et al: A national survey on the practice patterns of anesthesiologist intensivists in the use of muscle relaxants. Crit Care Med 1992; 20:1341–1345.
14. Ramsey FM: Basic pharmacology of neuromuscular blocking agents. Anesth Clin North Am 1993; 11:219–236.
15. Stanski DR, Watkins WD: Drug disposition in anesthesia. New York, Grune & Stratton, 1982.
16. Taylor P: Are neuromuscular blocking agents more efficacious in pairs? Anesthesiology 1985; 63:1–3.
17. Rama Sastry BV: Nicotinic receptor. Anaesth Pharmacol Rev 1993; 1: 6–19.
18. Berg DK, Hall ZW: Increased extrajunctional acetylcholine sensitivity produced by chronic post-synaptic neuromuscular blockade. J Physiol (Lond) 1975; 244:659–676.
19. Martyn JAJ, White DA, Gronert GA et al: Up-and-down regulation of skeletal muscle acetylcholine receptors. Anesthesiology 1992; 76: 822–843.
20. Prielipp RC, Coursin DB: Pharmacolog of neuromuscular blocking drugs. New Horizons 1994; 2:34–37.
21. Fisher DM, Canfell PC, Fahey MR, et al: Elimination of atracurium in humans: contribution of Hofmann elimination and ester hydrolysis versus organ-based elimination. Anesthesiology 1986; 65:6–12.
22. Yate PM, Flynn PJ, Arnold RW et al: Clinical experience and plasma laudanosine concentrations during the infusion of atracurium in the intensive therapy unit. Br J Anaesth 1987; 59:211–217.
23. Parker CJR, Jones J, Hunter JM: Disposition of infusions of atracurium and its metabolite laudanosine in patients in renal and respiratory failure. Br J Anaesth 1988; 61:531–540.
24. Kopman AF: Onset of action of neuromuscular blockade: contributing factors. Curr Opin Anaesthesiol 1992; 5:561–567.
25. Puhringer FK, Khuenl-Brady KS, Koller J et al: Evaluation of endotracheal intubating conditions of rocuronium (ORG 9426) and succinylcholine in outpatient surgery. Anesth Analg 1992; 75:37–40.

26. Scott RPF, Savarese JJ: The cardiovascular and autonomic effects of neuromuscular blocking agents. Semin Anesthesiol 1985; 3:319–322.
27. Basta SJ, Savares JJ, Ali HH et al: Histamine releasing potencies of atracurium and dimethyl-tubocurarine. Br J Anaesth 1983; 55:105S-111S.
28. Coursin DB: Neuromuscular blockade: should patients be relaxed in the ICU? Chest 1992; 102:988–989.
29. Hudes E, Lee KC: Clinical use of peripheral nerve stimulators in anaesthesia. Can J Anaesth 1987; 34:525–534.
30. Brull SJ: An update on monitoring of neuromuscular function. Curr Opin Anaesthesiol 1992; 5:577–583.
31. Viby-Magensen J: Clinical assessment of neuromuscular transmission. Br J Anaesth 1982; 54:209–203.
32. Witt NJ, Zochodne DW, Bolton CF et al: Peripheral nerve function in sepsis and multiple organ failure. Chest 1991; 99:176–184.
33. Gregory TK, Pettus DC: An electroencephalographic processing algorithm specifically intended for analysis of cerebral electrical activity. J Clin Monit 1986; 2:190–197.
34. Pichlmayr L, Lips U: EEG monitoring in anesthesiology and intensive care. Neuropsychobiology 1983; 10:239–248.
35. Borel C, Hanley D: Neurologic intensive care unit monitoring. Crit Care Clin 1985; 1:223–239.
36. Partridge B, Abrams J, Bazemore D et al: Prolonged neuromuscular blockade after long-term infusion of vecuronium bromide in the intensive care unit. Crit Care Med 1990; 18:1177–1179.
37. Segredo V, Matthay MA, Sharma ML et al: Prolonged neuromuscular blockade after long-term administration of vecuronium in two critically ill patients. Anesthesiology 1990; 72:566–570.
38. Legasse RS, Katz RJ, Peterson M et al: Prolonged neuromuscular blockade following vecuronium infusion. J Clin Anesth 1990; 2:269–271.
39. Op de Coul AAW, Lambregts PCLA, Koeman J et al: Neuromuscular complications in patients given Pavulon (pancuronium bromide) during artificial ventilation. Clin Neurol Neurosurg 1985; 87:17–22.
40. Margolis B, Khachikian D, Friedman Y et al: Prolonged reversible quadriparesis in mechanically ventilated patients who received long-term infusions of vecuronium. Chest 1991; 100:877–878.
41. Sitwell LD, Weinshenker BG, Monpetit V et al: Complete ophthalmoplegia as a complication of acute corticosteroid and pancuronium associated myopathy. Neurology 1991; 41:921–922.
42. Bolton CF: The polyneuropathy of critical illness. J Intensive Care Med 1994; 9:132–138.
43. Danon MJ, Carpenter S: Myopathy with thick filament (myosin) loss following prolonged paralysis with vecuronium during steroid treatment. Muscle Nerve 1991; 14:1131–1139.
44. Gooch JL, Suchyta MR, Balbierz JM et al: Prolonged paralysis after treatment with neuromuscular junction blocking agents. Crit Care Med 1991; 19:1125–1130.
45. MacFarlane I, Rosenthal F: Severe myopathy after status asthmaticus. Lancet 1977; 2:615–617.
46. Segredo V, Caldwell JE, Matthay MM et al: Persistent paralysis in critically ill patients after long term administration of vecuronium. N Engl J Med 1992; 327:524–528.

Index